Spinal Cord Injury

Functional Rehabilitation

Third Edition

SPINAL CORD INJURY

FUNCTIONAL REHABILITATION

Third Edition

Martha Freeman Somers, MS, DPT

Department of Physical Therapy
Duquesne University

Institute for Rehabilitation and Research
University of Pittsburgh Medical Center

Pittsburgh, PA

Pearson

Boston   Columbus   Indianapolis   New York   San Francisco   Upper Saddle River
Amsterdam   Cape Town   Dubai   London   Madrid   Milan   Munich   Paris   Montreal   Toronto
Delhi   Mexico City   Sao Paulo   Sydney   Hong Kong   Seoul   Singapore   Taipei   Tokyo

Library of Congress Cataloging-in-Publication Data

Somers, Martha Freeman.
    Spinal cord injury: functional rehabilitation / Martha Freeman Somers.—3rd ed.
        p. ; cm.
    Includes bibliographical references and index.
    ISBN-13: 978-0-13-159866-9 (alk. paper)
    ISBN-10: 0-13-159866-X (alk. paper)
    1. Spinal cord—Wounds and injuries—Patients—Rehabilitation.   2. Spinal cord—Wounds
and injuries—Physical therapy.   I. Title.
[DNLM: 1. Physical Therapy Modalities.   2. Spinal Cord Injuries—rehabilitation. WL 400 S694s 2010]
RD594.3.S63 2010
617.4'82044—dc22

                                                                                            2009028571

Publisher: Julie Levin Alexander
Publisher's Assistant: Regina Bruno
Editor-in-Chief: Mark Cohen
Associate Editor: Melissa Kerian
Assistant Editor: Nicole Ragonese
Development Editor: Cathy Wein
Manufacturing Buyer: Renata Butera
Director of Marketing: Karen Allman
Executive Marketing Manager: Katrin Beacom
Marketing Specialist: Michael Sirinides
Marketing Assistant: Judy Noh
Creative Art Director: Jayne Conte
Cover Art: Photos courtesy of CCaetano/iStockphoto;
    Eraxion/iStockphoto; Martha Freeman Somers
Manager, Rights and Permissions: Zina Arabia
Manager, Visual Research: Beth Brenzel
Manager, Cover Visual Research & Permissions: Karen Sanatar
Image Permission Coordinator: Silvana Attanasio
Full-Service Project Management/Composition: Karpagam Jagadeesan/
    GGS Higher Education Resources, A Division of PreMedia Global, Inc.
Printing and Binding: Edwards Brothers
Cover Printer: Lehigh-Phoenix Color Corp.

Notice: The author and the publisher of this volume have taken care that the information and recommendations contained herein are accurate and compatible with the standards generally accepted at the time of publication. Nevertheless, it is difficult to ensure that all the information given is entirely accurate for all circumstances. The publisher disclaims any liability, loss, or damage incurred as a consequence, directly or indirectly, of the use and application of any of the contents of this volume.

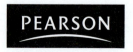

www.pearsonhighered.com

10 9 8 7 6 5 4 3 2
ISBN-13: 978-0-13-159866-9
ISBN-10:   0-13-159866-X

To Dave and Jess, still and always my two greatest blessings

~ and ~

to Connie and Dave Freeman, my first and best teachers.

Contents

Preface

Spinal cord injury causes a host of physical and psychosocial problems that can interfere with an individual's health, feelings of well-being, and participation in activities and relationships within the family and community. The goal of rehabilitation after spinal cord injury is to enable and empower the person to resume and then continue a lifestyle that is healthy, fulfilling, and integrated with his or her family and community. Physical therapists play a central role in this process, working with recently injured people and their families to maximize physical capabilities and mobility and to develop the knowledge and skills needed to remain healthy. Three major elements are required for a therapist to fulfill this role most effectively.

The first requirement is a basic understanding of spinal cord injuries and issues relevant to disability. Pertinent areas of knowledge include neuropathology and neurological return, physical sequelae, medical and surgical management, the prevention and management of complications, psychosocial impact, disability-related civil rights, functional potentials, equipment options, and wheelchair-accessible architectural design. These areas of knowledge are integrated with an understanding of the relationships between functioning, disability and health. This foundation of knowledge and understanding is needed for optimal program planning and implementation.

The second requirement is knowledge of the physical skills involved in functional activities and the process involved in acquiring these skills. It is not enough merely to know the eventual outcome, which may take months to accomplish. The therapist must know how to design and implement therapeutic programs to develop the needed strength, flexibility, and motor skills involved in functional activities. Many a therapist has been baffled when faced, on the one hand, with a text that explains the maneuvers that a person with a spinal cord injury performs during functional tasks and, on the other hand, with a newly injured person who can barely remain conscious while sitting upright, much less even begin to perform the skills shown in the book.

The third major element required for effective rehabilitation is an approach to the individual that promotes self-respect and encourages autonomy. Unfortunately this element is easily overlooked. Although we health professionals have as our stated goals the independent functioning of our patients, we can unwittingly encourage dependence. Many practices in health care serve to encourage "compliance" and to discourage autonomous behavior. If the rehabilitation effort is to be successful, the social environment of the rehabilitation unit must be structured in a way that fosters the development of self-reliant attitudes and behaviors.

In order to prepare readers to work effectively with people who have had spinal cord injuries, a text must encompass all of the elements described above. *Spinal Cord Injury: Functional Rehabilitation* was written to provide such a comprehensive treatment of the subject. The reader will gain a broad knowledge base relevant to spinal cord injuries and will develop an understanding of both the physical skills required for functional activities and the therapeutic strategies for achieving these skills. As importantly, the reader will gain an appreciation for the importance of psychosocial adaptation after spinal cord injury and will develop some insight into the impact that rehabilitation professionals can have in this area.

CHANGES IN THE THIRD EDITION

In the years since the second edition went to press, a number of developments have occurred in health care in general and rehabilitation in particular. An overarching goal in writing a third edition has been to make revisions as were needed to ensure that the text would continue to reflect current best practice. To this end, an exhaustive search of the literature was performed before each chapter was revised. Revisions were then made to reflect available evidence and current clinical practice guidelines. Revised chapters were reviewed by academic faculty and expert clinicians and additional revisions were made based on their feedback.

One of the developments in health care that is reflected in this edition is a change in the way that disability and disablement are conceptualized. In 2001, the member states of the United Nations adopted the International Classification of Functioning, Disability and Health (ICF) to provide a standard language and framework for descriptions of health and health-related states. The ICF is now used widely around the world to conceptualize the manner in which functioning and disability reflect an interaction between health conditions (disorders, diseases, injuries, etc.) and contextual (environmental and personal) factors. This edition of *Spinal Cord Injury: Functional Rehabilitation* uses the ICF as a conceptual framework for understanding both the impact of spinal cord injury and the role of rehabilitation. The ICF is introduced in Chapter 1. Each subsequent chapter uses language and concepts consistent with the ICF and begins with an image that illustrates how the content of that chapter relates to the ICF.

Another change that has occurred over the years is a shift in our understanding of neuroplasticity in the central nervous system. Basic science and clinical research have demonstrated a capacity for neural adaptation after spinal cord injury. Therapeutic approaches targeting the potential for restoration of function, particularly locomotor function, have gained prominence in the field of rehabilitation after spinal cord injury. In a closely related issue, questions have been raised about whether patients undergoing rehabilitation should work to regain functional independence using compensatory strategies or through restoration of more normal movement patterns. This edition includes information on neuroplasticity and therapeutic approaches to restoration of locomotor function through body weight–supported treadmill training (therapist-assisted and robotic-assisted) and addresses questions related to compensation versus restoration: Is there still a place for compensation in rehabilitation? If so, when is compensation appropriate and when should interventions stress restoration of normal movement patterns?

What does research tell us about the relative efficacy of the different approaches to restoration of ambulation?

Additional topics that have been added or expanded in this edition include pain, medications, cardiovascular disease and fitness, sleep apnea, standardized assessment tools appropriate for patients with spinal cord injury, strategies for preserving upper extremity function, and power-assist wheelchairs. Furthermore, images have been updated and added throughout the text and lists of suggested resources have been provided.

Perhaps the most welcome feature of the third edition will be the new organization of Chapters 9 through 12, which contain detailed descriptions of functional skills and strategies for functional training. The descriptions of skills and training are now more closely linked within the chapters; each skill is followed directly by strategies for developing that skill. It is hoped that this arrangement will make it easier for readers to use the information in program planning. In another change designed to make the new edition more user-friendly, Chapters 14 and 15 have been brought back from exile on the web.

Over the years, I have been gratified to hear from many physical and occupational therapists who have let me know what a useful resource this text was for them as they learned how to work with patients with spinal cord injuries. It is my hope that the third edition will continue to provide practical information and guidance for effective practice in today's health care environment.

Martha Somers

A Few Words about Words

"What's in a name? A rose by any other name would smell as sweet."

William Shakespeare

Maybe so, Bill, but I bet if you labeled that rose "radioactive," not too many people would get close enough to take a whiff.

Language has a profound impact on attitudes and values. Our perceptions of and judgments about others are both expressed and perpetuated by the words that we use. Despite the best efforts of proponents of person-first language, dehumanizing language remains in common use in the U.S. health care system. Many health professionals continue to label people by their diagnoses, calling them "paras," "quads," "cords," and so on. When we do this, we define people by their health conditions, reducing them to mere one-dimensional shadows. (How can a *person* be a *spinal cord*?)

Another common practice among health professionals involves referring to people as "patients" when this term no longer applies. Most of us think of ourselves as *patients* only while we are utilizing the services of another clinician. As soon as we walk out of the health professional's office, we cease being *patients* and revert to our accustomed roles. In thinking/writing/speaking about people with disabilities, however, we often refer to them as *patients* whether or not they are utilizing the services of health professionals. The implication is that they remain *dependent* on health professionals indefinitely. Once a patient, always a patient.

In writing this text, I have attempted to avoid language that dehumanizes people who have spinal cord injuries. Instead of labeling people by their diagnoses, I have chosen language that affirms their personhood. Thus rather than referring to "a C6 tetraplegic," for example, I have referred to "a person (or individual) with C6 tetraplegia."

In like manner, I gave much thought to eliminating the word *patient* from the text because it has implications of dependency and powerlessness. Another word might more appropriately convey the role of the person undergoing rehabilitation. But what word to use? *Client* evokes images of business suits and impersonal, formal interactions. I personally like *student*, but I didn't think it would fly. Readers, especially health professional students, may find the term confusing. For lack of a better term, I have retained the word *patient* but have attempted to avoid its overuse.

And then there's gender. The world is inhabited by both males and females. Both genders sustain spinal cord injuries, and both genders are involved in their rehabilitation. But hundreds of pages of "he or she," "himself or herself," and "his or her" would have been confusing in many places and tiresome throughout. I know, because I tried it. I also tried achieving gender neutrality by using plural pronouns, only to find that this approach rarely yields acceptable results. In the interest of retaining clarity and readability, I settled on the following solution: Each chapter contains either male or female pronouns, and the chapters alternate between the two. The one exception is Chapter 13, which addresses sexuality and sexual functioning. There, I chose to refer to both genders throughout the chapter in an attempt to counteract the tendency of some rehabilitation professionals to ignore or to minimize the impact of spinal cord injury on the sexual functioning of women.

As a result of my attempts to minimize the use of the word *patient*, achieve gender neutrality, and affirm the sexuality of women with spinal cord injuries, I may at times have resorted to some verbal gymnastics. I beg the reader's indulgence if I did so.

Martha Somers

Acknowledgments

I am deeply grateful to the following people for their assistance and support:

- Friends and colleagues who reviewed portions of the manuscript and provided extremely useful suggestions. Included in this group are Kim Atkinson, Rich Barbara, Sharon Caine, Sue Collins, Teresa Foy, Randy Huzenic, Isa McClure, Paige Moore, Chris Newman, Patricia Pasch, Sue Perry, Nate Schomburg, Anne Thompson, and Laura Wehrli.

- Paul Rockar, Beth Matcho, and Shelbey Rojik, who have provided me with the opportunity to return to my roots and practice in an inpatient SCI rehab unit.

- The physical and occupational therapists at the University of Pittsburgh Medical Center Institute for Rehabilitation and Research, for welcoming me into their midst every Tuesday afternoon.

- The participants at the 30th Annual Model Systems PT/OT Leadership Forum, dinosaurs and freshies and all in between, for sharing their wisdom and passion for this field.

- The numerous family, friends, and colleagues who provided suggestions, information, reference material, technical assistance, and encouragement in the writing of this edition. In this group are included Dave and Jess Somers, Elyn Tovey, Diane Borello-France, Rick Clemente, Leesa Dibartola, Mary Eberle, Ken Havrilla, Cathy Hramika, Greg Marchetti, Mary Marchetti, Cliff Pohl, Kate Baxter, Cathy Carver, Kristine Driscoll, Mark Drnach, Gina Mazure, Kim Eberhart, Susie Kim, Robert Somers, Dave and Connie Freeman, Patty Dineen, Annie Larsen, Sue Barton, Lynn Davidson, Sarah Gilmour, Karen Schmidt, and Helen Richards.

- Former students who provided feedback on the second edition. These include Jessica Blystone, Joni Brier, Jeff Bucci, Michele Calhoun, Kim Favara, Kelly Graham, Amy Greaney, Stephanie Gullace, Megan Holland, Amy Jarmul, Sara Parrish, Jessica Shattuck, Aaron Lanzel, Andrea Valigosky, Susan Wheeler, Holly Williams. A special thanks to Katie Demario and Gina Albright, who reviewed portions of the manuscript for this edition.

- Mark Cohen, Melissa Kerian and Cathy Wein of Pearson Health Science, who kept this project going.

- Steve Merchant and Corey Fuller, who spent countless hours adding references to the bibliographic files.

- Susan Gilbert, whose illustrations are still among the best features of the book.

- Most of all, thanks to Dave Somers for his endless patience and support.

Reviewers

Charlotte Chatto, PT, PhD
Assistant Professor, Physical Therapy
Medical College of Georgia
Augusta, Georgia

Susan Cromwell, MS, PT, NCS
Assistant Professor, Rehabilitation and Movement
    Sciences
University of Vermont
Burlington, Vermont

Steven Fehrer, PT, PhD
Assistant Professor, Physical Therapy and Rehabilitation
    Science
The University of Montana
Missoula, Montana

George Fulk, PT, PhD
Assistant Professor, Physical Therapy
Clarkson University
Potsdam, New York

Anne Hart, PT, PhD
Associate Professor, Physical Therapy
Northern Arizona University
Flagstaff, Arizona

Carolyn Kelley, PT, DSc, NCS
Associate Professor, Physical Therapy
Texas Woman's University
Houston, Texas

Karen McCulloch, PT, PhD, NCS
Associate Professor, Physical Therapy
University of North Carolina-Chapel Hill
Chapel Hill, North Carolina

Susan B. Perry, PT, DPT, NCS
Associate Professor, Physical Therapy
Chatham University
Pittsburgh, Pennsylvania

Anne W. Thompson, PT, EdD
Associate Professor, Physical Therapy
Armstrong Atlantic State University
Savannah, Georgia

Diana Veneri, EdD, PT
Assistant Professor, Physical Therapy
University of Hartford
West Hartford, Connecticut

Petra Williams, PT, MS, NCS
Assistant Professor, Physical Therapy
Ohio University
Athens, Ohio

Daniel Young, PT, DPT
Assistant Professor, Physical Therapy
University of Nevada, Las Vegas
Las Vegas, Nevada

Leslie Zarrinkhameh, MPT, DPT
Lecturer, Physical Therapy
California State University - Fresno
Fresno, California

Clinical Reviewers

Kimberly N. Atkinson, PT, CCCE
Program Director, Neurologic Physical Therapy
    Residency Program
TIRR Memorial Hermann
Texas Medical Center
Houston, Texas

Richard Barbara, PhD, MS Ed
Licensed Psychologist, Clinical Faculty, Department
    of Physical Medicine and Rehabilitation
UPMC Institute for Rehabilitation and Research
    at Mercy Hospital
Pittsburgh, Pennsylvania

Sharon Caine, PT
Clinical Team Leader
Thomas Jefferson University Hospital
Philadelphia, Pennsylvania

Sue Collins, PT, CWS
Senior Physical Therapist/Coordinator of Clinical
    Education
Advanced Wound Healing and Lymphedema Center
Allegheny General Hospital
Pittsburgh, Pennsylvania

Teresa Foy, OTR/L
Therapy Manager, Spinal Cord Injury Program
Shepherd Center
Atlanta, Georgia

Randall Huzinec, PT
UPMC Institute for Rehabilitation and Research
    at Mercy Hospital
Pittsburgh, Pennsylvania

Isa A. McClure, MA, PT
Clinical Specialist, Spinal Cord Injury
Inpatient Physical Therapy Department
Kessler Institute for Rehabilitation
West Orange, New Jersey

Paige C. Moore, OTR/L
Senior Occupational Therapist
Occupational Therapy Department
Woodrow Wilson Rehabilitation Center
Fishersville, VA

Christopher P. Newman, MPT
Physical Therapy Clinical Coordinator
Spinal Cord Injury & Specialty Rehab Program
TIRR Memorial Hermann
Texas Medical Center
Houston, Texas

Patricia Pasch, OTR/L
Occupational Therapist, Spinal Cord Injury
Shepherd Center
Atlanta, Georgia

Nathan Schomburg, PT, NCS
Team Leader
UPMC Institute for Rehabilitation and Research,
    Montefiore
Pittsburgh, Pennsylvania

Laura S. Wehrli, DPT, ATP
Physical Therapy Supervisor, SCI
Craig Hospital
Englewood, Colorado

1

Introduction

Damage to the spinal cord can have profound and global effects. Paralysis of voluntary musculature can lead to reduced mobility as well as impairment of vocational, avocational, and self-care abilities. Spinal cord injury can also affect the functioning of the sensory, respiratory, cardiovascular, gastrointestinal, genitourinary, and integumentary systems. A host of debilitating and potentially life-threatening secondary conditions can result.

The psychosocial sequelae of spinal cord injury are equally important. Bodily changes, impaired mobility, functional dependence, altered sexual functioning, and incontinence all constitute seemingly overwhelming losses with which people with spinal cord injuries must come to terms. Moreover, these problems can interfere with the social roles and activities that are central in each person's life and identity. Finally, spinal cord injuries cause previously "normal" people to become "handicapped" and thus to become subject to society's prejudices regarding people with disabilities.

The physical sequelae of damage to the spinal cord vary widely, depending on the level and completeness of the lesion. Regardless of the severity of injury, it is possible to return to a healthy, fulfilling, and productive life. Achieving this outcome, however, can be a monumental task. To the health professional unfamiliar with spinal cord injuries, it may seem daunting. With such a broad array of physical and psychosocial problems that can result from spinal cord injury, where should the health care team focus its attention? Perhaps the process of rehabilitation following spinal cord injury can be better understood using a conceptual framework of functioning, disability, and health.

Functioning, Disability and Health

Over the past several decades, a variety of models have been proposed to conceptualize disability and the process of disablement. Each model presents a different understanding of the nature of disability and the factors that affect it. In addition, the various models contain conflicting terminology. The lack of consensus on a conceptual framework and terminology related to disability has interfered with communication in clinical and research contexts.[1] In 2001, the member states of the United Nations adopted the International Classification of Functioning, Disability and Health (ICF) to provide a standard language and framework for descriptions of health and health-related states.[2,3] The ICF is now used widely around the world[4] and has the potential to enhance communication across disciplines and national boundaries, supporting progress in research, clinical practice, and social policy.[1,5]

In contrast to earlier models, the ICF emphasizes health and functioning rather than disability. "Previously, disability began where health ended; once you were disabled, you were in a separate category. We wanted to get away from this kind of thinking. . . . This is a radical shift. From emphasizing people's disabilities, we now focus on their level of health."[3]

The ICF is based on a biopsychosocial model[a] in which functioning and disability reflect an interaction between health conditions (disorders, diseases, injuries, etc.) and contextual (environmental and personal) factors (Figure 1–1). Functioning occurs at the level of the body or body part (body functions and structures), the whole person (activity), and the whole person in a social context (participation).[2,3] The term *disability* refers to dysfunction at any of these levels: impairment in body function or structure, activity limitation, or participation restriction.[2,3] Table 1–1 presents the ICF terminology.

One important feature of the model is that functioning and disability reflect an interaction of a number of

---

[a] The ICF conceptual framework includes biological, psychological, and social elements. The main concepts in the ICF are similar to those of the Nagi model of disablement,[1] which has been used widely in the United States.[6-10]

1

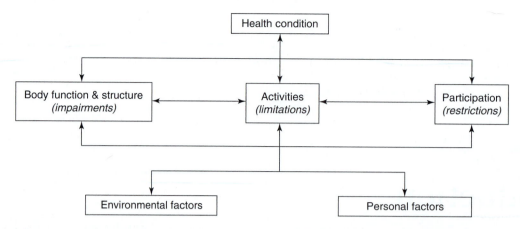

Figure 1–1 Schematic representation of the International Classification of Functioning, Disability and Health (ICF). The bidirectional arrows represent dynamic interactions; all components interact and influence one another.[11] (Adapted from www.who.int/classifications/icf/training/icfbeginnersguide.pdf. from the World Health Organization.)

factors, including the health condition, characteristics of the individual, and the physical and social milieu in which he functions.[1] Because of the many factors that modify functioning, identical pathologies in different people can result in widely divergent levels of disability. For example, one individual with a spinal cord injury could eventually return to full participation in life activities, including living at home and resuming the roles of spouse, parent, and breadwinner. Another person with identical damage to his spinal cord could wind up with severely restricted participation in life activities: living in a skilled nursing facility, divorced from his wife, estranged from his children, and unable to return to work (Figure 1–2).

Health professionals have a powerful influence on functioning, disability, and health. Applying the ICF framework to program planning, rehabilitation professionals investigate the relationships between the individual's impairments, activity limitations, and participation restrictions, and identify contextual factors that act as barriers or facilitators to functioning.[5,13] In collaboration with their patients, they establish goals and then work to enhance body function and structure (reduce impairments), maximize functional capacity (reduce activity limitations), and facilitate performance and participation in life situations (reduce participation restrictions). Some interventions directly address impairments, activity limitations, or participation restrictions. Others focus on contextual factors. Because of the interactions between the different elements of the system, interventions that address one area can influence others[13] (Figure 1–3). All interventions should be directed toward enhancing the health and functioning of the individual undergoing rehabilitation.[5] Table 1–2 provides examples of rehabilitative strategies that address the various factors associated with functioning, disability, and health.

REHABILITATION FOLLOWING SPINAL CORD INJURY

Goals of Rehabilitation

The ultimate goal of rehabilitation after spinal cord injury is to optimize functioning and health. This involves enabling the person with a spinal cord injury to return to as healthy, fulfilling, and independent a lifestyle as possible. It also involves facilitating his return to participation in accustomed tasks and roles in his family and in society. Accomplishing these outcomes requires psychosocial, sexual, vocational, and avocational adjustment; the acquisition of functional skills, appropriate equipment, and the knowledge and behaviors required for health maintenance; and the appropriate adaptation of the person's environment.

Psychological and Social Adjustment

To return to a happy and fulfilling life following spinal cord injury, an individual who experiences significant neurological damage must come to terms with his losses, formulate a new identity, and learn how to cope in a society in which he is now a member of a devalued minority. In terms of disability and quality of life, this psychological and social adjustment may be the most crucial area of growth after spinal cord injury.

Sexual Adjustment

Many of the social roles that are typically performed in the family and in society include an element of sexuality. To return to full participation in social and sexual relationships, a person with a spinal cord injury must adjust to the changes in sexuality and sexual functioning that the cord injury brings.

TABLE 1–1   ICF Terminology[2,3,12]

Neutral or Positive Term	Related Terms	Examples
Body functions: physiological functions of body systems (including psychological functions). **Body structures:** anatomical parts of the body such as organs, limbs, and their components.	**Impairments:** problems in body function or structure such as significant deviation or loss.	**Impairments:** paralysis, altered sensory function, abnormal muscle tone, joint contractures, pain, depression, cardiopulmonary deconditioning.
Activity: execution of a task or action by an individual.	**Activity limitations:** difficulties an individual may have in executing activities. **Qualifiers:** **Capacity:** the individual's ability to execute a task or action. *(Optimal performance in a neutral environment, without assistance of another person or equipment.)* **Performance:** what an individual does in his or her current environment. *(Actual performance in the overall societal context, including available assistance and equipment.)*	**Activity limitations:** limitations in performance of tasks such as walking, climbing, reaching, transfers, or other physical tasks such as using public transportation. **Capacity:** capability and amount of difficulty in rolling from supine to side-lying in a standard bed without adaptive equipment or assistance from another person, or walking on a linoleum floor without orthoses, assistive devices, or assistance from another person. **Performance:** capability and amount of difficulty in rolling from supine to side-lying in bed using a bed rail, or walking in the community using an ankle–foot orthosis and canes.
Participation: involvement in a life situation.	**Participation restrictions:** problems an individual may experience in involvement in life situations. **Qualifiers: Capacity** and **Performance** qualifiers (defined above) are also used in reference to participation.	**Participation restrictions:** restrictions in ability to return to work, participate in social activities, function as a parent or spouse, participate in sports.
Environmental factors: physical, social, and attitudinal environment in which people live and conduct their lives.	**Facilitators:** factors that improve functioning and reduce disability. **Barriers:** factors that limit functioning and create disability.	**Facilitators:** accessible buildings and public transportation; available assistive technology; positive social attitudes; services, systems and laws that foster involvement. **Barriers:** inaccessible buildings and public transportation; lack of access to assistive technology; negative social attitudes; services, systems, and laws that hinder involvement.
Personal factors: attributes of the person that influence how disability is experienced by that individual.		Age, behavior patterns, coping styles, education, gender, lifestyle, past experiences, profession, race, social background.

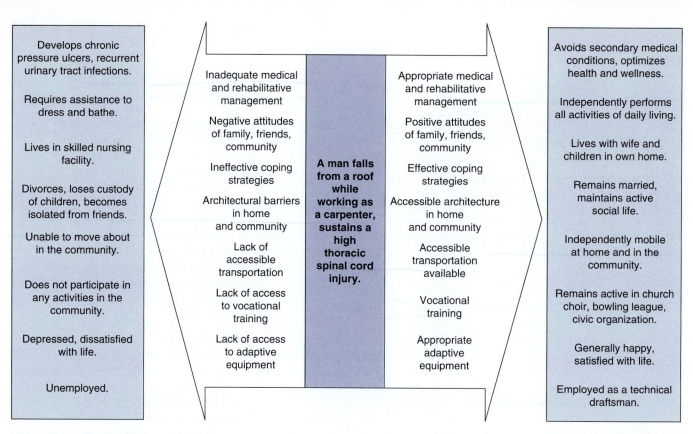

Figure 1–2   Example showing the impact of personal and environmental factors on health and function after spinal cord injury.

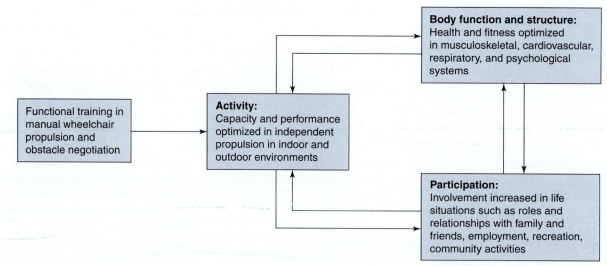

Figure 1–3   Example of intervention affecting health and function at several levels, due to the interaction between the levels. Functional training in manual wheelchair propulsion and obstacle negotiation enhances the person's ability to propel a manual wheelchair independently in indoor and outdoor environments (**activity**). These skills enhance **body structure and function**: manual wheelchair propulsion provides exercise that improves muscle strength, cardiovascular endurance, and respiratory function. This enhanced fitness can, in turn, lead to improved capacity for wheelchair propulsion (**activity**), as well as allowing greater involvement in life situations (**participation**). Wheelchair skills (**activity**) also make it possible to participate in social, recreational, civic, and vocational activities (**participation**). This participation can, in turn, improve the individual's wheelchair skills (**activity**) through increased practice of the skills, and can benefit his physical fitness and psychological well-being (**body structure and function**).

TABLE 1–2   Application of the ICF Framework to Rehabilitation

Focus of Interventions	Examples of Rehabilitation Strategies
Body function and structure (impairments)	Prevent secondary conditions, reduce impairments, and enhance health and function through exercise, education, training, provision of equipment, medical management, and psychological interventions.
Activities (activity limitations)	Maximize functional capacity through functional training, locomotor training, and provision of equipment.
Participation (participation restrictions)	Facilitate participation through community reintegration programs, advocacy, and provision of equipment.
Environmental factors	Optimize functioning though architectural adaptation; education, training, and support of family and others in social milieu; as well as access to social support resources in the community.
Personal factors	Facilitate participation through vocational and avocational training and cognitive behavioral therapy.

Vocational and Avocational Adjustment

In many instances, paralysis makes it impossible or impractical to return to the job one held prior to the spinal cord injury. Recreational activities enjoyed prior to the injury may also now be impossible or impractical. Return to an independent and fulfilling lifestyle with full participation in life situations requires adaptation in both of these areas.

Functional Independence

During rehabilitation, a person with a spinal cord injury learns how to perform a variety of physical activities. Through functional training, he gains the skills required for self-care and mobility in the home and community. By maximizing his functional skills, he can enhance his capacity to participate in various life situations. Depending on the severity of the cord injury, functional gains can occur as a result of compensatory strategies, restoration of more normal movement patterns, or a combination of both.[b]

Acquisition of Equipment

Following spinal cord injury, equipment can have a significant impact on function and health. Thus, equipment acquisition is an important aspect of rehabilitation. Following spinal cord injury, the rehabilitation team and the patient work together to identify and obtain the equipment needed to maintain health, maximize functional independence, and enhance participation in life situations.

Health and Wellness

Health maintenance is an active process after spinal cord injury. Virtually constant vigilance is required to avoid

---

[b] Chapter 8 addresses the topic of compensation versus recovery in rehabilitation.

Problem-Solving Exercise 1–1

Your patient has come to your facility for outpatient rehabilitation. During your initial examination, you find that she has the following problems:

- She has no voluntary motor function in her lower extremities.
- She is unable to walk.
- She has not been able to return to her job as a hair stylist.
- She has limited knee extension range of motion.
- She requires assistance to transfer in and out of bed, is unable to perform uneven transfers, and cannot negotiate uneven terrain, ramps, or curbs in her wheelchair.
- She cannot take care of her infant son.
- She cannot live in her own home with her husband and son because there are steps at the home's entrance and the bathroom door is too narrow for a wheelchair.

Classify each of the problems listed above as impairment, activity limitation, participation restriction, or environmental barrier. (Some of the bullets include more than one level of problem.)

complications such as pressure ulcers and urinary tract infections. Spinal cord injury also brings vulnerabilities and challenges in the areas of cardiovascular fitness and orthopedic integrity. If an individual is to stay healthy after spinal cord injury, he must learn how his body works, how to prevent and detect complications and maximize fitness, and what to do when complications occur.

Architectural Adaptation

The presence of architectural barriers in the physical environment increases disability by limiting mobility and function. By providing guidance and advocacy regarding architectural adaptations, the rehabilitation team can enhance a person's ability to participate in life situations in his home and community.

Services Required

Spinal cord injury necessitates specialized and comprehensive rehabilitation services; a multidisciplinary team is required to enable people to achieve their optimal levels of health and functioning. Rehabilitation involves the coordinated efforts of counselors, nurses, occupational therapists, physical therapists, physicians, recreation therapists, rehabilitation engineers, respiratory therapists, speech therapists, and vocational counselors. To maximize outcomes, each of these professionals should have expertise in rehabilitation after spinal cord injury. Because of the specialized services required, general hospitals are not able to provide the comprehensive care needed for rehabilitation following spinal cord injury. For this reason, patients who receive care in specialized centers are likely to have better outcomes.[14–17]

Fostering Independence Following Spinal Cord Injury

One of the major ways in which a rehabilitation program reduces disability is by maximizing the individual's capacity to function independently. Independent, or autonomous, functioning involves living without undue reliance on others.

Requirements for Independent Functioning

There are three basic requirements that must be met for a person to function independently: knowledge, ability, and attitude.

Knowledge is critical to self-direction. Knowledge in the following areas will promote independence after spinal cord injury: the body's functioning following spinal cord injury, prevention and management of secondary conditions, treatment alternatives, legal rights, equipment options, architectural accessibility, and the services and resources available in the community. Armed with this knowledge, a person with a spinal cord injury can be self-reliant.

A variety of abilities are required for independent functioning. Physical abilities enable people to perform functional tasks without assistance. If a person lacks the physical capacity to perform a given activity, autonomous functioning requires the ability to gain and direct assistance from another person. Other abilities involved in

independent functioning include skills in problem solving, social interaction, and self-advocacy.

Finally, an independent attitude is essential for autonomy. This attitude involves a sense of personal competence, control, and responsibility. It provides the foundation for independent functioning, undergirding the individual's drive for and achievement of self-reliant living.

Fostering Independence

A rehabilitation program must address each of these areas—knowledge, ability, and attitude—if the person with a spinal cord injury is to function as independently as possible. The first two requirements, knowledge and ability, may be most readily achieved. Educational and training programs can be implemented to provide information and develop skills.

The development of an independent attitude can be more problematic; it is an area more likely to be neglected and most easily undermined. By virtue of the types of people who enter the health professions, and the training that we receive, health professionals tend to be good at taking care of people. Because of this, we can inadvertently develop a *dependent attitude* in our patients. This happens when we feed them, bathe them, dress them, and push their wheelchairs even when they are capable of doing these things for themselves. It happens when we make decisions for them or "protect" them from full knowledge of their physical conditions. When we do these things, we communicate to our patients that they are dependent and that they need our help.

To foster an independent attitude, the rehabilitation team must emphasize the patient's autonomy and personal responsibility. From the day of injury onward, the person with a spinal cord injury should be included in decision making and self-care as much as possible. He should be provided with all relevant information and work as a partner with clinicians to set goals, solve problems, and make decisions. To the extent possible, the patient should be responsible for the rehabilitation program—taking initiative, directing, and participating fully in it.

Autonomous behaviors do not always appear spontaneously when a patient is given the opportunity to direct his care. A variety of factors can cause initial reluctance or inability to participate actively in rehabilitation. Some people learn dependence after their injuries when they are placed in the role of dependent and passive patient. Some feel incapable of self-direction because of their preexisting beliefs about people with disabilities. Others may simply feel overwhelmed. Finally, a certain number may have been passive and dependent prior to their injuries. Whatever the cause of a patient's reluctance or inability to participate actively in his program, the rehabilitation team must work with him to encourage and develop his sense of empowerment and self-sufficiency.

ON YOUR MARK, GET SET, GO

One of the greatest challenges facing health professionals today is that of adapting to a rapidly changing health care environment. The reduction of time allotted to inpatient care is one of the more profound changes that have occurred in health care. In the not-too-distant past, a person who sustained a spinal cord injury could spend months in an acute care hospital, followed by months in an inpatient rehabilitation facility. The process of recovery and adaptation began in the acute care hospital and continued in the rehabilitation setting when the patient was determined to be ready for the rigors of rehabilitation. Inpatient rehabilitation continued until the patient reached, or at least approached, his maximal functional potential. Prior to discharge, there was time for physical and psychological healing, comprehensive patient and family education, and extensive training in functional skills. The procurement of equipment could be delayed until significant time had been spent in rehabilitation and the patient's definitive equipment requirements could be determined.

In today's health care environment, a person who becomes injured or ill moves as rapidly as possible through intensive care, floor-level care, and rehabilitation.[c] People with spinal cord injuries now often arrive at inpatient rehabilitation facilities while they remain medically and orthopedically unstable, and have not had adequate time to begin the process of adapting psychologically to their losses. Although they may not be ready to participate fully in rigorous therapeutic programs when they arrive, they are expected to complete their rehabilitation in as short a time as possible. As a result, people with spinal cord injuries may leave inpatient rehabilitation facilities without having reached their full potentials.[19]

Health professionals must accommodate to the time constraints imposed by funding sources. With shortened time

---

[c] This reduction of time spent in rehabilitation is particularly evident in the United States. Significantly longer lengths of stay have been reported in other countries.[16,18]

allotted to inpatient stays in hospitals, more emphasis must be placed on rehabilitation in outpatient clinics, extended care facilities, and homes. The inpatient stay should be seen as the beginning phase of rehabilitation, with significant continued progress expected in appropriate alternative settings following discharge. Immediately after discharge from inpatient rehabilitation, therapy in the home will allow patients to continue to develop skills and utilize them in their home environments. Patients can continue their rehabilitation in outpatient therapy, and utilize their developing functional skills between therapy sessions. Their performance at home and in the community can provide information that is helpful in program planning. Months or years after patients have been discharged from outpatient therapy, subsequent episodes of therapy can enhance physical capacity, independence, and quality of life.[20,21]

Although therapy at home and in outpatient settings can be beneficial, the inpatient phase of rehabilitation remains critical. It is during inpatient rehabilitation that the foundation is laid for physical, functional, psychological, and social adaptation. Patients who have orthopedic or medical restrictions that temporarily prevent full participation in rehabilitation may benefit from discharge to other settings (home or extended care facility, as indicated), with readmission to rehabilitation facilities when they are ready to participate in their programs.

In the face of shrinking lengths of stay, goals must be prioritized carefully during each phase of rehabilitation, with the highest priority being given to those goals that are critical to survival. When patients are discharged home prior to achieving independent functioning, it is imperative to give them and their caregivers the education and training needed to enable them to remain healthy and continue to progress after discharge.

Summary

- Spinal cord injury can have a profound impact on a person's ability to care for himself, move from place to place, and participate in his accustomed social, vocational, and avocational activities. Injury to the spinal cord also makes a person vulnerable to social discrimination and a variety of physical complications.
- The International Classification of Functioning, Disability and Health (ICF) provides a conceptual framework that can be useful in rehabilitation. In this framework, functioning and disability reflect an interaction between health conditions (disorders, diseases, injuries, etc.) and contextual (environmental and personal) factors. Functioning occurs at the level of the body or body part (body functions), the whole person (activity), and the whole person in a social context (participation). Using the ICF, health professionals can minimize disability through a variety of interventions at each level of functioning while also addressing relevant environmental and personal factors.

- The ultimate goals of rehabilitation after spinal cord injury are to optimize functioning and health. Interventions are aimed at enhancing psychological, social, sexual, vocational, and avocational adjustment; maximizing functional independence; and developing the knowledge, skills, and behaviors that the individual will need in order to remain healthy in the years to come.
- During rehabilitation, *how* things are done can be as important as *what* is done. Services should be delivered in a manner that affirms and fosters the autonomy of patients undergoing rehabilitation.
- Spinal cord injury necessitates specialized and comprehensive rehabilitation services. In the past, these services were delivered primarily in inpatient settings. In recent years, inpatient stays have been shortened dramatically. This change has necessitated a continuation of the rehabilitation process in outpatient clinics and in the home.

2

Spinal Cord Injuries

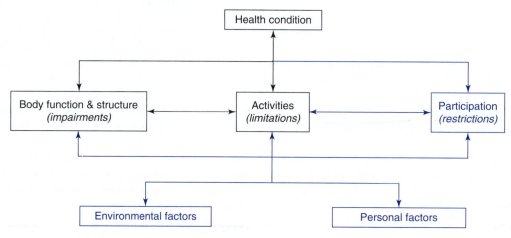

Chapter 2 presents information on spinal cord injury, the physical impairments that result, and secondary conditions.

Every year an estimated 12,000 people[a] in the United States sustain spinal cord injuries. Today, there are approximately 255,702 people with spinal cord injuries alive in this country.[1]

In the United States, motor vehicle accidents are the most common cause (42%) of spinal cord injury, followed by falls (27.1%), acts of violence (15.3%), and sports injuries (7.4%). The remaining 8.1% of spinal cord injuries result from either unknown or other causes.[1] The incidence of the different causes of cord injury changes over time[1] and varies with gender, race, age, employment status, and marital status, being influenced by the activities and hazards prevalent in each population.[2-5] A large majority of spinal cord injuries (approximately 80%) are sustained by males. Injury occurs most frequently between 16 and 30 years of age.[2,3]

---

[a] This number does not include people who die at the scene of the accident.

Anatomy Review

Vertebral Column

Most spinal cord injuries are the result of trauma to the vertebral column, which contains 7 cervical, 12 thoracic, 5 lumbar, 5 sacral, and 4 coccygeal vertebrae. The cervical, thoracic, and lumbar vertebrae are separated by intervertebral disks. The sacral and coccygeal vertebrae are fused.

A typical vertebra consists of a body, located anteriorly, and an arch. The spinal cord is encased within the vertebral foramen, which is formed by the vertebral bodies and arches. Figure 2–1 illustrates the components of a vertebra.

The vertebral column is stabilized by ligaments (Figure 2–2). The anterior longitudinal ligament is attached to the anterior aspect of the vertebral bodies and intervertebral disks; it limits extension. The posterior longitudinal ligament is attached to the posterior aspect of the vertebral bodies and intervertebral disks; it limits flexion.[4,5] The ligamenta flava, supraspinous ligament

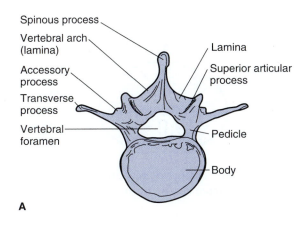

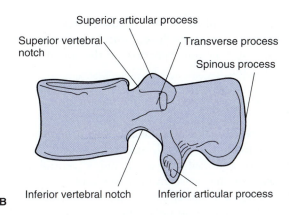

Figure 2–1   Components of a vertebra. (A) Superior view. (B) Lateral view.

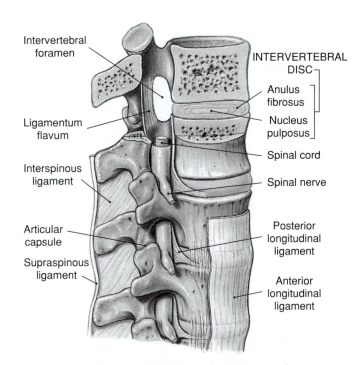

Figure 2–2   Ligaments stabilizing the spinal column. *Fundamentals of Anatomy and Physiology,* 5/e by Frederic H. Martini. © 2001 by Frederic Martini, Inc. Reprinted with permission of Pearson Education, Inc.

(C7 and below), ligamentum nuchae (cervical region), interspinous ligaments, and articular capsules stabilize the posterior arch.[4,6,7]

Spinal Cord

The spinal cord extends from the medulla oblongata just above the foramen magnum to the level of the L1 or L2 vertebra.[8] Its tapered caudal end is called the conus medullaris. The spinal cord contains long axons of upper motor neurons descending from the brain, lower motor neurons (somatic motor neurons) with axons that travel to the periphery to innervate skeletal muscles, sympathetic and parasympathetic visceral motor neurons, long axons of sensory neurons ascending to the brain, and interneurons (segmental and intersegmental) that interconnect neurons within the cord itself. Normal voluntary and reflexive motor function, sensory function, and autonomic control involve complex interactions between supraspinal systems, lower motor neurons, visceral motor neurons, peripheral afferents, and networks of interneurons. The spinal cord also contains glial cells, nonneuronal cells that are essential to the neurons' functioning and survival.

Seen in transverse section, the spinal cord has an H-shaped area of gray matter centrally (Figure 2–3). This gray matter is composed of the cell bodies of neurons, their

dendrites, and the initial segments of their axons; the terminals of axons that synapse on these neurons; and glial cells.[8] The dorsal (posterior) horn of the gray matter is predominately sensory. The ventral (anterior) horn contains the bodies of lower motor neurons innervating skeletal muscles. From T1 to L2 or L3, a small lateral horn contains the cell bodies of sympathetic visceral motor neurons.[9]

The gray matter of the spinal cord is surrounded by white matter consisting of ascending and descending fibers—the axons of sensory and motor neurons. Fibers carrying similar sensory information or motor functions travel together in tracts (Figure 2–4 and Table 2–1). Additionally, the fibers within at least some tracts are organized somatotopically: they are grouped with others

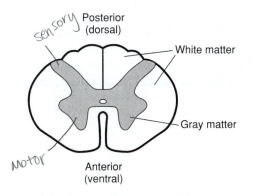

Figure 2–3   Schematic cross section of the spinal cord.

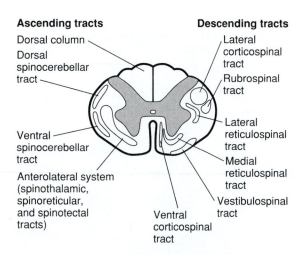

Figure 2–4   Major ascending and descending fiber tracts in the spinal cord. Ascending tracts are shown on the left; descending tracts are shown on the right.

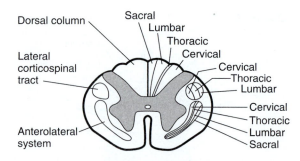

Figure 2–5   Somatotopic organization of the spinal cord (depicted on the right).

traveling to or from the same cord segment (Figure 2–5).[6,10] In addition to the long fiber tracts, the white matter contains the axons of interneurons (propriospinal neurons) that project between cord segments.[8]

Vascular Supply

The spinal cord receives its blood supply from a single anterior spinal artery and two posterior spinal arteries. In the cervical region, the anterior spinal artery is supplied primarily by the vertebral arteries and the intracranial vessels from which they arise. The posterior spinal arteries in this region are supplied by the vertebral arteries or the posterior inferior cerebellar arteries. In the thoracic, lumbar, and sacral regions, the anterior and posterior spinal arteries are fed by segmental arteries arising from the aorta.[8]

The anterior and posterior spinal arteries travel the length of the cord.[10] They supply circulation to the cord through the centrifugal and centripetal arterial systems. Figure 2–6 illustrates the distribution of blood supply in the cord.

Centrifugal System

The anterior spinal artery gives rise to small branches, called sulcal arteries, that enter the anterior median fissure of the spinal cord and supply the central portion of the cord. This area includes most of the gray matter and approximately the inner half of the posterior, lateral, and anterior white matter.[13] Adjacent sulcal arteries alternate between the right and left sides of the cord.[14]

Centripetal System

The anterior spinal artery also gives rise to pial arteries. The pial arteries and branches of the posterior spinal arteries travel circumferentially around the outer surface of the cord and supply its peripheral regions. The area of the

spinal cord supplied by the pial and posterior spinal arteries includes part of the dorsal horns, most of the posterior columns, and the outer portions of the lateral and anterior white matter.[13]

Spinal Nerves

There are 31 pairs of spinal nerves: 8 cervical, 12 thoracic, 5 lumbar, 5 sacral, and 1 coccygeal. Each spinal nerve has a dorsal (sensory) and a ventral (primarily motor) root that arise from a single cord segment. The C1 through C7 spinal nerves exit the vertebral foramen above the correspondingly numbered vertebrae. The C8 spinal nerve exits below the C7 vertebra. (There are 8 cervical nerves and only 7 cervical vertebrae.) The spinal nerves of T1 and below exit below the correspondingly numbered vertebrae.[8]

Because the spinal cord is shorter than the vertebral column, the nerve roots travel caudally before exiting the vertebral canal. Distal to the conus medullaris, the nerve roots form the cauda equina (Figure 2–7).

VERTEBRAL INJURIES

Most spinal cord injuries occur as the result of trauma to the vertebral column. This trauma is usually indirect, involving forces that create violent motions of the head or trunk. These forces cause flexion, extension, axial loading, distraction, or shearing.[15,16] Injury often occurs as a result of a combination of forces that occur simultaneously or in rapid succession. The magnitude and direction of the traumatic forces, combined with the characteristics of the region of the spine subjected to these forces, determine the pattern and severity of the injury (Figure 2–8). The extent and location of the bony and ligamentous damage determines the injured spine's stability.[17,18] Spinal cord damage occurs when vertebral injury leads to compression (transient or persistent), traction, or transection of the cord[19] or disrupts its vascular supply. Spinal nerve damage also frequently occurs.

Most injuries of the vertebral column involve either a single level or a limited number of contiguous vertebrae.

TABLE 2–1   Major Spinal Pathways

Motor Tracts		
Name	**Travels in cord ipsilateral or contralateral to muscles it innervates**	**Type of control**
Lateral corticospinal	Ipsilateral	Voluntary motion, especially precisely controlled movements of the distal limbs
Ventral corticospinal	Contralateral	Voluntary motion of axial musculature; minimal clinical significance due to small size
Rubrospinal	Ipsilateral	Voluntary motion of the upper extremities, especially precisely controlled movements of the distal musculature
Vestibulospinal	Bilateral	Posture and balance
Lateral and medial reticulospinals	Ipsilateral	Posture, balance, modulation of spinal reflexes, axial and proximal limb motions; in performance of motor tasks, complements actions driven by corticospinals

Sensory Tracts		
Name	**Travels in cord ipsilateral or contralateral to areas it innervates**	**Type of control**
Anterolateral system (spinothalamic, spinoreticular, and spinotectal tracts)	Contralateral	Pain, temperature, and crude touch
Dorsal column	Ipsilateral	Proprioception, vibratory sense, deep touch, and discriminative touch
Dorsal spinocerebellar	Ipsilateral	Unconscious proprioception from trunk and lower extremities
Ventral spinocerebellar	Bilateral	Unconscious proprioception from trunk and lower extremities

Sources: References 8 and 10 to 12.

In a small number of cases,[b] however, the spinal column sustains damage at two or more levels that are separated by undamaged vertebrae. These multiple noncontiguous vertebral injuries are associated with severe trauma. Noncontiguous injuries rostral to a known injury are a matter of concern because, if undetected and not treated properly, they may cause paralysis and sensory loss at a higher level. Caudally located noncontiguous injuries can affect muscle tone and bowel, bladder, and genital functioning.[20]

Spinal cord injuries occasionally occur without any vertebral injury that can be detected on plain radiographs or computed tomography scans.[c] This condition is called spinal cord injury without radiographic abnormality, or SCIWORA. In adults, SCIWORA is most likely to occur in individuals with preexisting narrow spinal canals or degenerative changes.[21,22] It may occur in children due to the flexibility of their spinal columns.[23,24]

Cervical Injuries

Because of its relatively poor mechanical stability, the cervical spine is more vulnerable to trauma than are other areas of the vertebral column.[25] Moreover, injury to the spine in this region is likely to result (40% incidence) in damage to

---

[b] Estimates range from 1.6% to 23.8%,[240] with most estimates ranging from 3% to 8%.[241]

[c] Magnetic resonance imaging typically reveals neural or extraneural damage.[23]

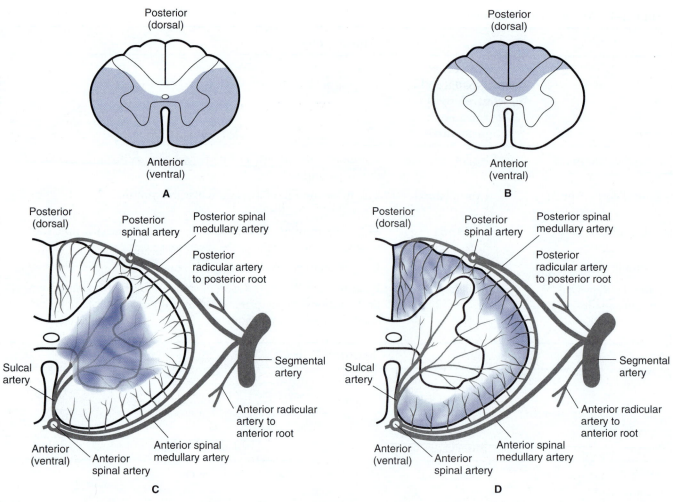

Figure 2–6   Blood supply to the spinal cord. (A) Area supplied by the anterior spinal artery. (B) Area supplied by the posterior spinal arteries. (C) Area supplied by the centrifugal system. (D) Area supplied by the centripetal system.

the cord.[22] As a result of these factors, a disproportionate number (approximately 52%) of spinal cord injuries occur in the cervical region.[1]

Most survivors of cervical spinal cord injuries have cord damage at the lower cervical levels; vertebral fractures at C1 and C2 are rarely associated with significant neurological deficits.[22] This is largely due to a combination of two factors. The vertebral canal is large at the craniovertebral junction, with the spinal cord occupying only 50% of the available space. Thus it is possible for 50% of the canal's area to be intruded upon by displaced bony elements without damage to the spinal cord. In addition, when the spinal cord is injured at this level, the injury is not likely to be survived. Complete cord injuries at C1 and C2 interrupt the innervation of the diaphragm, making survival possible only if resuscitation is provided immediately.[26,27]

The forces most frequently causing vertebral injury in the cervical spine are flexion, axial loading, distraction, and extension. These forces may be accompanied and modified by rotation, lateral flexion, or shear.[16,17]

Thoracic Injuries

The rib cage provides the T1 through T10 spine with great stability. As a result, extreme violence is required to injure the spine in this region. Thoracic spinal cord injuries are less common than cervical injuries, but are more likely to be complete[26,28,29] and are less frequently associated with any subsequent return of motor or sensory function below the lesion.[29,30] These findings are probably due to the magnitude of force required to injure the thoracic spine, the small size of the vertebral foramen in this region, and the relatively poor vascular supply of the upper thoracic cord.[26,27] Trauma to the lower thoracic spine can injure the vessel of Adamkiewicz, a radicular artery that is a major source of the thoracolumbar cord's vascular supply. The resulting neurological damage can ascend as high as T4.[27]

Thoracic injuries are often caused by gunshot wounds, vehicular accidents, and falls.[27] The most common site of injury to the thoracolumbar spine is the T12-L1 junction.[5] This is where the relatively rigid thoracic spine meets the relatively flexible lumbar spine.[22,31]

combination of flexion and rotation.[7,22,27] Isolated extension or lateral flexion forces rarely cause injury in the thoracic spine.[5,22,27]

Lumbar Injuries

The lumbar region of the spinal column is of intermediate stability: it is more flexible than the thoracic spine but less flexible than the cervical spine. Although it lacks the stability provided by the thoracic cage, the lumbar spine is supported by strong paraspinal and abdominal musculature.[22]

Common causes of injury to this region include falls, vehicular accidents, gunshot wounds, and direct impact from heavy objects.[27,32] Injury occurs most frequently at the thoracolumbar junction.[33]

Neurological damage resulting from trauma to the lumbar spine is usually incomplete.[26] This fact is due in part to the relatively good vascular supply and large vertebral foramen in this region. In addition, caudal to L1 or L2, the cord is not present in the vertebral foramen. The cauda equina, the sole neurological element in this region, is less sensitive than the spinal cord to trauma.[5,27] It can be damaged, however, by compression, stretching, avulsion, or tearing.[33]

Lumbar injuries are commonly caused by flexion, axial loading, or flexion combined with distraction or rotation. Shear forces, such as occur when a person is struck from behind by a heavy object or falls onto an uneven surface, are less commonly responsible for vertebral injuries.[34]

Associated Injuries

Traumatic spinal cord injuries often occur with additional injuries sustained at the same time. Some of the more common associated injuries include fractures, pneumothorax, hemothorax, head injury, brachial plexus injury, and peripheral nerve injury.[35] These injuries can delay and prolong rehabilitation and, in some cases, limit patients' ultimate functional outcomes.

Neuropathology

When spinal cord injury is caused by vertebral injury, the cord typically sustains damage due to impingement by bony or soft tissue structures. This occurs, for example, when vertebrae dislocate or a vertebral body bursts. The spinal cord can also be damaged by traction[19,36] or by direct insult from a foreign body such as a bullet or knife. Gunshot wounds can damage the cord even if the bullet does not enter the spinal canal; in these cases, a concussive shock wave damages the cord. In both penetrating and nonpenetrating injuries, more severe disruption of the spinal canal leads to more severe neurological damage.[37]

The spinal cord does not have to be severed for irreversible damage to occur. In fact, anatomic transection of the cord is rare.[38,39] This is an important point to remember

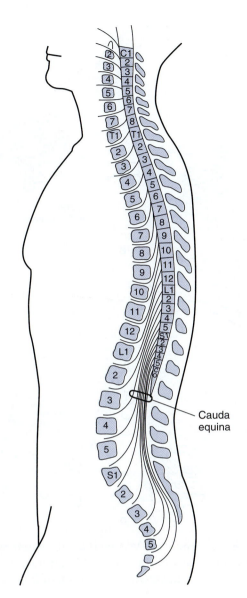

Figure 2–7   Schematic diagram of the spatial relationship of the vertebrae, spinal cord, nerve roots, and cauda equina.

The spatial arrangement of bony and neural tissue in the low thoracic and upper lumbar regions is such that vertebral injury can result in diverse patterns of neurological damage. All of the lumbar and sacral cord segments lie between the upper border of the T10 vertebral body and the level of L1 or L2. Additionally, spinal nerves from higher levels lie adjacent to the cord within the vertebral canal in this region as they travel caudally before exiting. As a result, the vertebral foramen at a given level may enclose more than one cord level as well as spinal nerves from several higher levels. Vertebral damage can result in trauma to any or all of this neural tissue, or in no neurological damage.

Thoracic injuries are most commonly caused by flexion forces. Injury can also result from axial loading or a

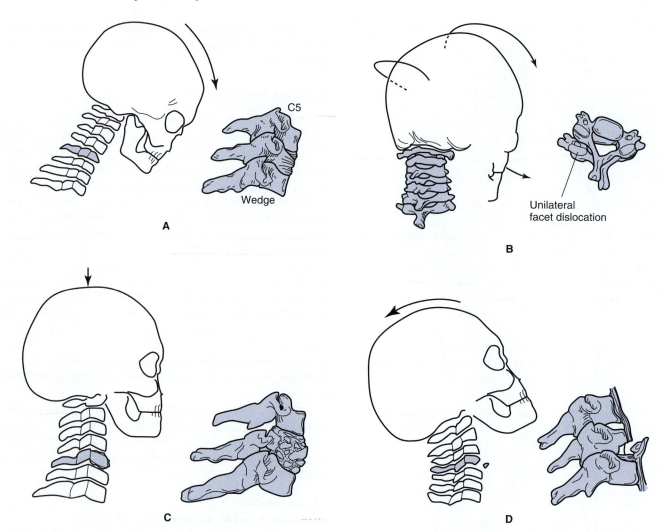

Figure 2–8   Examples of direction of traumatic force influencing pattern of injury. (A) Wedge fracture caused by flexion. (B) Unilateral facet dislocation caused by combined flexion and rotation. (C) Burst fracture caused by compression (axial loading). (D) Ruptured anterior longitudinal ligament and avulsion of fragment from anterior vertebral body caused by extension.

when educating people about their injuries. Often, patients are told that their spinal cords were "bruised" instead of severed, and they interpret this fact to mean that they will recover from their paralysis. Trauma that results in "bruising" or hemorrhaging in the spinal cord, however, can (and often does) cause neurological damage that is just as complete and permanent as when the cord is severed.

Not all spinal cord damage occurs as the result of trauma to the cord itself. The spinal cord can also be damaged when its vascular supply is disrupted by vertebral trauma, gunshot or knife wounds, or various other causes. In addition, there are a variety of nontraumatic causes of spinal cord damage. Examples include spinal hematoma, infection, transverse myelitis, arachnoiditis, radiation, spondylosis, rheumatoid arthritis, neoplasm, and interruption of the cord's vascular supply due to surgery, cardiac arrest, or aortic aneurysm.[5]

Pathological Changes

Blunt trauma to the spinal cord results in some primary destruction of neurons at the level of injury. This neuronal damage (primary injury) is most severe in the cell bodies but can also occur in the axons.[40] Much of the damage to the cord, however, is caused by sequelae (secondary injury) of the initial trauma.[41–44]

Typically, the spinal cord sustains a contusion[d] as the result of impingement by displaced bone, soft tissues, or

---

[d] The following description of the pathological changes associated with spinal cord injury is based primarily on studies of blunt trauma to the cord, as occurs when bony elements impinge on the cord as a result of vertebral injury. However, research indicates that the same process of secondary progressive tissue destruction occurs with any injury to the spinal cord, including damage from ischemia, slow compression,[52] contusion, or transection.[48]

both. Within hours following the initial trauma, a process of progressive tissue destruction is initiated within the cord. These secondary reactions lead to ischemia, edema, demyelination of axons, and necrosis of the spinal cord.[39,45]

The injured spinal cord can look undamaged on visual examination soon after injury.[5] Microscopic examination within the first few hours, however, reveals patchy hemorrhage, tissue laceration, edema, and necrosis; these are most prevalent in the central gray matter. Tissue destruction spreads outward into the white matter as time passes, as well as rostrally and caudally.[5,13,46] The resulting area of cord necrosis is commonly spindle-shaped, tapering in its rostral and caudal extensions.[40] The area of maximal cord damage usually spreads over one to three segments; however, the tissue destruction can spread over several segments.

The process of secondary tissue destruction may last from several days[47] to 4 weeks[48] after the initial trauma. The extent of destruction that ultimately occurs is dependent on the severity of the initial trauma,[49] with some modification by the therapeutic interventions administered to limit progression of the lesion. Axons located peripherally in the cord are most likely to survive. Of those that survive, many remain nonfunctional as a result of demyelination.[47]

Gross edema of the spinal cord can also occur following trauma. As the cord swells, it becomes compressed within the meninges, and further damage to the cord occurs.[40]

As the primary and secondary reactions to trauma subside, the necrotic region of the spinal cord is gradually resorbed and replaced by scar tissue, cysts, or cavities.[15,40,50,51]

Underlying Mechanisms of Secondary Tissue Destruction

Despite extensive research in recent years, the mechanisms underlying the secondary tissue destruction initiated by spinal cord injury remain only partially understood. Initial trauma to the cord appears to set off a multifactorial process that expands the area of cell death and damage. The mechanisms involved in this process include ischemia, inflammation, disruption of ion concentrations in the injured tissues, and apoptosis (Figure 2–9). Each of these pathologic processes, and the cell damage and death that they cause, leads to the release of substances that stimulate additional secondary tissue damage, creating an escalating cycle of tissue destruction.

Ischemia

Blood flow diminishes in the traumatized area of a spinal cord following injury. This reduction in circulation occurs rapidly in the gray matter. In severely traumatized cords, blood flow in the white matter falls after a 2- to 3-hour delay. It may not diminish at all in the white matter of less severely traumatized cords.[52]

One of the primary causes of interrupted blood supply to the damaged segment of the cord appears to be injury

to the anterior sulcal arteries and arterioles. These vessels provide circulation to the central part of the spinal cord, including the gray matter and the adjacent ascending and descending tracts (Figure 2–6C).[13]

Blood supply to the spinal cord is disrupted by mechanical trauma, including rupture or compression of blood vessels, and intravascular thromboses.[13,53] Vasospasm also plays a significant role: the arterioles arising from the anterior sulcal arteries constrict progressively during the first 24 hours after injury.[53] Vasoconstrictive substances such as norepinephrine, serotonin, histamine, and prostaglandins in the injured cord may contribute to this vasospasm and the resulting ischemia.[53,54] Additional possible causes of vasospasm include mechanical stimulation and the presence of vasoconstrictive substances formed during the breakdown of erythrocytes following hemorrhage.[53]

Disruption of the venous system in the damaged region of the cord may also contribute to ischemia.[13,53] Other possible causes of ischemia in the injured spinal cord include metabolic disturbances and elevated pressure due to edema.[52]

The central nervous system is very intolerant to ischemia; as little as 15 to 30 seconds of anoxia can cause irreversible damage in the neurons.[55] When the blood supply to the injured portion of the spinal cord is interrupted, lack of oxygen and nutrients interferes with normal cellular functioning in this area. Ion derangement (described later in this chapter) quickly follows, initiating a cascade of metabolic events that lead to cell death.[56]

Inflammation

Inflammation plays a significant role in the process of secondary tissue destruction, apparently contributing to the expansion of the lesion for 24 to 48 hours after the injury. Cells that are damaged in the initial trauma release proinflammatory substances that attract neutrophils to the injured area within a few hours of the injury. Activated microglia and macrophages arrive[e] slightly later.[43,55,57] Inflammatory cells have been found in injured spinal cords as early as 4 hours and as late as 1 year after injury.[43]

Neutrophils, activated microglia, and macrophages phagocytose debris in the damaged area. Early after injury, they release reactive oxygen species and a variety of other substances that damage surrounding tissue, thus expanding the area of necrosis.[42–44,57,58] Reactive oxygen metabolites damage cells by attacking cellular components such as nucleic acids, proteins, and phospholipids.[56] The breakdown products of these reactions can further disrupt cell functioning, contributing to the development of ion imbalance.[42]

Although inflammation contributes to the process of tissue destruction that follows spinal cord injury, it may also play a role in protecting some of the surviving neurons and promoting tissue repair.[43,44,48,55,57]

[e] Microglia already present in the tissue are activated and transformed into macrophages. Macrophages also infiltrate from the bloodstream.[43]

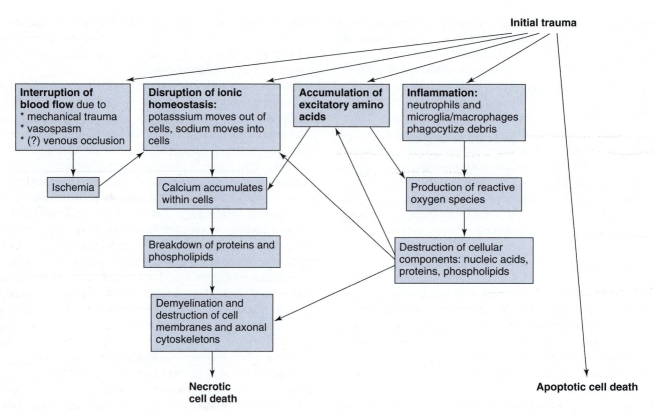

Figure 2–9   Secondary tissue destruction initiated by spinal cord injury.

Ion Derangement

Disruption of cell membranes in the injured area of the spinal cord results in abnormal concentrations of potassium and sodium: potassium moves out from the neurons into the extracellular space, and sodium accumulates within the cells. This derangement causes a loss of neuronal excitability because neurons require a normal ion balance to generate action potentials.[56] More importantly, a high concentration of sodium within the neurons results in a shift in calcium, a key factor in secondary tissue destruction following spinal cord injury.[f]

Calcium ions accumulate in injured cells after a spinal cord is traumatized. The influx of calcium results from the abnormally high sodium concentration within the neurons and the collapse of the membrane potential.[56] Neurotoxic transmitters, particularly glutamate, contribute to this shift of calcium into the neurons.[39,42,44,49,59–62]

Concentration of calcium within neurons is one of the most important contributors to secondary tissue destruction following spinal cord injury.[56, 63, 64] The abnormal concentration of calcium within the damaged cells disrupts their functioning and causes breakdown of protein and phospholipids, with resulting demyelination, destruction of the cell membrane and axonal cytoskeleton, and

cell death.[41,52,56,64–67] The metabolic by-products of this deranged cell functioning and membrane destruction may contribute to further membrane destruction and the development of ischemia and edema.[52]

Apoptosis

Apoptosis is a form of cell death (programmed cell death) that occurs normally during embryonic development and also as a pathological process following central nervous system damage. It is an active process performed by individual cells, in contrast to the passive death of groups of cells as occurs in necrotic[g] cell death.[68,69]

Both neurons and supporting cells within the spinal cord tissue undergo apoptotic cell death.[69] It is not yet known what initiates this "intrinsic suicide mechanism."[68] It begins at the level of the initial injury within 4 to 6 hours of the trauma and runs its course at this level within 24 hours.[69]

Apoptosis occurs for a more prolonged time (up to 3 weeks) in areas of the spinal cord rostral and caudal to the site of the initial injury.[68,70] It occurs in oligodendrocytes[h] associated with the myelin sheaths of degenerating ascending white matter tracts rostral to the site of the injury, and in descending tracts caudal to the injury.[68,70] Apoptotic

---

[f] Calcium overload is involved in cell death of both glial cells and neurons.[56]

[g] Mechanical disruption of injured cells and the secondary pathological processes described in the preceding paragraphs lead to necrosis.
[h] Oligodendrocytes are glial cells that form the myelin sheaths surrounding axons.

oligodendrocyte cell death may cause demyelination of surviving axons, thus interfering with their subsequent functioning.[44,68,70]

Effect of Compression on Recovery of Function

Spinal cord trauma does not always result in complete disruption of the cord at the level of lesion. Incomplete lesions are common, with surviving neurons passing through the damaged portion of the cord. If this undamaged neural tissue is subjected to chronic compression, however, it may survive but not resume functioning while subjected to the compression.[71]

Spinal Shock

Spinal shock is a transient phenomenon that occurs after trauma to the spinal cord. Spinal reflexes, voluntary motor and sensory function, and autonomic control are absent or depressed caudal to the lesion after the cord is injured.[72,73] The cause is unknown. Neurons below the lesion may become hyperpolarized, losing their excitability due to the absence of facilitation from descending tracts.[72,74] Reflex functioning gradually returns as spinal shock resolves. The timing of this resolution is a matter of debate. In one model, spinal shock is conceptualized as occurring in four phases, starting with absent or depressed reflexes (phase 1, from 0 to 1 day), followed by an initial return of some reflexes (phase 2, from 1 to 3 days), further return of reflexes and early hyper-reflexia (phase 3, from 1 to 4 weeks), and finally spasticity/hyper-reflexia (phase 4, from 1 to 12 months).[72]

Spinal Cord Function Below the Lesion

As spinal shock passes, the cord gradually resumes functioning below the lesion. This return of function is evidenced by resumption of spinal reflexes caudal to the lesion. Sensorimotor interneuronal networks below the lesion also resume functioning. These circuits are normally involved in the mediation of both reflexive and voluntary motion,[75] and are thought to include central pattern generators that can produce complex patterns of motor output for repetitive rhythmic actions such as locomotion[76] and possibly ejaculation.[77]

As spinal shock resolves, voluntary motor function, sensation, and supraspinal influences on the spinal autonomic centers may also resume. This return of function can occur if the brain and the spinal cord caudal to the lesion remain "connected" by some surviving and functioning neurons that span the damaged segment of the cord.[i] If this "connection" does not exist, the portion of the cord

caudal to the lesion will function but will not communicate with the brain. In these cases, the individual will exhibit spinal reflexes below the lesion but will lack voluntary motor control, autonomic control, and sensation below the lesion. Interneuronal circuitry caudal to the lesion will function in response to afferent input but will not be subject to activation or modulation by supraspinal centers.

Neurological Return

Neurological return refers to a resumption of voluntary motor function or sensation that has been lost as the result of a spinal cord injury. For example, individuals may regain the ability to voluntarily contract one or more muscles that had been paralyzed, or regain the ability to feel a pin or cotton ball contacting the skin in one or more areas that had been anesthetic. This resumption of motor or sensory function below the level of the lesion is evidence of at least some "connection" between the brain and the muscles or dermatomes that resume functioning. In contrast, the return of reflexive functioning below the lesion is not considered to be neurological return. For example, the onset of spasticity[j] below the lesion without any gains in sensory ability or voluntary motor function is not classified as neurological return. The presence of spasticity gives evidence of functioning of the spinal cord below the lesion, but it does not demonstrate a "connection" between the brain and the muscles.

Most neurological return occurs in the first year after spinal cord injury, most rapidly during the first 3 months.[78-86] Additional return can take place for 2 or more years, but improvements in motor function after the first year typically are minimal.[78,79,81-83,85,86] In unusual cases, neurological return can occur for 5 or more years after injury.[87]

Mechanisms of Neurological Return

Neurological return after spinal cord injury can occur as a result of resumed functioning within either the nerve roots or the spinal cord itself. The first of these is referred to as nerve root return, or root recovery. It may be the most common source of neurological return, possibly occurring after all traumatic spinal cord injuries.[61] The reason that nerve root return occurs so frequently is that the nerve roots are more resistant to trauma and have a greater capacity for recovery and regeneration than do neurons within the spinal cord.[61]

The mechanisms of neurological return are not fully understood. In addition to root return, possible causes include remyelination of surviving neurons, and resolution of pathologic processes such as hemorrhage, vasoconstriction, and edema.[61,74,88-91] Adaptive alteration in the structure and functioning of surviving neurons (injury-induced plasticity) throughout the central nervous system may also play a role

---

[i] In many cases, a small number of surviving axons span the level of the lesion, but the patient has no motor or sensory sparing. This may be due to demyelination or hypomyelination of the spared neurons[114] or insufficient numbers of surviving axons traversing the injured segment. This is sometimes referred to as a "discomplete" injury.[15,167]

[j] Spasticity, an involuntary motor response, is discussed later in this chapter.

in neurological return following incomplete injuries. A discussion of neuroplasticity follows later in this chapter.

Predictors of Motor Return

Perhaps the most central question for patients, their families, and health professionals is how much recovery of motor function will occur after a spinal cord injury.[k] Unfortunately it is not possible to predict with certainty the neurological return that any individual will experience. Predictions within the first 24 hours after injury are the least likely to be accurate. During that time, motor function commonly improves or deteriorates[92] due to resolution or progression of ongoing pathological processes within the spinal cord. Predictions based on the patient's motor function at 72 hours to 1 week after injury are more reliable.[78,93] During the months and years that follow, the probability of additional neurological recovery diminishes. Because of this, predictions regarding future return made at later times are even more likely to be accurate.

Most patients experience at least some neurological recovery after spinal cord injury,[61,84] but the amount of motor return varies widely. At one extreme, some individuals regain normal strength in all of their musculature. At the other extreme are patients who do not experience any improvement in motor function, or regain strength only in muscles innervated just caudal to their lesions. An examination of the patient's motor and sensory function can be used to predict the extent of neurological recovery that will occur.[94] Several factors, presented in the following paragraphs, have been found to be associated with a better prognosis for neurological return. Table 2–2 presents examples of research findings on motor return after spinal cord injuries.

Degree of Impairment

The probability of future motor return varies with the degree of completeness of the lesion; people with incomplete injuries experience more motor return than do those with complete injuries.[78,95,98–102] This is true both with paraplegia and tetraplegia, and for return in myotomes innervated either near to or distant from the lesion.[78,85,86,98,101]

Extensive motor recovery rarely occurs after complete spinal cord injury. However, even individuals who have injuries that remain complete frequently experience return in muscles innervated just below the neurological level of injury.[82] In patients with complete tetraplegia, this motor recovery can significantly improve the capacity to perform functional skills.[78]

Preserved Motor Function

Preserved motor function after a spinal cord injury is the best predictor of future motor return. This is true both

with paraplegia and tetraplegia, and for return in myotomes innervated either near or distant from the lesion.[82–84,86,91,103] Moreover, in muscles that initially test 0/5, return is more common in those that are innervated one level below innervated musculature.[82,83,85,86]

Preserved Pin Prick Sensation

Preserved pin prick sensation[l] in the sacral region[86,104] or the extremities[96] is associated with a greater likelihood of significant motor return. This finding has been reported in studies with various degrees of impairment and levels of injury, and in muscles innervated either close to or distant from the lesion.[86,96,103,104]

Pattern of Neurological Injury

Among people with incomplete spinal cord injuries, the pattern of injury is a predictive factor for motor return. Individuals with either central cord or Brown–Séquard syndrome have a better prognosis for motor return than do those with anterior cord syndrome.[81, 105]

Early Neurological Return

Motor return is associated with better long-term outcomes if it occurs soon after the injury rather than later.[79,91,105,106] For example, if a muscle's strength converts from 0/5 to 1/5, the significance of this return depends on the time that has elapsed since the injury. If this change occurs during the first month after injury, it will be more predictive of future return than a similar improvement that occurs at 6 months. Likewise, a person who has a spinal cord injury that converts from complete to incomplete more than a month after injury is not likely to experience extensive motor return.[82]

Age

Younger age at the time of injury is associated with greater motor return.[81,102,106,107] This association has been found in studies that compared groups of patients older and younger than 65,[108] 50,[102] and 18[81] years of age.

Neurological Deterioration

Deterioration of neurological function, evidenced by reduced sensation or muscle strength, can also occur soon after injury. This deterioration, which is exhibited by approximately 2% to 5% of people with spinal cord injuries, has been associated with sepsis, intubation, early surgical intervention, and ankylosing spondylitis.[109] Additional causes of neurological deterioration include vertebral instability and the development of a posttraumatic cyst.[110]

---

[k] A closely related question is the prognosis of regaining the capacity for functional ambulation. This issue is addressed in Chapter 12.

[l] The association between spared pin prick and subsequent motor return may stem from the fact that the lateral spinothalamic tract (carrying pain information) and the corticospinal tract (carrying motor commands) lie relatively close to each other in the white matter of the spinal cord.[242] The corticospinal tract is essential to voluntary motor control in humans.[114]

TABLE 2–2 Factors Associated with Motor Return

Factor	Subjects	Outcomes
ASIA Impairment Scale (AIS) grade* at time of admission	842 patients with spinal cord injury admitted to Regional Spinal Cord Injury Centers within 7 days of injury[95]	Percent progressing to higher AIS grade by 1 year after injury**

Initial Grade	Percent progressing to Higher Grade	Percent progressing to AIS D or E
A	15.4	2.3
B	72.8	34.8
C	70.5	70.5
D	4.2	4.2 (E)

Factor	Subjects	Outcomes
Presence or absence of early motor return in muscles initially testing 0/5	32 patients with tetraplegia, Frankel† A and B[91]	Motor return in zone of partial preservation‡ • ≥1/5 strength regained by 1 month after injury: 86% regained ≥3/5 by 1 year. • ≥2/5 strength regained by 3 months after injury: 100% regained ≥3/5 strength by 1 year.
Motor function at 1 month after injury	54 patients with traumatic incomplete paraplegia[85]	Strength in individual lower extremity muscles • 1/5 to 2/5 strength at 1 month after injury: 85% recovered to ≥3/5 by 1 year. • 0/5 strength at 1 month after injury: 26% recovered to ≥3/5 by 1 year.
Motor function at 1 month after injury	50 patients with traumatic incomplete tetraplegia[86]	Strength in individual upper extremity muscles • 2/5 strength at 1 month after injury: 100% recovered to ≥3/5 by 1 year. • 1/5 strength at 1 month after injury: 73% recovered to ≥3/5 by 1 year. • 0/5 strength at 1 month after injury: 20% recovered to ≥3/5 by 1 year. Strength in individual lower extremity muscles • 2/5 strength at 1 month after injury: 97% recovered to ≥3/5 by 1 year. • 1/5 strength at 1 month after injury: 77% recovered to ≥3/5 by 1 year. • 0/5 strength at 1 month after injury: 24% recovered to ≥3/5 by 1 year.
Pin prick sensation at the time of initial examination	59 patients with complete and incomplete tetraplegia and paraplegia[96]	Return of functional strength in muscles initially testing 0/5 • Dermatomes with spared pin prick sensation: 85% of the corresponding myotomes regained ≥3/5 strength. • Dermatomes without spared pin prick sensation: 1.3% of the corresponding myotomes regained ≥3/5 strength.

* The ASIA Impairment Scale is presented in Figure 2–11.
** Progress from A to B, C, or D; from B to C, D, or E; etc.
† The Frankel Scale is similar to the ASIA Impairment Scale.
‡ Note that the definition of "zone of partial preservation" was changed in the 1996 version of the International Standards for Neurological and Functional Classification of Spinal Cord Injury to include sparing in complete injuries only. Previous definitions included motor and sensory sparing in both complete and incomplete injuries.[97]

In many cases, the lost function is regained within a year. This is particularly true when the deterioration was relatively minor.[109]

Plasticity

Plasticity is the capacity of neurons throughout the central nervous system to change their structure and function in support of normal development and learning, as well as in response to injury or disease.[111–113] After spinal cord injury, plastic changes occur at all levels of the central nervous system, including the cerebral cortex and other areas of the brain as well as the spinal cord both rostral and caudal

to the lesion.[38,111,112,114] Both spontaneous and activity-dependent plasticity can occur.

Spontaneous plasticity after spinal cord injury includes structural changes such as axonal sprouting in both damaged and undamaged neurons projecting to and from the brain, axonal sprouting in spared intersegmental interneurons, creation of new synapses, and synaptic remodeling.[111,114] Figure 2–10 illustrates some of the structural remodeling that may occur in the motor system. Plasticity also involves alterations in neuronal functioning, including activation (unmasking) of latent pathways and changes in conduction velocity and responsiveness to neurotransmitters.[111,114] Spontaneous plasticity is thought to contribute to neurological

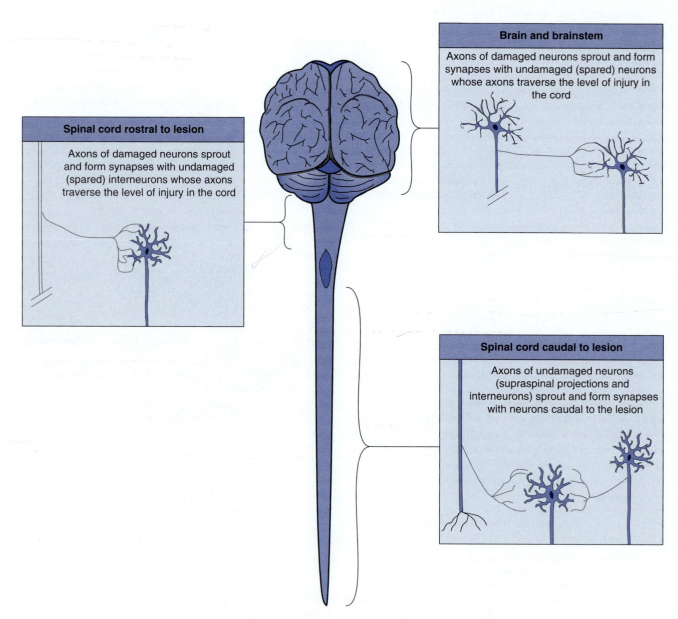

Brain and brainstem

Axons of damaged neurons sprout and form synapses with undamaged (spared) neurons whose axons traverse the level of injury in the cord

Spinal cord rostral to lesion

Axons of damaged neurons sprout and form synapses with undamaged (spared) interneurons whose axons traverse the level of injury in the cord

Spinal cord caudal to lesion

Axons of undamaged neurons (supraspinal projections and interneurons) sprout and form synapses with neurons caudal to the lesion

Figure 2–10   Structural changes in neurons possibly contributing to motor recovery after incomplete spinal cord injury.

return[112,114] and improvements in respiratory[114] and possibly sexual[115] functioning. It may also have maladaptive effects, such as elevated muscle tone, autonomic dysreflexia (described later in this chapter), and pain.[111,112,114]

Activity-dependent plasticity occurs in response to afferent input. Sensory input from the periphery, typically arising from repetitive limb activity, causes adaptive neuronal changes.[116] Activity-dependent plasticity is task-specific, meaning that the plastic changes that occur in response to a particular activity can enhance the performance of that activity but will not generalize to others. (For example, stepping practice will enhance stepping but not standing.)[111,116] The motor responses associated with activity-dependent plasticity fade over time if practice of the activity is discontinued.[112] The mechanisms of activity-dependent plasticity after spinal cord injury remain to be determined,[116] but appear to involve functional and structural changes at all levels of the central nervous system.[112]

Although the central nervous system exhibits significant plasticity in response to spinal cord injury, its inherent capacity for axonal regeneration (regrowth of axons) *through an injury site* is limited.[114] This limitation is reflected in the small amount of neurological recovery associated with complete spinal cord lesions.[m]

CLASSIFICATION OF SPINAL CORD INJURIES

In the past, communication regarding spinal cord injuries was hampered by the lack of a universally accepted system of terminology.[117] This problem has been reduced with the use of the classification system published by the American Spinal Injury Association (ASIA) and endorsed by the International Medical Society of Paraplegia.[n] A worksheet for this classification system is presented in Figure 2–11.

Tetraplegia Versus Paraplegia

Damage to the nervous tissue contained within the cervical region of the spinal canal causes tetraplegia.[o] *Tetraplegia* refers to impairment or loss[p] of motor and/or sensory function in the upper and lower extremities, trunk, and pelvic organs.[118]

Damage to the nervous tissue contained within the thoracic, lumbar, or sacral regions of the spinal canal causes paraplegia. Depending on the level of lesion, paraplegia can involve impairment or loss of motor and/or sensory function in the trunk, lower extremities, and pelvic organs.[118] Motor and sensory function is normal in the upper extremities.

Neurological Level of Injury

The neurological level of injury is defined as the most caudal level of the spinal cord that exhibits intact sensory and motor functioning bilaterally. To determine an individual's neurological level of injury, the clinician tests sensitivity to light touch and pin prick at key points in each dermatome, and strength in key muscles that are representative of specific cord segments. Key sensory points and key muscles are included in Figure 2–11.

The key sensory points are well demarcated; each is innervated by a single spinal cord segment. As a result, the sensory ability at a key point provides a good representation of the functioning in the sensory portions of its corresponding cord segment. In contrast, muscles receive innervation from more than one spinal cord level (Figure 2–12). Thus, the strength of a given muscle is a reflection of the functioning of two or more cord segments. A lesion in the caudal segment innervating a muscle will cause reduced strength in that muscle.[q]

For the purposes of identifying the neurological level of injury, a key muscle is defined as demonstrating intact innervation from the cord segment that it represents[r] if (1) it exhibits 3/5 or greater strength and (2) the next more rostral key muscle exhibits 5/5 strength. If the next more rostral key muscle tests less than 5/5 but the examiner judges that its reduced performance in the manual muscle test is due to factors such as pain or disuse rather than spinal cord damage, this muscle can be assigned a grade of 5/5 for the purposes of determining neurological level.[118]

Certain spinal cord levels do not have myotomes that are readily testable using a manual muscle test. When classifying a spinal cord injury within these levels of the spinal cord (C1 through C4, T2 through L1, and S2 through S5), the motor level is presumed to be the same as the sensory level.[118]

---

[m] Extensive ongoing research is likely to lead, in the future, to advances in medical, surgical, and rehabilitative management resulting in greater neurological and functional recovery.[38,114]

[n] The International Standards for the Neurological and Functional Classification of Spinal Cord Injury[118] is revised periodically. Clinicians and researchers should use the most current version.

[o] *Quadriplegia* is synonymous with *tetraplegia*.

[p] In this context, *loss* refers to an absence of motor function (0/5 strength) or sensory function (anesthesia). *Impairment* refers to a reduction in motor or sensory function or altered sensory function, such as hyperesthesia. This is not to be confused with *impairment* as defined in the International Classification of Functioning, Disability, and Health—a broader definition that would include all of the above.

---

[q] For example, the biceps brachii receives C5 and C6 innervation, and normal functioning of this muscle involves intact innervation from both of these cord segments. A cord lesion that disrupts the functioning of the C6 level of the cord will result in a reduction of biceps strength.

[r] Key muscles are identified with the more rostral of the spinal cord segments from which they receive innervation. For example, the biceps brachii, which is the C5 key muscle, receives innervation from both C5 and C6.

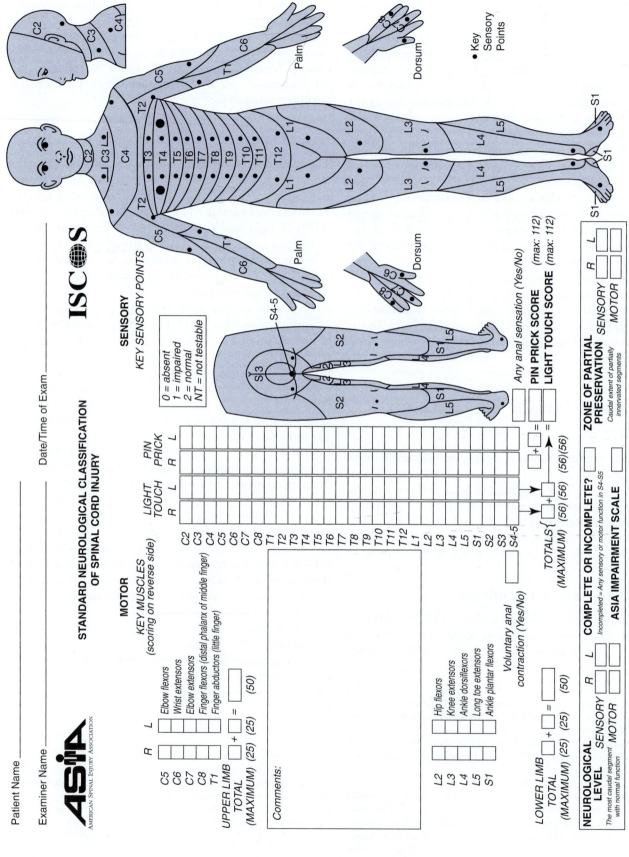

STANDARD NEUROLOGICAL CLASSIFICATION
OF SPINAL CORD INJURY

Patient Name _____

Examiner Name _____ Date/Time of Exam _____

ISC♦S

MOTOR

KEY MUSCLES
(scoring on reverse side)

	R	L
C5			Elbow flexors
C6			Wrist extensors
C7			Elbow extensors
C8			Finger flexors (distal phalanx of middle finger)
T1			Finger abductors (little finger)

UPPER LIMB
TOTAL
(MAXIMUM) (25) (25) ☐ + ☐ = ☐ (50)

Comments:

	R	L
L2			Hip flexors
L3			Knee extensors
L4			Ankle dorsiflexors
L5			Long toe extensors
S1			Ankle plantar flexors

Voluntary anal
contraction (Yes/No) ☐

LOWER LIMB
TOTAL ☐ + ☐ = ☐
(MAXIMUM) (25) (25) (50)

SENSORY

KEY SENSORY POINTS

0 = absent
1 = impaired
2 = normal
NT = not testable

	LIGHT TOUCH		PIN PRICK	
	R	L	R	L
C2				
C3				
C4				
C5				
C6				
C7				
C8				
T1				
T2				
T3				
T4				
T5				
T6				
T7				
T8				
T9				
T10				
T11				
T12				
L1				
L2				
L3				
L4				
L5				
S1				
S2				
S3				
S4-5				

TOTALS { ☐ + ☐ (56) (56) = ☐ ☐ + ☐ (56)(56) = ☐
(MAXIMUM) LIGHT TOUCH (56) (56) PIN PRICK

Any anal sensation (Yes/No) ☐

PIN PRICK SCORE ☐ (max: 112)
LIGHT TOUCH SCORE ☐ (max: 112)

COMPLETE OR INCOMPLETE? ☐
Incomplete = Any sensory or motor function in S4-S5

ASIA IMPAIRMENT SCALE ☐

NEUROLOGICAL
LEVEL
The most caudal segment
with normal function
	R	L
SENSORY	☐	☐
MOTOR	☐	☐

ZONE OF PARTIAL
PRESERVATION
Caudal extent of partially
innervated segments
	R	L
SENSORY	☐	☐
MOTOR	☐	☐

• Key Sensory Points

Palm   Dorsum

This form may be copied freely but should not be altered without permission from the American Spinal Injury Association.

ASIA
AMERICAN SPINAL INJURY ASSOCIATION

MUSCLE GRADING

0 total paralysis

1 palpable or visible contraction

2 active movement, full range of motion, gravity eliminated

3 active movement, full range of motion, against gravity

4 active movement, full range of motion, against gravity and provides some resistance

5 active movement, full range of motion, against gravity and provides normal resistance

5* muscle able to exert, in examiner's judgment, sufficient resistance to be considered normal if identifiable inhibiting factors were not present

NT not testable. Patient unable to reliably exert effort or muscle unavailable for testing due to factors such as immobilization, pain on effort or contracture.

ASIA IMPAIRMENT SCALE

☐ A = **Complete:** No motor or sensory function is preserved in the sacral segments S4–S5.

☐ B = **Incomplete:** Sensory but not motor function is preserved below the neurological level and includes the sacral segments S4–S5.

☐ C = **Incomplete:** Motor function is preserved below the neurological level, and more than half of key muscles below the neurological level have a muscle grade less than 3.

☐ D = **Incomplete:** Motor function is preserved below the neurological level, and at least half of key muscles below the neurological level have a muscle grade of 3 or better.

☐ E = **Normal:** Motor and sensory function are normal.

CLINICAL SYNDROMES (OPTIONAL)

☐ Central Cord
☐ Brown-Sequard
☐ Anterior Cord
☐ Conus Medullaris
☐ Cauda Equina

STEPS IN CLASSIFICATION

The following order is recommended in determining the classification of individuals with SCI.

1. Determine sensory levels for right and left sides.

2. Determine motor levels for right and left sides.
   Note: in regions where there is no myotome to test, the motor level is presumed to be the same as the sensory level.

3. Determine the single neurological level.
   This is the lowest segment where motor and sensory function is normal on both sides, and is the most cephalad of the sensory and motor levels determined in steps 1 and 2.

4. Determine whether the injury is Complete or Incomplete. (sacral sparing).
   *If voluntary anal contraction = **No** AND all S4-5 sensory scores = **0** AND any anal sensation = **No**, then injury is COMPLETE. Otherwise injury is incomplete.*

5. Determine ASIA Impairment Scale (AIS) Grade:

   Is injury Complete?   If **YES**, AIS=A Record ZPP
         NO → (For ZPP record lowest dermatome or myotome on each side with some (non-zero score) preservation)

   Is injury motor incomplete?   If no, AIS=B
         YES → (Yes=voluntary anal contraction OR motor function more than three levels below the motor level on a given side.)

   Are at least half of the key muscles below the (single) neurological level graded 3 or better?
      NO → AIS=C   YES → AIS=D

If sensation and motor function is normal in all segments, AIS=E
Note: AIS E is used in follow up testing when an individual with a documented SCI has recovered normal function. If at initial testing no deficits are found, the individual is neurological. ASIA Impairment Scale does not apply.

Figure 2–11   Standards for Neurological Classification of SCI Worksheet. This form is available from http://www.asia-spinalinjury.org/publications/store.php. (Reproduced with permission from the American Spinal Injury Association [2008]. International Standards for Neurological Classification of Spinal Cord Injury.)

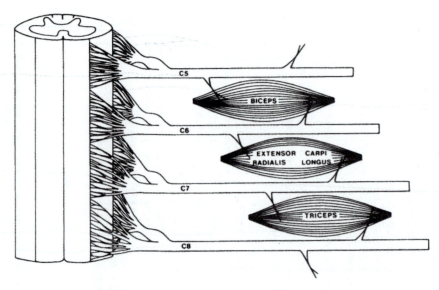

Figure 2–12   Schematic depiction of innervation of each of three key muscles by two nerve segments. (Reproduced with permission from the American Spinal Injury Association [2000]. International Standards for Neurological Classification of Spinal Cord Injury.)

Sensory and motor examinations often reveal differences in the lowest level of intact cord functioning. For example, an individual may exhibit intact motor function through the C5 myotome bilaterally but intact sensory function only through the C4 dermatomes. In cases such as this, it is more appropriate to report separate motor and sensory levels rather than a single neurological level of injury.[118] In this example, the patient exhibits a C5 motor level and a C4 sensory level.

Frequently, the motor function, sensory function, or both differ between the right and left sides of the body. When this is the case, it is best to report right and left motor and sensory levels[s] rather than a single neurological level.[118] This reporting gives a more complete picture of the patient's neurological functioning.[t]

Complete Versus Incomplete Lesion

A person is said to have an incomplete spinal cord injury if some sensory and/or motor function is preserved below the level of the lesion, and includes preserved function in the lowest sacral segments of the spinal cord (S4 and S5). Preserved sensory function is evidenced by the ability to detect pin prick or light touch at the anal mucocutaneous junction, or to detect touch or pressure during a digital

examination of the rectum. Motor function is evidenced by the ability to contract the anal sphincter voluntarily during a digital examination.[118]

With a complete spinal cord injury, both sensory and motor function are absent in S4 and S5. (Motor and sensory function are defined as described above.)

Zone of Partial Preservation

The term *zone of partial preservation* is used only with complete injuries. It refers to partial preservation (sparing) of function in dermatomes and myotomes caudal to the neurological level.[118]

ASIA Impairment Scale

Varying degrees of sensory and voluntary motor function can be seen caudal to incomplete spinal cord lesions. At one end of the spectrum, an individual with an incomplete injury can have sparing of sensation or motor function in the lowest sacral segments with no other sensory or motor function below the lesion. At the other end of the spectrum, an individual can retain near-normal motor and sensory function caudal to the lesion. Thus two people with incomplete C6 tetraplegia, for example, could have markedly different motor and sensory function preserved below their lesions. The ASIA impairment scale (AIS), included in Figure 2–11, allows clinicians and researchers to communicate more effectively about the clinical presentations of people with spinal cord injuries.

---

[s] This will involve reporting four levels: right sensory, left sensory, right motor, and left motor.

[t] Additional documentation involves generating motor and sensory scores. These scores, as well as additional components of an examination, are presented in Chapter 7.

Problem-Solving Exercise 2–1

Your patient sustained a T10 fracture 2 weeks ago. His motor and sensory function have not changed since he was admitted to the hospital: his strength is normal (5/5) in both upper extremities and absent (0/5) in his lower extremities. On the right side of his body, his sensation (pin prick and light touch) is intact in the C2 through the T11 key sensory points, impaired in T12, and absent below. On the left, his sensation is intact in the C2 through the T12 key sensory points, impaired in L1 and L2, and absent below. He does not have any sensation around his anus and cannot contract the anal sphincter voluntarily.

- Classify the injury: neurological level of injury, complete versus incomplete, and ASIA Impairment Scale. (Suggestion: download a worksheet from http://www.asia-spinalinjury.org/publications/store.php to assist with this process.)
- This patient wants to know about his potential for regaining the use of his legs. What is the likelihood that he will experience motor return? Should you give him a definite answer about whether his legs will resume functioning?

CLINICAL SYNDROMES

Incomplete lesions of the spinal cord can result in a variety of patterns of motor and sensory loss. The clinical presentation is determined by the location and pattern of neurological damage. The three incomplete spinal cord injury syndromes are central cord, Brown-Séquard, and anterior cord. Two additional syndromes result from lesions of the conus medullaris and the cauda equina.

Central Cord Syndrome

Central cord syndrome (Figure 2–13) results from damage to the central aspect of the spinal cord with sparing of the peripheral portions of the cord. This syndrome almost always occurs in the cervical region. People with central cord syndrome exhibit more pronounced weakness in their upper extremities than in their lower extremities as well as sparing of sensation in the sacral region.[118] Many also have sparing of sacral motor function.[119]

Central cord syndrome may result when the process of central hemorrhage and necrosis (secondary tissue destruction) described earlier in the chapter does not progress peripherally to full destruction of the cord segment. An alternative explanation for the pattern of central damage with peripheral sparing is that it results from damage to the sulcal arteries, which supply the central portion of the spinal cord.[13]

This syndrome is most common in older people following extension injuries to the neck.[27,119] It can occur at any age, however, and can follow flexion injury. This syndrome often results from relatively minor trauma (especially in older adults) with no evidence of vertebral trauma.[27]

People with central cord syndrome are likely to experience neurological return and achieve functional independence during rehabilitation.[119]

Brown–Séquard Syndrome

When one side of the spinal cord is damaged, the resulting clinical picture is called Brown–Séquard syndrome (Figure 2–14). True hemisection of the spinal cord is rare. With incomplete lesions, however, it is common in for one side of the cord to sustain more damage than the other.

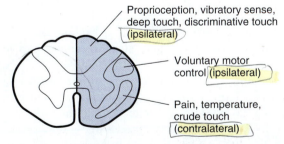

Proprioception, vibratory sense, deep touch, discriminative touch (ipsilateral)

Voluntary motor control (ipsilateral)

Pain, temperature, crude touch (contralateral)

Figure 2–14 Area of spinal cord damage in Brown–Séquard syndrome. Proprioception, vibratory sense, deep touch, discriminative touch, and voluntary motor control are lost ipsilateral to the lesion. Sensation of pain, temperature, and crude touch are lost contralateral to the lesion.

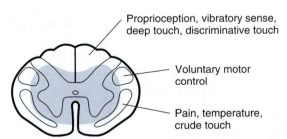

Proprioception, vibratory sense, deep touch, discriminative touch

Voluntary motor control

Pain, temperature, crude touch

Figure 2–13 Area of spinal cord damage in central cord syndrome. The clinical picture resulting from central damage in the cord is due to the somatotopic organization of fibers within the tracts (see Figure 2–5).

People with Brown–Séquard syndrome exhibit more severe motor and proprioceptive deficits on the side of the lesion and more severe loss of sensitivity to pin prick and temperature on the contralateral side.[118] At the level of the lesion, the skin is anesthetic ipsilaterally. Spasticity is likely to be present below the lesion ipsilaterally.[5,6,120]

Brown–Séquard syndrome frequently occurs as a result of traffic accidents or penetrating (stab or gunshot) injuries.[121] When it is caused by vertebral injury, this syndrome is often associated with unilateral facet locks or burst fractures.[122]

People with Brown-Séquard syndrome are likely to experience neurological return and achieve functional independence during rehabilitation.[121]

Anterior Cord Syndrome

Anterior cord syndrome (Figure 2–15) includes preserved proprioception combined with variable loss of motor function and pain and temperature sensation.[118] It results from damage to the anterior and anterolateral areas of the cord, with preservation of the posterior columns. This damage can occur due to trauma to the cord itself, damage of the anterior spinal artery, or both.[5] This syndrome results most often from flexion teardrop fractures and burst fractures.[122,123]

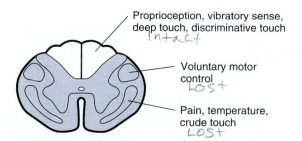

Figure 2–15   Area of spinal cord damage in anterior cord syndrome.

Conus Medullaris Syndrome

Conus medullaris syndrome results from damage to the sacral cord and lumbar nerve roots within the spinal canal. Most people with conus medullaris syndrome exhibit flaccid paralysis of their lower extremities and have areflexic bowels and bladders. Some individuals retain sacral reflexes.[118]

Cauda Equina Syndrome

Cauda equina syndrome results from injury to the cauda equina, the lumbar and sacral nerve roots within the spinal canal caudal to the spinal cord. People with cauda equina injuries exhibit flaccid paralysis of their lower extremities and have areflexic bowels and bladders.[118] The pattern of lower extremity paralysis, sensory loss, and bowel and bladder impairment varies.[33]

Problem-Solving Exercise 2–2

You have three patients who have spinal cord injuries with a C5 neurological level of injury. Their clinical presentations are as follows:

Patient 1 has (bilaterally) normal strength in her biceps, 2/5 strength in her radial wrist extensors, and 0/5 strength in all other key muscles. Pin prick and light touch are intact in the C2 through C5 key sensory points, impaired in C6 and C7, and absent below. She can detect pressure during a digital rectal examination but is not able to contract her anal sphincter voluntarily. Proprioception is normal in the upper and lower extremities.

Patient 2 has normal strength in her biceps bilaterally. Her radial wrist extensors test 2/5 on the right and 1/5 on the left. Her triceps test 1/5 on the right and 0/5 on the left. All other key muscles in the upper extremities test 0/5. All key muscles in both of her lower extremities test 4/5 to 5/5. Pin prick and light touch are intact (bilaterally) in the C2 through C5 key sensory points, impaired in C6, absent in C7 through T3, and impaired in T4 and below. Anal sensation and voluntary contraction are present.

Patient 3 has 5/5 strength in his right biceps, and 4/5 to 5/5 strength in all other key muscles of his right upper and lower extremities. His left biceps exhibits normal strength. All other key muscles in the left extremities test 1/5 to 3/5. Pin prick and light touch are intact in C5 and higher key sensory points bilaterally. Below C5, pin prick is impaired or absent in all key points on the right, and intact on the left. Light touch is intact on the right but impaired on the left. Proprioception is intact in the right extremities and impaired on the left. Anal sensation and voluntary contraction are present.

- Classify each patient's injury: complete versus incomplete, and ASIA Impairment Scale. (Suggestion: download worksheets from http://www.asia-spinal-injury.org/publications/store.php to assist with this process.)
- Does the term *zone of partial preservation* apply to these patients?
- What are the names of the clinical syndromes exhibited by the three patients?
- Explain the neuroanatomical bases of each patient's clinical presentation.

PHYSICAL EFFECTS OF SPINAL CORD INJURIES

The location and extent of damage to neural tissue determines the motor, sensory, and autonomic effects produced by spinal cord injury. Complete spinal cord injury effectively disconnects the brain from the body below the lesion, disrupting supraspinal control of all of the various systems innervated below the lesion (Figure 2–16).

Primary Effects

Voluntary Motor Function

Paralysis of the voluntary musculature is the most obvious effect of a spinal cord injury. Damage of descending motor tracts, anterior horn cells, or nerve roots leads to an impaired capacity to contract the skeletal muscles at or below the level of the lesion. This paralysis results in a loss of control over the trunk and extremities, affecting the ability to manipulate the environment and move in space.

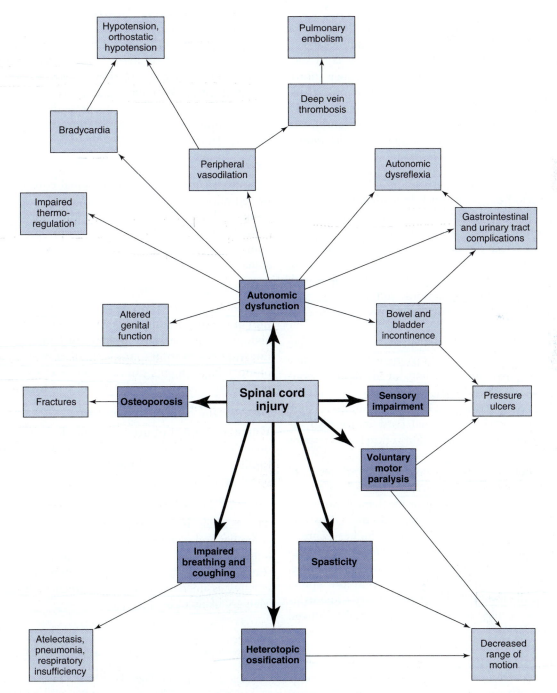

Figure 2–16   Schematic representation of the physical effects of spinal cord injury. Cardiovascular effects are presented in more detail in Figure 2–17.

Wellness and Fitness

Wellness is a multidimensional concept that encompasses physical, psychological, social, and spiritual well-being.

Physical fitness is part of the physical dimension of wellness. Cardiovascular and respiratory functioning, muscle strength, endurance, flexibility, and body composition are aspects of physical fitness.[124]

The physical sequelae of spinal cord injury, both primary effects and secondary conditions, can significantly affect all areas of wellness and fitness.

Damage that occurs at or peripheral to the anterior horn cell is a lower motor neuron lesion and results in flaccid paralysis of muscles innervated by that cord segment. Damage to descending tracts is an upper motor neuron lesion and results in spastic paralysis of muscles innervated by cord segments caudal to the lesion.[6] Most spinal cord injuries are a combination of upper and lower motor neuron lesions because both gray and white matter are disrupted at the level of the lesion.[120]

Muscle Tone

During the period of spinal shock immediately following cord injury, muscles innervated below the lesion are areflexive. As time passes and spinal shock resolves, reflexes return. Reflexive functioning is weak at first but becomes stronger with time,[72,125] commonly progressing to spasticity. Spasticity is more prevalent in people with cervical and upper thoracic lesions and in those with incomplete lesions,[126–129] particularly those classified as ASIA B and C.[128,130]

Spasticity is a velocity-dependent increase in muscle tone in response to passive movement.[131,132] (Passive stretching of a spastic muscle elicits an involuntary contraction of that muscle, with higher-velocity motion eliciting stronger contraction.)[u] The elevated muscle tone that frequently occurs after spinal cord injury also includes clonus, increased deep tendon reflexes, and spasms elicited by cutaneous or proprioceptive stimuli.[125,132–134] Spasticity, clonus, increased deep tendon reflexes, and spasms result from upper motor neuron damage. The underlying neurological mechanism or mechanisms of these hyperreflexive responses are as yet unknown. Possible causes include a loss of inhibition from higher centers, loss of descending facilitation of afferents from Golgi tendon organs, loss of afferent input from limb loading, sprouting of new synaptic terminals within the spinal cord caudal to the lesion, and hypersensitivity of neurons caudal to the lesion in response to their reduced input.[5,74,116,125,126,132,134–137]

Spinal cord injury can also result in flaccid paralysis, with deep tendon reflexes and reflexive response to passive stretch diminished or absent. Flaccid paralysis frequently occurs with more caudal lesions, due to lower motor neuron damage of the conus medullaris or cauda equina.[128] Flaccid paralysis can also occur with higher lesions in muscles innervated by anterior horn cells or nerve roots that are damaged.[138]

Sensation

Sensation is disrupted in most spinal cord injuries. A loss of sensation can lead to discoordination of body movements, vulnerability to trauma, and impaired body awareness. As is true with voluntary motor function, sensory ability usually improves with the passage of time after spinal cord injury.[52]

Breathing and Coughing

Normal breathing and coughing involve coordinated action of the diaphragm, accessory muscles, intercostals, and abdominal musculature. Spinal cord injuries above T12 interrupt innervation to some or all of these muscles. Respiratory impairments can range in severity from difficulty in clearing secretions to the inability to breathe.[v]

Bowel and Bladder Function

Voluntary control of urination and defecation requires an intact sacral cord in communication with the brain. As a result, most spinal cord injuries lead to a loss of voluntary bowel and bladder control.[w]

Genital Function

The genitals receive their innervation from the thoracolumbar and sacral regions of the spinal cord. Spinal cord injury alters the functioning of the genitals, disrupting sexual responses mediated by the brain and spinal cord. Fertility is unchanged among women with cord injuries. Men are likely to be infertile.[x]

---

[u] There is no universally agreed upon definition of spasticity. Some authors use broader definitions that include other manifestations of hypertonicity, such as hyperactive deep tendon reflexes, clonus, and spasms.[126,133,135,243]

[v] Chapter 6 addresses the respiratory sequelae of spinal cord injuries in depth.

[w] Complete descriptions of bowel and bladder function, complications, and care following spinal cord injury are presented in Chapter 14.

[x] Sexuality, sexual functioning, and sexual rehabilitation strategies are addressed in Chapter 13.

TABLE 2–3   Cardiovascular Responses to Autonomic Stimulation

	Response to Parasympathetic Stimulation	Response to Sympathetic Stimulation
Heart	Reduced heart rate	Increased heart rate
	Reduced contractility	Increased contractility
	Reduced cardiac output	Increased cardiac output
Peripheral vasculature supplying		
Skeletal muscles	——	Variable effect
Skin	Face: vasodilation	Vasoconstriction
Viscera	Vasodilation	Vasoconstriction

Sources: References 140 and 141.

Cardiovascular Function

Vasomotor centers in the medulla normally control the cardiovascular system. By reflexively adjusting the sympathetic and parasympathetic outflow to the heart and peripheral vasculature, the vasomotor centers control blood pressure, heart rate, and the distribution of blood flow.[10,139] Sympathetic outflow, arising from spinal segments T1 to L2 or L3, causes increases in heart rate, strength of cardiac contraction, and vasoconstriction in peripheral arterioles. Parasympathetic outflow, transmitted through the vagus nerve (cranial nerve X) from the brainstem, slows the heart and slightly reduces ventricular contractility.[140–142] Table 2–3 presents the effects of sympathetic and parasympathetic stimulation on the heart and peripheral vasculature.

When spinal cord injury blocks communication between the brainstem and the thoracic spinal cord, sympathetic input to the heart is lost and parasympathetic input remains (Figure 2–17). This disruption of the normal balance of sympathetic and parasympathetic control results in bradycardia and bradyarrhythmias. Loss of sympathetic outflow also causes dilation of the peripheral vasculature below the level of the lesion, resulting in hypotension.[27,139,143,144]

The loss of sympathetic reflexes that normally modulate blood pressure during postural changes causes orthostatic hypotension: blood pressure drops when the individual moves from a horizontal to an upright position. Symptoms of orthostatic hypotension include loss of vision, dizziness, ringing in the ears, nausea, and loss of consciousness.[5,145,146]

Bradycardia, bradyarrhythmias, hypotension, and orthostatic hypotension are usually significant only in people with lesions above T6.[5,143,145] These cardiovascular effects are transient, resolving[y] within a few weeks of injury.[5,143,145,147,148] Both a compensatory reduction in parasympathetic outflow[149] and the return of sympathetic spinal reflexes[139] may contribute to the return of more normal cardiovascular function.

Although the parasympathetic/sympathetic imbalance that follows spinal cord injury resolves to some degree within a few weeks of the injury, cardiovascular control does not return to normal. Injuries that lie rostral to or within the region of thoracolumbar sympathetic outflow

---

[y] Hypotension frequently continues[223] but does not tend to be as severe as during the early phase after injury.[139]

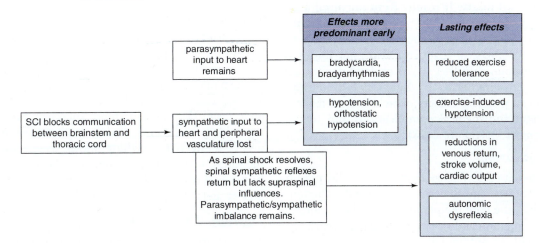

Figure 2–17   Schematic representation of the cardiovascular effects of spinal cord injury.

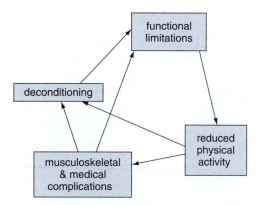

Figure 2–18   Cycle of decline, which can cause increasing deconditioning, functional limitations (activity limitations), and inactivity.

interfere with the brain's communication with sympathetic neurons caudal to the lesion, disrupting normal cardiovascular reflexes.[148] Cardiovascular responses to exercise are impaired, resulting in reduced exercise tolerance and, in some cases, exercise-induced hypotension.[139,150–153]

Another lasting effect of cervical and high thoracic spinal cord injury is reduced venous return to the heart. This probably results from a combination of reduced tone in the peripheral vasculature due to lower sympathetic input, loss of reflexive redistribution of blood flow during exercise, loss of the normal muscular pumping action in the lower extremities due to paralysis, and altered intrathoracic and intraabdominal pressures due to impaired respiratory musculature.[139,148,152,154] The reduction in venous return to the heart leads to reduced stroke volume and cardiac output in people with tetraplegia. Exercise capacity is reduced, and the left ventricle of the heart atrophies.[139,151,154,155] People with paraplegia also exhibit a reduction in stroke volume. Their cardiac output tends to be lower than normal,[150] but it can be adequate during exercise due to a higher heart rate.[139,152,154]

Reduced cardiovascular fitness typically occurs following spinal cord injury. It results from impaired autonomic control (described in the preceding paragraphs) combined with limited skeletal musculature available for exercise.[150,151,156] Physical inactivity also contributes to this deconditioning.[148,150,151,157–159] A cycle of decline can result: deconditioning leads to functional limitations, causing reduced physical activity, which in turn leads to musculoskeletal and medical complications and further deconditioning[158,160] (Figure 2–18).

Thermoregulation

Normally, when a person's core temperature falls, peripheral vasoconstriction and shivering serve to raise the temperature. When the core temperature rises above normal, peripheral vasodilation and sweating cause greater dissipation of heat, with a resulting fall in core temperature.[10,161]

Thermoregulation involves both the autonomic and somatic nervous systems. The sympathetic nervous system (T1 to L2 or L3) is involved in the regulation of body temperature through its influence on peripheral vascular tone and sweating.[140] The somatic system controls shivering.

Spinal cord injury that interrupts the cord's communication with the hypothalamus disrupts thermoregulation. Soon after injury, hypothermia is likely to occur as a result of peripheral vasodilation, which allows loss of heat through the superficial vessels. When reflexive tone eventually returns in the peripheral vasculature, this problem resolves.[27] Although shivering remains absent below the level of lesion,[161] the tendency toward hypothermia is replaced by a tendency toward hyperthermia. This is because sympathetic control of the apocrine (sweat) glands is lost. Below the level of lesion, sweating does not occur in response to a rise in body temperature.[27] Impairment of thermoregulation varies with the level of lesion; higher injuries result in greater impairment of thermoregulatory responses.[162]

Complications

A variety of secondary conditions can result from spinal cord injury. With proper management, the incidence and severity of most of these complications can be minimized.

Pressure Ulcers

Pressure ulcers are among the most common complications of spinal cord injury.[163–166] They are localized areas of tissue necrosis that can occur when soft tissues are subjected to prolonged unrelieved pressure. People with spinal cord injuries are prone to developing this complication because of a combination of (1) motor and sensory impairments that cause the skin to be subjected to prolonged unrelieved pressure and other damaging forces, plus (2) skin and circulatory changes that make the skin more vulnerable to these damaging forces.

Vulnerability to the development of pressure ulcers begins at the time of injury and continues for the remainder of the individual's lifetime. A variety of serious medical, functional, and social problems can result from this complication. Chapter 5 addresses pressure ulcers in greater depth.

Respiratory Complications

Respiratory complications are the most common cause of death following spinal cord injury.[3,28,167–170] These complications occur as a result of a reduction in both inspiratory and expiratory ability. Impaired functioning in the muscles of inspiration causes reduced ventilation of the lungs and atelectasis. Weakness in these muscles also makes them more likely to fatigue, which can lead to ventilatory failure.[171] Ineffective coughing allows secretions to build in the lungs, with atelectasis, pneumonia, and respiratory insufficiency resulting.[5,172] Chapter 6 addresses the respiratory sequelae of spinal cord injuries in greater depth.

Decreased Range of Motion

Any condition that causes joint immobilization can result in reduced joint range of motion and muscle flexibility. People with motor paralysis are vulnerable to contractures due to the simple fact that their muscles do not actively move their joints. Range limitations are especially likely to develop when muscle strength imbalance, spasticity, gravity, or a habitual posture causes one or more joints to remain in a particular position for extended periods without intermittent motion out of the position. Contractures tend to develop more rapidly when edema is present.[173]

Reduced range of motion can seriously impair a person's functional capacity and create cosmetic problems. Moreover, deformity can increase vulnerability to pressure ulcers by altering pressure distribution in sitting and by limiting the number of postures available for pressure relief when lying in bed.

Heterotopic Ossification

Heterotopic ossification, the formation of new bone within soft tissue, occurs following 10% to 53% of all spinal cord injuries. It is always located below the neurological level of injury, most frequently in the hips, knees, and elbows. Heterotopic ossification usually first appears from 1 to 6 months after the injury and matures 6 to 18 months later.[174] It can restrict joint motion and lead to activity limitations, pressure ulcers, and increased spasticity.[5,130,174–177] The cause of heterotopic ossification following spinal cord injury is unknown. Complete lesions and microtrauma have been identified as risk factors.[174]

Osteoporosis and Fractures

Following spinal cord injury, osteoporosis develops in the extremities innervated below the lesion. It does not develop in the spine.[178–180] The reduction in bone mass is the result of loss of both calcium[145] and collagen[181] from the bones. The etiology of osteoporosis following spinal cord injury is poorly understood. Likely causes include the loss of muscular action and weight bearing, as well as circulatory, endocrine, and immune system changes.[178,182,183]

Bone mass is lost most rapidly in the first few months after spinal cord injury.[158,184,185] The rate of decline in bone mineral density slows after this point, but it can continue for many years.[180,186,187] Osteoporosis tends to be more severe in the lower extremities and with complete injuries and flaccid paralysis.[184]

Osteoporosis is of concern because it increases the likelihood of fractures. Estimates of the incidence of pathologic fracture rates among people with spinal cord injuries range from 1% to 46%.[158] The following characteristics are associated with a higher incidence of fractures due to osteoporosis after spinal cord injury: motor complete injuries (ASIA A or B), paraplegia, white race, greater time since injury, advanced age, female gender, and low body mass index.[130,158,188]

Pain

Pain is a problem for the majority of people with spinal cord injuries, occurring during the acute phase after injury or as a chronic problem in the months and years that follow. It can negatively affect rehabilitation potential, activities of daily living, work, community reintegration, and quality of life.[189–194] Pain after spinal cord injury can have a nociceptive (musculoskeletal or visceral) or neuropathic origin.

Musculoskeletal Pain

This type of pain results from stimulation of nociceptors in musculoskeletal structures such as muscles, bones, and ligaments. Injury, mechanical stresses, inflammation, and muscle spasm are common causes of musculoskeletal pain after spinal cord injury.[193,195,196]

Soon after spinal cord injury, neck or back pain often results from vertebral column injury or surgery.[193,197] Shoulder pain is also common during the acute postinjury phase, particularly in people with tetraplegia. This pain can be caused by abnormal stresses on the joints and soft tissues during activity, resulting from impaired functioning in the upper extremity and shoulder girdle musculature.[130,198,199] Poor positioning in bed may also contribute to shoulder pain.

Overuse injuries are a common cause of musculoskeletal pain in individuals with long-standing spinal cord injuries. Chronic repetitive stresses during manual wheelchair propulsion; weight-bearing activities such as transfers, crutch-walking, and pressure reliefs; and repetitive or static shoulder flexion and abduction are thought to be the main contributors to chronic upper extremity pain and injury.[186,193,200–204] The incidence of upper extremity pain and injury increases with time after spinal cord injury.[186,203–205] Common conditions include arthritis, bicipital tendinitis, capsulitis, impingement syndrome, recurrent dislocations, and rotator cuff tears in the shoulders; arthritis, lateral epicondylitis, olecranon bursitis, and ulnar nerve entrapment at the elbows; and arthritis, carpal tunnel syndrome, and tendinitis in the wrists.[200] Lower extremity pain increases with age in individuals with incomplete spinal cord injuries, presumably due to mechanical stresses during ambulation.[186] The increases in upper and lower extremity pain over time may be caused by a combination of chronic overuse and age-related degenerative changes.

Visceral Pain

This type of pain results from stimulation of nociceptors in visceral structures such as the kidneys, bladder, or bowel. Individuals with paraplegia typically experience visceral pain in the same manner as they did before their injuries. In contrast, individuals with tetraplegia may experience visceral pain as a vague unpleasant sensation.[196]

Neuropathic Pain

Neuropathic pain arises from the nervous system itself. At or near the level of injury, this pain can be caused by damage or impingement of nerve roots or the spinal cord, or by a syrinx[z] in the cord.[196] Neuropathic pain below the level of injury results from spinal cord rather than peripheral nerve damage.[196] It can be constant or fluctuating, and can occur spontaneously or in response to sensory stimulation.[195,196,206] Neuropathic pain can also occur above the level of injury in individuals with peripheral nerve compression (carpal tunnel

---

[z] A syrinx, or syringomyelia, is a fluid-filled cyst in the spinal cord that can be associated with spinal cord trauma, tumor, or arachnoiditis.

syndrome, for example) or complex regional pain syndromes (reflex sympathetic dystrophy).[195,196]

Gastrointestinal Complications

From 2.2% to 22% of people with spinal cord injuries develop stress ulcers in the stomach or duodenum during the acute phase following injury.[207–209] The cause of this complication is unknown. Possible contributing factors include shock, emotional stress, circulating catecholamines, steroid therapy, mechanical ventilation, and unopposed parasympathetic input to the stomach causing increased gastrin production.[145,208,210]

Stress ulcers and gastrointestinal (GI) bleeds are most likely to occur during the first month after injury.[5,94,211] Additional GI complications of spinal cord injury include paralytic ileus, gastric dilation, fecal impaction, bowel obstruction, superior mesenteric artery syndrome,[aa] pancreatitis, esophagitis, gallstone disease, chronic constipation, and hemorrhoids.[5,94,145,167,210,212–214]

Urinary Tract Complications

For many years, urinary tract complications were the leading cause of death after spinal cord injury. Advances in urologic management practices have significantly reduced the mortality rate in recent decades.[1,28,167,168] Abnormal bladder function following spinal cord injury, combined with improper management, can lead to urinary retention, bladder infection, and reflux of urine into the ureters. Kidney and bladder stones, hydronephrosis, pyelonephritis, kidney failure, septicemia, and death can result.[110,212,215] Moreover, chronic use of indwelling catheters is associated with an elevated risk of bladder cancer.[167]

Deep Vein Thrombosis and Pulmonary Embolism

Deep vein thrombosis (DVT) is a common complication following spinal cord injury, particularly in the acute phase after injury. Various studies have reached conflicting conclusions about the frequency of this complication, with DVT being found in 23% to 100% of subjects tested with current diagnostic techniques (venography and I-fibrinogen scanning).[216]

Several factors combine to promote the development of blood clots in the deep veins after spinal cord injury. Peripheral vasodilation, absent or reduced lower extremity muscular function, and immobility lead to venous stasis. Hypercoagulability, increased blood viscosity, endothelial damage, and sepsis may also play a role.[5,217–220] Factors associated with a higher risk for the development of DVT[bb] include male gender, flaccid paralysis, complete lesions, and paraplegia.[167,220,221] The incidence of this complication is highest between 72 hours and 2 weeks after a spinal cord injury.[218] It is rare in chronic spinal cord injury.[221]

Thrombi in the deep veins are of great concern because of their potential to embolize. Pulmonary embolism is one of the leading causes of death during the first year following spinal cord injury. These thrombi are also problematic because they can progress to postthrombotic syndrome, which includes chronic edema, induration, pain, and skin ulceration.[218]

Autonomic Dysreflexia

People with spinal cord lesions above the T6 level[cc] can experience autonomic dysreflexia due to a "disconnection" between the brain and the sympathetic neurons in the thoracolumbar spine.[222,223] This phenomenon, also called autonomic hyperreflexia, occurs in 10% to 85% of people with spinal cord injuries above T6.[224–226] It is characterized by a sudden increase in blood pressure, bradycardia, a pounding headache, and flushing and profuse sweating above the level of the lesion (Figure 2–19). It is often accompanied by anxiety. Additional signs and symptoms that can occur include flushing or sweating below the lesion, piloerection ("goose bumps") above or sometimes below the lesion, blurred vision, spots in the visual fields, nasal congestion, muscle spasm, paresthesias in the neck and shoulders, and cardiac arrhythmias.[73,227] Occasionally autonomic dysreflexia occurs without any symptoms.[227]

Autonomic dysreflexia occurs when a noxious stimulus below the lesion triggers an excessive sympathetic response. Possible causes of this exaggerated sympathetic response include loss of descending inhibition from the medulla, sprouting of new synaptic terminals in the spinal cord caudal to the lesion, and hypersensitivity of the sympathetic neurons.[161,224,228] Hypertension results when increased sympathetic outflow causes an increase in cardiac output and peripheral vasoconstriction. The hypertension stimulates baroreceptors in the aortic arch and carotid sinus, triggering an increase in parasympathetic activity, which slows the heart.[dd] Vasodilation above the lesion also occurs as a compensatory mechanism in response to the elevated blood pressure.[148,161,222,226,227]

Typically, autonomic dysreflexia first appears 6 or more months after the injury. This complication is more prevalent with tetraplegia than with paraplegia and is more likely to occur in people with complete lesions.[147,161,221,222,229]

Any noxious stimulus below the lesion can cause autonomic dysreflexia. Common origins of this noxious stimulus include bladder or rectal distention, urinary tract infection, and bowel impaction. A large variety of other stimuli have been reported to trigger autonomic dysreflexia, including but not limited to range-of-motion exercises, cutaneous stimulation, muscle spasm, pressure ulcers, fractures,

---

[aa] In this syndrome, the superior mesenteric artery compresses the duodenum.
[bb] Risk factors not specific to spinal cord injury include advanced age, cancer, congestive heart failure, obesity, pelvic or lower extremity trauma, and a previous history of thromboembolism.[167,216]

[cc] Autonomic dysreflexia has been reported in patients with lower lesions. However, it is more typically associated with lesions above T6.[148,161,230]
[dd] In some cases, tachycardia (increased heart rate) occurs instead of bradycardia. The different clinical pictures occur because both parasympathetic and sympathetic stimulation to the heart are increased in autonomic dysreflexia.[161]

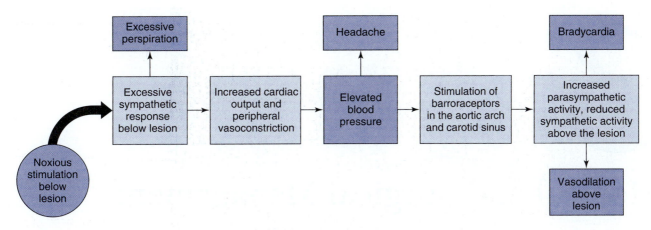

Figure 2–19   Schematic representation of autonomic dysreflexia. Clinical signs and symptoms are in darkened boxes.

heterotopic bone formation, ingrown toenails, functional electrical stimulation, electroejaculation, epididymitis or vaginitis, scrotal compression, sexual intercourse, labor, surgical and diagnostic procedures, and abdominal conditions such as appendicitis.[145,147,161,222,224,227,230,231] The elevation in blood pressure that occurs with autonomic dysreflexia can lead to renal failure, cardiopulmonary failure, loss of consciousness, seizures, hypertensive encephalopathy, retinal hemorrhage, apnea, aphasia, cerebrovascular accidents, coma, and death.[161,224,226,230,231]

Cardiovascular Disease

In recent decades, advances in medical management and rehabilitation have led to a reduction in deaths from complications of spinal cord injury. As people with spinal cord injuries are living longer, cardiovascular disease has become more prevalent in this population.[139,148,159] The risk of morbidity and mortality from ischemic heart disease is now comparable to[169,232,233] or higher than[158,168,186,234–236] that of the general population. Cardiovascular disease has become the most frequent cause of death among individuals who survive more than 30 years after having a spinal cord injury, as well as among those who are over 60 years old.[157]

Several factors may contribute to the development of cardiovascular disease following spinal cord injury. These include a sedentary lifestyle, a higher than normal proportion of body fat relative to lean body mass, lipid abnormalities, altered glucose metabolism, insulin resistance, and the increased prevalence of diabetes.[139,148,157–159,167,183,186,235,237–239]

Summary

- Most spinal cord injuries occur when direct or indirect forces applied to the vertebral column cause violent motion, resulting in failure of the ligamentous or bony elements or both. With disruption of the vertebral column, the spinal cord is traumatized.
- The neurological damage resulting from spinal cord injury is due only in part to the initial trauma to the neurons themselves. Most of the damage to the cord is caused by secondary sequelae of the initial trauma—an escalating cycle of tissue destruction involving ischemia, inflammation, ion derangements, and apoptotic cell death.

- The motor, sensory, and autonomic effects of spinal cord injury vary widely, depending on the level of lesion and pattern of neurological damage. The American Spinal Injury Association and International Medical Society of Paraplegia have developed and adopted a classification system to facilitate communication about spinal cord injuries.
- Depending on the site and extent of a spinal cord lesion, it can result in paralysis, abnormal muscle tone, and sensory loss as well as impaired control of the respiratory, gastrointestinal, genitourinary, cardiovascular, and thermoregulatory systems. A variety of debilitating and potentially fatal complications can result.

Suggested Resources

American Spinal Injury Association: *www.asia-spinalinjury.org*
International Spinal Cord Society: *www.iscos.org.uk*
Model Systems Knowledge Translation Center: *www.mscisdisseminationcenter.org*

National Institute of Neurological Disorders and Stroke: *www.ninds.nih.gov*
Spinal Cord Injury Information Network: *www.spinalcord.uab.edu*

3

Medical and Surgical Management

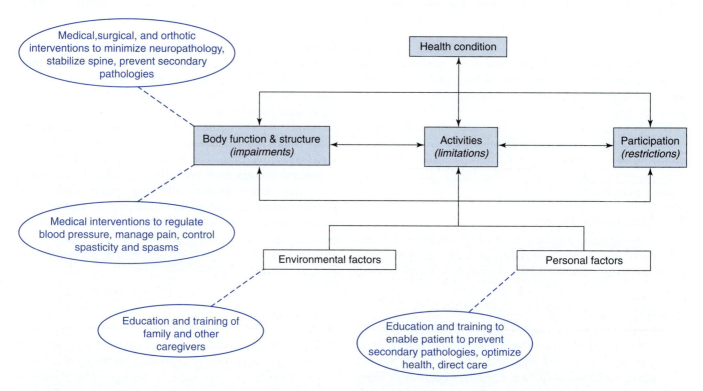

Chapter 3 presents information on medical, surgical, and orthotic interventions as well as education and training following spinal cord injury.

Following injury to the vertebral column or spinal cord, specialized management is imperative. The effects of spinal trauma can be lessened or worsened by the first aid and subsequent medical and surgical interventions provided. At the accident site, care must be taken to avoid causing additional neurological damage. At the hospital, operative or nonoperative measures or both are taken to stabilize the spine to preserve neurological functioning. From the time of injury on, proper management is required to prevent a host of secondary complications. In the absence of appropriate fracture management and medical care, a cycle of worsening impairments in body

function and structure is virtually inevitable, resulting in unnecessary disability or death.

EMERGENCY MANAGEMENT

Prehospital Care

The first aid treatment that people receive following spinal cord injury is crucial to their health and neurological integrity. Stabilization of the injured spine is of particular importance: if the vertebral column is allowed to move, the cord can sustain additional damage. In an emergency situation, if there is any indication of a possible injury of the spinal cord or spinal column, a person should be treated as though a spinal injury has occurred. After a traumatic event such as a vehicular accident, fall, physical attack, diving accident, and so on, an individual who exhibits any of the following characteristics should be assumed to have a possible spinal injury: spinal pain or tenderness; motor or sensory deficits, however minor; paresthesias; altered mental status; evidence of intoxication[a]; or concomitant painful injury that may be distracting her from the pain of a spinal injury.[1–4] Proper handling of the person displaying any of these characteristics may prevent unnecessary neurological damage. Currently accepted practice[b] in cases of potential spinal injury is immobilization of the entire spine at the scene, and continued immobilization during transport and emergency treatment until spinal column injury has been ruled out or, if injury is detected, definitive care has been provided.[1,5] The spine can be effectively immobilized for transport

---

[a] Although drug- or alcohol-induced impairment is not a sign of spinal injury, it can make these signs difficult or impossible to detect.
[b] Because this practice has not been investigated in randomized controlled trials, and because it increases the risk of a variety of serious complications, spinal immobilization in emergency management has been questioned in recent years.[5,179] The spine should be immobilized only when the mechanism of injury or the patient's clinical presentation indicates the potential for a spinal injury, and the period of immobilization should be minimized by "clearing" the spine expeditiously.[180]

using a combination of rigid cervical collar, supportive blocks, rigid backboard, and straps (Figure 3–1).[1]

In addition to stabilizing the spine, emergency medical personnel must ensure that ventilation and circulation are adequate, avoiding unnecessary motion of the spine while doing so.[3,6] Intubation or ventilation with an air-mask-bag unit may be necessary if either associated injuries or cord damage above C5 significantly impairs breathing. Once the patient's spinal column has been stabilized and adequate ventilation and circulation have been assured, the injured person can be taken by ambulance or helicopter to a trauma center. Ideally, the patient is taken to a center that specializes in the care of spinal cord injuries, as these centers have better outcomes.[1,7–13]

Hospital Care

When someone with a known or suspected spinal injury arrives at the hospital, the trauma team works to discover and treat any life-threatening conditions and to preserve neurological function. During all procedures, care is taken to avoid motion in the spine.

The establishment of adequate ventilation, oxygenation, and circulation are of highest priority. Respiratory status is evaluated and arterial blood gases are monitored. Intubation and ventilation are performed if indicated.[14–16] The trauma team controls hemorrhaging from associated injuries and monitors for and treats cardiac arrhythmias or

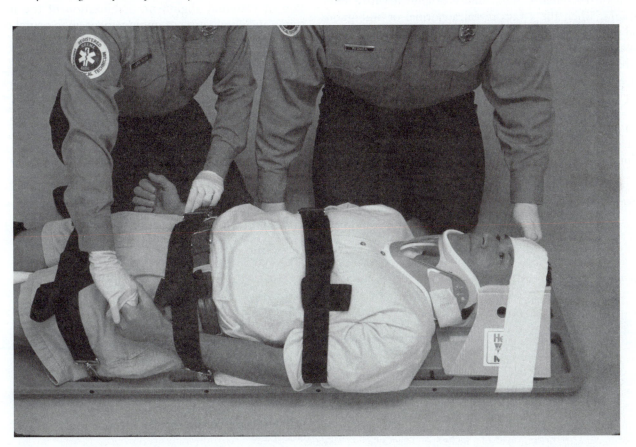

Figure 3–1   Patient immobilized and ready for transport to hospital. (Source: Pearson Education/PH College.)

hypotension.[1,16–18] In addition to enhancing the patient's survival, these measures may help to prevent additional neurological damage from inadequate perfusion of the spinal cord with oxygenated blood.[1,16,19–21]

Once the priority survival needs have been addressed, a neurological examination can be performed. This should include assessment of level of consciousness and cranial nerve function, because the patient may have sustained a head injury during the accident. Sensation, voluntary motor function, and reflexes should also be evaluated thoroughly.[6,16,22,23] This baseline data will influence decisions regarding fracture management and make it possible to detect any future improvement or deterioration in neurological status. Neurological examination results can also be used to determine the patient's neurological and functional prognosis.

Imaging studies are performed to detect damage in the spinal column and cord. Consensus is lacking regarding protocols for this examination.[24] The Consortium for Spinal Cord Medicine recommends computed tomography (CT) of the entire spine in patients with signs or symptoms of spinal cord injury, and plain radiographs when CT is not available.[1] CT frequently reveals injuries that are not evident on radiographs.[1] CT scans are often performed in trauma patients thought to be at risk for spinal cord injury when altered mental status interferes with the clinical examination, when there is continued suspicion of spinal column injury despite negative radiographs, when the x-rays reveal abnormal or ambiguous findings, or when these studies do not provide adequate visualization of the spine.[1,6,16,25–28] The Consortium for Spinal Cord Medicine also recommends magnetic resonance imaging (MRI) of areas that are known or suspected to have spinal cord damage.[1] MRI provides superior visualization of spinal cord compression as well as morphologic changes in ligamentous, hematologic, intervertebral disk, and spinal cord tissue following trauma to the vertebral column.[1,5,17,26,29–31]

Additional emergency procedures include evaluation and initial management of the gastrointestinal and urinary systems, a complete evaluation for associated injuries,[1] and initial management of these injuries as indicated. Finally, methylprednisolone is often administered[32,33] as a neuroprotective agent, but its use has been challenged in recent years.[c]

FRACTURE MANAGEMENT

The primary goal of spinal fracture management is minimization of the neurological damage caused by vertebral injury. At the scene, during transport, and in the emergency room, extreme care is taken to avoid moving the spine while evaluations and treatments are being administered. The spine is evaluated as soon as is feasible in the hospital, and any vertebral column injuries found are reduced and stabilized. This early detection, reduction, and stabilization of vertebral injuries serves to optimize the ultimate neurological outcome of the injured person.

In addition to the preservation of neurological function, fracture management interventions are aimed at minimizing deformity and stabilizing the injured spine to optimize the patient's functional outcome and prevent the late development of spinal deformity.[12,44] Fracture management regimens include the use of traction, positioning, surgery, orthoses, or any combination thereof for restoration of vertebral alignment, stabilization of the injured spine, and elimination of impingement upon neural tissue.

---

[c] Treatment with high doses of methylprednisolone, initiated within 8 hours of injury, was found to enhance the recovery of motor and sensory function in patients with nonpenetrating injuries.[35,181–185] Concerns have been raised, however, regarding methodological flaws in the research, treatment effects that were statistically significant but not clinically relevant, and significant complications.[1,17,20,33,186] General agreement is currently lacking regarding the use of methylprednisolone after spinal cord injury.[20,33]

Research on interventions for optimizing neurological outcomes

Research is ongoing on interventions that could enhance neurological functioning after spinal cord injury. Blood volume augmentation and elevation of patients' mean arterial blood pressure may improve outcomes by enhancing blood flow to the spinal cord, thus reducing posttraumatic ischemia of the neural tissue.[20,34] A variety of pharmacologic therapies aimed at reducing secondary tissue destruction and enhancing axonal regeneration within the spinal cord are also under investigation.[20,33,35] Local and systemic hypothermia have been studied in animals, with mixed results.[36] Another area of research is transplantation: tissues or cells are inserted into or near the damaged portion of the cord. Depending on the type of transplantation performed, the transplanted material can provide a bridge for axonal regeneration, create chemical and mechanical conditions conducive to this regeneration, create conditions beneficial to surviving neurons, and even provide new neurons to the damaged portion of the cord.[20,35,37–39] Additional lines of research include enhancing neuronal survival and regeneration using neurotrophic and growth factors, antiapoptotic molecules, hormones, antibodies for inflammatory cells or growth-inhibiting factors, and electrical stimulation.[20,33,35 40–43]

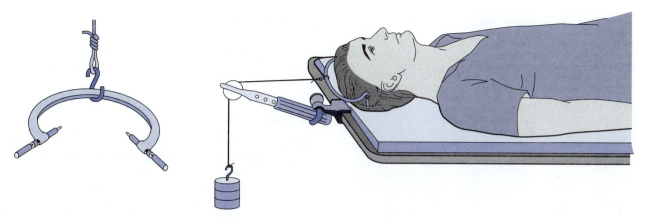

Figure 3–2   Cervical skeletal traction using tongs.

Nonsurgical Management

When radiologic examination reveals vertebral angulation or subluxation in the cervical region, the spine is usually realigned as soon as possible using skeletal traction.[45,46] Since this alignment decompresses the spinal cord, it may increase the patient's chances of neurological recovery.[22] In the cervical region, skeletal traction is achieved with a halo device or tongs affixed to the skull (Figure 3–2). The halo or tongs are attached through a pulley system to weights that apply traction to the cervical vertebrae. Reduction is confirmed by x-ray. Failure to achieve optimal alignment through traction may make surgery necessary.[14,19] In some instances, a cervical spine that will not reduce with traction can be realigned through nonsurgical manipulation.[16] In the treatment of thoracic and lumbar injuries, initial conservative (nonoperative) management generally involves careful positioning in a standard[d] or rotating bed (Figure 3–3).[14]

In some cases, the injured spine is managed definitively through nonsurgical reduction and stabilization. Conservative management is particularly appropriate in instances of either stable or multiple-level vertebral injuries. Surgical stabilization of multiple-level injuries results in severe restriction of spinal motion, potentially interfering with functional status.[44]

When nonsurgical management techniques are used as the definitive treatment, the patient may be immobilized initially in traction or with bed positioning.[e] This treatment is followed by immobilization of the vertebral column in a spinal orthosis for a period of weeks or months. The length of time that a patient spends in traction, positioned in bed, or immobilized in an orthosis varies with the nature of the injury and the physician's philosophy.[47–49] At the end of the period of orthotic sta-

bilization, the injured region of the patient's spine is evaluated radiologically. Persistent instability may make surgical stabilization necessary.[48,50,51]

Surgical Management

Indications for surgical intervention include an unstable fracture, a fracture that will not reduce without surgery, gross spinal malalignment, evidence of continued cord compression in the presence of an incomplete injury, deteriorating neurological status, and continued instability following conservative management (Figure 3–4). Open reduction and internal fixation may be done to restore optimal vertebral alignment and stabilize the injured portion of the spine. Surgery may also be performed for decompression of neural

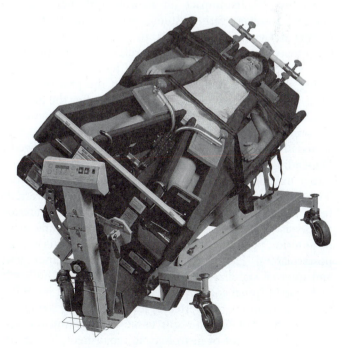

Figure 3–3   Roto-Rest™ Delta Advanced Kinetic Therapy™ System. (Courtesy of KCI Licensing, Inc. 2009.)

---

[d] Positioning in a standard bed is controversial, as significant vertebral motion can occur during repositioning, including log rolling.[187,188]
[e] Certain *stable* fractures without neurological deficit can be managed without these restrictions, with the patient allowed out of bed without an orthosis and participating in activities as tolerated.[189]

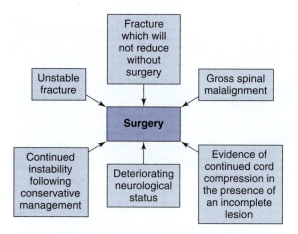

Figure 3–4   Indications for surgical management of spinal injury.

tissue through removal of any bony fragments, soft tissue structures, or foreign bodies impinging on the cord. Finally, surgery is often performed to enable the patient to get out of bed earlier, thus reducing hospitalization time and avoiding the physical and psychological deterioration that can come from prolonged bed rest.[14,45,52,53]

Surgery may be performed within the first 24 hours after admission to the hospital, or following a period of days or weeks of skeletal traction or positioning in bed. The optimal timing of surgery is a matter of debate. Early surgery (<72 hours after injury) makes it possible for patients to begin out-of-bed activities and rehabilitation earlier, resulting in a lower incidence of complications and morbidity.[53–55] Its impact on neurological outcomes is unclear, however; various studies have found that early (versus delayed) surgery leads to superior, inferior, or equivalent outcomes.[33,53,55–59] Regardless of its timing, cervical spine surgery is often preceded by closed reduction (using skeletal traction, as described in the previous section), which is achieved as soon as possible after the injury.

During surgery, bone fragments, soft tissue structures, or foreign bodies that are impinging on neural tissue are removed and the spinal column is aligned and stabilized. Depending on the type of surgery performed, various internal fixation devices may be used to enhance stability. The spine is often fused, using a graft with bone harvested from an iliac crest or fibula or from vertebral spinous processes.[46,60–63] The surgical approach to the spine may be anterior, posterior, combined anterior and posterior, or posterolateral. Factors influencing the surgical approach and internal stabilization device chosen include the level and type of spinal column injury, extent of spinal instability present, number of vertebral levels requiring stabilization, location of bone or soft tissue encroaching on the spinal canal, extent of neurological impairment, length of time that has passed since the injury, and preference of the surgeon.[27,52,58–60,62–65] Postsurgical management depends on the nature of the injury, the surgery performed, and

physician preference.[66] In some instances, orthotic stabilization is not necessary.[52,60] In other cases, an orthosis is used postsurgically to provide stability to the spine while it heals. The time of postoperative orthotic stabilization varies.[52,66]

Spinal Orthoses

Spinal orthoses are often used to stabilize the spine for a variable period of time following injury. This stabilization promotes fusion, prevents deformity, reduces pain, and protects neurological tissue from further damage. Spinal orthoses may be used either after or in lieu of surgical stabilization.

The various designs of spinal orthoses differ in the degree to which they stabilize the vertebral column and the direction of motion they can control. The selection of an orthosis is influenced largely by the motion restriction that the spine requires. This, in turn, will depend on the nature of the injury and surgery performed.[60,67,68] In recent years, advances in instrumentation have reduced the need for orthotic stabilization following surgery. In many cases, either no orthotic stabilization is required postoperatively or less restrictive orthoses can provide adequate stability.[44,52,54,60]

Cervical Orthoses

An assortment of cervical orthoses is available. The halo, Minerva, poster-type, and a number of different collars are commonly used for stabilization of the cervical spine.

Halo

A halo orthosis consists of a metal ring that encircles the skull and is attached via metal bars to a prefabricated adjustable plastic vest lined with sheepskin (Figure 3–5).

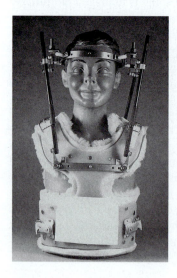
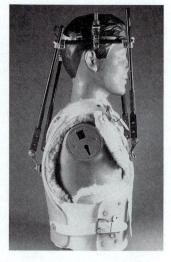

Figure 3–5   Halo orthosis. (Courtesy of RSNA Journal, http//www.rsnajnls.org. Figures 19a and 19b Hunter, TB, Yoshino, MT, Dzoiba, RB, *et al.* Medical Devices of the Head, Neck, and Spine. *RadioGraphics* 2004; 24:257–285)

The "halo" portion of the orthosis is attached to the skull with screws, which are called "pins."

With the possible exception of the Minerva, the halo is the orthotic device that is most effective in preventing cervical motion. It is particularly effective in limiting rotation and lateral flexion of the entire cervical spine and flexion and extension in the higher cervical levels.[69–72] The halo provides maximal stabilization, but not complete immobilization, of the cervical spine. It allows some gross motion as well as "snaking" – flexion or extension at one cervical level with compensatory opposite motion in adjacent segments.[71,73–75] Halo orthoses are appropriate for people who require maximal cervical stabilization to allow healing. Unfortunately these orthoses make functional training more difficult because they limit shoulder motion and raise the wearer's center of gravity.[76,77]

Complications experienced by people wearing halo devices include loss of reduction, pin loosening, infection at the pin sites (in turn occasionally resulting in septicemia, osteomyelitis, and subdural abscess), pressure ulcers in the skin underlying the vest, skin rash under the vest, injury of the supraorbital or supratrochlear nerve, dural penetration, dysphagia, disfiguring scars, pin discomfort, and temporomandibular joint dysfunction.[54,60,73,78–86] Proper application, care, and monitoring can minimize the occurrence and severity of these complications.

The majority of complications associated with halo orthoses originate at the pins. Pin loosening is of concern for two reasons: it can result in loss of stability and it often precedes infection at the pin site. Pins that loosen should be tightened or replaced with pins in different sites. Proper hygiene at the pin sites will minimize the occurrence of infection. When an infection occurs, it should be treated early.[51,79,82,83,87]

Complications involving the skin underlying the vest can also be minimized with proper care and monitoring. The skin over the scapulae, ribs, acromion processes, and spinous processes is at greatest risk. These areas should be checked frequently when possible. The liner between the skin and vest should be kept dry and changed monthly.[77]

A halo should be comfortable. If pain occurs, the health care team should investigate the cause. Pain at the pin sites is likely to be caused by loosening or infection. Pain in the trunk is likely to be due to excessive pressure from the vest.

Minerva

The thermoplastic Minerva body jacket (TMBJ) is a custom-molded orthosis that encases the chin and the posterior aspect of the skull and extends caudally either to the inferior costal margin or to enclose the pelvis, depending on the stability required. A headband encircles the skull to hold the head in place. Prefabricated Minerva orthoses are also available (Figure 3–6).

Like the halo, the Minerva restricts cervical motion in all planes.[71,88] Neither the halo nor the Minerva provides perfect immobilization of the cervical vertebrae; both

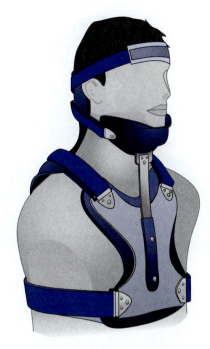

Figure 3–6   Prefabricated Minerva orthosis.

allow some gross motion and "snaking." The custom-molded Minerva orthosis has been reported[f] to provide better stabilization of the cervical spine than does the halo except between C1 and C2.[74]

As is true with halo orthoses, the excellent stability afforded by Minerva orthoses allows early initiation of functional training. Because the Minerva allows good range of motion in the shoulders, it does not interfere as much with functional progress. Minervas are also reported to be more comfortable and cosmetically acceptable than halos.[74,76]

Fewer complications are associated with Minerva orthoses than with halos. Since a Minerva is not screwed into the wearer's skull, it does not cause any pin-related problems. The Minerva's design may also reduce skin complications. Custom molding can result in better pressure distribution than is achieved with the prefabricated halo vest. Additionally, half of a Minerva can be removed at a time (with the wearer positioned in prone or supine) for skin inspection, bathing, and cleaning of the orthosis. If an area of excessive pressure is noted, the orthosis can be modified.[76]

Poster-Type Orthoses

Several different designs of poster-type orthoses are used for restriction of cervical motion. These orthoses consist of pads at the chin and occiput, supported by two to four posts that are attached to anterior and posterior thoracic components.

The SOMI (sterno-occipital-mandibular immobilizer) is an example of a poster-type orthosis. It is made of a

---

[f] In the study cited, the measurement of cervical motion allowed by the Minerva was done 3 weeks after measurement with the halo.[74]

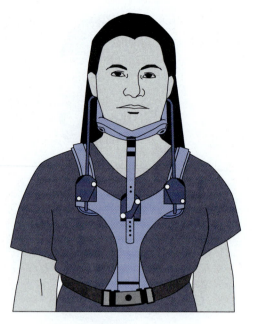

Figure 3–7   SOMI orthosis.

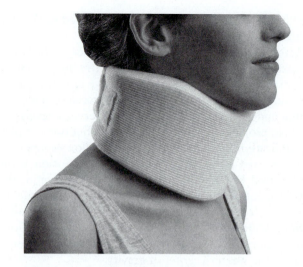

Figure 3–8   Soft collar, not suitable for cervical stabilization. (Reproduced with permission from PROCARE, DJO, LLC.)

padded metal sternal plate to which are attached three adjustable uprights connected to occipital and mandibular supports (Figure 3–7). It is most effective in restricting flexion between C1 and C5.[71] The motion restriction provided by the SOMI orthosis is less than that provided by halo and Minerva orthoses.[46,70]

When someone wearing a SOMI moves between supine and upright postures, the position of the mandibular support should be adjusted. Proper adjustment is required for both comfort and optimal restriction of cervical motion.[77]

Cervical Collars

A number of different cervical collars can be used to stabilize the spine. Most are made of either rigid plastic or semirigid foam reinforced by rigid plastic struts. A typical cervical collar consists of two halves that encircle the neck and are joined by Velcro straps. The anterior portion of the collar cups the mandible and extends to the upper chest. The posterior portion cups the occiput and extends to the upper back.

Cervical collars limit cervical spine motions to varying degrees, depending on their design. Soft collars, made of foam rubber (Figure 3–8), do not limit motion to any significant degree.[69,73] Other collars, such as Philadelphia (Figure 3–9) or Miami J (Figure 3–10) collars, provide some restriction of motion. This restriction is provided primarily in flexion and extension of the middle and lower cervical spine. No cervical collar can effectively immobilize the spine.[67,71,73,78,89–91] Orthotic designs that include thoracic extensions provide superior stabilization (Figure 3–11).[92]

Thoracolumbosacral Orthoses

There are several different types of thoracolumbosacral orthoses. Three designs are described in this section: molded plastic body jackets, Jewett orthoses, and Knight-Taylor orthoses.

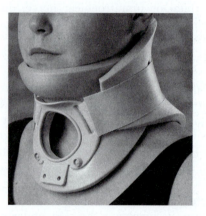

Figure 3–9   Philadelphia collar. (Reproduced with permission from Medline Industries, Inc.)

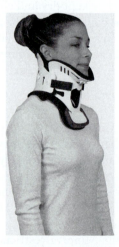

Figure 3–10   Miami J collar. (Reproduced with permission from Ossur Americas, Orthopaedics.)

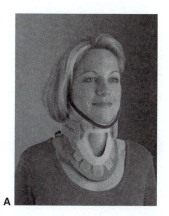
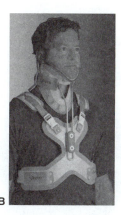

A   **B**

Figure 3–11   Thoracic extensions enhance stability.
(A) Aspen collar. (B) Aspen CTO (cervical–
thoracic orthosis) includes thoracic extensions.
(Reproduced with permission from Aspen
Medical Products.)

Molded Plastic Body Jacket

A molded plastic body jacket encases virtually the entire
trunk (Figure 3–12). It is made of two pieces of rigid plastic that are molded to fit the individual[g] and attached to
each other with Velcro straps. The abdominal area may be
covered or exposed. (A window in the abdominal region
makes assisted coughing possible.)

Molded plastic body jackets provide maximal stability
to the trunk, limiting motion in all planes.[88,93,94] A thigh
extension (spica) may be included in the orthosis if immobilization is required at L5 or lower levels,[51,67,71] although
the effectiveness of this extension has been questioned.[95]
Immobilization of vertebral levels higher than T7[67] or T8[71]
requires the inclusion of anterior shoulder outriggers[67] or a
cervical extension (Figure 3–13).[71]

The locations of the inferior and superior borders of the
anterior portion of the jacket determine the degree to which
the orthosis restricts hip and shoulder motion. If the jacket is
shaped appropriately in these regions, hip flexion should be
possible to at least 90 degrees[h] and shoulder motion should
be unrestricted. As rehabilitation progresses, hypertrophy of
the shoulder musculature may necessitate trimming of the
jacket's superior border.[77] A cotton T-shirt worn under the
orthosis will absorb perspiration to increase comfort and
prevent skin maceration. When the wearer is prone or
supine, half of the orthosis can be removed to allow inspection and washing of the skin and cleaning of the orthosis.[77]

Jewett

A Jewett orthosis is a prefabricated orthosis made of a metal
frame to which pads are attached (Figure 3–14). The suprapubic, sternal, and thoracolumbar pads exert forces on the

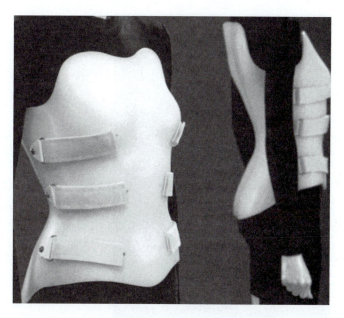

Figure 3–12   Molded plastic body jacket. (Reproduced
with permission from Spinal Technology,
Inc.)

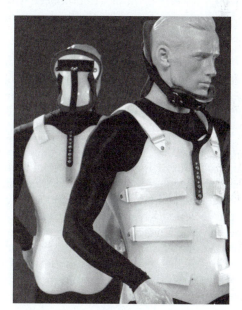

Figure 3–13   Molded plastic body jacket with cervical
extensions. (Reproduced with permission
from Spinal Technology, Inc.)

trunk that restrict flexion and encourage hyperextension of
the lower thoracic and upper lumbar spine.[71,88,93] Extension
is free at all levels. Rotation and lateral flexion are controlled
to an intermediate degree at best, depending on the amount
of hyperextension[i] that the orthosis maintains.[88,93] Improper
adjustment of the orthosis can result in loss of vertebral stabilization and pressure on the throat or genitals when sitting.

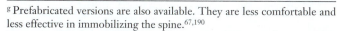

[g] Prefabricated versions are also available. They are less comfortable and
less effective in immobilizing the spine.[67,190]
[h] In some instances, the inferior trim line needs to be lower in order to
provide adequate immobilization of the spine. Hip flexion may then be
limited to a greater degree. A thigh extension will also restrict hip motion.

[i] The hyperextension of the spine places the vertebrae in a close-packed
position. With the vertebrae "locked" in this manner, lateral flexion and
rotation are restricted to some degree.[88,93]

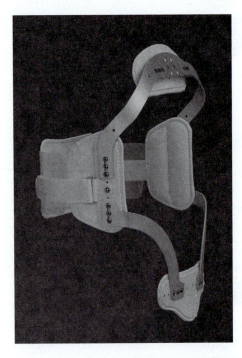

Figure 3–14   Jewett® orthosis. (Reproduced with permission from Florida Brace Corporation.)

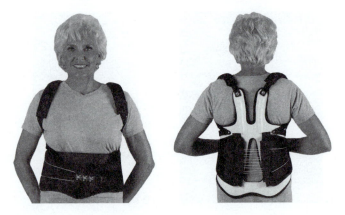

Figure 3–15   Prefabricated Knight-Taylor orthosis. (Courtesy of Orthomerica Products, Inc. © 2008.)

Management Differences

There is no generally agreed-upon protocol for the management of spinal column injuries. Decisions regarding surgical versus nonsurgical management, surgical procedure, timing of surgery, choice of orthoses, and duration of orthotic wear are influenced by the philosophy of the institution and the surgeon involved.[59,60,66,96,97]

Jewett braces are less effective than molded body jackets in preventing flexion, extension, rotation, and lateral flexion.[67] For this reason, they are not appropriate orthoses for unstable spines.[71]

Knight-Taylor

The Knight–Taylor orthosis consists of a rigid frame, worn posteriorly, to which are attached axillary straps that encircle the shoulders, and an abdominal support. Figure 3–15 shows a prefabricated Knight–Taylor orthosis.

In the thoracic region, Knight–Taylor orthoses allow unrestricted rotation and provide an intermediate degree of restriction of flexion, extension, and lateral bending. A cervical extension should be added if motion restriction is required above T8.[71] Lumbar rotation is restricted to an intermediate extent. Motions in other planes are effectively restricted in the lumbar spine. In the lumbosacral region, flexion and extension are essentially unrestricted, rotation is limited to an intermediate degree, and lateral flexion is effectively restricted.[88,93]

MEDICAL MANAGEMENT

Spinal cord injury can affect the functioning of virtually every system in the body. A variety of debilitating and potentially lethal complications can result. With proper medical management involving the coordinated efforts of a multidisciplinary team, many of these secondary conditions can be prevented. Without proper management, unnecessary morbidity and mortality are virtually inevitable. For this reason, specialized care is essential.

Bladder Care

Beginning at the time of injury, appropriate bladder care is required to prevent a variety of complications. This topic is discussed in Chapter 14. Table 3–1 includes information on medications commonly used for management of the urinary and other systems after spinal cord injury.

Problem-Solving Exercise 3–1

Your patient wears a thermoplastic body jacket to stabilize his lower thoracic spine. He is on a mat in therapy when you notice that the anterior portion of his orthosis is on upside-down. (You are familiar with this type of orthosis and are certain that this one has been put on wrong.)

- What should you do about this?
- How can you prevent this problem from reoccurring?

Gastrointestinal Care

During spinal shock, gastric dilation and paralytic ileus may develop. This is of particular concern because of the potential threat to the patient's already compromised respiratory system: diaphragmatic movements are inhibited by this distention, and vomiting and aspiration may occur. To avoid these complications, the stomach can be decompressed using a nasogastric or orogastric tube.[14,19,105,106]

Stress ulcers may also occur during the acute stage after spinal cord injury. Prophylactic treatment includes the use of histamine H2 receptor antagonists or proton pump inhibitors to reduce gastric acid secretion, or sucralfate to enhance gastric mucosal microcirculation and defensive mechanisms.[1,14,19,105,107,108] Stress ulcer prophylaxis can be discontinued 4 weeks after injury unless other risk factors are present.[1]

After spinal cord injury, a bowel program is required to induce bowel movements at regularly scheduled intervals and to avoid incontinent episodes between times. This regulation can prevent a variety of complications. Bowel management is presented in Chapter 14.

Skin Care

People with spinal cord injuries are vulnerable to the development of pressure ulcers. This complication can be prevented with proper care. A critical component of such prevention is the avoidance of prolonged periods of unrelieved pressure on the skin, particularly over bony prominences. Immediately after the injury, as the patient is transported to a hospital and undergoes an initial evaluation and emergency interventions, immobilization is necessary. Prolonged periods of immobility during this time, however, can lead to the development of pressure ulcers.[109,110] To avoid this problem, health professionals should provide pressure relief to the patient's skin as soon as it is possible to do so without compromising the patient's vertebral stability, and then reposition the patient at least every 2 hours to provide pressure relief.[1] Additional strategies to prevent skin damage during emergency care include insertion of pressure-distributing gel pads under the patient's bony prominences while the patient remains immobilized[17]; minimizing the time involved in transportation, waiting in the emergency room, and x-ray procedures; and admission to the nursing unit as soon as possible.[110]

The prevention of pressure ulcers remains an important focus for the remainder of the patient's life. Chapter 5 addresses the prevention and treatment of pressure ulcers.

Respiratory Care

When spinal cord injury disrupts the functioning of the diaphragm, intercostals, or abdominals, the resulting impaired ability to breathe and cough can lead to atelectasis, pneumonia, and death. Respiratory care should be initiated soon after spinal cord injury and continue throughout acute and postacute rehabilitation. Chapter 6 presents respiratory management in detail.

Cardiovascular Care

When spinal cord injury interrupts communication between the brain and the sympathetic preganglionic neurons in the spinal cord, peripheral vasodilation and bradycardia result. These effects are usually significant only in people with lesions above T6; they generally resolve within a few weeks of injury. Placement of a temporary pacemaker or treatment with anticholinergic or inotropic medication may be indicated for severe bradycardia.[105,111,112] Intravenous fluids and vasopressor medication may be indicated to maintain an adequate blood pressure.[1,105]

Vasovagal Response

Acutely after spinal cord injury, tracheal suctioning can cause a precipitous fall in heart rate and cardiac arrest. This problem may be avoided by administering oxygen prior to and after these procedures. Atropine may be given prophylactically or to correct the problem if it develops.[113]

Orthostatic Hypotension

People with recent spinal cord injuries frequently exhibit orthostatic hypotension when upright activities are first initiated. Strategies for developing tolerance to upright sitting are presented in Chapter 11. In some cases, medication is required.[1]

Autonomic Dysreflexia

Autonomic dysreflexia is a potentially life-threatening exaggerated sympathetic response to noxious stimulation below the lesion. This condition occurs almost exclusively among people with lesions at or above T6. It usually first appears 6 or more months after the injury but can occur earlier.[114,115]

Because autonomic dysreflexia can develop rapidly and is potentially life-threatening, immediate response is necessary when it occurs. The signs and symptoms of autonomic dysreflexia[j] include systolic and diastolic blood pressure elevated 20 mm Hg or more above the individual's normal postinjury level; a pounding headache; heart rate slower than the individual's normal postinjury rate; profuse sweating or skin flushing above the lesion, particularly in the face, neck, and shoulders; piloerection above the level of the lesion; paresthesias in the head, neck, and upper chest; visual deficits; nasal congestion; anxiety; and cardiac arrhythmias.[100,112,116,117] When a patient exhibits signs and symptoms of autonomic dysreflexia, her blood pressure should be assessed. If an individual's blood pressure is above her postinjury normal, she should immediately be placed in the sitting position (head and torso elevated and lower extremities lowered). This may lower the blood pressure and

---

[j] Atypical signs and symptoms include tachycardia[118]; sweating, flushing, or piloerection below the lesion; or a significant elevation in blood pressure without any symptoms.[100]

TABLE 3–1   Medications Commonly Used Following Spinal Cord Injury

Body System	Medication	Therapeutic Effect	Examples
Urinary system			
Enhancement of urine storage	Anticholinergics	Increase bladder storage capacity through detrusor relaxation	Oxybutynin, propanthelene, tolterodine
Enhancement of reflexive voiding	Alpha-adrenergic blockers	Lower resistance to voiding by relaxing smooth muscle at base of bladder	Doxazosin, prazosin, tamsulosin, terazosin
Gastrointestinal system			
Prevention of stress ulcers	H2 receptor antagonists	Inhibit gastric acid secretion	Cimetidine, famotidine, nizatidine, ranitidine
	Proton pump inhibitors	Inhibit gastric acid secretion	Esomeprazole magnesium, lansoprazole, omeprazole, pantoprazole sodium
	Sucralfate	Protect mucosal lining, inhibit pepsin activity	Sucralfate
Bowel regulation	Rectal stimulants	Suppositories or mini-enemas trigger defecation by stimulating peristalsis	Bisacodyl, glycerin
	Bulk-forming agents	Optimize stool consistency	Calcium polycarbophil, psyllium, methylcellulose
	Stool softeners	Optimize stool consistency	Docusate sodium
	Laxatives	Stimulate peristalsis by drawing fluid into colon	Magnesium salts, lactulose, polyethylene glycol
Cardiovascular system			
Hypotension, orthostatic hypotension	Vasopressors	Increase blood pressure through peripheral vasoconstriction	Ephedrine, midodrine hydrochloride, phenylephrine hydrochloride
	Mineralocorticoids	Increase intravascular volume through retention of sodium and water	Fludrocortisone acetate
Autonomic dysreflexia	Antihypertensive medications	Reduce blood pressure through peripheral vasodilation	Diazoxide, hydralazine, nifedipine, nitroglycerine

promote cerebral venous return.[100] Clothing and other devices that may be constricting should be loosened.[100,116,117] During the episode, blood pressure and heart rate should be monitored frequently.[100,116,117]

The underlying source of the noxious sensation causing the dysreflexia should be investigated and eliminated as quickly as possible. Since bladder distention is the most common stimulus for autonomic crisis, the individual should be catheterized if an indwelling urinary catheter is not in place. If she has an indwelling catheter, it should be checked along its entire length for anything that could be obstructing it, and the obstruction should be corrected immediately by unkinking, flushing or replacing the catheter as appropriate. If the blood pressure remains elevated after the bladder has been emptied, it may be brought under control using antihypertensive medication.[k] A rectal examination can then be

---

[k] Antihypertensive medication should be considered if the systolic pressure remains at or above 150 mm Hg. A rapid-onset short-duration medication should be used, and the patient should be monitored for hypotension.[100]

TABLE 3–1   (*continued*)

Body System	Medication	Therapeutic Effect	Examples
Prevention of deep venous thrombosis	Low-molecular-weight heparin	Prevent coagulation	Dalteparin sodium, danaparoid sodium, enoxaparin, tinzaparin
	Adjusted-dose unfractionated heparin	Prevent coagulation	Heparin sodium
Neuromuscular and musculoskeletal systems			
Management of spasticity	GABA agonists	Reduce spasticity through effect on GABA receptors in the central nervous system	Baclofen, diazepam
	Imidazolines	Reduce spasticity through effect on alpha-2 receptors in the spinal cord	Clonidine, tizanidine
	Dantrolene sodium	Reduces spasticity through effect on muscle contractility	Dantrolene sodium
Management of pain	Nonsteroidal anti-inflammatory drugs	Reduce musculoskeletal pain and inflammation	Aspirin, ibuprofen, indomethacin, naproxen
	Narcotics	Cause analgesia, euphoria, sedation; used for musculoskeletal or neuropathic pain	Codeine, fentanyl, hydrocodone, meperidine, morphine, oxycodone, propoxyphene
	Anticonvulsants	Reduce neuropathic pain	Carbamazepine, gabapentin, pregabalin
	Tricyclic antidepressants	Reduce neuropathic pain	Amitriptyline, doxepin, nortiptyline
Prevention of osteoporosis	Bisphosphonates	Decrease bone resorption	Alendronate, clodronate, etidronate, tiludronate
Prevention of heterotopic ossification	Nonsteroidal anti-inflammatory drugs	Prevent ectopic bone formation	Indomethacin
	Bisphosphonates	Inhibit progression of ectopic bone growth	Etidronate

Sources: References 1 and 98 to 104.

performed, and fecal impaction removed if present. Topical anesthetics should be used during both catheterization and rectal examination and evacuation, in order to avoid exacerbating the dysreflexic response.[100,116–118]

If bladder and rectal emptying do not stop the dysreflexic response, other possible sources of the dysreflexia should be investigated. If the patient's blood pressure remains elevated after the underlying cause has been removed, it can be controlled using antihypertensive medication.[100,117] If the source of the autonomic dysreflexia cannot be removed immediately (if it is caused by a pressure ulcer, for example), the patient may be treated prophylactically until the underlying problem has resolved.[119]

The underlying cause of an individual's dysreflexic episode should be noted. To some degree, future episodes can be prevented by avoiding the development of the precipitating condition. For example, better urinary management practices may prevent the development of bladder distention and resulting autonomic dysreflexia. Individuals who experience recurrent episodes of autonomic dysreflexia may benefit from prophylactic medication.[117,118] In

Problem-Solving Exercise 3–2

Your patient, who has C8 tetraplegia, has been practicing rolling from supine to prone on a mat. She states that she has a pounding headache, and you notice that her face is flushed and damp with perspiration.

- What do you suspect as a likely cause of the patient's signs and symptoms?
- How should you respond?

addition, these individuals and their families should be taught how to minimize the risk of autonomic dysreflexia, and to recognize and respond to its symptoms.[100]

Deep Venous Thrombosis and Thromboembolism

Deep venous thrombi (DVTs) are common in the early weeks after spinal cord injury and can lead to pulmonary emboli. A variety of measures are typically taken during the acute phase after injury to prevent this potentially lethal complication. Thromboprophylaxis is initiated soon after injury and continues for 8 weeks or more, depending on the individual. After the acute phase of injury, an event such as surgery or a period of prolonged bed rest may necessitate the reinstitution of thromboprophylaxis.[99] Table 3–2 presents interventions used for the prevention of thromboembolism following spinal cord injury.

In addition to providing thromboprophylactic interventions, clinicians should monitor patients for signs of DVT. Swelling in one calf or thigh, discoloration, pain, local or systemic temperature elevation, and dilation of the superficial veins are indications of possible DVT.[99,120,121] These symptoms are often present without DVT, however, and thrombus formation often occurs without recognizable symptoms.[121–123] Because DVTs are both common and relatively difficult to detect in people with spinal cord injuries, the index of suspicion for DVTs should be high.[18,19,106]

A variety of procedures can be used to diagnose DVT, including contrast venography, impedance plethysmography, ultrasound, I-fibrinogen scans, and magnetic resonance venography.[99,106,111,120,122] When venous thrombosis is detected, anticoagulant therapy is indicated.[111,112,120] Out-of-bed activity and lower extremity exercise should be suspended for 48 to 72 hours.[99]

Patients with recent spinal cord injuries should be monitored for signs of pulmonary embolus: chest pain, shortness of breath, tachycardia, sweating, apprehension, fever, and cough.[19,99,112,120] As is true with DVTs, pulmonary embolism can be difficult to detect in people with spinal cord injuries. Diagnostic tests for pulmonary embolism include ventilation/perfusion scans and pulmonary angiography.[19,106] Treatment involves anticoagulation therapy and placement of a vena cava filter.[19]

Cardiovascular Disease and Fitness

Spinal cord injury causes a variety of physiologic changes as well as a significant reduction in physical activity. An elevated risk of cardiovascular disease results[1]; cardiovascular disease has become one of the leading causes of death in this population.[116,124–130] Because of this, long-term cardiovascular wellness has become a focus of rehabilitation.

The prevention of cardiovascular disease in people with spinal cord injuries involves many of the same strategies as it does in the general population: smoking cessation, low-fat diet, weight control, and aerobic exercise.[112] Cardiovascular conditioning through exercise, a critical component of wellness programs, can be problematic following spinal cord injury. Both altered autonomic control of the cardiovascular system and limited skeletal muscle mass available for exercise make it difficult to stress the heart enough to effect adaptive changes.[116,128,131–134] Additional problems associated with spinal cord injury that can interfere with exercise include autonomic dysreflexia, exertional hypotension, exercise-induced hyperthermia, and overuse injuries of the upper extremities.[128,134]

Despite the challenges associated with exercise following spinal cord injury, fitness training can occur. Twenty to 60 minutes of moderate exercise, performed 3 days per week,

---

[1] Chapter 2 contains additional information on cardiovascular function and cardiovascular disease.

Problem-Solving Exercise 3–3

You are about to help your patient, who has T3 paraplegia (ASIA A), transfer from his wheelchair to a mat in therapy. You notice that his left lower extremity appears to be swollen below the knee. The right lower extremity is not swollen. Closer examination reveals pitting edema and slight redness distal to the left knee. The patient denies feeling any pain.

- What should you suspect as a likely cause of the swelling and redness in the left lower extremity?
- How should you respond?

TABLE 3–2   Thromboembolism Prophylaxis Following Spinal Cord Injury

Interventions	Indications	Precautions and Contraindications	Timing
Anticoagulant prophylaxis with low-molecular-weight heparin or adjusted-dose unfractionated heparin	• All patients acutely after injury unless contraindicated	Contraindications • Active or potential bleeding that cannot be controlled. • Head injury. • Coagulopathy. Precautions • May be withheld for 24 to 48 hours postinjury due to potential for bleeding and for neurological deterioration. • Withheld on day of surgery.	Initiated within 72 hours of injury. Duration varies with completeness of lesion, presence of additional risk factors for thromboembolism, access to medical care.
Compression hose or pneumatic compression devices	• All patients acutely after injury unless contraindicated	Precautions • Proper placement of hose and compression devices, and frequent skin inspections. • When thromboprophylaxis is delayed more than 72 hours after injury, testing for leg thrombi should precede initiation of compression.	First 2 weeks after injury.
Vena cava filter placement (possibly removable filters)	Indicated for patients who have • Failed anticoagulant prophylaxis • A contraindication to anticoagulation Should be considered for patients who have: • C2 or C3 complete motor paralysis • Poor cardiopulmonary reserve • Thrombosis in the inferior vena cava despite anticoagulant prophylaxis	Precautions • May become dislodged during assisted coughing with abdominal compression. • May increase risk of future DVTs.	Upon detection of failure of anticoagulation prophylaxis.
Mobilization and active or passive extremity exercises	• All patients unless contraindicated	Contraindications • Any orthopedic or medical condition that would make mobilization and passive exercise potentially harmful. • Presence of DVT: suspend activity and passive exercise during first 48 to 72 hours of anticoagulation therapy. Precautions • Avoid motions or activities that will cause movement in unstable area(s) of spine. • Protect skin from damaging forces.	Range-of-motion exercise, out-of-bed activities, and active use of functioning musculature should be initiated as soon as is medically and orthopedically feasible. Should continue indefinitely.

Sources: References 18, 19, 99, 111, 112, and 120.

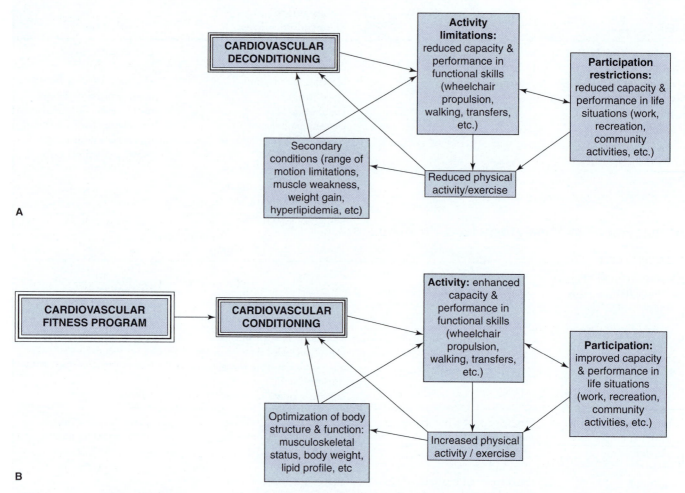

Figure 3–16 Cardiovascular fitness program reduces disability. (A) Cardiovascular deconditioning causes cycle of worsening activity limitations, impairments, and participation restrictions. (B) Cardiovascular fitness program enhances cardiovascular fitness, initiating a cycle of improving activity, body structure and function, and participation in life situations.

has been shown to enhance cardiovascular fitness and exercise capacity.[130] This can be accomplished through any of the following activities and interventions: electrically stimulated leg cycling or ambulation, body-weight–supported treadmill training, walking with crutches, arm ergometry training, combined arm ergometry and electrically stimulated leg cycling, wheelchair ergometry training, circuit resistance training, wheelchair propulsion, swimming, or participation in wheelchair sports.[90,116,127,128,130,132,134–144] Exercise can also improve glucose homeostasis and blood lipid profiles in individuals with spinal cord injury, which may reduce the risk of cardiovascular disease.[130]

In addition to preventing cardiovascular disease, fitness programs may enhance quality of life. Physical deconditioning can lead to an escalating cycle of disability. Fitness programs, by increasing tolerance for physical activity, can make more independent functioning and integration into the community (participation in life situations) possible. (Figure 3–16)[131,145,146]

Cardiovascular fitness training should be a standard component of rehabilitation following spinal cord injury.

Patients should participate in individualized exercise programs appropriate to their abilities, impairments, functional capacities, and cardiovascular status.[133,145,147] Unfortunately, the physical benefits of these programs will not last if the exercise is discontinued.[138] To achieve a lasting benefit to the patient's health, the rehabilitation team should focus on developing a physically active lifestyle that can continue long after rehabilitation is over. The exercise regimen most suited to the individual will depend on her preferences, physical abilities, financial resources, support systems, and access to exercise facilities, equipment, and organized sports. Compliance is likely to be higher if the activities are practical and enjoyable.[127,131]

In designing and implementing fitness programs, clinicians should keep in mind the cardiovascular and musculoskeletal changes associated with spinal cord injuries. Appropriate precautions include gradually increasing the intensity, duration, and frequency of exercise sessions; closely monitoring the patient's response to exercise; avoiding exercise when the bladder or rectum is full; avoiding exercise when episodes of autonomic dysreflexia are increasing; ensuring adequate hydration and clothing appropriate to the ambient temperature; and limiting the time spent exercising in warm or humid environments.[128,134,148] Additionally, care should be taken to minimize the risk of overuse injuries and pain in the upper extremities.[131,149] Cardiovascular conditioning activities that are varied[148] and involve movement patterns that are both biomechanically normal[150] and different from those used during daily activities[127] may help with this problem. An exercise program that develops appropriate flexibility and balanced strength in the shoulders will also help prevent overuse injuries.[150]

Management of Musculoskeletal Problems

Osteoporosis

Osteoporosis develops after spinal cord injury in the extremities innervated caudal to the lesion, leading to increased vulnerability to fractures. Bisphosphonates, which inhibit bone resorption, can be used to preserve or restore bone mass after spinal cord injury.[98] Ambulation, prolonged standing, and electrical stimulation have also been investigated; none of these interventions have been shown to be effective in reducing or reversing the development of osteoporosis in the lower extremities,[98,151–156] with the possible exceptions of early weight-bearing,[157] and electrical stimulation creating large compressive forces.[98]

Heterotopic Ossification

Although the causes of heterotopic ossification (HO) are unknown, microtrauma is a likely contributor. This microtrauma can occur during vigorous stretching exercises. Gentle, passive range-of-motion exercise of joints below the lesion, initiated on the day of injury, may help to prevent HO by preventing the development of joint contractures and thereby reducing the need for stretching.[104]

The signs and symptoms of HO include pain, swelling, erythema, warmth, and restricted range of motion in the affected area.[104,111,158] HO may be seen on x-ray, but can be detected earlier using a bone scan.[104,159]

Interventions for HO include gentle range-of-motion exercise to preserve joint range of motion, and treatment with either bisphosphonate or nonsteroidal anti-inflammatory agents to minimize ossification.[104,111,158,159] Despite these interventions, HO can progress to the point where it significantly impairs the individual's ability to function. When this occurs, the patient may undergo resection of the ectopic bone, often followed by radiation therapy and pharmacologic treatment.[158,160]

Pain

Pain is a common problem both during the acute phase after spinal cord injury and in the years that follow. It can have a musculoskeletal, visceral, or neuropathic cause.[161,162] Psychosocial and environmental factors can contribute to the problem.[162] The first step in the management of existing pain is an examination and evaluation to determine its source and contributing factors. Appropriate interventions can then be implemented.

Musculoskeletal Pain

Some musculoskeletal pain arises from conditions that require medical or surgical intervention. Examples include pain caused by heterotopic ossification or vertebral instability.[163] In contrast, acute or chronic pain arising from soft tissue injury, inflammation, or mechanical stress can often be addressed through a variety of physical therapy interventions. The nature of the pathology or dysfunction will influence the choice of interventions, which can include any of the following: exercise, electrical or thermal modalities, massage, correction of postural abnormalities, activity or equipment modification, or adaptation of the environment. Pharmacotherapy may also be indicated to control pain.[163,164] Pain should be addressed quickly when it develops, in order to prevent it from becoming chronic.[163,164]

Although treatment of pain is important, prevention is preferable. Because upper extremity overuse injuries are a common cause of pain in individuals with long-standing spinal cord injuries, upper extremity preservation is an essential focus of rehabilitation. Strategies include exercise, functional training, equipment selection and adjustment, education, and environmental adaptation.[m]

Visceral Pain

Management of visceral pain involves treatment of the underlying cause. Examples include antibiotic therapy for a bladder infection, or evacuation of a bowel impaction.

Neuropathic Pain

If pain is caused by a spinal cord syrinx or compression of a nerve root or peripheral nerve, surgical intervention may provide relief.[162] When it is not caused by these conditions, neuropathic pain originating at or below the lesion is less amenable to intervention and is typically managed with medication.[162,165,166] Some individuals respond to transcutaneous electrical nerve stimulation (TENS), acupuncture, or spinal cord stimulation.[162]

Psychological Interventions

Patients with chronic pain, regardless of the etiology, can benefit from psychological interventions to help manage the pain and reduce its impact on their lives. Cognitive-behavioral therapy or training in self-hypnosis or relaxation may be beneficial.[164,166,167] Antidepressant or anxiolytic medications are also utilized in some cases.[162,166]

Spasticity and Spasms

Spasticity and spasms[n] occur frequently in people with spinal cord injuries, particularly in those who have lesions

---

[m] Strategies for preventing overuse injuries in the upper extremities are presented in Chapter 8 and throughout the text.
[n] Spasticity is a velocity-dependent increase in muscle tone in response to passive movement.[191,192] Spasms are involuntary muscle contractions that occur spontaneously or are elicited by stimuli such as tactile stimulation.[193]

in the cervical or upper thoracic cord. Although elevated muscle tone is not always problematic and occasionally is useful, it often causes pain, interrupts sleep, interferes with independent functioning, and makes it difficult for others to provide assistance. It can also contribute to the development of contractures and pressure ulcers.[168]

When elevated muscle tone is problematic, a variety of management strategies are available. Physical therapy interventions include passive stretching and positioning, rhythmic passive movements, prolonged standing, hydrotherapy, neuromuscular electrical stimulation, and TENS.[169–172] Nonpharmacological interventions should be tried before resorting to medication.[168,171] When spasticity remains problematic despite these measures, pharmacotherapy should be considered. Baclofen, clonidine, diazepam, tizanidine, or dantrolene sodium can be taken orally. Clonidine can be administered using a transdermal patch. Each of these systemic medications has potential side effects, ranging in severity from drowsiness to liver toxicity.[168,170–175] Baclofen or clonidine can be administered intrathecally by a surgically implanted pump (Figure 3–17).[171] Because the medication is delivered directly into the subarachnoid space surrounding the spinal cord, spasticity and spasms can be controlled with fewer systemic effects. Potential side effects include withdrawal symptoms or potentially lethal[172, 176] overdose, which can occur when the pump does not function properly.[168,174]

Regardless of the mode of delivery, pharmacotherapy is generally started with low doses, which are increased gradually until the desired clinical outcome is achieved.[171,172,174] Optimal dosing reduces the patient's muscle tone enough to decrease discomfort and permit safe functioning, with minimal side effects.

A variety of conditions such as bladder infections, fractures, pressure ulcers, or hangnails can cause temporary increases in spasticity and spasms. Such sources of increased muscle tone should be investigated and treated before medications are initiated or adjusted.[171,173,174,177]

When problematic spasticity exists in a limited number of muscles, alternative locally acting agents may be utilized. These agents include botulinum toxin, which is injected into muscles, and phenol or ethyl alcohol, which are injected into peripheral nerves. These interventions cause temporary[o] reductions in spasticity.[168,171,172,175,177]

EDUCATION

Education is a critical component of any rehabilitation program. It has become even more critical as hospital stays have shortened. People are leaving rehabilitation centers earlier, before they have had time for full physiological, functional, and psychosocial adaptation to their injuries. If they are to survive and stay healthy after discharge, they must gain knowledge and skills in a variety of areas, including pressure ulcer prevention, skin inspection, bowel and bladder care, assisted coughing, and use of medications and orthoses. During rehabilitation, patients should learn about how their bodies function, the complications they may experience, how to avoid these complications, and what to do if they occur. For long-term health and wellness, they should also learn strategies for enhancing cardiovascular fitness and preventing overuse injuries in the upper extremities.[P]

Many people with spinal cord injuries require assistance when they leave rehabilitation, either because they have not yet reached their full functional potential or because their impairments are such that independent functioning is not possible. When individuals are likely to require assistance after discharge, their educational programs should include the people who will provide this assistance. This group may include family members, friends, attendants, or other caregivers. In addition to addressing the topics already mentioned, the educational programs for patients and caregivers should include instruction and practice in training and directing others in the safe performance of the tasks that will require assistance. This will prepare them to train future caregivers.

In addition to "survival skills," instruction should address the individual's potential for neurological return. Although definitive predictions are often not possible, patients can be apprised of the range of possibilities for neurological return and the likely time course of any return that may occur. They should also be informed about the rehabilitation team's best estimate of their ultimate outcomes. People with incomplete lesions should be encouraged to inform the rehabilitation team if significant change occurs.

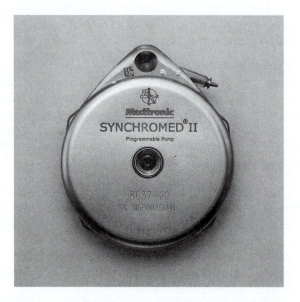

Figure 3-17   Baclofen pump. (Reproduced with permission from Medtronic, Inc. ©2009.)

---

[o] Three to 6 months for botulinum toxin, 2 to 36 months for ethyl alcohol or phenol.[177]
[P] Additional information related to these topics is presented throughout the text.

Finally, the education program should work to develop the self-reliance and communication skills that patients will need to direct their care following discharge. Unfortunately, many members of the general medical community are ignorant about the special health needs of people with spinal cord injuries. As a result, someone who places total trust in the system may not get adequate care. People with spinal cord injuries need to learn to manage their own care if they are to stay healthy through the years.

"I realized that no one would know my needs or wants unless I knew what they were and could tell people. I learned about my care so I could teach it to others. Now that I have to be my own best advocate, I'm much better at communicating."

Steve Ferguson
band director, mentor, father,
C5 SCI survivor[178]

Follow-Up

Follow-up is another important component of health care after spinal cord injury. After discharge, periodic checkups make it possible to monitor and respond to changing physical and psychosocial needs, promote health, detect and treat complications early, and gather feedback on the effectiveness of the rehabilitation program. These postdischarge evaluations should continue indefinitely, because many of the sequelae and potential complications of spinal cord injury continue for the remainder of the individual's life.

Follow-up has added significance for people who experience neurological return. As lengths of stay in rehabilitation diminish, the chance of motor return occurring after discharge increases. Significant motor return that is evident at follow-up may indicate the need for further rehabilitation to maximize functional gains made possible by the return. This additional rehabilitation can take place in inpatient, outpatient, or in-home settings as appropriate.

Summary

- Following injury of the spinal column, motion of the spine may result in trauma to previously undamaged neural tissue. Appropriate fracture management is required to preserve neurological function.
- Fracture management starts with immobilization of the spine at the scene of the accident. Definitive management involves operative and/or nonoperative restoration of the spine's alignment, decompression of the neural tissue, and stabilization of the injured structures.
- An orthosis may be used to immobilize the injured spinal column, either in lieu of or following surgery. A variety of orthoses are available for each region of the spine.

- Spinal cord injury leaves an individual susceptible to a variety of serious complications. During acute care and rehabilitation, specialized medical management is necessary to avoid these complications.
- In order to stay healthy, a person with a spinal cord injury must learn strategies for enhancing fitness and wellness, including the prevention, detection, and management of complications. The educational component of rehabilitation addresses these areas with both the patient and those who will be involved in her care.
- Because spinal cord injury causes lifelong vulnerability to a variety of problems, postdischarge follow-up is critical.

Suggested Resources

ORGANIZATIONS

Christopher and Dana Reeve Paralysis Foundation:
  www.christopherreeve.org
Model Systems Knowledge Translation Center:
  http//msktc.washington.edu/sci/index.html
National Rehabilitation Information Center: *www.naric.com*
National Spinal Cord Injury Association: *www.spinalcord.org*
Paralyzed Veterans of America: *www.pva.org*

PUBLICATIONS

Clinical practice guidelines published by Paralyzed Veterans of America, available free; download from *www.pva.org*:

- *Acute Management of Autonomic Dysreflexia: Individuals with Spinal Cord Injury Presenting to Health-Care Facilities,* 2nd ed, 2001.
- *Early Acute Management in Adults with Spinal Cord Injury,* 2008.
- *Prevention of Thromboembolism in Spinal Cord Injury,* 2nd ed, 1999.

Spinal Cord Injury Rehabilitation Evidence:
  www.icord.org/scire

4

Psychosocial Issues

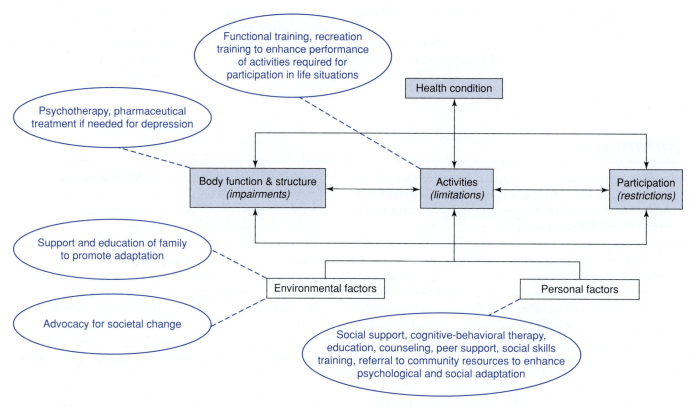

Chapter 4 presents information on psychosocial issues following spinal cord injury and strategies for facilitating adaptation.

Spinal cord injury brings sudden and profound life changes. The person who sustains a cord injury may be swimming, playing football, driving, or earning a living one minute, and the next minute be incapable of moving his extremities. Over the next days and weeks he finds himself paralyzed, incontinent, immobile, dependent, and isolated. As his rehabilitation progresses and he ventures out from the rehabilitation center, he is faced with a social and physical environment that seems almost hostile in its inaccessibility.

"My world was constructed of obstacles and barriers that other people could not see, even though they stared at me all the time."

John Hockenberry
journalist, author, advocate,
T5 SCI survivor[1]

Despite the magnitude and scope of the problems that spinal cord injury can cause, most people who sustain a cord injury are able to adjust. For some, the injury ultimately results in psychological and spiritual growth.[2] Others never fully recover psychologically from their loss. The outcome depends partly on the individual and partly on the psychosocial support he receives. To maximize their patients' potential for adaptation and growth following spinal cord injury, the rehabilitation team must address itself to their psychosocial needs.

PSYCHOSOCIAL IMPACT OF SPINAL CORD INJURY

Losses Associated With Spinal Cord Injury

The physical losses engendered by spinal cord injury are perhaps the most obvious. Depending on the completeness and level of the injury, a person can lose control of some or all of his limb and trunk musculature. His physique changes dramatically as his muscles atrophy. Where sensation is affected, the individual loses the ability to perceive the presence, position, and motion of his limbs or to experience the myriad pleasant and unpleasant sensations from the environment. He is likely to lose bowel and bladder control, and his sexual functioning will be altered.[a]

The person with significant neurological damage from spinal cord injury loses the ability to care for himself and to move from place to place. Dependent on others to care for him, and placed in an environment where power and self-direction are taken away, he loses his autonomy. Additionally, he is unable to participate in the recreational, social, educational, and vocational activities that previously filled his days. With rehabilitation, he may regain the capacity to do some of these things, but his manner of doing them will be altered.

Spinal cord injury also threatens financial security and disrupts plans for the future. Unemployment is extremely common[b] following injury.[3–9] Financial difficulties are also created by the expenses of medical care, attendant care, and equipment.[10,11]

During acute hospitalization and rehabilitation, a person is likely to experience separation from loved ones. Even after discharge, relationships with friends and family members are likely to be different. Roles may be altered, and patterns of communication and levels of intimacy are likely to change.[12–14] Old friends tend to drift away.[15–17]

> "It was as if that old Tim Gilmer, the athlete, the one who had all this promise – it was almost as if he had died. And now there was this ghost in his place."
> Tim Gilmer
> professor, author, editor, husband,
> T11–T12 SCI survivor[18]

Faced with the changes in his physique, physical functioning, functional capacity, accustomed activities, financial status, relationships, and plans for the future, the individual's previous self-concept no longer fits. Thus, personal identity can be added to the list of losses brought on by spinal cord injury.[16, 19]

Finally, spinal cord injury challenges a person's notions about how the world functions. Each of us has illusions about the world and our place in it. These irrational beliefs, left over from early childhood, may include feelings of invulnerability, immortality, or a sense of total control over one's life.[20] Spinal cord injury can make these and other illusions untenable.

> "I think with a spinal cord injury, one realizes that one is not going to live forever, that you are mortal."
> Don Rugg
> engineer, husband, peer counselor,
> C5 SCI survivor[21]

Social Impact of Spinal Cord Injury

People with disabilities are devalued in society. As a group, they are seen as substantially different from and less desirable than able-bodied people; as a result, they are subject to discrimination.[22–25]

Discrimination against people with disabilities manifests itself in many ways. Architectural and transportation barriers interfere with activities and participation. People with disabling conditions encounter discriminatory treatment when seeking education, employment, medical insurance, and housing.[24,26,27] Financial disincentives within public assistance programs can make it difficult to break out of a cycle of unemployment and poverty; in some cases, employment can result in a loss of medical insurance[c] and funding for attendant care, meaning that some people with disabilities simply cannot afford to work.[3,16,28]

People with disabilities are also subject to discrimination in their interpersonal relationships. When meeting someone with a disability, an able-bodied person's perception of that person is likely to be dominated by the disability; people focus on the disabling characteristics rather than other qualities.[12] People with disabilities are viewed as fundamentally different from "normal" people and are afforded less esteem and status.[29] They are often perceived as dependent and helpless,[30,31] tragic victims who remain bitter about their misfortune.[32]

> "I felt stuck in a box people placed me in, categorized and labeled disabled. I felt like nothing in society's eyes, which was a terrible blow for a twelve-year-old who already believed she was something."
> Kris Ann Piazza
> writer, editor, community board member, public speaker,
> C5 SCI survivor[33]

---

[a] Chapter 13 addresses the impact of spinal cord injury on sexuality and sexual functioning and presents strategies for promoting adjustment in this area.

[b] The rate of unemployment varies with many factors, including age at injury, time since injury, and country of residence.[3,68,154]

[c] The Ticket to Work and Work Incentives Improvement Act, passed in 1999, has reduced these financial disincentives in the United States.[155]

Because of the devaluation and stereotyping of people with disabilities, able-bodied people are likely to be uncomfortable talking with them and tend to avoid contact.[12,30,34] This discomfort, in combination with architectural barriers in the community, creates a formidable obstacle to community integration. As a result, social isolation is common following spinal cord injury.[16,35]

After sustaining a spinal cord injury, a person soon discovers that he is a member of a disadvantaged minority, "the disabled." The demoralizing effects of the stereotyping and discrimination that he experiences are likely to be compounded by his own preexisting prejudices regarding people with disabilities.[25]

Additional Factors Affecting Behavior

During the acute phase following spinal cord injury, a person is likely to experience sensory deprivation, social isolation, lack of time cues, sleep deprivation, and pain. He is likely to be on medications that have psychoactive effects, and may undergo surgery with general anesthesia. He may have sustained a head injury or experienced a period of anoxia at the time of the accident. Particularly if he has a cervical lesion, he may have periods of hypoxia due to sleep-disordered breathing.[36,37] Any of these conditions alone can have a profound impact on cognitive functioning, emotions, and behavior.[16,17,37–39] When faced with a recently injured person, it is difficult, if not impossible, for the health professional to determine which behaviors are the result of the patient's psychological reaction to spinal cord injury and which are due to other circumstances and physical variables.

Many of the conditions just described—particularly medication, sleep deprivation, oxygen desaturation during sleep, and the sequelae of brain injury—can persist throughout and beyond rehabilitation. Additionally, during inpatient rehabilitation, the person may be bored[40] and may find himself in an environment that encourages complacency and inactivity.

Cautionary Note

Many health professionals are quick to interpret any of a variety of behaviors as psychological reaction to spinal cord injury. Before making this judgment, they should keep in mind the multiple factors that can affect a recently injured person's cognitive functioning, emotions, and behavior. If the person who has recently sustained a spinal cord injury seems confused, is it the result of a psychological response to overwhelming loss? Is it a result of pain, medication, brain injury, social isolation, or sensory deprivation? If he expresses anger, is this a manifestation of inner turmoil brought on by the injury, or could it be a reaction to demeaning treatment? Before assuming that a patient's behavior stems from his psychological response to spinal cord injury, health professionals should consider other possible explanations. Most importantly, they should try to determine whether anything in the physical or social environment could be contributing to the behavior in question.

Health professionals should also keep in mind the following humbling fact: research has demonstrated that as a group, we are not very good at determining our patients' moods. There is a strong tendency to overestimate the emotional and social problems of patients with spinal cord injuries[41–44] and to underestimate their coping ability.[41] Many people with spinal cord injuries report that they do not view their injuries as tragic or even as the worst thing that ever happened to them.[17,45] Health professionals who view spinal cord injury in an overly catastrophic light are more likely to convey a defeatist and pitying attitude that could, in turn, affect their patients' ability to adjust.

PSYCHOLOGICAL ADJUSTMENT AND ADAPTATION FOLLOWING INJURY

Spinal cord injury causes significant losses in many areas: physical, functional, social, financial, personal identity, and world view. In general, the process of adjustment to these losses takes years.[13,16,20,46] As evidence of continuing adjustment over the years, both life satisfaction and quality of life increase with time after injury.[3,47–50]

In the past, it was believed that people who sustained spinal cord injuries went through a specific series of mood states as they adjusted. Typically, each patient was expected to experience shock, denial, depression, anger, dependency, and finally adjustment.[17,19] Although various theorists described slightly different stages of adjustment, it was generally agreed that adjustment required progression through these stages. Research, however, has shown the stage theory of adjustment to be inaccurate.[16,17,28,51–53] People do not progress through a neat series of mood states in lockstep fashion as they adapt to life following spinal cord injury. Each adapts in his own way. Moreover, an individual may adjust to different aspects of spinal cord injury at different rates and with varying success. For example, emotional adjustment to using a wheelchair may precede adaptation to altered bowel functioning.

If people do not pass through a predictable and universal series of stages, what do they do? After spinal cord injury, as after any significant loss, people grieve and adjust. Each individual does so, however, in his own way and pace. A variety of factors influence the manner in which an individual responds and adjusts to spinal cord injury and the success of this adjustment. These include personal characteristics such as personality; cognitive style; coping style; problem-solving skills; verbal learning ability; values, attitudes, and psychological health prior to the injury; prior loss or trauma experiences; and age.[2,16,49,52,54–64] The social support provided by loved ones, health professionals, and others also has a strong influence on adaptation and participation following cord injury.[16,40,52,56,60,65–67] Finally, factors such as cultural context, financial security, education, and access to transportation also affect adjustment.[16,50,60,68,69]

Contrary to common assumptions, level of injury is not a significant factor; people with tetraplegia adjust as successfully as those with paraplegia.[5,60,63,70–81] Moreover, individuals with less profound neurological damage can have greater adjustment problems[d] than those with more severe injuries.[82] Although people with relatively good motor function (Frankel D and E, comparable to ASIA D and E) are likely to function with a high degree of independence, they can also experience many of the same difficulties as those with more complete lesions: orthopedic problems, bowel and bladder dysfunction, pain, medical complications, sexual problems, neurological deterioration, spasticity, depression, and unemployability.[83] Unfortunately these difficulties may be overlooked or minimized by health professionals, family members, friends, other patients, and others in the community. As a result, individuals with minimal residual neurological deficits may not receive the "permission" and support they need to grieve their losses and adjust to their injuries.[82]

Finally, adjustment after spinal cord injury may best be viewed as an ongoing, lifelong process rather than a static endpoint. Although an individual may succeed in "adjusting" after his injury, this adjustment can be disrupted years later. His emotional equilibrium may be upset by something seemingly minor such as realizing that he is unable to play "catch" with his child. It can also be disturbed by bodily changes such as chronic shoulder pain that interferes with his functional capacity. Repeatedly over the years, various changes in events or circumstances are likely to trigger the need for continued adjustment.

> "To this day, I mourn for my losses. Not that I cry and feel sorry for myself everyday—just every now and then. This past spring, as I was driving to work by the river, I watched a couple jogging, and I just burst into tears—what I wouldn't give to be jogging with somebody I loved by the river on a spring day."
>
> Daniel H. Gottlieb
> family therapist, radio show host, newspaper columnist,
> public speaker, grandfather,
> C5–C6 SCI survivor[33]

Tasks of Grieving and Adaptation

Grieving involves more than a passive acceptance, more than "getting used to" a loss. It is an active process by which a person lets go of what has been lost and formulates a life without it.

Following spinal cord injury, a person may feel that he has literally lost everything. It may seem that all aspects of his life, his relationships, himself, and his future have been destroyed. But in grieving, he gradually gains perspective on his loss. One task of grieving involves sorting through his losses, identifying what aspects of his life and himself he has truly lost, and what remains. He can then let go of what has been lost and reclaim what remains.[64]

In response to the loss of his old self-image, a person with a spinal cord injury forges a new identity.[23,25] This identity is "an amalgamation of all of the 'I am's' from pre-injury that are still relevant with the new 'I am's' that are consonant with the physical disability."[16]

In addition to finding a new identity, the individual discovers and develops a new lifestyle, with new goals and sources of satisfaction.[84] By creating a new existence rather than holding onto the old, the person with a spinal cord injury can feel good about himself and his life. As time passes and life circumstances change, the individual's identity, lifestyle, goals, and sources of satisfaction will continue to evolve.

Early Reactions to Spinal Cord Injury

After spinal cord injury, people commonly go through a period of confusion and forgetfulness. Often, a newly injured person appears to have difficulty processing information. For example, he may ask a question that he has already asked on several occasions and seem to have no memory of discussing the topic. A newly injured health professional may ask questions or express beliefs that are inconsistent with his medical expertise.

In the past, the period of confusion that often follows spinal cord injury was assumed to be a sign of denial. Research findings have challenged this assumption. Sensory deprivation, social isolation, lack of time cues, sleep deprivation, pain, and medications are other possible explanations.[16,17,38,39,85]

Research has not demonstrated that denial is the cause of the confused behavior commonly seen after injury. By the same token, research has not ruled it out. If people do, in fact, grieve after sustaining spinal cord injuries, denial remains a possibility. When grieving a profound loss, denial serves a purpose: it allows people to rally their psychological and social resources and prepare themselves for their loss. It can be a normal, healthy psychological response that makes it possible for the reality of a loss to sink in gradually as the person becomes able to cope.[19,20,31] On the other hand, denial can be maladaptive if it prevents the person from progressing in the process of adjustment,[86] or leads to self-neglect.[87]

Grief

After an initial period of confusion, whatever the source, people tend to grieve following spinal cord injury. Grief is a normal, healthy process by which a person adapts to a significant loss. People vary widely in the emotions

---

[d] In one study, people with injuries classified as Frankel E (comparable to ASIA E) had higher suicide rates than did those with more complete injuries.[82]

that they experience after spinal cord injuries as well as in the order, intensity, and length of time experiencing the various emotions associated with grieving. An individual may alternate rapidly between moods or "move past" a particular mood state, only to return to it at a later time.[20,88]

A variety of emotions and behaviors are associated with grief. During normal grief following spinal cord injury, a person may experience any of the following: sadness, anger, hostility, anxiety, panic, and feelings of inadequacy, shame, helplessness, and vulnerability.[84,89] He may have periods of regression and self-neglect.[84,90] Many consider suicide, although most do not attempt it.[25,82,91]

It is important to make the distinction between grief, which is a normal and healthy response to loss, and clinical depression, which is pathological. True depression involves a specific, fairly global, and persistent pattern of emotions and behaviors.[e] Whereas most grieve after spinal cord injury, the majority do not exhibit true depression.[16,17,43,49,52,79,81]

Outcomes

Most people adapt well following spinal cord injury. After a period of adjustment, the majority have positive self-concepts[7,60] and are generally satisfied with life,[7,47,72] neither more anxious[63,68,92] nor more depressed[11,63,68,93] than noninjured people. The majority of long-term survivors rate their quality of life as good to excellent.[94]

> "I am not the same man as that twenty-year-old boy who was so sure his life was over so many years ago. . . . Today, I continue to lead a good, full life."
>
> Bill Hiser
> bed and breakfast owner, Sunday school teacher,
> husband, father,
> T10 SCI survivor[33]

Spinal cord injury is not a devastating catastrophe that creates victims who are forever bitter and psychologically impaired. In fact, for many it is a powerful stimulus for growth. Because it brings such profound losses, a spinal cord injury can shatter a person's identity and basic assumptions about himself and his world. In the aftermath of this disruption, it is possible for him to examine and alter his self-image and world view. Thus, he has an opportunity to grow in ways in which he might otherwise

never have grown, as these assumptions are rarely questioned except during times of crisis.[95]

> "I believe I'm a better person because of my disability, because of the way it has forced me to adjust to different situations, and the way I live my life. I think I'm more patient, more tolerant, and more understanding of other people. I'm more compassionate, and more able to relate to people of differing abilities and from different walks of life."
>
> Larry Nitz
> woodworker, camper, husband, father,
> T12 SCI survivor[33]

People often report that they have grown as a result of spinal cord injury.[40,96] Some even state that they would not opt for a cure if one were available.

> "This changed my life for the better. I was pretty miserable just before and after my injury. Now my life is pretty much straightened out. . . . I'm stronger than I thought and more patient, more ambitious, more humble. I wouldn't take the cure if it meant losing all I've learned."
>
> Joel Lorentz
> 911 dispatcher, NASCAR enthusiast,
> T12–L1 SCI survivor[97]

Although the majority of individuals with spinal cord injury adapt well, many do not.[f] Depression, though not universal, is more common among people with spinal cord injuries than it is in the general population.[49,98,99] Findings on the prevalence of depression vary widely, likely because of differences in research methodology. Estimates of its incidence range from 11% to over 30%.[100] In addition to depression, the following problems are more common in individuals with spinal cord injuries than in the general population: posttraumatic stress disorder,[101] anxiety, and feelings of helplessness.[102] A small percentage exhibits self-neglect, even years after injury.[90] A few find themselves unable to adapt to their disability and never regain a sense of happiness and satisfaction with their lives. The suicide rate among people with spinal cord injuries is 3.3 to 5 times higher than that of the general population.[6,82] Most of these suicides occur within the first 5 years of injury.[6]

---

[e] The diagnosis of a major depressive episode requires that the individual exhibits at least five of the following almost every day for at least 2 weeks: (1) depressed mood most of the day, (2) loss of interest or pleasure in activities, (3) significant weight loss or gain, (4) insomnia or hypersomnia, (5) psychomotor retardation or agitation, (6) fatigue or energy loss, (7) feelings of worthlessness or excessive or inappropriate guilt, (8) diminished ability to think or concentrate, or indecisiveness, (9) recurrent thoughts of death or suicide, or a suicide attempt or specific plan for suicide.[156]

---

[f] At first glance, the information that follows may appear to contradict the statements made earlier that the majority of individuals with spinal cord injury do not exhibit problems such as depression and anxiety. However, there is no contradiction: although *the majority* do not experience these problems after a period of adjustment, their incidence is higher than in the general population.

Problem-Solving Exercise 4–1

Try to imagine what your life would be like if you had a spinal cord injury. A few years down the road, would you feel that the quality of your life was good? Would you feel like a person of worth?

- If you could not breathe on your own, would you want to be placed on a ventilator or would you rather die than live with high tetraplegia?
- What do your answers tell you about your perceptions about life after a spinal cord injury?

COMMUNITY REINTEGRATION

Humans are social beings. Our relationships with families, friends, neighbors, coworkers, and members of the community at large are important aspects of our lives. Through these relationships, we can gain a sense of belonging and well-being. The roles that we play within these social groups help to define us and give us a sense of purpose.

One important focus of rehabilitation is community reintegration, the return to full participation in all aspects of the life of the community. In this context, "community" refers to social groups in a variety of settings: home, neighborhood, work or school, place of worship, and geographic region. Community reintegration includes the performance of age-, gender-, and culture-appropriate roles and activities in natural settings,[g] with normative status, rights, and responsibilities.[103] A high degree of community integration is associated with greater levels of life satisfaction.[104]

STRATEGIES FOR GROWTH AND REINTEGRATION

The purpose of rehabilitation after spinal cord injury is to maximize health, autonomy, and participation, enabling the person to return to full involvement in life. Teaching the physical skills needed to function independently is not enough to meet this end; living is more than getting in and out of bed and regulating bowels. These activities are not life; they are things that we do in order to live. To prepare a person to live with the sequelae of spinal cord injury, the rehabilitation team must focus beyond mere functional training and promote psychological and social adaptation as well. This involves providing the needed support as the individual mourns his losses and develops a new identity, lifestyle, future, and world view. It also involves preparing him to meet the social, environmental and logistical challenges that he will face after discharge.

The development of self-advocacy skills is a critical task of social adjustment after spinal cord injury. People with disabilities are protected by law against discrimination in housing, transportation, employment, and access to businesses and public facilities. Unfortunately, these laws are not always enforced. If they are to function in society, people with spinal cord injuries must be aware of their rights and know how to ensure that these rights are not violated.

Adaptation after spinal cord injury involves more than the injured individual; family members have significant adjustments of their own to make.[12,37] When someone becomes disabled, changes are likely to occur in his family's lifestyles, roles, communication patterns, and finances. The rehabilitation team can support the family as they learn to cope with these changes. In turn, the family will be better able to provide needed social support to the injured person as he adjusts to the injury and its consequences.

Destructive Practices in Rehabilitation

Most, if not all, rehabilitation professionals would agree that they should (and do) work to prepare people with physical impairments to live as independently as possible and to develop positive attitudes toward themselves and their lives. In practice, however, this is all too often not the case. While we teach the physical skills needed for independent functioning, we can also, inadvertently, teach people that they are second-class citizens, incapable or unworthy of self-direction or independence.

Dependence

From the moment a person sustains a spinal cord injury, he loses control of his life. He is handled, poked, prodded, examined, treated, and "done to" by an endless stream of health professionals as they care for his physical needs. Even after he reaches a rehabilitation unit, he may not be treated in ways that would enable him to regain control of his life. He may not be given any real choices, being expected to conform to the goals and practices of the rehabilitation team.[40] If his desires do not coincide with those of the team, and if he asserts himself, he is likely to be labeled "noncompliant" and a "difficult patient." Passive, compliant behavior is expected and rewarded.[16,25,31]

---

[g] An example of a natural setting is a standard workplace rather than a sheltered workshop.

Another harmful practice involves assisting people who are capable of performing an activity independently. This is often done for the sake of expedience. ("Yes, you worked hard in OT to learn how to dress yourself, but I'm going to dress you so that you won't be late for your appointment.") The underlying message is that the person can do the activity in therapy, but in real life he needs others to help him. In addition to receiving this negative message, the person is deprived of practice of the activity. His skill, then, does not develop as it should. Ultimately, he will not be able to perform the task as well or as quickly as he should, and does in fact end up needing assistance.

Negative Attitudes

Many health professionals, being products of society at large, have negative attitudes about people with disabilities.[42,105,106] These attitudes influence their behavior as they interact with patients and can have a detrimental effect on their patients' adjustment.[4] Health professionals who are overly pessimistic or defeatist can convey these attitudes to patients and their families.[42] Negative attitudes can also cause health professionals to treat their patients as second-class citizens. They may disregard their privacy needs and interact with them in ways that are demeaning.[40] By talking to adult patients as though they were children or by talking about them in their presence as though they were unable to hear, health professionals dehumanize and infantilize them. We also dehumanize patients by labeling them by their disabling conditions. This practice focuses attention on the disability rather than on the person, making it easier to lose sight of the person himself.

Medical Model

The practices just described are symptomatic of the medical model of health care. In systems operating according to this model, there is a rigid hierarchy of power, with physicians at the top, other health professionals in the middle, and patients and family members at the bottom. The job of the staff is to "fix" patients, and the patients are expected to accept that treatment passively.[16,26,107,108] Health professionals are firmly in control. Rounds are likely to be conducted either in the patient's absence or at bedside, with the patient lying down.[109] Clearly, a unit functioning according to the medical model does not provide an atmosphere that encourages those undergoing rehabilitation to exercise their autonomy.

Inherent in the medical model is the inferior, powerless status of the patient. Health professionals dominate all interactions. These practices and values are so ingrained in the medical community that the demeaning domination and subjugation inherent in these interactions is seen by many as appropriate professional–patient relations.

During rehabilitation, people are often exposed to practices and attitudes that convey to them that they are dependent, sick, incapable of running their own lives, and less than fully human. These messages of dependence and dehumanization may be particularly destructive to a newly injured person. At a time when he is piecing together a new identity, he is likely to be more vulnerable to feedback from others about who he is now that he has a disabling condition. This may be especially true when the feedback comes from health professionals.

> "In the first weeks after my injury, I was like a child and the doctors seemed like parents, while the nurses became older brothers and sisters. I hung on every word and tried to interpret the expressions on their faces. Everything they said and did had an enormous impact on me. I remembered all of it; sometimes I replayed scenes over and over in my head."
>
> Christopher Reeve
> actor, director, activist, author, husband, father,
> C2 SCI survivor[110]

Constructive Practices in Rehabilitation

Within the social environment of a hospital or rehabilitation center, there is a massive potential for breaking patients' spirits. There is also great potential for healing and growth. For the latter to occur, the health care team must consciously and consistently pursue this goal. From day one, from the scene of the accident on, the person with a spinal cord injury must be treated as the thinking, feeling, autonomous person that he is. Instead of relentlessly stripping him of his power and dignity, all members of the team must treat him with respect and support his right to self-determination.

Independence and Autonomy

In people with spinal cord injuries, perceived control is strongly associated with life satisfaction.[74] To adapt successfully after spinal cord injury, people must gain (or retain) a sense of personal effectiveness and control over their lives. For this to occur, they must be given opportunities to make choices throughout the period of acute care and rehabilitation. They should be given true control, not just the opportunity to choose between compliance and noncompliance. From the day of injury onward, patients should be kept informed about their condition and treatment options and should be given a voice in setting goals, scheduling activities, and making decisions about their care.

To promote independence, the rehabilitation team should include patients in problem solving. With guidance and encouragement, patients can participate in analyzing problems, coming up with possible solutions, and evaluating outcomes. This can be done while they are learning functional skills, deciding on bowel and bladder management practices, choosing between equipment options, and determining virtually any aspect of their programs. By participating in problem solving in this manner, patients can develop the ability to solve problems on their own. This skill will prove invaluable to independent functioning during and after rehabilitation.

Problem-Solving Exercise 4–2

It is time to begin the process of selecting a wheelchair to purchase for a patient.

- Describe a process for wheelchair selection that would reinforce the patient's sense of independence and autonomy.

- In addition to empowering the patient, are there other potential benefits that could result from using the process that you propose?

Independent functioning also requires a sense of personal responsibility. To live independently, a person must know what to do and when to do it, and must take the initiative to get things done. For this sense of responsibility to develop during rehabilitation, the patient should be given as much responsibility as possible for his rehabilitation. He should know his schedule and be accountable for getting to the various therapies and activities, either under his own power or by asking for assistance when needed. Once in therapy, he should be encouraged to initiate exercises or functional practice without waiting to be told what to do. The same kind of initiative can be encouraged in his personal care practices, such as pressure reliefs, morning hygiene, and bowel and bladder programs. From the time of his initial hospitalization onward, he should be expected to take as much responsibility for himself as he can, with increasing expectations of independent functioning as he progresses in his rehabilitation.

> "After an accident like mine, it is easy to say, 'My whole life's been destroyed.' But the idea is to decide 'I can do anything. Now, how can I do it?'"
>
> Steve Soper
> airplane pilot,
> L1 SCI survivor[18]

Positive Atmosphere

While a person is adapting to the sequelae of a spinal cord injury, the physical and social environment of the rehabilitation center can have a powerful impact. A prevailing climate of gloom and tragedy conveys a sense of hopelessness and despair to all involved: those undergoing rehabilitation, family members, friends, and health professionals. A more positive atmosphere will encourage the development of a more optimistic outlook.[53]

The physical environment in a rehabilitation setting is important. Dark corridors and institutional decor convey a feel of sickness and debilitation. At the other extreme, a saccharine and childlike atmosphere communicates a sense of dependence and childishness. Upbeat, age-appropriate decor and music will provide a more positive environment for rehabilitation.

Staff attire also contributes to the atmosphere of a rehabilitation center. Uniforms and laboratory coats help create a hospital-like atmosphere, with all of its connotations of illness and power hierarchies. Likewise, the dress of those undergoing rehabilitation is important. Pajamas are appropriate attire for people who are either sick or asleep. Certainly they are inappropriate for conferences, therapies, or any other activities that take place outside of an individual's room.

Another element in a rehabilitation setting's atmosphere is the activity level of those undergoing rehabilitation. Long, empty hours in the days and evenings can deaden the spirit. Meaningful activity can provide a sense of purpose and personal control.[23] Active participation in therapies and recreational activities can also reduce boredom, promote better sleep at night,[17] and facilitate the grieving process.[20]

In working to create a positive atmosphere, the rehabilitation team should focus on abilities rather than limitations. Too often, health practitioners concern themselves with the problems while ignoring the strengths of those whom they serve.[106] To convey a greater sense of optimism, the rehabilitation team should emphasize what a person can do rather than dwelling on what he cannot do. In discussions during conferences, problem-solving sessions, and informal interactions, the focus can be placed on abilities and accomplishments. During therapies and other activities, patients should perform meaningful tasks that are structured in such a way that they can experience success and see their accomplishments. Success experiences can help improve motivation[23] and develop a sense of mastery and control.[25]

Although success experiences during rehabilitation can have beneficial effects, it does not follow that all experiences of failure will be detrimental. In physical and occupational therapy, for example, people with significant motor impairments learn new ways to move their bodies and perform various tasks. This functional training inevitably involves a certain number of unsuccessful attempts as they gradually master new motor skills. These unsuccessful attempts can be positive learning experiences.

People undergoing rehabilitation should be encouraged to take risks.[111] If an individual's goals and activities are limited to those in which he is certain to succeed, functional progress will be limited. Perhaps more importantly, this overprotectiveness communicates to the individual and others that he is not capable of coping with possible failure. A person who is "protected" from risk may never develop the self-confidence and experience the psychological growth that comes from challenging one's limits.[h]

"Most everything that's good in life requires taking risks. Being in a chair doesn't change that."

Pat McGowan
economist,
C5-6 SCI survivor[97]

Interactions With Staff

Interactions with the staff are critical in rehabilitation; the attitudes and behaviors of rehabilitation professionals have a powerful influence on patients and their families at this time.[112] To foster the development of a positive self-image, all members of the rehabilitation team must treat the patient as an equal, worthy of respect. This respect should be evident in interactions with patients and their families in formal situations such as conferences, as well as in informal daily communication.

Demeaning language should be avoided at all times, even when only health professionals are present. Referring to groups or individuals by their diagnoses serves to reinforce a negative attitude among those present.

Finally, it is imperative for rehabilitation personnel to maintain appropriate "professional" relations with people undergoing rehabilitation.[53] This does not mean that interactions should be cold and formal or patterned on the dominance and submission relations inherent in the medical model. Rather, relationships should have clearly defined and mutually understood boundaries. A newly injured person who becomes too attached to a health professional may grow dependent on that person. Likewise, a health professional who becomes overly involved with someone undergoing rehabilitation may not act in that person's best interests, prolonging rehabilitation unnecessarily and encouraging dependence.[84] In an appropriate professional relationship, mutual respect, caring, and enjoyment can coexist with an understanding of the relationship's limits.

Social Support

Social support can enhance a person's capacity to cope and recover following loss.[20,113] The rehabilitation team can promote emotional recovery and growth after spinal cord

injury by providing this support. Health professionals should listen to patients as they air their feelings, helping them to clarify their emotions and reassuring them that their feelings are normal. Staff should listen with empathy, not pity, and avoid judging what they hear.[20,23,25,114] This support should be available from all members of the team, not just from the psychiatric or counseling staff.

Each individual should be allowed to grieve and adapt in his own way; staff members must not impose their own notions of how people should feel and act following spinal cord injury. The recently injured person should neither be required to mourn nor be rushed to complete the grieving process prematurely.

In addition to enhancing psychological adaptation, social support is an important contributor to participation in community-dwelling individuals with spinal cord injury.[15,66] One focus of rehabilitation should be to investigate and develop the social support from family, friends, and others that will be available to the individual following discharge.

Hope and Truth

Health professionals have conflicting attitudes about hope and truth. On the one hand, expressions of hope may be labeled as "denial" and seen as signs of failure to cope with reality. On the other hand, health professionals are often reluctant to provide newly injured people with information,[40] fearing that the truth will crush all hope.

Neither hope nor denial are necessarily bad as long as they do not interfere with an individual's progress in psychosocial and functional adaptation after injury. In fact, hope can help a person cope with his injury.

"When we have hope, we discover powers within ourselves we may never have known – the power to make sacrifices, to endure, to heal, and to love. Once we choose hope, everything is possible."

Christopher Reeve
actor, director, activist, author, husband, father,
C2 SCI survivor[110]

Whereas hope has its benefits, information is critical to adjustment after a spinal cord injury. Knowledge, even if unpleasant, can help a person with an illness or disability regain a sense of control of his life.[115,116] Anyone who asks a question has the right to get an honest answer; feigned ignorance and vague or inaccurate answers are not helpful responses.[40]

Although health professionals should provide honest information, they should do so in a way that does not destroy all hope.[17,117] Perhaps it is best to speak in terms of probabilities rather than absolutes. In truth, we rarely have definitive answers anyway. Who can predict with certainty whether a particular individual will experience neurological return, father a child, or walk again?

---

[h] The risks referred to in this discussion involve stretching one's limits and striving to accomplish goals that may be difficult to achieve. It is not meant to imply that we should encourage behaviors that are physically hazardous, such as performing transfers or practicing "wheelies" without guarding before one has learned to do so safely.

Educational Model

Many of the constructive practices just described are inherent in an educational model of rehabilitation. Using this model, health professionals and people undergoing rehabilitation work as partners in pursuit of mutually agreed-upon goals. The model relationship is one of teacher–student[i] rather than healer–patient. This nonmedical orientation conveys the attitude that those undergoing rehabilitation are not sick—an understanding crucial to coping with a disabling condition.[118]

In the educational model, people undergoing rehabilitation are expected to be active participants in designing, carrying out, and evaluating their programs. Respect for the individual is inherent in this model. Emphasis is placed on consumerism and autonomous functioning rather than on compliance. Clearly, this approach is superior to the medical model in fostering independence and growth.[16,17]

A rehabilitation team attempting to implement a program consistent with the educational model should keep in mind the fact that it is likely to run counter to their natural tendencies. Having grown up in a society in which disabilities are strongly stigmatized, health professionals are likely to hold negative attitudes about people undergoing rehabilitation. In addition, most of their professional training and practice is likely to have been in delivery systems based on the medical model. Thus many practices inherent in the medical model (and contrary to the educational model) may go unquestioned.

Because the educational model is likely to run counter to the natural tendencies of health professionals, its implementation requires careful scrutiny and vigilance. All members of the team, as well as the team as a whole, must take a close look at their own behavior and practices. In all formal and informal interactions, health professionals must approach the individuals undergoing rehabilitation with an attitude of respect and equality. All aspects of the social and physical environment should be examined for consistency with the educational model.

Formal Strategies

Personal control, a positive atmosphere, and supportive and respectful interaction provide the necessary foundation for rehabilitation. Additional strategies that can be used to promote growth and adaptation after spinal cord injury are presented in the following sections. These include various approaches to dealing with the personal loss and changes in family dynamics, as well as strategies aimed at successful reintegration into society.

Evaluation

Individuals and their families are highly variable in their responses to the life changes brought on by spinal cord injury. Thus, the psychosocial interventions that are most appropriate will vary. For this reason, evaluation is the logical starting point of planning the psychosocial component of a rehabilitation program.[79,118,119] An initial evaluation should be performed soon after injury, because many may benefit from intervention during their acute hospitalization.[89] Once an evaluation has been completed, a program can be designed that best meets the needs of a particular individual and his family. Subsequent evaluations will make it possible to alter the program as needs change.

The psychosocial evaluation can address the patient's personality structure and behavioral style; social problem-solving skills; cognitive abilities; coping styles and ability to cope with the cord injury; current level of anxiety, distress and depression; and past history of interpersonal relations, loss, trauma, psychiatric illness, and substance abuse. The assessment can also include an investigation of the patient's social support network and its communication patterns, coping styles, and level of distress. Finally, the evaluation should investigate whether there is a family history of depression or suicide attempts.[79,118–123]

The evaluation results can provide the patient, family, and health professionals with a better understanding of the individual's and family's reactions to the injury and its sequelae. It can also alert them to potential areas of future difficulty. They can then all work together to identify problems, set goals, and develop a plan of action.

Education

Education provides a critical foundation for psychosocial rehabilitation. To maintain or regain control of his life following spinal cord injury, a person must first have an understanding of his body's altered functioning and of strategies for avoiding complications and promoting health. Without this understanding, he will be unable to participate fully in the planning of his rehabilitation program or to take responsibility for his self-care.

Education regarding the physical sequelae of spinal cord injury is just a start. To function in society, a person with a disability needs to know about his legal rights and available resources in the community. He will also require financial management skills and the knowledge and skills required to obtain needed funding from insurance companies and government agencies. Those who require attendant care must know how to obtain and manage attendants.[10,16,23,68]

Education can take the form of lectures, discussions, audiovisual presentations, and printed material. Inclusion of family members can enhance their capacity to provide constructive support to the person with a spinal cord injury during rehabilitation and after discharge.[10,12,124]

Counseling

Recovering, adapting, and growing after spinal cord injury involves coming to terms with a host of losses, developing a new self-concept, and often redefining one's roles within the family. Social support can facilitate this process. For many, counseling is an important source of this support.

Group counseling provides an arena for people to discuss their experiences with others who have sustained spinal cord

---

[i] Teacher–adult student.

injuries. In this exchange, there are opportunities for the expression of emotions, enhancement of self-awareness, mutual encouragement, exchange of information, role modeling, examination and expansion of values and perceptions, feedback, and problem solving. Participation in group work may enhance motivation, normal grief resolution, and overall adjustment to the spinal cord injury.[23,53,125,126]

Family members can be included in group counseling, either in "family groups" with other families or in family or marital therapy. In group settings, they can gain information, express and come to grips with their emotions, give and receive support, grow in their attitudes regarding disability, develop more constructive communication patterns, and learn new coping strategies.[13,23,25,119,126] Group counseling need not be limited to people with disabilities and their families; other members of the social support system may be included.[114]

Some people with spinal cord injuries and their family members also benefit from individual counseling. In one-on-one counseling, a person may receive more individualized support and more assistance with grieving, clarification of intrapsychic and interpersonal conflicts, and the development of new coping skills. Individual counseling is especially (but not exclusively) indicated when a person feels overwhelmed by his emotions, exhibits signs of pathology, or has a personal or family history of early or unresolved loss, psychiatric illness, substance abuse, or difficulty with interpersonal relations.[64,90,113,114,117,119]

Peer Support

Contact with others who have experienced spinal cord injury can be very helpful in the adjustment process. Peer mentors, or peer supporters, are volunteers who have adapted well to their spinal cord injuries and have reintegrated into the community. The shared experience of spinal cord injury enables them to serve as role models and provide credible and practical information to people with recent injuries as well as their families. A peer mentor can be a source of reassurance, hope, and empowerment, and can help reduce stress and fear of the future.[127,128] Peer mentoring can occur during any phase after injury, from acute care through rehabilitation and after discharge.[127]

> "The biggest help was talking to someone already in a chair who was making it. I figured if he could do it, so could I. Peers made a huge impact on me. Seeing positive people who are doing well is so important those first few weeks."
>
> Matthew Seals
> customer service assistant, outdoorsman, husband,
> father,
> T12 SCI survivor[97]

Social Skills Training

Following spinal cord injury, an individual is likely to find that people are uncomfortable around him. As a result, he may find it difficult to meet people or to maintain old friendships. Fortunately, there are things that a person can do to lessen the negative impact of his disability on interactions with others. By projecting a positive self-image and putting others at ease, he can enhance the quality of his interactions with nondisabled people and facilitate a positive change in their attitudes.[16,34,129,130] These behaviors can be acquired in social skills training.

Social skills training involves learning stigma management strategies: verbal and nonverbal behaviors that can improve the quality of interactions with others. These communication techniques center primarily around putting others at ease and establishing rapport during initial encounters. Typical strategies include acknowledging the disability, legitimizing curiosity, providing information, answering questions, behaving assertively, and projecting a positive self-image and acceptance of the disabling condition.[16,30,129–131]

A variety of approaches to social skills training can be used. Through videotapes, lectures, and discussions, people can be introduced to the concept of stigma management and can gain some understanding about behaviors that will help or hinder their interactions with others. Actual practice of communication techniques is helpful in the development of these skills. Feedback from others can alert people to behaviors that they display that may impede interactions. This feedback can also help them to hone their communication skills.[16,22]

Cognitive Behavioral Therapy

Cognitive behavioral therapy is a therapeutic approach aimed at developing more adaptive behaviors, feelings, and thinking patterns.[102] It can include relaxation techniques; visualization; self-hypnosis; cognitive restructuring[j] ; increasing levels of pleasant events; training in coping strategies, social skills, and assertiveness; and education and discussion of sexual issues.[102,132,133] Participation in group cognitive behavioral therapy during rehabilitation is associated with higher levels of self-reported adjustment, lower rates of hospital readmission,[k] and lower rates of drug use for at least 2 years after injury.[102] It also reduces depressive mood in individuals who have high levels of depressive mood prior to initiation of therapy, and this benefit continues for at least 2 years after treatment.[132,134]

Functional Training

Activity limitations can interfere with the performance of a variety of roles and tasks involved in participation in life situations. For example, a person who cannot negotiate environmental barriers or manipulate objects will have difficulty

---

[j] Cognitive restructuring involves learning to isolate negative thoughts, mentally eliminate them, and replace them with rational and positive thoughts, as well as learning positive coping statements, distracting attention, and techniques for the reinterpretation of pain.[132]
[k] Hospital readmissions frequently occur as a result of preventable secondary conditions such as pressure ulcers. Thus a reduced rate of hospital readmission probably reflects better self-care practices (less self-neglect).

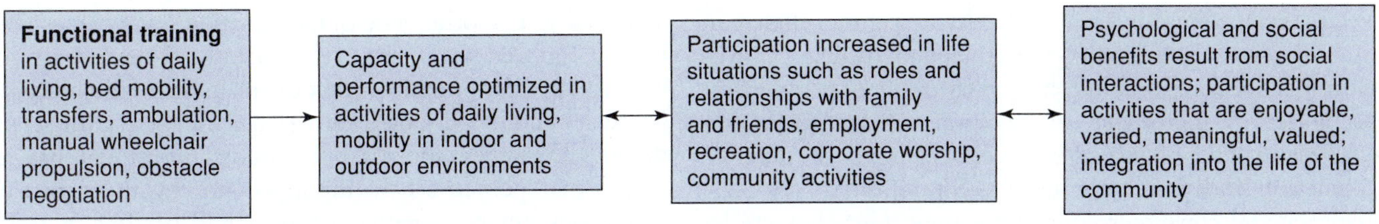

Figure 4–1   Schematic diagram of functional training that enhances psychosocial adaptation by improving activity and participation. Bidirectional arrows represent the reciprocal nature of the interactions.

performing the activities inherent in the roles of breadwinner, homemaker, or student.[135] Functional training can aid in psychosocial adaptation following spinal cord injury by increasing the individual's ability to function independently: improved capacity and performance in various activities can in turn enhance participation (Figure 4–1). Greater independence enables the person to resume or assume a variety of social roles,[135] and is associated with less anxiety and depression[81] and a higher perceived quality of life.[5,62,136]

Recreation Training

Many people who acquire disabling conditions find themselves unable to participate in the recreational activities to which they were previously accustomed. This represents a significant loss; leisure activities are an important source of pleasure, personal pride, relaxation, physical wellness, and social support. Through recreation training, people can learn ways to resume many of their previous activities or find alternative leisure activities. Resumption of an active leisure life can promote physical and psychological health and provide an avenue for reintegration into society.[85,137] By including spouses in leisure training, the team can help couples find activities that they can enjoy together. This may, in turn, have a beneficial effect on marital relations.[14]

Pharmaceutical Treatment

People exhibit a variety of emotions as they mourn their losses following spinal cord injury. Often, these emotions are unpleasant, both to experience and to witness. For this reason, it can be tempting to medicate people to lessen their (and our) discomfort.[117] Although pharmaceutical treatment can be beneficial in cases of clinical depression or psychosis,[16,52,90] it is not indicated for normal grief reactions. Medication aimed at ameliorating emotional pain can impede the ability to work through loss.[20,138]

Postdischarge Strategies

When a recently injured person leaves a rehabilitation center, his adjustment has just begun. Although this has probably always been the case, it has become more so in recent years. Because of shorter inpatient stays, "recently injured individuals are usually back in the home and in the community before confronting the full impact of their losses."[120] Moreover, discharge from inpatient rehabilitation brings a new set of challenges and adjustments. Although, during rehabilitation, people with spinal cord injuries gain some of the knowledge and skills required for

living in the community, they typically find that they have more to learn when they leave. In addition, they are faced with the challenging task of applying their new knowledge and skills in daily life at home and in the community.

Because adaptation and growth after spinal cord injury do not end at discharge, people can benefit from continued psychosocial support after completing their initial rehabilitation. Any of the strategies described previously can be used either during inpatient rehabilitation or in alternative settings following discharge. Additional strategies specific to people living in the community are presented in the following paragraphs.

One approach that can be beneficial is to put a recently injured person in contact with an individual who lives in the same community and has adjusted successfully following spinal cord injury. The "veteran" can share information and coping strategies, provide support to the person and his family[16] and help create a sense of acceptance and belonging.[15] Contact with a peer mentor can have lasting beneficial effects on life satisfaction and occupational involvement.[139]

Self-help groups are another potential source of social support after discharge. These groups can be helpful both for people with spinal cord injuries and their families. True self-help groups are made up of and run by people with common experiences[140]—in this case, spinal cord injuries. The focus and structure of self-help groups vary, depending on the needs and priorities of the membership. Groups may concern themselves with any or all of the following: education (of members, health professionals, or society at large), fund raising, sharing emotions, mutual social support, recreation, or social action. Individuals participating in self-help groups can gain information, new coping skills, and an increased sense of personal responsibility for their health and social well-being. Self-help groups can also be a source of affirmation, foster a sense of belonging, and provide motivation and reinforcement for successful coping. Perhaps most importantly, self-help groups can be empowering for the participants as individuals and as a group.[26,113,114,140,141]

Independent living centers located throughout the United States offer a variety of services to people with disabilities. These services can include provision of information and logistical assistance with equipment, home modification, accessible housing, attendant services, transportation, and community resources. Independent living centers can also provide legal advocacy, peer counseling, and financial counseling.[16,107,142–144] Many centers engage in disability rights activism.[144] The independent living movement focuses on improving the quality of life of people with disabilities by increasing architectural and transportation accessibility and obtaining services that make it possible to function independently in the community.[107,142] Self-advocacy and consumer control are important characteristics of the independent living model.[142,144,145]

Vocational rehabilitation and formal education can also facilitate psychosocial adjustment after spinal cord injury. Education and vocational training can enhance a person's self-confidence, increase his chances of obtaining gainful employment, and promote social interaction.[3,60,146] Among people with spinal cord injuries, education and employment are associated with higher quality of life,[3,5,62,147] life satisfaction and social integration,[148] and lower levels of depression[71,148] and psychological distress.[81] Typically, years elapse between the time of injury and return to work.[149] Opportunities for career counseling, formal education, and vocational training should be available both soon after injury and in the years that follow.[3,149,150]

Psychological healing and growth as well as social adaptation can continue for years after a spinal cord injury. In essence, they continue for the remainder of a person's life[16,46] as new issues and challenges continue to surface. Rehabilitation professionals can aid the process following discharge by including a psychosocial evaluation in routine follow-up visits[35,119,151] and by referring people to appropriate services and resources available in the community. Routine screening for depression is particularly important because of the prevalence of depression and its impact on health, relationships, social integration, and daily living.[71,120]

THE BIGGER PICTURE: OUR IMPACT ON THE COMMUNITY

As rehabilitation professionals, our function is to facilitate adjustment and reentry into society after the acquisition of a disabling condition. Traditionally, to reach this end we have placed our focus exclusively on patients themselves, teaching them various physical and social skills needed for living with a disability. The other side of the equation, society, has been largely ignored until relatively recently. The assumption underlying this approach is that the problem of disability lies in those who are disabled rather than in society. In recent decades, however, the disability rights movement has asserted that people are handicapped not by their physical conditions but by negative attitudes and barriers in transportation, architecture, employment, and public assistance programs.[28,107,142,152] Current rehabilitation practice reflects the International Classification of Functioning, Disability and Health (ICF), which is based on a biopsychosocial model that synthesizes elements of both perspectives: functioning, disability, and health are influenced both by characteristics of the individual and by the social and physical environment.[153] It follows that we should expand our focus to include societal change rather than concerning ourselves solely with providing services to individuals with disabilities.

One area with which we must concern ourselves is the devalued status of people with disabilities. Our attention to this area is imperative because of the powerful impact that rehabilitation professionals have on society's attitudes. By our actions and inactions, by what we say and do, and by the nature of our service delivery systems, we can strengthen or weaken the stigmatizing attitudes of those around us and of society at large.

As health care professionals, we are seen as experts on people with spinal cord injuries and other disabling conditions. Our communications about people with disabilities can influence others' attitudes. This communication occurs in a variety of situations, from casual social encounters ("You work with cripples? You must be soooo patient.") to interviews with television or newspaper reporters. Any discussion relating to people with disabilities presents an opportunity to either reinforce devaluing attitudes and beliefs or to portray a more positive picture.

Professional responsibility dictates that rehabilitation professionals direct attention to their impact on society's perceptions of people with disabilities. Additionally, some may choose to promote change through political action. Much work is needed in the areas of architectural barriers in the community, accessible housing, accessible transportation, and discriminatory practices and legislation.[16,22,106]

Problem-Solving Exercise 4–3

Often, unconscious motivations can taint services that are well meaning and, on the surface, good.[29] The following true story is an example.

A rehabilitation unit sponsored a race that included both able-bodied runners and athletes using wheelchairs. (So far so good.) At the awards ceremony after the race, the able-bodied runners received such prizes as athletic equipment and gift certificates from athletic stores. The winning athlete in the wheelchair division received a lap blanket.

- What message did the nature of the awards convey about the participants in the wheelchair division of the race?
- Why does that matter?
- How could the organizers of the race convey a more positive message?

Summary

- Anyone who sustains a spinal cord injury is faced with major losses, ranging from changes in physique and functional ability to the disruption of personal relationships, financial security, and future plans. His former self-image no longer fits. He has become a member of a devalued and disadvantaged minority—"the disabled."

- Psychosocial adjustment after spinal cord injury involves coming to terms with these losses, formulating a new identity, and learning communication skills needed to return to life within his family and the community.

- Most people with spinal cord injuries are able to adjust satisfactorily, and many even grow from the experience. A minority remains unable to adapt.

- Whether an individual grows from or succumbs to his disability can be influenced by the support that he receives during and after rehabilitation. To promote growth and adaptation following spinal cord injury, the rehabilitation team must support the individual as

he comes to terms with his injury and its consequences. Attention must also be directed to empowering him; therefore all interactions should be based on respect, equality, and mutuality.

- Formal strategies for enhancing psychosocial adaptation include education, counseling, peer mentoring programs, social skills training, cognitive behavioral therapy, functional training, recreation training, pharmaceutical treatment, and a variety of postdischarge strategies.

- Because spinal cord injuries affect family members as well as those who are injured, and reintegration into family life will require adaptation by all involved, families should be included in the psychosocial component of rehabilitation programs.

- Rehabilitation professionals should strive to have a positive impact on the community at large, working to increase its inclusiveness of people with spinal cord injuries and other disabling conditions.

Suggested Resources

ORGANIZATIONS

Disability Rights Education and Defense Fund: *www.dredf.org*

Disabled Sports USA: *www.dsusa.org*

Independent Living Centers USA: *www.ilusa.com/links/ilcenters.htm*

National Center on Physical Activity and Disability: *www.ncpad.org*

National Council on Independent Living: *www.ncil.org*

National Disability Rights Network: *www.napas.org*

Paralyzed Veterans of America: *www.pva.org*

U.S. Government
- Department of Health and Human Services, Office on Disability: *www.hhs.gov/od*

- Department of Justice, ADA Homepage: *www.ada.gov*
- Department of Labor, Office of Disability Employment Policy: *www.dol.gov/odep*
- National Council on Disability: *www.ncd.gov*

PUBLICATIONS

Depression Following Spinal Cord Injury: A Clinical Practice Guideline for Primary Care Physicians. (1998). Published by the Paralyzed Veterans of America. Available for free download from *www.pva.org*

Spinal Network: *The Total Wheelchair Resource Book*, 4th ed. (2009) Published by No Limits Communications. Available for purchase from *www.newmobility.com*

5

Skin Care

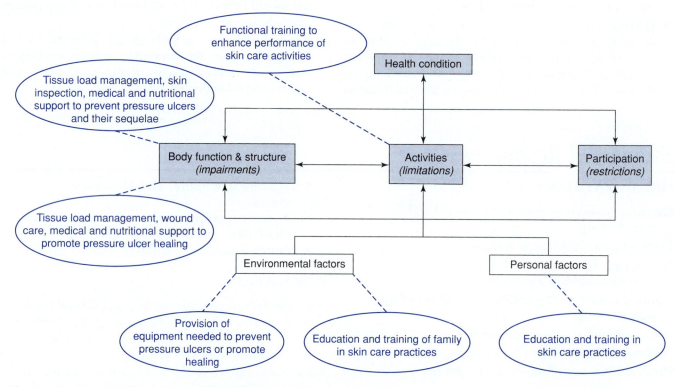

Chapter 5 presents information on the prevention and management of pressure ulcers after spinal cord injury.

Spinal cord injury brings with it a lifelong vulnerability to the development of pressure ulcers—localized areas of tissue necrosis that can occur when soft tissues are subjected to prolonged unrelieved pressure. Pressure ulcers—also called pressure sores, decubitus ulcers, decubiti, or skin breakdown—are among the most common complications of spinal cord injury.[1-7] It has been estimated that as many as 85% of people with spinal cord injuries develop at least one pressure ulcer at some point after injury.[8,9]

A number of risk factors are associated with the development of pressure ulcers following spinal cord injury (see Table 5–1). Pressure ulcers are more prevalent among people with complete lesions.[5,7,10–12] Level of injury may or may not be a contributing factor; some studies report a higher incidence of pressure ulcers in people with paraplegia,[10,12] whereas others report higher rates among people with tetraplegia[7,11] and still others report no relation between the incidence of pressure ulcers and level of lesion.[6,13–15]

Pressure ulcers occur almost exclusively over bony prominences. The areas over the sacrum, coccyx, heels, ischium, and greater trochanters are the most common sites of skin breakdown in individuals with spinal cord injury.[3,7,12,28,30,31]

TABLE 5–1   Factors Associated With The Occurrence And Severity Of Pressure Ulcers Following Spinal Cord Injury

	Factors Associated With Higher Risk
Completeness of injury	Complete injury (ASIA A)
Impairments resulting from spinal cord injury	Autonomic dysreflexia
	Excessive perspiration
	Fecal or urinary incontinence
	Lower ASIA motor score*
	Muscle tone abnormality: hypotonia or severe spasticity
	Sensory impairment
Emergency management	Prolonged immobilization after injury
Functional status	Bed-confined > mobile in wheelchair > ambulatory
	Lower level of independence
Medical conditions	Cardiovascular disease
	Diabetes
	Hypertension or hypotension
	Urinary tract infections
	Malnutrition (anemia, hypoalbuminemia)
	Previous pressure ulcer
	Pulmonary disease
	Renal disease
Psychological and social factors	Impaired cognitive function
	Inadequate social support
	Psychological disorders
	Ineffective problem-solving ability
	Inadequate financial resources
Behavioral factors	Noncompliance with skin care regimen
	Smoking
	Substance abuse
Demographics	Advanced age
	Longer time since injury
	Lower educational level
	Male gender
	Nonwhite race
	Residence in nursing home or hospital

* The ASIA motor score is presented in Chapter 7.

Sources: References 6, 7, 9, 10, 12, and 14 to 29.

ETIOLOGY OF PRESSURE ULCERS

A variety of factors are thought to make people with spinal cord injuries vulnerable to the formation of pressure ulcers. Skin collagen degradation after spinal cord injury makes the skin more fragile.[16,32] In addition, spinal cord injury leads to compromised peripheral blood flow, with resulting reduction in oxygen and nutrient supply to the tissues.[33] The skin and subcutaneous tissues are more vulnerable to trauma; the interruption of skin blood flow caused by external stresses is more pronounced in people with spinal cord injuries than in those with intact nervous systems.[33]

In addition to having skin that is more vulnerable to external stresses, people with spinal cord injuries develop higher interface pressures[a] in sitting than do people without such injuries.[34-36] These higher pressures may be due in part to uneven loading on the ischial tuberosities resulting from pelvic obliquity.[35] Atrophy also contributes to the elevated interface pressures by reducing the soft tissue "padding" over bony prominences.[16,35]

The problems listed above are compounded by the increased likelihood of trauma to the skin following spinal cord injury. Combined paralysis and sensory impairment result in areas of the skin being subjected to pressure for prolonged periods. Wherever external pressure on soft tissues is greater than capillary pressure, the capillaries in that region are occluded.[b] This condition exists in tissues compressed between bony prominences and the supporting surface (for example, over the ischial tuberosities when sitting).

Local capillary occlusion does not normally present a problem for people with intact motor and sensory function because these people shift their positions frequently throughout the day, redistributing pressure long before tissue damage occurs. In contrast, people who have sensory impairments resulting from spinal cord injuries lack the sensation that would stimulate protective weight shifts. Moreover, motor paralysis results in more static positioning. The combination of reduced motion and loss of protective sensation results in compression of the tissues between the bony prominences and supporting surfaces or other objects (such as orthoses) for long periods of time. The resulting prolonged ischemia can lead to necrosis of the skin and underlying tissues.[c]

Prolonged unrelieved pressure is the most common cause of pressure ulcers after spinal cord injury.[37] High pressure applied for a short duration can also cause pressure ulcers.[38,39] In addition to pressure, shear forces play a significant role in the development of many pressure ulcers.[38-40] Shearing occurs when tissue is subjected to oppositely directed parallel forces. For example, the skin overlying the sacrum is subjected to shear forces when a person lies supine in bed with the head of the bed elevated. In this position, the skin is stabilized against the bed while the deeper tissues slide caudally due to the effects of gravity pulling the person downward toward the foot of the bed.[39,41] Shear forces increase the skin's vulnerability to pressure by disrupting the tissues' vascular supply. In the presence of shear stresses, vascular occlusion can occur at lower pressures.[35,40]

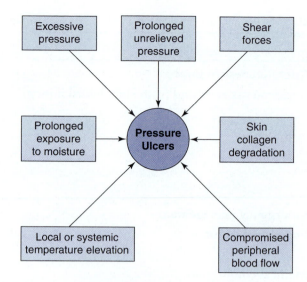

Figure 5–1   Factors that contribute to the development of pressure ulcers.

Several additional conditions can increase the skin's vulnerability to the damaging effects of pressure. Local or systemic elevations in temperature can make the skin and subcutaneous tissue more prone to ischemia because they increase the tissues' oxygen requirements.[8,38] Prolonged exposure to moisture, as can occur with incontinence or excessive sweating, softens the skin and increases its vulnerability to trauma.[38,39,42] Both low blood pressure and smoking can reduce peripheral circulation and increase the likelihood of breakdown. Factors that contribute to the development of pressure ulcers are illustrated in Figure 5–1.

Sequelae

Pressure ulcers can lead to osteomyelitis, sepsis, and even death.[2,7,43-45] Additionally, a pressure ulcer that heals leaves a scarred area that remains highly vulnerable to breakdown in the future.

Depending on the location of the pressure ulcer, it may be necessary to limit activities to avoid damaging forces and allow healing. This limitation can interfere with participation in work, recreation, and other life situations. If prolonged bed rest is required, a variety of physical problems—including deconditioning, pulmonary complications, joint contractures, additional pressure ulcers, and reduced functional status—can result.

Pressure ulcers are costly in terms of the expense of hospitalization and surgery, time lost from vocational and avocational activities, and postponement of physical rehabilitation and reintegration into the community.[11,16,22,30,38,46,47] The prevalence of pressure ulcers among people with spinal cord injuries is most tragic when one considers that this complication can usually be avoided with proper care.

---

[a] Interface pressures are the pressures at the interface between the person and the supporting surface.

[b] Capillary closure is commonly considered to occur at 25 to 32 mm Hg, but a variety of factors can affect capillary closure.[68] Research has demonstrated that tissue blood flow can occur despite significantly higher pressures.[42] Conversely, capillary occlusion can occur at lower pressures.[72]

[c] Ischemia is thought to occur in human skin after it is subjected to 60 mm Hg of pressure for 1 hour.[97] Higher pressures take less time to cause ischemia.

PREVENTION

A lifelong process of skin care beginning at the time of injury is required to prevent pressure ulcers and their sequelae. During the initial postinjury phase encompassing acute care and inpatient rehabilitation, meticulous preventive care is particularly important because it sets the stage for future care. The prevention of pressure ulcers should remain a focus during postacute rehabilitation in outpatient settings and in the home. This continued emphasis on skin care is particularly important in the light of shrinking hospital stays in both acute care and rehabilitation. Postdischarge follow-up care is also critical, as indicated by the fact that pressure ulcers occur with increasing incidence as time passes after injury.[6,14,21,25]

The prevention of pressure ulcers involves avoiding prolonged unrelieved pressure on the skin, particularly over bony prominences. This is accomplished through periodic repositioning when the individual is in bed and by the performance of pressure reliefs when sitting. Specialized equipment (beds, mattresses, mattress overlays, and wheelchair cushions) helps prevent skin breakdown by distributing the pressure on the person's skin when in bed or in a wheelchair. (By distributing forces over a greater surface area on the body, these support surfaces can reduce pressure on vulnerable areas such as the skin overlying bony prominences.)

In addition to pressure management, proper care involves regular skin inspection and measures to minimize other conditions that cause breakdown.[d] The patient and those involved in his care should protect his skin from shear forces, friction, blunt trauma, and exposure to hot objects. Clothes, shoes, and orthoses should fit properly; if too tight, they exert prolonged pressure on the skin. The person's skin should be kept clean and dry,[e] with special attention given to preventing prolonged contact with urine, feces, and excessive perspiration.[16,41,48,49]

The patient's overall health should also be a focus of the preventive skin care program. Exercises to enhance cardiovascular fitness should be included in the patient's rehabilitation and postrehabilitation wellness programs,[16] and medical conditions that increase the risk of developing pressure ulcers or interfere with wound healing should be brought under control to the extent possible. Additionally, a balanced diet must be ensured, as nutritional deficiencies are important contributors to skin breakdown.[16,41]

Risk Assessment

All people with spinal cord injuries should be considered to be at risk for developing pressure ulcers and therefore should be included in pressure ulcer prevention programs.

It is appropriate, however, to identify those who are at highest risk so that they and the health care team can exercise an even greater level of diligence in pressure ulcer prevention.[16] Figure 5–2 presents a pressure ulcer risk-assessment tool appropriate for individuals with spinal cord injuries.[f]

Prevention While in Bed

Acutely following spinal cord injury, patients on standard hospital beds must be turned every 2 hours around the clock to avoid the development of pressure ulcers.[41,48–51] This repositioning should occur whether or not the spine is stable.[52] The skin should be inspected each time the patient is turned. Although 2 hours is the standard interval, some patients require more frequent turning.[40,53] On the other hand, the time spent in each position may in some cases be increased gradually as skin tolerance improves.[7,50,54] When the time between position changes is increased, the skin over the bony prominences should be monitored especially closely.

Specially designed beds, mattresses, and mattress overlays can help to maintain the skin's integrity by reducing pressure over bony prominences. These devices should be used in addition to regular position changes, not in their place.[50,52,53,55] Ring-shaped donut cushions are not appropriate for either the prevention or management of pressure ulcers, as they create ischemia in tissues encircled by the donut.[16,49]

When a person lies in bed, his position will determine which areas of his body receive the most pressure and are thus most vulnerable to skin damage. In the supine position, breakdown is most likely to occur in the skin overlying the occiput, scapulae, sacrum, posterior iliac crests, and heels. In side-lying, breakdown is most common over the greater trochanters and both the medial and lateral aspects of the knees and ankles. In the prone position, the breasts, anterior iliac spines, knees, and toes are vulnerable.[56,57]

Proper bed positioning after spinal cord injury involves more than regular turning. In each position, care should be taken to prevent excessive pressure and shear.[g] Pillows or blocks of foam rubber can be used to relieve pressure on the bony prominences and to prevent skin surfaces from contacting each other.[16,40,41,58] A variety of commercially available devices can be used to protect the heels from pressure and shear (Figure 5–3).

Side lying with direct pressure on the greater trochanter should be avoided, as this places excessive pressure over this bony prominence.[16,41] Positioning the patient reclined 30 degrees back from sidelying will provide better pressure distribution.[16,40,59,60]

---

[d] Strategies for protecting the skin during functional activities and functional training are presented in Chapters 9 to 12.

[e] The skin should be dry but not excessively so. Topical moisturizers may be used if flaking or cracking of the skin occurs.[41]

[f] A self-rating scale, the Pressure Ulcer Risk Assessment Scale for Persons with Paralysis, is more appropriate for people with spinal cord injuries who live in the community.[27]

[g] Proper bed positioning also involves positioning the extremities to preserve range of motion. For example, the elbows should be placed in extension and the ankles dorsiflexed to neutral.

Risk factor	Coded value		Score
1. Level of activity[a]	0 [ ] ambulatory 2 [ ] wheelchair 4 [ ] bed		
2. Mobility[b]	0 [ ] full 1 [ ] limited 2 [ ] immobile		
3. Complete SCI	0 [ ] no	1 [ ] yes	
4. Urine incontinence or constantly moist[c]	0 [ ] no	1 [ ] yes	
5. Autonomic dysreflexia or severe spasticity	0 [ ] no	1 [ ] yes	
6. Age (years)	0 [ ] ≤ 34 1 [ ] 35-64 2 [ ] ≥ 65		
7. Tobacco use/smoking	0 [ ] never 1 [ ] former 2 [ ] current		
8. Pulmonary disease	0 [ ] no	1 [ ] yes	
9. Cardiac disease or abnormal EKG	0 [ ] no	1 [ ] yes	
10. Diabetes or glucose ≥ 110 mg/dl	0 [ ] no	1 [ ] yes	
11. Renal disease	0 [ ] no	1 [ ] yes	
12. Impaired cognitive function	0 [ ] no	1 [ ] yes	
13. In a nursing home or hospital	0 [ ] no	1 [ ] yes	
14. Albumin < 3.4 or t. protein < 6.4	0 [ ] no	1 [ ] yes	
15. Hematocrit < 36.0% (HGB < 12.0)	0 [ ] no	1 [ ] yes	
Total score			

Risk: Low 0–2, Moderate 3–5, High 6–8, Very high 9–25

[a] **Level of activity**
0 - ambulatory - can walk with/without assistance
2 - wheelchair mobile - sits out of bed only, cannot bear own weight and/or must be assisted into chair or wheelchair
4 - bed mobile - confined to bed during entire 24 hours of the day

[b] **Mobility**
0 - full - independent in moving, no limitations, able to control and move all extremities at will
1 - limited - (slightly to very) requires assistance when moving
2 - immobile - complete immobility, unable to change position. Does not make even slight changes in body or extremity position without assistance, completely dependent on others for movement.

[c] **Minimally controlled urinary bladder** - incontinent of urine at least once a day, absence of control.
Constantly moist - skin is kept moist almost constantly by perspiration, urine, etc. Dampness is detected every time patient is moved or turned

Figure 5–2   Pressure ulcer risk assessment scale for the spinal cord injured. (From Salzberg C, Byrne D, Cayten C, et al. A new pressure ulcer risk assessment scale for individuals with spinal cord injury. *Am J Phys Med Rehabil.* 1996, 75(2), 96–104. Reproduced with permission from Lippincott Williams & Wilkins.)

To prevent skin damage from shear forces over the sacrum when the patient is supine, the head of the bed should not be elevated above 30 degrees.[40,49,61] Time spent with the head of the bed elevated should be kept to a minimum.[16,41,58]

In the prone position, pillows are used to bridge areas vulnerable to pressure. One advantage of lying prone is that the hips and knees are extended in this position, preventing the development of flexion contractures. In addition, the time spent in this position can be increased to several hours because bridging with pillows eliminates pressure over bony prominences. The person can then sleep uninterrupted through the night.[62] Prone positioning may be contraindicated at first because of spine precautions.[16]

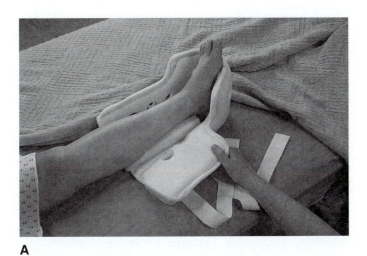
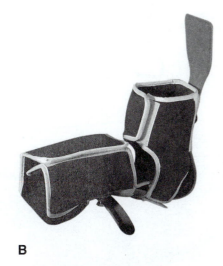

A   **B**

Figure 5–3   Devices designed to protect heels from friction and sheer by preventing contact between bed and heels. (A) Soft foam boot. (B) Padded plastic splint. (Reproduced with permission from AliMed.)

When repositioning patients, health professionals should take care to avoid subjecting the skin to undue stretching, folding, shear forces, and friction.[16,41] Draw sheets make it possible to move patients (turn, move laterally, or reposition them toward the head of the bed) without dragging their skin across the supporting surface.[h]

In addition to turning and positioning, pressure ulcer prevention while in bed involves keeping the sheets clean and dry. Sheets should also be free of wrinkles where they come in contact with the patient's skin.[48]

Beds, Mattresses, and Mattress Overlays

Integrated bed systems, mattresses, and mattress overlays can be used to distribute pressure on the skin, both to prevent pressure ulcers and to promote healing when skin breakdown has already occurred. In the past, these support surfaces were classified as providing either pressure reduction or pressure relief. This distinction has been questioned in recent years, but there remains a lack of agreement in the literature about appropriate terminology. The terms "pressure relief"[63] or "pressure redistribution"[64] are utilized as umbrella terms for all these support surfaces.

Beds

An integrated bed system (specialty bed) includes a support surface and frame designed to function together as a unit.[64] Low-air-loss, air-fluidized, and rotating beds are integrated bed systems, all of which require electricity to function.

A low-air-loss bed (Figure 5–4) supports the patient on a number of inflated cushions. Air is pumped into these cushions continually and leaks out of small holes in the cushions. The continual filling/leaking airflow allows the

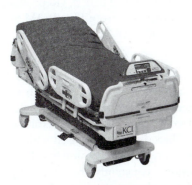

Figure 5–4   Low-air-loss bed. (Courtesy of KCI Licensing, Inc., 2009.)

support surface to conform to the patient's body, minimizing interface pressures by distributing the supporting forces. The flow of air can also keep the skin from overheating and prevent the harmful buildup of moisture, but it can also cause harmful drying of existing wounds. This type of bed typically has a multizoned surface, allowing adjustment of the maximal and minimal pressures in different areas.[65,66] Low-air-loss mattresses and mattress overlays are also available.[66] Low-air-loss systems are used with loose-fitting, low-friction covers[65] that help to reduce friction and shearing on the patient's skin.

An air-fluidized bed is filled with ceramic microspheres. The patient "floats" on the supporting surface as air is pumped continually through the beads. Air-fluidized beds provide constantly changing supporting forces and distribute pressure by conforming to the patient's body. The constant flow of air has a drying effect on the skin, which can be helpful in preventing skin damage from body fluids,[65, 66] but can also cause harmful drying of existing wounds. The air-fluidized feature requires a specialized bed (Figure 5–5); it is not available in mattresses or mattress overlays.[66]

---

[h] Draw sheets have the added benefit of making it easier to move the patient with less physical strain on the people providing this assistance.

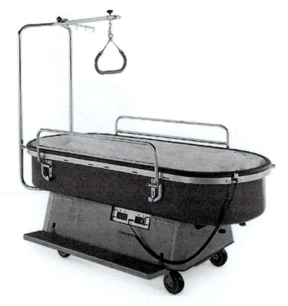

Figure 5–5   Air-fluidized bed™. (Reproduced with permission from Hill-ROM Services, Inc., © 2009. All rights reserved.)

Low-air-loss beds and air-fluidized beds can be used by people with stable spines.[55] A patient with an unstable spine may be placed on a rotating bed (also called an oscillating support surface or kinetic treatment table) to prevent pressure ulcers.[i] These beds can be used while the patient is in traction.[48] Rotating beds rock slowly side to side in a continuous motion, constantly redistributing the weight-bearing forces on the patient's skin. A rotating bed must be adjusted properly; otherwise it will allow the patient to slide back and forth as the bed rocks, subjecting the skin to shear forces and *causing* skin breakdown instead of preventing it.[55] These beds are most practical for patients who are restricted to bed, as transfers in and out are difficult.

Mattresses and Mattress Overlays

Pressure-distributing mattresses and mattress overlays are less costly alternatives to integrated bed systems. They utilize foam, water, gel, air, or a combination of these materials to distribute pressure on the skin.[40,67,68] Each type of mattress or overlay comes in a variety of models made by different manufacturers. Mattresses and overlays tend to deteriorate over time,[40] so their condition should be monitored.

Mattress overlays are placed on top of standard mattresses. Most function without power.[67] Some have been shown to significantly reduce[j] interface pressures.[69] One

disadvantage of mattress overlays is that they can "bottom out," compressing excessively when people are positioned on them. Caregivers should check beneath patients' bony prominences as they lie in the various positions to ensure that bottoming out does not occur.[k 16,58]

Pressure-reducing mattresses are designed to replace standard hospital bed mattresses. A study comparing several brands of pressure-reducing mattresses found large differences in interface pressures over bony prominences.[68]

Most mattresses and mattress overlays provide static pressure distribution. These support surfaces reduce interface pressure by maximizing the contact area between the support surface and the person. The pressure on any given area remains constant until the patient moves. In contrast, alternating pressure mattresses and mattress overlays provide dynamic pressure relief. They are made of air-filled cells that inflate and deflate asynchronously, subjecting the patient's skin to fluctuating pressure.[64,66]

Selecting an Appropriate Support Surface

There is a large variety of beds, mattresses, and mattress overlays designed to prevent pressure ulcers and promote healing of existing ulcers. The various support surfaces differ in their effectiveness in reducing pressure over the user's bony prominences. They also differ in the degree to which they reduce shear, provide alternating (dynamic) pressure, and cause or prevent the buildup of moisture and heat. Each of these factors is relevant to the prevention and treatment of pressure ulcers; an ideal support surface would minimize shear and pressure, and prevent the buildup of moisture and heat on the skin.[16,40] Table 5–2 summarizes the performance characteristics of the different types of support surface. The various brands of similar types of support surface can be very different in the degree to which they reduce interface pressures. Moreover, the performance of a particular support surface can vary. For example, the interface pressures on air-filled mattresses and mattress overlays are determined by their inflation. Under- or over-inflation will result in high interface pressures.[70]

Selection of an appropriate support surface should be based on the user's unique needs. Factors to consider include the presence or absence of pressure ulcers, history of pressure ulcers, the skin's tolerance to pressure, feasibility of regular turning with positioning on skin free of breakdown, and the presence of moisture from sources such as excessive perspiration, incontinence, or wound drainage. One consideration unique to the needs of people with spinal cord injury is spinal stability. When the spine is unstable, some options such as low-air-loss beds and alternating pressure mattresses are unsuitable[73] because of the potential for motion at the site of vertebral instability. Another important consideration is the impact

---

[i] The constant turning provided by rotating beds (Figure 3-3) reduces the risk of pressure ulcers, pneumonia, atelectasis, and pulmonary emboli; it also enhances pulmonary status.[55,153,154]

[j] For example, one study found that the RoHo dry flotation mattress overlay significantly reduced interface pressures in patients with spinal cord injuries who had undergone myocutaneous flap surgery. The pressure reduction was slightly less than that provided by air-fluidized beds, but both surfaces prevented flap breakdown.[69]

---

[k] Bottoming out is detected by placing a hand beneath the mattress overlay while it is underneath the patient. If the support material has compressed to less than an inch at any point, it has bottomed out.[40]

TABLE 5–2   Performance Characteristics Of Mattresses, Mattress Overlays, And Beds

	Pressure Redistribution Greater than Standard Mattress	Shear Reduction	Low Moisture Retention	Reduced Heat Build-up	Dynamic	Requires Power Source	Cost per Day*	Interferes with Functional Skills
Standard mattress							Low	No
Foam	■						Low	Minimal
Static air or water flotation	■	■					Low	Yes
Alternating air mattress or overlay	■	■			■	■	Moderate	Yes
Low-air-loss bed	■		■	■	■	■	High	Yes
Air-flu-idized bed	■	■	■	■	■	■	High	Yes
Rotating bed	■				■	■	High	Yes

Key: ■ = characteristic present.

* Cost per day reflects cost of equipment only. Support surfaces that allow less frequent turning may be less costly overall, because of the reduced cost of labor.[71]

Sources: References 58, 66, 68, 71, and 72.

of the support surface on activity. Many of the pressure-reducing support surfaces increase the difficulty of both independent functioning and dependent handling. Finally, cost should be considered when selecting a bed, mattress, or mattress overlay. The most appropriate support surface will facilitate the prevention of pressure ulcers (and healing if ulcers are present) without unnecessarily interfering with activity and with minimal cost per day.

Prevention While Using a Wheelchair

The skin overlying the ischial tuberosities, sacrum, and coccyx is susceptible to the development of pressure ulcers in sitting.[57] Proper positioning, an appropriate wheelchair and cushion, periodic relief of pressure on the skin, and a gradual buildup of sitting tolerance can prevent this problem.

Positioning

Appropriate positioning in a wheelchair will reduce the risk of pressure ulcers. During prolonged sitting, the patient's buttocks should be located well back in the chair and the pelvis should be positioned in a slight anterior tilt.[74] In this position, the skin overlying the sacrum and coccyx will not be subjected to excessive pressure.[75] The pelvis should be horizontal, without a right or left lateral tilt. This horizontal orientation will result in equal weight bearing on the right and left ischial tuberosities, reducing the maximal pressure in this area.[35,76] The patient's buttocks should be centered on the seat. If the pelvis is off center, the patient is likely to sit with his trunk leaning laterally, resulting in increased pressure on one ischial tuberosity.

Because improper positioning can increase the risk of skin breakdown, health professionals should ensure that patients sit with good posture whenever they are in a chair. During acute care and early rehabilitation, most patients require assistance to transfer and position themselves in their wheelchairs. Health professionals should take the time to check patients' positions after they transfer, and make adjustments as needed. They should also make adjustments as needed if patients' postures shift during periods of prolonged sitting.

During rehabilitation, patients who have the physical potential to do so should learn how to position themselves optimally in their wheelchairs.[1] Those who are unable to position themselves should learn how to direct others in assisting with this task.

---

[1] Chapter 10 presents methods for independent positioning in a wheelchair and therapeutic strategies for teaching these skills.

TABLE 5–3   Wheelchair Characteristics Relevant To Positioning and Prevention of Pressure Ulcers

Wheelchair	Characteristics	Impact on Positioning and Skin
Seat dimensions	Too wide	Promotes the development of a lateral trunk lean, resulting in increased pressure on one ischial tuberosity.
	Too narrow	Skin overlying the greater trochanters may be subjected to pressure from armrests or clothing guards, or friction from wheels.
	Too deep (too long from front to back)	Can cause the wheelchair user's buttocks to slide forward on the seat, causing a posterior pelvic tilt with resulting increased pressure on the sacrum and coccyx.
	Too shallow (too short from front to back)	Reduces the area over which sitting forces can be distributed, increasing the pressure on the buttocks.
Footrest height	Too high	Reduces weight bearing on thighs, increasing pressure on buttocks.
	Too low	Does not provide adequate postural support. Allows buttocks to slide out (anteriorly) on the wheelchair seat, resulting in a posterior pelvic tilt and increased pressure on the sacrum and coccyx.
Armrests	Present on wheelchair	May reduce the risk of developing skin breakdown because of (1) reduced seating pressure due to partial support of body weight; (2) promotion of upright sitting posture; and (3) enhanced stability, encouraging the performance of more pressure reliefs.
	Absent from wheelchair	May increase the risk of skin breakdown due to absence of the benefits listed above.
	Too low or uneven	Encourage wheelchair user to sit with a lateral lean, increasing pressure on one ischial tuberosity.
Seat and back construction	Upholstered	Stretches over time, reducing postural support. Seat upholstery (sling seat) can also increase shear forces on the back and buttocks and promote sitting with a pelvic obliquity and posterior pelvic tilt.
	Solid back and solid seat or seat insert	Provides superior postural support, promoting optimal distribution of pressure.
Seating system (power wheelchairs)	Tilt-in-space	Allows pressure reliefs without causing potentially harmful shear forces.
	Reclining	Allows pressure reliefs, but creates shear forces on the buttocks and sacrum and can cause sitting posture to shift.

Sources: References 16, 54, 74, and 76 to 83.

Proper posture in a wheelchair requires that the wheelchair user or those providing assistance place the buttocks and trunk appropriately on the seat. The wheelchair's components, size, and adjustment are also critical for appropriate positioning and pressure distribution in a wheelchair. Table 5–3 presents wheelchair characteristics that are relevant to positioning and the prevention of pressure ulcers.[m]

Wheelchair Cushions

People with spinal cord injuries who utilize wheelchairs require wheelchair cushions[n] to aid in the prevention of pressure ulcers. These cushions are specifically designed to reduce the pressure on the buttocks (the ischial tuberosities in particular) by distributing the supporting forces over a greater area. Cushions that minimize shear forces also help to maintain skin integrity.

Selection

Selecting an appropriate cushion is critical because of its enormous impact on the individual's health and function. Cushions vary in their effectiveness in reducing pressure and shear forces and in providing postural support. They also differ in the degree to which they cause buildup of heat and moisture on the skin, as well as in their weight, durability, maintenance requirements, cost, and the amount of difficulty that they cause during transfers. Likewise, people with spinal cord injuries vary widely in their skin tolerance, pressure relief habits and abilities, functional capacity, and

---

[m] Chapter 11 provides additional information on wheelchair components, adjustment, and selection.

[n] People with spinal cord injuries should use wheelchair cushions designed specifically for the prevention of pressure ulcers in high-risk populations. Standard foam rubber cushions and donut-type cushions are inappropriate.

willingness or ability to provide regular cushion maintenance. When selecting a cushion, the wheelchair user and the rehabilitation team should work together to determine which cushion will be most suitable to the individual's needs and preferences.

The most critical factor in cushion selection is its effect on skin integrity. A cushion that is not adequate in this respect is inappropriate for the individual in question. A wheelchair cushion should reduce the pressure and shear on the buttocks enough to enable the wheelchair user to function in a normal day (sitting and performing his accustomed activities all day, with pressure reliefs) without skin breakdown.

People with spinal cord injuries are highly variable in the degree to which their skin can tolerate pressure without breaking down. Moreover, people differ in the degree to which cushions distribute pressure on their skin; different people with spinal cord injuries sitting on identical cushions exhibit large variation in the pressure found at their ischial tuberosities.[76] As a result, cushion selection must be individualized.

Because pressure reduction/redistribution is a critical feature of wheelchair cushions, pressure-measuring devices are often used as a part of the cushion selection process. These devices can be used to compare the interface pressures that occur on different cushions. Seating pressures should not, however, be the sole factor considered in selecting a cushion.[8,84,85] The only way to determine a given cushion's appropriateness for an individual is to have him use the cushion (or an identical model) for a period of time. If at all possible, he should use a cushion for several days before one is ordered. During the trial period, sitting time on the cushion should be increased progressively and the skin checked frequently[85] to determine whether the cushion provides adequate pressure distribution, shear reduction, and heat and moisture dissipation to meet the individual's needs. The patient should participate in activities such as wheelchair propulsion during the trial period, as these activities alter interface pressures.[86,87]

A second important consideration in cushion selection is posture. A cushion that supports the wheelchair user in a good posture will enhance breathing capacity[o] and functional status, and can help prevent the development of skeletal deformity[41,79] and overuse injuries of the upper extremities.[88]

In addition to pressure distribution and posture, the cushion's influence on the patient's functional status must be considered.[41] Unfortunately, the cushions that distribute pressure most effectively tend to be heavier and interfere more with transfers. Heavy cushions add to the overall weight that wheelchair users must push when propelling their chairs and can be difficult or impossible for some

individuals to take in and out of their chairs independently. Cushion selection involves finding the cushion that provides adequate pressure reduction/redistribution for the individual in question while interfering the least with his functioning.

The maintenance required by a cushion should also be considered. Those that need frequent maintenance to retain their effectiveness are appropriate only for people who will take the responsibility to provide or obtain this maintenance.[89]

Expense may also be considered when selecting a cushion. This factor should be of the lowest priority, however, since wheelchair cushions have such a significant impact on health and function. The cost of even the most expensive cushion is negligible compared with the potential cost of a single pressure ulcer. Because funding sources (insurance companies, government agencies) are often reluctant to purchase expensive equipment, health professionals should be prepared to lobby for these purchases.

Options

The four classes of commonly used wheelchair cushions are polymer foam, air-filled, gel flotation, and flexible matrix cushions.[p] Different brands are available in the various types, and each brand offers a variety of designs.

Foam cushions are made from various types of relatively dense viscoelastic foam.[q] They come in different densities, thicknesses, and seat dimensions. Density and thickness are chosen according to the user's weight and skin tolerance. Options include contoured cushions and cushions composed of two or more layers of different densities (Figure 5–6). Foam cushions are the least effective type of cushion in distributing pressure but are adequate for some people with spinal cord injuries. Custom-contoured foam cushions and those made of softer foam provide better pressure distribution than do planar (flat) cushions (Figure 5–7) and those made of stiffer foam.[16,90] The advantages of foam cushions are that they are light, do not greatly inhibit function, are relatively inexpensive and easily modified, and can absorb moisture. The disadvantages of foam cushions are that they cannot be washed, they tend to cause elevated skin temperatures, and they may need to be replaced as often as every 6 months.[74,79,81,89,91]

Gel, or fluid, cushions (Figure 5–8) are typically made of gel-filled pouches supported on firm, contoured foam bases.[74,79] Gel cushions provide better

[p] Dynamic cushions, which provide alternating pressure, are less commonly used because they are cumbersome and require a power source.[94] These cushions may be beneficial for some individuals who are either unable to perform pressure reliefs or are noncompliant with pressure reliefs.[85]
[q] These foams are not to be confused with standard foam rubber, which provides virtually no pressure distribution. The foam rubber cushions that often come with wheelchairs do not provide adequate pressure distribution for people with spinal cord injuries.

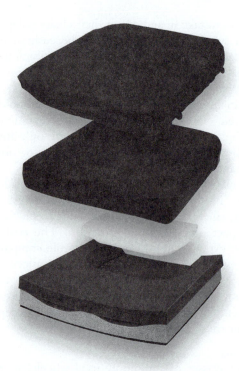

Figure 5–6   Multilayer foam cushion. (Reproduced with permission from Sunrise Medical, ©2009.)

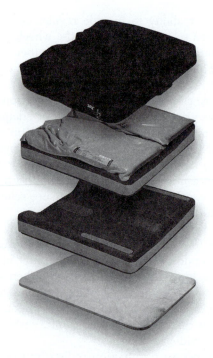

Figure 5–8   Fluid cushion. Images show (from top to bottom) cushion with cover, cover removed, base only, and optional wood seat insert. (Reproduced with permission. Sunrise Medical, © 2009.)

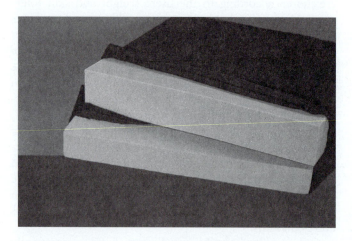

Figure 5–7   Planar foam cushions. (Reproduced with permission from AliMed.)

pressure distribution than do foam cushions.[92] They can reduce heat buildup[89, 91] and may be the most effective type of cushion in minimizing shear forces on the skin. This characteristic is particularly advantageous for the active person, who is more likely to have skin problems due to shearing. The disadvantages of gel cushions are that they tend to be heavy and can cause moisture

buildup on the skin, elevation of local skin temperature after prolonged sitting, reduced sitting stability, and difficulty in transfers.[57,77,89,93]

Air-filled cushions (Figure 5–9) can provide excellent weight distribution. When an air-filled cushion is properly inflated, the person's buttocks are "immersed" in the cushion: the buttocks sink into the cushion as far as they can without bottoming out. This immersion maximizes the area of contact between the person and the cushion, which minimizes the interface pressures.[94] Thus, on properly inflated air-filled cushions, interface pressures are lower than those that occur on either foam or gel cushions.[76,85,92] The disadvantages of air-filled cushions include the following: they are heavier than foam cushions, are easily punctured, can reduce sitting stability, and make transfers much more difficult. Some designs can cause the buildup of moisture on the skin.[74,76] Perhaps the greatest disadvantage of air-filled cushions is that they are ineffective in pressure reduction if they are either overinflated or underinflated. To optimize pressure reduction, the inflation pressure should be checked daily.[95] Combination foam–air cushions are also available (Figure 5–10).

Flexible matrix cushions are made of thermoplastic urethane that is formed into open cells. Research on flexible matrix cushions is lacking in the literature. For this

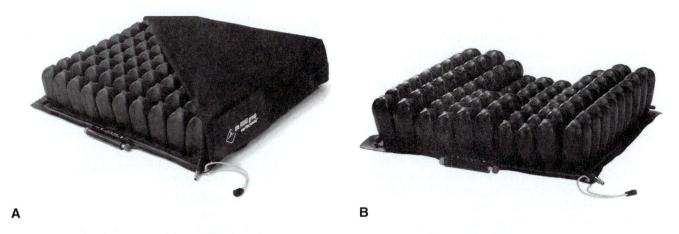

A   **B**

Figure 5–9   Air-filled cushions. (A) Planar air-filled cushion. (B) Contoured air-filled cushion. (Reproduced with permission from the ROHO Group.)

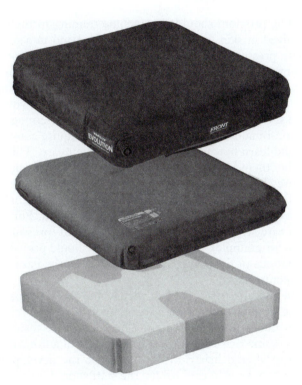

Figure 5–10   Combination foam- and air-filled cushion. (Reproduced with permission from VARILITE®.)

reason, it is unknown how their performance in pressure relief and shear reduction compares with other types of cushions.

Wheelchair cushions are typically used with protective covers. Cushion covers should be selected carefully, as they can influence cushions' effectiveness in pressure distribution. Covers can also increase or decrease moisture and heat buildup on the skin.[81,89,96]

Pressure Relief

When a person with a spinal cord injury sits for a prolonged period of time, a properly fitting and adjusted wheelchair, good sitting posture, and an appropriate wheelchair cushion are required to protect the skin over the buttocks and sacrum. These precautions, however, are not sufficient to prevent the development of pressure ulcers. Even an optimal wheelchair and cushion will reduce interface pressures to only a limited degree. When a wheelchair user sits, his skin is subjected to pressures that are high enough to occlude capillary circulation. This is particularly true of the skin overlying the ischial tuberosities. Regardless of the cushion used, periodic relief of pressure is necessary to prevent tissue necrosis.[16,97]

Starting at the time of injury and continuing through the remainder of their lives, people with spinal cord injuries must perform pressure reliefs whenever they sit for prolonged periods of time. This can be accomplished by lifting the buttocks from the seat or by shifting the trunk forward or to the side. These maneuvers can be performed with assistance or independently, depending on the individual's ability. Alternatively, the wheelchair can be tilted or reclined to shift weight off the ischial tuberosities.[r]

When out-of-bed activities are initiated, pressure reliefs should be performed every 15 to 20 minutes when sitting.[51,54,57] Sitting time should be limited at first, and the skin's status should be monitored closely to determine its tolerance to sitting.[7,16,98] Some individuals are able to tolerate longer times between pressure reliefs without developing pressure ulcers.[42] If the patient's skin tolerance allows, sitting time can be increased slightly every few days.[16] When the time between pressure reliefs

---

[r] Techniques for independent pressure reliefs, strategies for teaching these skills, and power tilt and recline wheelchair features are presented in Chapter 11.

is increased, frequent skin checks should be performed to determine whether the individual's skin is able to tolerate the longer periods of unrelieved pressure. The skin over the ischial tuberosities, sacrum, and coccyx in particular should be monitored closely for early signs of breakdown or potential breakdown.

Skin Inspection

Following spinal cord injury, insensitive areas of the skin should be inspected at least daily. More frequent skin checks are indicated in high-risk patients or when there is a change in conditions that could increase the risk of pressure ulcers. For example, the skin should be inspected each time the patient is turned during the early postinjury phase and during periods of bed rest when a patient is ill or has a pressure ulcer. The skin should be checked after each sitting session when sitting is first initiated during the acute hospitalization, when a new cushion is utilized, or when sitting is resumed after a period of prolonged bed rest.

During skin inspection, particular attention should be given to bony prominences. Skin overlying the sacrum, coccyx, ischial tuberosities, greater trochanters, heels, medial and lateral malleoli, knees, scapulae, and elbows should be examined carefully.[16] The person inspecting the skin should look for redness, discoloration, blisters, cracks, rashes, scabs, or areas that are dry, raised, or shiny. He should also palpate for areas of the skin that are hard, soft, warm, or wet.[16]

Skin inspection is a critical component of pressure ulcer prevention because the skin's status provides feedback on the effectiveness of the individual's skin care program. Redness[s] that does not resolve within 30 minutes[7,98] of removal of pressure from the skin may indicate a problem with the wheelchair cushion, bed support surface, turning or pressure relief schedule, pressure relief techniques, wheelchair components or adjustment, orthotic fit, or any other source of damaging forces on the skin. If skin inspection reveals early signs of skin breakdown or potential breakdown, the patient and health care team should attempt to determine the source of the problem and take measures to eliminate it.

In addition to providing feedback on the pressure ulcer prevention program, skin inspections allow for early detection of imminent or actual breakdown. This early detection makes it possible to intervene before undue damage occurs.

Education and Training

People with spinal cord injuries, particularly those who have significant motor and sensory impairments, are at high risk for developing pressure ulcers. This risk starts at the time of injury and continues for the rest of their lives. During the initial hospitalization after a spinal cord injury, the health care team bears the responsibility for providing the constant vigilance and meticulous care required to prevent pressure ulcers. By discharge, however, this responsibility must shift to the individual with a spinal cord injury and (if assistance will be required) those who will be involved in his care.

The skin care educational program should be individualized to accommodate differences in learning style[16] and ability. It should provide information about pressure ulcers: what they are, why they develop, and how to prevent them, detect them, and respond if breakdown occurs. The program should emphasize the severity of pressure ulcers and their sequelae, to underscore the importance of prevention. Individuals who perceive pressure ulcers as being a severe problem may be more likely to comply with their skin care.[99]

The program should also include training in the skills involved in skin care: positioning in bed and in a wheelchair, pressure reliefs, skin inspection, and any equipment maintenance required. If the patient will not achieve independence in his care by the time of discharge from inpatient rehabilitation, those who will be assisting with his care should be included in the education and training program.[t] In addition, individuals who will require assistance should learn how to instruct others in their care. This will enable them to continue their skin care programs despite future changes in their support systems.

Table 5–4 summarizes the content of an education and training program for pressure ulcer prevention. For each skin care strategy presented in the program (pressure reliefs, for example), the health care team should provide explanations of the purpose of the action and the hazards of not complying.

In addition to gaining knowledge and skills, the patient must develop good skin care habits prior to discharge from inpatient rehabilitation. The health care team cannot assume that education and training will automatically lead to altered behavior. To encourage the development of preventive skin care habits, the staff should involve patients in their care as much as possible. Although patients' physical capacity to participate in their care may be limited during acute care and early rehabilitation, health professionals can involve them by explaining the measures designed to prevent pressure ulcers as these measures are used. Patients can also be encouraged to take responsibility for their care. For example, they can be encouraged to remind others to assist them with pressure reliefs at the appropriate intervals. As patients become more physically able, they can gradually increase their participation in skin care activities. They may require frequent reminders at

---

[s] People with darkly pigmented skin may not exhibit redness as an early sign of skin breakdown. Early signs of skin damage include discoloration, warmth, edema, induration, and hardness.

[t] All members of the health care team should also receive education and training in the prevention of pressure ulcers.[41,63,98]

TABLE 5–4   Content of The Education And Training Program For The Prevention Of Pressure Ulcers

	Program Content
General information	General information on causes, risk factors and sequelae of pressure ulcers.
	Terminology for pressure ulcer location and stages.
Skin protection in bed	Positioning: appropriate positions, use of pillows or foam blocks to prevent excessive pressure over bony prominences.
	Turning: turning schedule, techniques for turning.
	Support surface (if specialized support surface is used): operation and maintenance of specialty bed, mattress, or mattress overlay.
	Bed linens: maintain clean, dry, wrinkle-free.
Skin protection in sitting	Positioning: beneficial sitting posture, methods (independent, assisted, or dependent) of obtaining and maintaining good sitting posture.
	Pressure reliefs: methods, frequency.
	Cushion: maintenance, schedule of use (use whenever sitting!), limitations (will not eliminate the need for pressure reliefs).
Skin inspection	Frequency: at least daily. More frequent under certain conditions, as during the initial use of new orthoses or shoes or when medical condition or activity level changes.
	Where to inspect: any surfaces subjected to external loads, with particular attention to bony prominences and weight-bearing surfaces.
	Signs of skin damage or potential breakdown.
	Techniques: visual inspection with mirror where needed, assistance if indicated.
Hygiene	Keep skin clean and dry, especially avoiding prolonged contact with feces or urine.
Response to signs of skin damage	Identify source of skin damage and take corrective action.
	Avoid pressure on damaged skin until it has healed.
	Indications for contacting health professional.
General health strategies	Maintain good nutritional status, hydration, and cardiovascular fitness.
	Avoid smoking and substance abuse.
Additional sources of skin trauma	Avoid clothes that exert excessive pressure on the skin, such as tight clothing or shoes, or pants with heavy seams over the sacrum or coccyx.
	Regularly inspect shoes and orthoses for wear that could result in increased pressure, friction, or shear on the skin.
	During transfers and other functional activities, avoid actions that subject the skin to excessive friction, shear, or high-impact forces.

first, but these reminders can decrease as they begin to assume responsibility for their own care.[u]

Patients' perceptions of the importance of skin care can be influenced by the degree to which health professionals comply with the recommended actions.[100] For this reason, all members of the rehabilitation team should model appropriate attention to and prioritization of pressure ulcer prevention. Even health professionals who do not normally focus on skin care (speech therapists, for example)

should ensure that the patient performs or is assisted with pressure reliefs at the appropriate intervals. If preventive skin care measures are implemented by some team members and not by others, the patient will receive mixed messages about the importance of these measures.

In some cases, poor psychological adjustment leads to self-neglect and lack of adherence to skin care guidelines. Counseling may help prevent or correct this problem.

One of the greatest challenges of rehabilitation following spinal cord injury involves preparing the patient to prevent pressure ulcers after discharge. With the current trend of shorter hospital stays, this challenge has become greater. Patients may be discharged from inpatient rehabilitation before they have developed the physical skills,

[u] A patient who has difficulty remembering to perform pressure reliefs at the appropriate intervals may benefit from a device that provides reminders.[8]

Problem-Solving Exercise 5–1

Your patient is a 68-year-old man who has complete T6 paraplegia resulting from anoxia to his spinal cord during recent surgery (coronary artery bypass graft). He moves his arms independently but requires assistance to move in bed. He remains in bed on a ventilator and has developed pneumonia.

- Identify the factors that make this individual highly susceptible to pressure ulcers.
- What measures would you suggest to prevent the development of pressure ulcers?

knowledge base, and level of psychological adaptation required to assume full responsibility for their skin care. For this reason, education and training should extend beyond the traditional inpatient rehabilitation program.[101] This education and training can continue in day hospital[102] or outpatient settings as well as in home-based rehabilitation and follow-up visits and phone calls.[103-105] During and after inpatient rehabilitation, the educational program should be designed to equip the patient with self-management, problem-solving, and information-gathering skills.[103,106] In order to enhance communication with health care providers after discharge, patients and their families should also be instructed in the terminology related to the location and staging of pressure ulcers.[16]

ASSESSMENT OF PRESSURE ULCERS

When a pressure ulcer is detected, its management should immediately become a priority. This should start with an examination of the ulcer and investigation of any factors that may have contributed to its development. A thorough assessment will make it possible to design an appropriate program of interventions and subsequently to determine the effectiveness of these interventions.[16,107]

After the initial assessment, pressure ulcers should be examined at least once a week; in addition, the status of the pressure ulcer should be monitored with each dressing change.[49,107] Examinations should be more frequent if either the patient's medical condition or the ulcer itself deteriorates.[58,107] Repeat assessments make it possible to evaluate the effectiveness of the interventions and to alter the program as indicated.[16,49] Several scales have been developed to assess and document pressure ulcer healing.[108-113] One such instrument is the PUSH tool (Figure 5–11), a scale for healing developed by the National Pressure Ulcer Advisory Panel (NPUAP).[114]

Characteristics of Pressure Ulcers

When examining pressure ulcers, health professionals should note their location, size (length, width, and depth), shape, and stage. (Staging is presented in the section that follows.) They should determine whether the ulcer extends under adjacent tissue in the form of sinus tracts,

undermining, or tunneling.[49,58] Health professionals should also note which of the following are present in the wound bed: exudate, eschar, slough, granulation tissue, or epithelial tissue.[58,114] Table 5–5 describes the characteristics of pressure ulcers the examination should address.[v] The condition of the periwound tissue is also relevant; any erythema, warmth, swelling, induration, or maceration should be noted. Wound margins should be examined for thickening or rolling under.[16] Color photographs on grid paper are useful for documenting the ulcer's initial and subsequent condition.[16,61] Digital images can readily be utilized in computerized documentation systems.

Staging of Pressure Ulcers

One important feature of pressure ulcers is their depth. Table 5–6 and Figure 5–12 present a classification system for grading or staging pressure ulcers according to their depth. This system was developed by the National Pressure Ulcer Advisory Panel[115] and updated in 2007.[116]

Clinicians should be aware of the following limitations of the staging system: (1) Deep tissue injuries and Stage I pressure ulcers are difficult to detect in patients with darkly pigmented skin; (2) Stage I pressure ulcers may be superficial or may indicate deeper tissue damage; and (3) the presence of eschar interferes with accurate staging of a pressure ulcer. Once eschar has been removed, the ulcer can be staged accurately.[41,52,58,116,118]

A pressure ulcer that deteriorates can be assigned a new stage (restaged) to reflect its increased depth. For example, an ulcer that originally appears as a blister or shallow crater extending into the dermis may progress to the point where it presents as a deeper crater extending into the subcutaneous fat. In this instance, it would be appropriate to change its classification from Stage II to Stage III. In contrast, ulcers should not be restaged (or "downstaged") to reflect healing, since normal tissue is not restored as ulcers heal.[61,113]

---

[v] If an ulcer is painful, clinicians should also note this fact, as the pain will have to be managed during ulcer care. Typically, however, people with spinal cord injuries develop pressure ulcers in areas that are insensitive to pain.

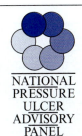

Pressure Ulcer Scale for Healing (PUSH)
PUSH Tool 3.0

NATIONAL
PRESSURE
ULCER
ADVISORY
PANEL

Patient Name _____ Patient ID# _____

Ulcer Location _____ Date _____

Directions:

Observe and measure the pressure ulcer. Categorize the ulcer with respect to surface area, exudate, and type of wound tissue. Record a sub-score for each of these ulcer characteristics. Add the sub-scores to obtain the total score. A comparison of total scores measured over time provides an indication of the improvement or deterioration in pressure ulcer healing.

	0	1	2	3	4	5	Sub-score
LENGTH X WIDTH	0	< 0.3	0.3 – 0.6	0.7 – 1.0	1.1 – 2.0	2.1 – 3.0	
		6	7	8	9	10	
(in cm²)		3.1 – 4.0	4.1 – 8.0	8.1 – 12.0	12.1 – 24.0	> 24.0	
EXUDATE AMOUNT	0	1	2	3			Sub-score
	None	Light	Moderate	Heavy			
TISSUE TYPE	0	1	2	3	4		Sub-score
	Closed	Epithelial Tissue	Granulation Tissue	Slough	Necrotic Tissue		
							TOTAL SCORE

Length x Width: Measure the greatest length (head to toe) and the greatest width (side to side) using a centimeter ruler. Multiply these two measurements (length x width) to obtain an estimate of surface area in square centimeters (cm²). Caveat: Do not guess! Always use a centimeter ruler and always use the same method each time the ulcer is measured.

Exudate Amount: Estimate the amount of exudate (drainage) present after removal of the dressing and before applying any topical agent to the ulcer. Estimate the exudate (drainage) as none, light, moderate, or heavy.

Tissue Type: This refers to the types of tissue that are present in the wound (ulcer) bed. Score as a "4" if there is any necrotic tissue present. Score as a "3" if there is any amount of slough present and necrotic tissue is absent. Score as a "2" if the wound is clean and contains granulation tissue. A superficial wound that is reepithelializing is scored as a "1". When the wound is closed, score as a "0".

4 – **Nectotic Tissue (Eschar):** black, brown, or tan tissue that adheres firmly to the wound bed or ulcer edges and may be either firmer or softer than surrounding skin.

3 – **Slough:** yellow or white tissue that adheres to the ulcer bed in strings or thick clumps, or is mucinous.

2 – **Granulation Tissue:** pink or beefy red tissue with a shiny, moist, granular appearance.

1 – **Epithelial Tissue:** for superficial ulcers, new pink or shiny tissue (skin) that grows in from the edges or as islands on the ulcer surface.

0 – **Closed/Resurfaced:** the wound is completely covered with epithelium (new skin).

www.npuap.org

11F

PUSH Tool Version 3.0: 9/15/98

©National Pressure Ulcer Advisory Panel

Figure 5–11 PUSH tool (version 3.0) for documenting pressure ulcer healing. (Reproduced with permission from the National Pressure Ulcer Advisory Panel.)

TABLE 5–5   Characteristics of Pressure Ulcers

Characteristic	Definition	Comments
Location	Anatomic location of ulcer.	Can be described in words or by mark on diagram of body.
Size	Length, width, and depth of the lesion.	Length can be measured as largest diameter, width can be measured perpendicular to length. Alternatively, length can be measured as greatest distance in a cephalad-to-caudal direction and width as greatest distance in line perpendicular to length. Depth can be measured at deepest point using sterile probe.
Shape	Configuration of wound's perimeter at the level of the skin surface.	Can be documented with drawing or (preferably) photograph.
Stage	Depth of ulcer.	Staging system presented in Table 5–6.
Nonblanchable erythema	Redness that persists when pressure is applied with a fingertip.	Indicative of Stage I pressure ulcer. Should not be confused with reactive hyperemia, which is a normal response of intact skin. Reactive hyperemia is redness that blanches (turns white or pale) when pressure is applied by a fingertip.
Sinus tract	Cavity or channel underlying a wound that involves an area larger than the visible surface of the wound.	Note presence or absence. If present, note location.
Undermining	A closed passageway under the surface of the skin that is open only at the skin surface; generally this appears as an area of skin ulceration at the margins of the ulcer with skin overlying the area.	Often develops from shearing forces.
Tunneling	Passageway under the surface of the skin that is generally open at the skin level; however, most of the tunneling is not visible.	Note presence or absence. If present, note location.
Exudate	Any fluid that has been extruded from a tissue or its capillaries, more specifically because of injury or inflammation.	Note presence or absence. If present, describe amount, color, opacity, consistency, odor.
Eschar	Thick, leathery, necrotic tissue.	Appearance: dark brown or black, adherent to ulcer bed.
Slough	Devitalized tissue in the process of separating from viable portions of the body.	Appearance: white or yellow, adherent to ulcer bed in clumps or loose strings.
Granulation tissue	Tissue that contains new blood vessels, collagen, fibroblasts, and inflammatory cells, which fills an open, previously deep wound when it starts to heal.	Appearance: pink or beefy red, moist, granular, shiny.
Epithelial tissue	Tissue made of epithelial cells that migrate across the surface of a healing wound.	Appearance: pink or red. Extends across wound bed in partial thickness wounds; starts at wound periphery and moves toward center of full-thickness wounds.

Sources: References 16, 58, 61, and 114.

TABLE 5–6   NPUAP Pressure Ulcer Staging System

Stage	Characteristics
Suspected deep tissue injury	Purple or maroon localized area of discolored intact skin or blood-filled blister due to damage of underlying soft tissue from pressure and/or shear. The area may be preceded by tissue that is painful, firm, mushy, boggy, warmer or cooler as compared to adjacent tissue.
I	Intact skin with nonblanchable redness of a localized area usually over a bony prominence. Darkly pigmented skin may not have visible blanching; its color may differ from the surrounding area.
II	Partial-thickness loss of dermis presenting as a shallow open ulcer with a red pink wound bed, without slough. May also present as intact or open/ruptured serum-filled blister.
III	Full-thickness tissue loss. Subcutaneous fat may be visible but bone, tendon or muscle are *not* exposed. Slough may be present but does not obscure the depth of tissue loss. *May* include undermining and tunneling.
IV	Full-thickness tissue loss with exposed bone, tendon or muscle. Slough or eschar may be present on some parts of the wound bed. Often include undermining and tunneling.
Unstageable	Full-thickness tissue loss in which the base of the ulcer is covered by slough (yellow, tan, gray, green or brown) and/or eschar (tan, brown or black) in the wound bed.

Source: Reference 117.

Comprehensive Examination

To treat a pressure ulcer effectively, the health care team must focus on the "whole picture" rather than on the ulcer alone. Their assessment must investigate the various factors that can contribute to the development of a pressure ulcer and its deterioration or healing, including the individual's medical and nutritional status, psychological and social factors, and possible sources of damaging forces or conditions affecting the skin.

Medical Status

The comprehensive examination should investigate the overall health of the patient, with emphasis on determining whether there are any conditions that could affect the healing of the ulcer. Such conditions include cardiovascular disease, diabetes, hypertension or hypotension, urinary tract infection, pulmonary disease, and renal disease.[w]

Nutritional Status

The examination should investigate whether the patient's diet is adequate to support healing of the ulcer. The diet should include adequate intake of protein (1.25 to 1.5 g protein/kg/day), calories (30 to 35 calories/kg/day), and vitamins and minerals. Laboratory tests may also be indicated. Serum albumin below 3.5 mg/dL or a total lymphocyte count of less than 1500/mm^3 is associated with pressure ulcers.[16] A drop in body weight of more than 15% is also significant.[58]

Psychological and Social Factors

The assessment should address psychological factors, since they can influence the patient's ability to participate in a skin care program. Impaired mental status, poor learning ability, or depression may limit an individual's capacity to learn or follow through with ulcer care and preventive measures.

Social support is also important. Particularly if the patient is staying at home, the health care team should assess the caregivers' ability to understand and implement the ulcer care and prevention program; they should also investigate the community resources that are available.[58] In addition, the patient's financial resources (insurance or other assets) should be determined to ensure that the intervention strategies planned are within the individual's means.[61]

Possible Sources of Skin Damage

When a pressure ulcer develops, the source of the problem must be identified. Discerning the cause(s) of skin damage is important because it enables the health care team to take corrective action. Eliminating damaging forces and conditions will enhance healing and reduce the likelihood of future breakdown.

One area to investigate is whether the individual's activities have subjected the skin to damaging pressure,

---

[w] The comprehensive examination should also investigate the presence of complications resulting from the pressure ulcer. These complications include amyloidosis, endocarditis, heterotopic bone formation, maggot infestation, meningitis, perineal–urethral fistula, pseudoaneurysm, septic arthritis, sinus tract or abscess, squamous cell carcinoma in the ulcer, systemic effects of topical treatments, osteomyelitis, bacteremia, sepsis, and advancing cellulitis.[58]

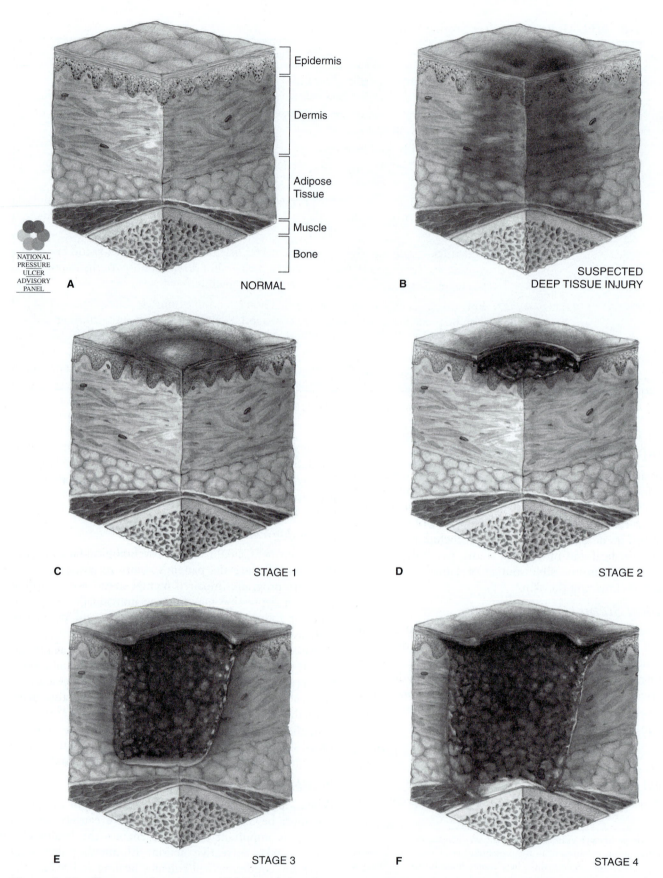

Figure 5–12   Pressure ulcer stages. (A) Normal skin. (B) Suspected deep tissue injury. (C) Stage I pressure ulcer. (D) Stage II pressure ulcer. (E) Stage III pressure ulcer. (F) Stage IV pressure ulcer. (G) Unstageable. (Reproduced with permission from the National Pressure Ulcer Advisory Panel.)

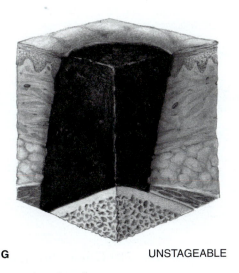

G   UNSTAGEABLE

Figure 5–12   *(continued)*

shear, or friction. Examples of activities that could cause pressure ulcers include lying in bed with the head of the bed elevated, sliding the buttocks across a transfer board, negotiating stairs on the buttocks, sitting for periods of time that are too long for the individual's skin tolerance, allowing too much time to pass between pressure reliefs, and utilizing inadequate pressure relief methods. This list is by no means complete—there are virtually limitless ways in which the skin may be traumatized during daily activities.

Faulty or inadequate equipment is another possible source of pressure ulcers. Skin damage can occur when equipment does not provide adequate pressure distribution to meet the patient's needs. This can happen when equipment has not been properly selected, when it is incorrectly adjusted or maintained, or when it has deteriorated over time. The equipment assessment should include the support surface of the individual's bed; the wheelchair cushion; the wheelchair's fit, components, and adjustment; and the fit and alignment of spinal or extremity orthoses.

In addition to assessing a patient's activities and equipment, the health care team should look for any other possible sources of damaging forces on the skin. Improper positioning in the bed or wheelchair can cause shearing and excessive pressure. Clothes that are too tight or have heavy seams can exert damaging pressure on the skin. Spasticity that causes repeated motions of the extremities can cause friction as the extremities rub against bedclothes or other objects in the environment.

Finally, the health care team should investigate whether any other conditions may have contributed to the development of the pressure ulcer. Prolonged exposure to urine, feces, or perspiration is an example of such a condition.

Health professionals should assess the individual's activities, equipment, and other potential sources of skin damage in an attempt to discern the most likely causes of

the pressure ulcer. The ulcer's location is often a good starting point for this analysis, since it provides a clue to the source of the damaging forces. For example, an ulcer over the ischial tuberosities most likely developed as a result of excessive tissue loads in sitting or during transfers. The individual's wheelchair, cushion, sitting posture, sitting time, pressure relief frequency and technique, and transfer technique are possible problem areas to investigate. In contrast, an ulcer over the posterior heel is likely to result from damaging tissue loads when the patient is supine in bed or when he uses lower extremity orthoses. The patient's position in bed and turning schedule as well as the bed's support surface should be evaluated. If the patient wears orthoses, the wearing schedule and the orthoses' fit and alignment should be evaluated.

*I*NTERVENTIONS

A comprehensive care program addresses both the ulcer itself and any factors that may contribute to its healing or the development of pressure ulcers in the future.[x] Interventions include prevention of additional pressure ulcers, managing tissue loads, wound cleansing and debridement, use of dressings, managing bacterial colonization and infection, adjunctive therapies to promote wound healing, surgery (if indicated), optimization of the patient's health and nutritional status, and education and training. If a pressure ulcer does not show evidence of healing within 2 to 4 weeks, the treatment program should be assessed and modified.[16,40]

Pressure Ulcer Prevention

Anyone with a spinal cord injury who has a pressure ulcer is at risk for developing additional ulcers. The limitations in activity and positioning necessary for ulcer or surgical flap healing result in greater time spent bearing weight on areas of unaffected skin, increasing the risk of breakdown in these areas. Moreover, once an ulcer heals, it leaves a scarred area that is vulnerable to trauma; the healed area will never be as strong as the original tissue.

To avoid both the development of new skin breakdown and the recurrence of healed or surgically repaired pressure ulcers, the patient and health care team should develop and institute a pressure ulcer prevention program. Based on the results of their initial assessment, the team should work with the patient to correct any factors that may have contributed to the development of the ulcer or could result in future breakdown.

---

[x] For complex wounds, clinicians should consider consulting with a wound specialist, such as a certified wound specialist (CWS) or a certified wound, ostomy, continence nurse (CWON). Specialists can be located through the American Academy of Wound Management (www.aawm.org) or the Wound, Ostomy and Continence Nursing Certification Board (www. wocncb.org).

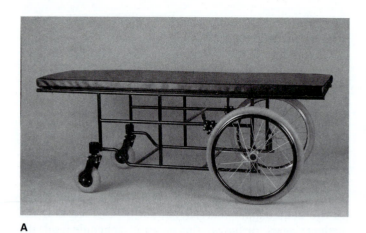
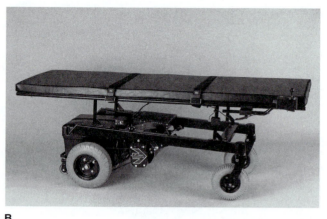

A   **B**

Figure 5–13   Prone carts. (A) Manual. (B) Power. (Reproduced with permission from 21st Century Scientific, Inc.)

Managing Tissue Loads

Tissue load management involves protecting both the ulcer and areas of intact skin from damaging pressure, shear, and friction. Minimization of these forces will make healing possible and will help to prevent the development of additional pressure ulcers.

First and foremost, damaging pressure over the affected area must be avoided.[52,58] A Stage I pressure ulcer may heal without any intervention other than this relief of pressure.[119] Depending on the source of trauma to the skin, pressure relief may involve adjusting an orthosis or avoiding a certain posture, such as supine or sitting. People who need to avoid sitting can utilize prone carts (Figure 5–13), which allow independent mobility in a prone position. Although these carts are not as comfortable or functional as wheelchairs, they make it possible to participate in out-of-bed activities without subjecting the buttocks and sacral area to pressure or shear. Using a prone cart, a person can avoid sitting while remaining active and mobile, thus preventing some of the social and physical sequelae of prolonged bed rest.[120,121] Alternatively, use of an appropriate wheelchair and cushion that

minimize pressure and shear to the affected area—combined with limited out-of-bed time, regular pressure reliefs, and close monitoring of the wound—may provide enough protection to allow healing.[49]

When a patient has multiple pressure ulcers, relief of pressure may be problematic: positioning in bed that avoids pressure on one ulcer is likely to involve weight bearing on another. When this is the case, an air-fluidized or low-air-loss bed may promote healing by reducing pressure over bony prominences.[49,55,58,122,123] Even if a patient has only one ulcer, it may limit the number of positions in which he can safely lie in bed. (For example, a sacral ulcer may necessitate the avoidance of the supine position.) This limitation will effectively increase the time spent in the remaining positions over the course of a day, increasing the risk of developing ulcers while in these positions. A specialized support surface is indicated to reduce the tissue loads on these areas.

The turning schedule in bed may also have to be adjusted as a part of a pressure ulcer management program.[58] It may be necessary for the patient to turn in bed more frequently in order to keep tissue loads low enough to promote healing and prevent new ulcers from developing.

Problem-Solving Exercise 5–2

Your patient is undergoing inpatient rehabilitation. She has been using a wheelchair for the past several weeks without exhibiting any problems with her skin. Yesterday, she began using a different wheelchair. All other relevant factors remained unchanged: the patient remained sitting for the same number of hours as usual, participated in her usual activities, continued performing pressure reliefs on the same schedule, and did not change cushions. When she went to bed and inspected her skin at the end of the day, she noticed redness over her ischial tuberosities. This redness blanched when touched with a finger. After 50 minutes, the redness disappeared. In the

past, redness over this patient's ischial tuberosities has always resolved within 15 to 20 minutes.

- Does the redness over the patient's ischial tuberosities indicate that she has a pressure ulcer? If so, what stage is the pressure ulcer?
- You suspect that the redness over the patient's ischial tuberosities was caused by the change in wheelchairs. What characteristics of the new wheelchair could have caused this problem?
- What actions should you take to ensure that the patient does not develop a more serious problem in the skin overlying her ischial tuberosities?

Cleansing and Debridement

Wound cleansing is a necessary component of any pressure ulcer care program. Ulcers should be cleaned initially and at every dressing change until they have healed. This cleansing reduces the potential for infection and enhances healing by removing nonadherent necrotic tissue, exudate, metabolic wastes, residual topical agents, and dressing residue.[16,58,118,124]

Cleansing is typically accomplished by irrigating the wound. Irrigation pressure should be between 4 and 15 pounds per square inch (psi). Pressures lower than 4 psi do not provide enough force to clean the wound adequately. Pressures higher than 15 psi can traumatize viable tissue and drive bacteria into the wound's tissues. Pressures in the 4 to 15 psi range can be achieved using a 35-mL syringe with a 19-gauge needle or angiocatheter,[58,107] or a pulsatile lavage system.

Normal saline is the cleansing solution of choice for most pressure ulcers. Irrigation with normal saline provides adequate cleaning in most cases, and this solution does not contain any potentially harmful chemicals. In contrast, many commercially available wound cleansers can be toxic to the wound's viable tissues.[16,58,61,107,118,124] Commercial wound cleansers containing surfactant may be indicated for wounds with adherent materials, but clinicians should take care to select solutions that do not contain harmful chemicals.[58]

Many pressure ulcers contain adherent necrotic tissue that cannot be removed by cleansing alone. Necrotic tissue prolongs inflammation, promotes bacterial growth, and interferes with wound healing. For this reason, it should be removed from pressure ulcers to enhance healing and reduce the risk of infection. Debridement of devitalized (necrotic) tissue can be achieved using sharp instruments, wet-to-dry dressings, whirlpool baths, pulsatile lavage, wound irrigation, dextranomers, enzymatic agents, or moisture-retentive dressings.[16,51,58,61,123,125–127] Different methods of debridement are often combined.

Dressings

Dressings are used to protect pressure ulcers and create conditions that are conducive to healing: a clean and moist ulcer bed, dry surrounding tissues, an absence of unfilled empty space within the wound, and protection from infection and trauma.[16,49,58,107,128] A large variety of dressings are available. These differ in their effects on the wound environment, cost per dressing, and the frequency with which they should be changed. Each type of dressing is available from a number of manufacturers. Clinicians should familiarize themselves with the characteristics and manufacturer's usage recommendations of the dressings that they utilize.

Clinicians should select dressings that are most appropriate for their patients. The most important factor in selecting dressings is the condition of the ulcer: the depth, presence or absence of infection, amount of exudate, and nature of the tissues (necrotic, granulation, or epithelial). Additional considerations include cost,[y] financial resources, caregiver time required for dressing changes, and (if the patient is at home) access to assistance and health care services.

Adjunctive Therapies to Promote Healing

In recent years, a number of adjunctive therapies have been utilized to promote the healing of pressure ulcers. Probably the most widely used of these is high-voltage electrical stimulation, which has been shown to increase the rate of pressure ulcer healing dramatically.[129-131] Low-intensity direct current can also enhance wound healing.[132,133] Studies demonstrating enhanced healing with electrical stimulation have done so using a variety of protocols. For this reason, no one protocol is used universally.[58,61]

Additional adjunctive therapies include pulsed nonthermal diathermy,[134] ultrasound,[135,136] hyperbaric oxygen therapy,[61,135] low-energy laser,[136,137] ultraviolet,[136] negative-pressure therapy,[138,139] and the application of growth factors.[140] Other than electrical stimulation and pulsed nonthermal diathermy, the efficacy of the various adjunctive therapies in promoting healing in pressure ulcers has yet to be demonstrated in controlled clinical studies.

Managing Bacterial Colonization and Infection

All open (Stages II to IV) pressure ulcers are colonized with bacteria.[58] As long as the number of bacteria remains relatively low, this colonization should not interfere with ulcer healing. When colonization progresses to infection, however, healing is slowed. A wound is considered to be infected (as opposed to colonized) when the bacterial count is greater than 100,000 organisms per gram of tissue.[126]

In addition to slowing healing, infection in a pressure ulcer can spread locally or systemically. Local spread of infection can cause cellulitis, osteomyelitis, infection of involved joints and bursae, and abscess formation.[141] Systemic spread of infection can be fatal.

One important facet of ulcer care is the prevention of infection. In most cases, this can be accomplished through debridement of necrotic tissue, regular cleansing, dressings, and standard infection-control practices.[58,118] Topical antiseptics should not be used to control bacterial levels within wounds because they are toxic to the wound's viable tissues and can have systemic toxic effects.[7,58,118]

Evidence of infection in a pressure ulcer includes purulence, a foul odor, and marked erythema in the tissues

---

[y] Cost estimates should reflect the cost per dressing, the frequency of dressing changes, and the cost of nursing care.

surrounding the wound. When these signs of local infection are present, the first response should be more frequent cleansing and debridement of any necrotic tissue left within the wound. If signs of infection continue or if the wound does not show evidence of healing within 2 to 4 weeks, topical antibiotics should be applied to the wound. If a 2-week course of topical antibiotics does not lead to improved wound healing, the wound should be cultured[z] and the patient evaluated for osteomyelitis in the bone underlying the ulcer.[16,58]

Although good wound care and topical antibiotics can control infection within a wound, they cannot control an infection once it has spread from the wound. Systemic antibiotics are indicated for anyone who develops advancing cellulitis, osteomyelitis, bacteremia, or sepsis.[49,58,107]

Surgery

Surgical closure of pressure ulcers is usually avoided if the wounds can heal satisfactorily with conservative management. One reason for this is that there is a high rate of ulcer recurrence over time after surgery.[aa] Another reason why pressure ulcers are managed conservatively when possible is that surgical closure utilizes healthy tissue. This can be problematic in the long run for patients who have recurring breakdown requiring multiple surgeries in the same area. A limited number of surgeries can be performed at a given site, since each surgery takes tissue from nearby areas of the patient's body, and there is a finite amount of such tissue.[52,142–144]

Despite its limitations, surgical closure of pressure ulcers remains an important treatment option for many patients. Although many pressure ulcers can heal with conservative management, this process can take weeks or months when the ulcers are large and deep. Moreover, the healed area will be scarred and therefore will remain vulnerable to future breakdown. For these reasons, surgical closure may be considered for Stage III and IV pressure ulcers. For surgical closure of large wounds, a myocutaneous flap procedure has the advantage of filling the wound cavity and creating a well-vascularized and padded area.[51,69,142,145]

When surgery is planned, it is typically preceded by a period of debridement and dressing changes. This period of preoperative management prepares the wound by ridding it of necrotic tissue and reducing the level of bacterial contamination.[146] Moreover, with good wound care during the preoperative period, the ulcer may shrink and as a result require less tissue coverage.[52]

Preoperative care also involves preparing the patient to heal optimally. Nutritional status should be optimized, and any medical conditions that could impede healing

should be treated.[16,61] Smoking cessation during the preoperative period can also enhance healing after surgery.[58] A course of antibiotics is frequently administered pre- and postoperatively.[141,146,147]

Postoperative care includes a prolonged period of bed rest, with avoidance of pressure on the grafted area through positioning and use of a pressure-reducing support surface.[58,69,145] In addition, care should be taken to avoid friction, shearing,[58] or tension on the grafted tissue until adequate healing has occurred. Range-of-motion exercises must be suspended,[148] and antispasmodic medications may be administered to prevent excessive motion caused by spasticity.[16,51]

Once the surgical site has healed adequately, range-of-motion exercises can resume[149] and the patient can begin bearing weight on the flap. Weight bearing on the surgical site should be undertaken cautiously, with a gradual buildup of weight-bearing time, frequent pressure reliefs, and assessment of the skin's status after each sitting session.[52,58,145] The physical therapist should assess the patient's wheelchair and cushion to ensure that pressure distribution is adequate. The team should also reinstruct the patient in ulcer prevention strategies.[16,52,150]

Health and Nutrition

In addition to treatment of the pressure ulcer itself, optimal management addresses the patient's general health. Treatment of anemia, hypoalbuminemia, and edema may promote the healing of pressure ulcers.[119] Systemic antibiotics are indicated for patients who develop abscesses, advancing cellulitis, osteomyelitis, bacteremia, or sepsis.[49,51,58,107,125]

The patient's nutritional status is also important. Wound healing requires an adequate intake of proteins, carbohydrates, fats, vitamins (A, C, and E), minerals, and fluids.[16,53,127,135,151,152] A high-calorie, high-protein diet may facilitate wound healing. Zinc, magnesium, and vitamin supplements may be indicated for people with deficiencies of these nutrients.[16,49,51,123,125]

Education and Training

Education and training are necessary components of every program for pressure ulcer care. This education and training should develop the knowledge and skills required to perform ongoing assessments of the ulcer's status, prevent the development of additional pressure ulcers, and facilitate healing through the management of external forces on the wound, wound cleansing, and dressing changes. The patient, family, and any others involved in the patient's care should be included in the education and training program for ulcer care.

---

[z] The culture should be obtained through tissue biopsy or needle aspiration. Swab cultures may not give reliable information on the organisms infecting the ulcer's tissues.[16,58]

[aa] Reported recurrence rates vary widely.[140] In one study, patients with traumatic paraplegia had a 79% recurrence rate within a mean of 10.9 months after surgical repair of their pressure ulcers.[145]

Summary

- Spinal cord injury leads to lifelong vulnerability to the development of pressure ulcers, a complication that can have profound medical, functional, and social consequences. Because pressure ulcers are both preventable and serious, skin care is a critical focus of medical management, rehabilitation, and health maintenance following spinal cord injury.

- Preventive skin care after spinal cord injury includes a balanced diet, proper management of bowel and bladder incontinence, avoidance of damaging forces on the skin, and close monitoring of the skin's status. Special attention is given to avoiding prolonged, unrelieved pressure on the skin, particularly over bony prominences.

- Pressure ulcer prevention while in bed involves positioning, regular turning, and the use of a support surface (bed, mattress, or mattress overlay) suitable to the individual's needs. Pressure ulcer prevention while in a wheelchair involves positioning, regular pressure reliefs, an appropriate wheelchair cushion, and the use of a wheelchair with dimensions, components, and adjustment that are suitable to the individual's needs.

- Skin inspection is a critical component of pressure ulcer prevention. Regular skin checks give feedback about the effectiveness of the individual's pressure ulcer prevention program and make it possible to detect early signs of potential breakdown and intervene before it progresses.

- Pressure ulcer care starts with an assessment of the ulcer and a comprehensive examination to identify factors that may have contributed to the development of the ulcer or that may interfere with wound healing.

- Once a comprehensive pressure ulcer assessment has been completed, a wound care program is designed to promote wound healing and prevent the development of additional ulcers. Interventions include correcting any factors that may have contributed to the development of the pressure ulcer, managing tissue loads, cleansing the ulcer, debriding all devitalized tissue, using dressings, managing bacterial colonization and infection, adjunctive therapies to promote wound healing, surgery (if indicated), optimization of the patient's health and nutritional status, and education and training.

- People with spinal cord injuries and everyone who will be involved in their care after discharge must learn all aspects of pressure ulcer prevention in order to maintain skin integrity. They must also learn wound care if the person has a pressure ulcer.

Suggested Resources

ORGANIZATIONS

American Professional Wound Care Association (APWCA): *www.apwca.org*

Association for the Advancement of Wound Care (AAWC): *www.aawconline.org*

National Pressure Ulcer Advisory Panel (NPUAP): *www.npuap.org*

Wound, Ostomy, and Continence Nurses Society (WOCN): *www.wocn.org*

PUBLICATIONS

Clinical practice guidelines published by Paralyzed Veterans of America, available for free download from *www.pva.org*:

- *Pressure Ulcer Prevention and Treatment Following Spinal Cord Injury: A Clinical Practice Guideline for Health-Care Professionals*, 2000.

Clinical practice guidelines published by the Royal College of Nursing, available for free download from *www.nice.org.uk*:

- *Pressure Ulcer Management*, 2005.
- *The Use of Pressure-Relieving Devices (Beds, Mattresses, and Overlays) for the Prevention of Pressure Ulcers in Primary and Secondary Care*, 2003.

Sussman C, Bates-Jensen B. *Wound Care: A Collaborative Practice Manual for Health Professionals*, 3rd ed. Philadelphia: Lippincott Williams & Wilkins, 2006.

6

Respiratory Management

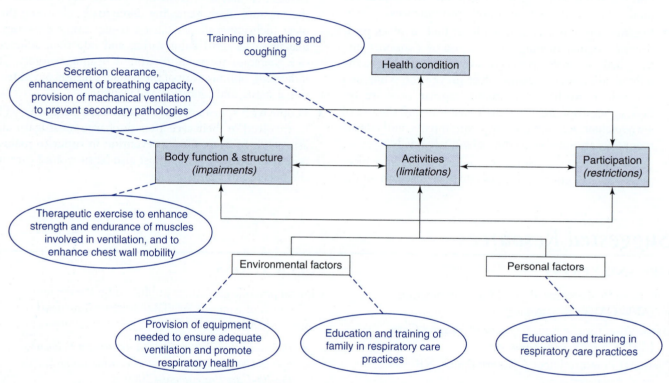

Chapter 6 presents information on respiratory function and respiratory care practices after spinal cord injury.

Respiratory complications are the most common cause of death after spinal cord injury.[1,2] Many of these secondary conditions can be avoided with proper care. Rehabilitation professionals should be familiar with the respiratory sequelae of spinal cord injury and should work with their patients to develop the ability to breathe and cough and to prevent complications.

Pulmonary function tests are used to examine breathing ability. Table 6–1 presents the various measures and their normal values.

REVIEW OF NORMAL BREATHING

Breathing, or ventilation, is achieved through motions of the ribs and diaphragm. These motions alter the volume of the thoracic cavity, a space bounded by the ribs, sternum, vertebral column, and diaphragm. When the volume within this cavity increases, intrathoracic pressure falls and air is drawn into the lungs. When the space within the thoracic cavity decreases, intrathoracic pressure rises and air moves out of the lungs. The motions involved are illustrated in Figure 6–1.

TABLE 6–1   Pulmonary Function Tests

Measure	Abbreviation	Definition	Normal Values*
Tidal volume	TV	The volume of air normally inhaled in one breath during quiet respiration.	~500 mL
Inspiratory reserve volume	IRV	The maximum volume of air that can be inhaled after a normal quiet inspiration.	~3000 mL
Expiratory reserve volume	ERV	The maximum volume of air that can be exhaled after a normal exhalation during quiet breathing.	~1100 mL
Residual volume	RV	The volume of air that remains in the lungs after a maximal exhalation.	~1200 mL
Vital capacity	VC	The maximum volume of air that can be exhaled by forceful exhalation following maximal inhalation. (Equal to the sum of the TV, IRV, and ERV.)	~4600 mL
Total lung capacity	TLC	The volume of air in the lungs at the end of a maximal inhalation. (Equal to the sum of TV, IRV, ERV, and RV.)	~5800 mL
Inspiratory capacity	IC	The maximum volume of air that can be inspired from the end of a normal quiet exhalation. (Equal to the sum of the TV and the IRV.)	~3500 mL
Functional residual capacity	FRC	The volume of air that remains in the lungs at the end of a normal quiet exhalation. (Equal to the sum of ERV and RV.)	~2300 mL
Forced expiratory volume in 1 second	FEV_1	The volume of air that can be expired in 1 second by forceful exhalation following maximal inhalation. (Often expressed as percentage of vital capacity.)	~80% of VC
Maximum positive expiratory pressure	PEP	The maximal positive pressure generated during forced expiration.	Male: 247 cm H_2O Female: 160 cm H_2O
Maximum negative inspiratory pressure	NIP	The maximal negative pressure generated during maximal inhalation.	Male: 132 cm H_2O Female: 94 cm H_2O
Peak cough flow	PCF	Maximum expiratory flow during cough maneuver.	360−1000 L/min

* Normal values vary with age, gender, and height. Most normal values were established in adult males. Reported normal values also vary between sources.

Sources: References 3 and 9 to 14.

Motions Involved in Inhalation

Movements that increase the cephalocaudal, anteroposterior, or transverse dimensions of the thoracic cavity cause inhalation.[3–5] The cephalocaudal dimension of the thoracic cavity increases when the diaphragm descends. The relaxed diaphragm is dome-shaped and extends superiorly into the thorax. When it contracts, it flattens and moves caudally. Because the diaphragm is the caudal boundary of the thoracic cavity, its descent increases the cavity's volume.[6]

Anteroposterior chest expansion occurs when the upper ribs are elevated. At rest, the upper ribs slope downward as they curve forward from the vertebral column to the sternum. When these ribs are elevated, their motion is similar to that of a pump handle: they pivot about an axis located posteriorly where the ribs articulate with the vertebrae. The sternum moves forward and rostrally when this occurs (Figure 6–2A), increasing the anteroposterior dimension of the thoracic cage.[4,5,7,8]

Transverse chest expansion occurs when the lower ribs are elevated. Like the upper ribs, the lower ribs in their resting position slope downward as they extend forward and around the chest from the vertebral column. Their motion during elevation is different, however, because they move about a different axis of rotation. When they elevate, the lower ribs pivot on an axis that runs through

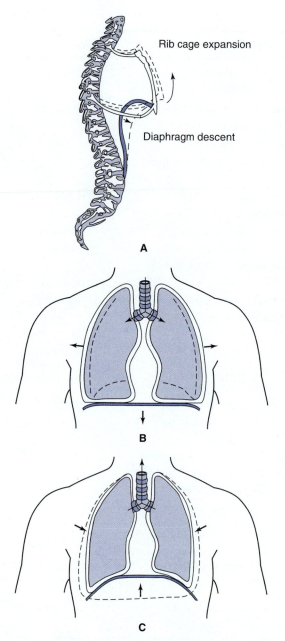

Figure 6–1   Mechanism of normal breathing. (A) Rib cage expansion and diaphragm descent cause inhalation. (B) During inhalation, rib cage expansion and diaphragm descent increase the volume within the thoracic cavity. Intrathoracic pressure falls and air is drawn into the lungs. (C) During exhalation, the rib cage contracts and the diaphragm ascends. Intrathoracic pressure rises and air is forced out of the lungs. (Adapted from *Fundamentals of Anatomy and Physiology*, 4th ed., by Martini. Reproduced with permission from Pearson Education, Inc.)

both their posterior and anterior attachments. As a result, the motion of the lower ribs during elevation is similar to that of a bucket handle when it is lifted (Figure 6–2B): when the ribs are raised, they swing up and out.[4,5,8]

Muscles Involved in Inhalation

During normal breathing, inspiration involves the coordinated action of a number of muscles. These muscles and their actions are illustrated in Figure 6–3A. Table 6–2 presents the innervation and actions of the muscles involved in inhalation.

Diaphragm

The diaphragm is the principal muscle used in inhalation, contributing most of the vital capacity[a] during normal breathing. It originates from the lumbar vertebrae, sternum, lower four ribs, and lower six costal cartilages and inserts into a central tendon.[3,8,17] When the diaphragm is relaxed, upward (cephalad) pressure from the abdominal contents pushes it into a dome-shaped resting position. The dome shape and superior position at rest contribute to the efficient functioning of this muscle. Its fibers are elongated in this position, enabling them to generate force more effectively because of the length–tension relationship of muscle contraction.[17,20] The diaphragm flattens and moves caudally when it contracts, increasing the volume within the thoracic cavity and drawing air into the lungs.

Because the diaphragm lies immediately cephalad to the abdominal cavity, it exerts pressure on the abdominal viscera when it descends. This descent causes the abdominal contents to protrude. When the abdominal contents have protruded as far as the abdominal wall will allow, further descent of the diaphragm is blocked. Continued diaphragmatic contraction results in elevation of the lower ribs. This elevation occurs as a result of two mechanisms. With the dome of the diaphragm "stabilized" as described above (caudal motion blocked), the angle of pull of its fibers is such that diaphragmatic contraction causes elevation of the lower ribs. Contraction of the diaphragm also causes an increase in intraabdominal pressure, and the resulting upward forces elevate the lower ribs. Rib elevation causes lateral chest expansion due to the bucket-handle action of the ribs.[7,8,21]

Intercostals, Scalenes, and Accessory Muscles

The intercostals, scalenes, and accessory muscles contribute significantly to normal breathing through their action on the ribs. These muscles stabilize the rib cage during inhalation, preventing the ribs from being drawn downward when the diaphragm descends. They also elevate the ribs, especially during deep inspiration. By stabilizing and elevating the ribs, these muscles contribute to the increase in intrathoracic volume required for inhalation.[17]

---

[a] Vital capacity and other measures of pulmonary function are defined in Table 6–1.

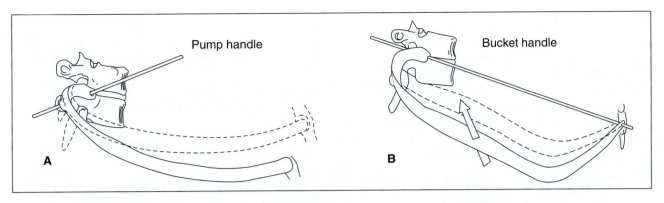

Figure 6–2   Rib motion during breathing. (A) "Pump-handle" motion of the upper ribs. (B) "Bucket-handle" motion of the lower ribs.

The intercostal muscles consist of three layers. From most superficial to deepest, they are the external intercostals, the internal intercostals, and the transversus thoracis. Contraction of the intercostals pulls the ribs closer together.[b] If the first rib is stabilized, this opposition of the ribs causes them to elevate.[3,5] The intercostals also aid in inspiration by preventing the tissues between the ribs from drawing inward when the intrathoracic pressure falls. By making the intercostal spaces more rigid, these muscles make it possible for rib and diaphragm motions to move air more effectively rather than causing distortion of the intercostal tissues.[5,8,18]

The scalenes[c] are active during quiet inhalation,[7,22] acting to stabilize and possibly elevate the rib cage.[6] During

---

[b] Some sources state that the intercostals stabilize the ribs during quiet inhalation and contract more forcefully to elevate them during deep inhalation.[6,17]

[c] Although the scalenes are often referred to as accessory muscles, they contract during every inhalation and therefore are primary muscles of inspiration.[7]

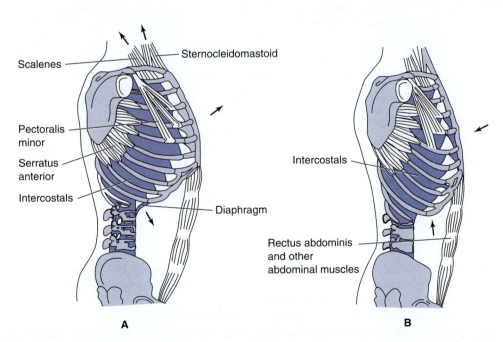

Figure 6–3   The respiratory muscles. The abdominal muscles are represented by the rectus abdominis. Muscles that stabilize or play a minor role in normal breathing are not shown. (A) Inhalation: The sternocleidomastoids, scalenes, pectoralis minor, serratus anterior, intercostals, and diaphragm contract to increase the volume within the thoracic cavity. (B) Forced exhalation: The abdominals and intercostals contract to decrease the volume within the thoracic cavity. (Adapted from *Fundamentals of Anatomy and Physiology*, 4th ed., by Martini. Reproduced with permission from Pearson Education, Inc.)

TABLE 6–2   Innervation and Actions of Muscles of Inspiration*

Muscles	Actions	Innervation
Primary muscles		
Diaphragm	Descends and moves caudally to increase the cephalocaudal dimension of the thoracic cavity. Elevates the lower ribs when abdominal viscera blocks further descent at the end of inhalation.	C3–C5
Scalenes	Stabilize and may help elevate ribs 1 and 2 during quiet inhalation. Elevate ribs 1 and 2 during deep or forced inhalation.	C3–C8
Intercostals	Stabilize the rib cage, and increase the rigidity of the intercostal spaces. Elevate the ribs when upper ribs are stabilized, especially during deep or forced inhalation.	T1–T11
Accessory muscles		
Sternocleidomastoid	Elevates the sternum during deep or forced inhalation.	Cranial nerve XI, C2–C3
Serratus anterior	Assists in rib elevation during deep or forced inhalation.	C5–C7
Pectoralis minor	Assists in rib elevation during deep or forced inhalation.	C6–T1
Pectoralis major, sternal portion	Assists in rib elevation during deep or forced inhalation.	C7–T1
Levatores costorum	Assist in rib elevation during deep or forced inhalation.	T1–T12
Serratus posterior superior	Assists in rib elevation during deep or forced inhalation.	T1–T3
Stabilizing and supporting muscles		
Trapezius	Stabilizes the head, neck, and scapula to enable accessory muscles to elevate the ribs during deep or forced inhalation.	Cranial nerve XI, C2–C4
Erector spinae	Stabilize the neck to enable accessory muscles to elevate the ribs and extend the trunk to enhance chest expansion during deep or forced inhalation.	C1–L4
Levator scapulae	Stabilize the scapula to enable accessory muscles to elevate the ribs during deep or forced inhalation.	C3–C5
Rhomboid major and minor	Stabilize the scapula to enable accessory muscles to elevate the ribs during deep or forced inhalation.	C4–C5
Abdominals	Provide support to the abdominal viscera, which support the diaphragm in its optimal position for functioning.	T6–L1

* This table presents spinal segment innervation and muscle actions of the muscles involved in inspiration. Because no two sources agree perfectly about either spinal segment innervation or muscle action, the table contains an amalgamation of the information from several different texts, presenting the points of greatest agreement among the various sources.

Sources: references 3, 4, 7, and 15 to 19.

deep or forced inspiration, the scalenes elevate the first two ribs.

The accessory muscles add force to the inspiratory effort during deep or forced inspiration, increasing the expansion of the thoracic cage. The sternocleidomastoids elevate the sternum, and the serratus anterior, pectoralis minor, levators costarum, and serratus posterior superior assist in rib elevation. The trapezius, erector spinae, rhomboids major and minor, and levator scapulae stabilize the head, neck, and scapulae so that the muscles listed above can act on the thoracic cage. The pectoralis major can assist in rib elevation when the arms are fixed. Finally, the erector spinae also aid in inspiration by extending the trunk.[3,5,6,8,18]

Abdominals

The rectus abdominis, internal and external obliques, and transversus abdominis aid in inhalation by providing support to the abdominal viscera, which in turn support the diaphragm in its optimal position for functioning. During inspiration, the abdominals relax to allow the viscera to protrude. This motion makes it possible for the diaphragm to descend.[8,17,20,23]

Motions Involved in Exhalation

Movements that reduce the anteroposterior, transverse, or cephalocaudal dimensions of the thoracic cavity cause exhalation. During quiet breathing, exhalation primarily involves the passive return of the rib cage and diaphragm to their pre-inspiratory positions. During forced expiration, as occurs in coughing or during heavy exercise, the ribs are drawn downward and the diaphragm is pushed upward to increase the intrathoracic pressure and force air out of the lungs.[3,5,6,8]

Muscles Involved in Exhalation

Exhalation during quiet breathing occurs as a result of passive recoil of the lungs and chest wall as the inspiratory muscles relax. Forced expiration is an active event in which the abdominals and intercostals contract to force air out of the lungs. The muscles involved are illustrated in Figure 6–3B. Table 6–3 presents the innervation and actions of the muscles involved in forced expiration.

Abdominals

The abdominals are the primary muscles of forced expiration. When the external and internal obliques, transversus abdominis, and rectus abdominis contract strongly, they push the abdominal viscera upward against the diaphragm. This upward force moves the diaphragm superiorly into the thoracic cage, pushing air out of the lungs.[3,6,8,17] Contraction of the external obliques also contributes to forced expiration by depressing the lower ribs.[8]

The abdominals can also add to the force of exhalation by flexing the trunk.[6-8] This motion aids in the upward movement of the abdominal viscera and diaphragm. Finally, the abdominals aid in forced expiration through their action on the ribs. The external obliques stabilize the twelfth rib, enabling the intercostals to perform their expiratory function.[5]

Intercostals

Contraction of the intercostals draws the ribs closer together. If the 12th rib is fixed caudally, intercostal contraction results in depression of the ribs.[5] This causes a reduction of the anteroposterior and mediolateral dimensions of the thoracic cavity due to the pump-handle and bucket-handle motions of the ribs, described above. Caudal fixation of the ribs is performed by the abdominal obliques, quadratus lumborum, and serratus posterior inferior.[4-6,18,19]

The intercostals also aid in expiration by preventing the intercostal tissues from bulging outward when intrathoracic

TABLE 6–3   Innervation and Actions of Muscles of Forced Expiration*

Muscles	Actions	Innervation
Primary muscles		
Rectus abdominis	Push abdominal viscera rostrally against the diaphragm to increase intrathoracic pressure during forced exhalation and coughing.	T6–T12
External obliques	Push abdominal viscera rostrally against the diaphragm to increase intrathoracic pressure during forced exhalation and coughing. Stabilize the 12th rib during forced exhalation and coughing, enabling intercostals to draw the ribs caudally.	T6–T12
Transversus abdominis	Push abdominal viscera rostrally against the diaphragm to increase intrathoracic pressure during forced exhalation and coughing.	T6–T12
Internal obliques	Push abdominal viscera rostrally against the diaphragm to increase intrathoracic pressure during forced exhalation and coughing.	T7–L1
Additional muscles		
Pectoralis major, clavicular portion	Can be used to depress the sternum and upper ribs during coughing.	C5–C6
Intercostals	Depress the ribs when the lower ribs are stabilized, and increase the rigidity of the intercostal spaces.	T1–T11
Serratus posterior inferior	Depresses the lower ribs during forced exhalation and coughing.	T9–T12
Quadratus lumborum	Depresses the 12th rib during forced exhalation and coughing.	T12–L4

* This table presents spinal segment innervation and muscle actions of the muscles involved in forced exhalation. Because no two sources agree perfectly about either spinal segment innervation or muscle action, the table contains an amalgamation of the information from several different texts, presenting the points of greatest agreement among the various sources.

Sources: references 3, 4, 7, and 15 to 19.

pressure rises. This stiffening of the intercostal spaces enables rib and diaphragm motions to move air more efficiently in and out of the lungs rather than causing bulging of the intercostal tissues.[5,8]

Diaphragm

Although it is primarily an inspiratory muscle, the diaphragm is also active during expiration. It contracts eccentrically for up to two thirds of expiration, working against the upward (cephalad) force of the abdominal contents. The effect of this eccentric contraction of the diaphragm is to slow the flow of air from the lungs.[20]

Influence of Postural Alignment

Breathing is effected by a variety of muscles working in concert to expand and contract the space within the thoracic cavity. The muscles of ventilation work optimally when they are in a slightly lengthened position, due to the length-tension relationship of muscle contraction. The alignment of the trunk, neck, and shoulder girdle determines the length of these muscles, and thus influences breathing ability. For example, the scalenes and sternocleidomastoids can work more effectively to expand the upper chest when the cervical spine is extended, as this position places these muscles on a slight stretch.[24]

Alignment of the trunk and shoulder girdle also influences breathing through its direct impact on movements of the thoracic cage and diaphragm. Postures that limit chest expansion or diaphragmatic motions interfere with pulmonary function.[25] For example, thoracic kyphosis and protracted scapulae make inhalation more difficult by impeding rib elevation.[24] Lumbar flexion, or a posteriorly tilted pelvis, can interfere with inhalation by limiting caudal displacement of the abdominal viscera, which in turn blocks diaphragmatic descent.

REVIEW OF NORMAL COUGHING

Coughing is an important action by which the airways are cleared when food or other foreign substances enter the trachea from the pharynx, or when respiratory secretions are too thick or copious to be cleared effectively by the normal action of the cilia lining the trachea.[26] During a respiratory tract infection, an inability to cough can lead to atelectasis, pneumonia, and ventilatory failure.[27]

Coughing involves coordinated action of the glottis and the muscles of both inhalation and exhalation. A cough occurs in stages: inhalation of an adequate volume of air, glottic closure, contraction of the muscles of forced exhalation with the glottis closed, and continued forced exhalation with the glottis open.[26,28,29] The motions and muscles involved in inhalation and forced exhalation are described in the previous section.

IMPACT OF SPINAL CORD INJURY ON THE ABILITY TO BREATHE AND COUGH

Neurological Level of Injury

After a spinal cord injury, a person's ability to breathe and cough depends largely on the functioning of her ventilatory muscles, which in turn is influenced by the level of her cord lesion.[11,17,30] Higher lesions affect breathing and coughing most profoundly because they interrupt innervation to muscles involved in both inhalation and exhalation. Lower lesions leave most of the muscles of inhalation intact but interfere with the functioning of the muscles used for forced exhalation. Figure 6–4 illustrates the innervation of the muscles of inspiration and forced expiration.

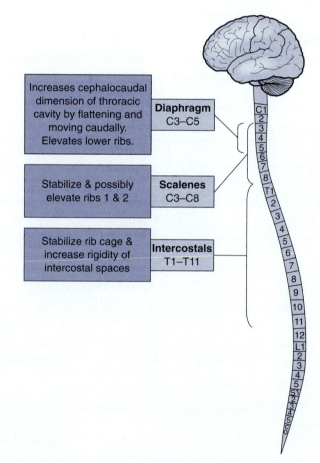

Figure 6–4   Schematic drawing showing innervation of respiratory muscles. Primary muscles are on the left of each image, accessory and additional muscles are on the right. Some supporting and stabilizing muscles are not shown. (A) Muscles of quiet inspiration. (B) Muscles of deep inspiration. (C) Muscles of forced expiration.

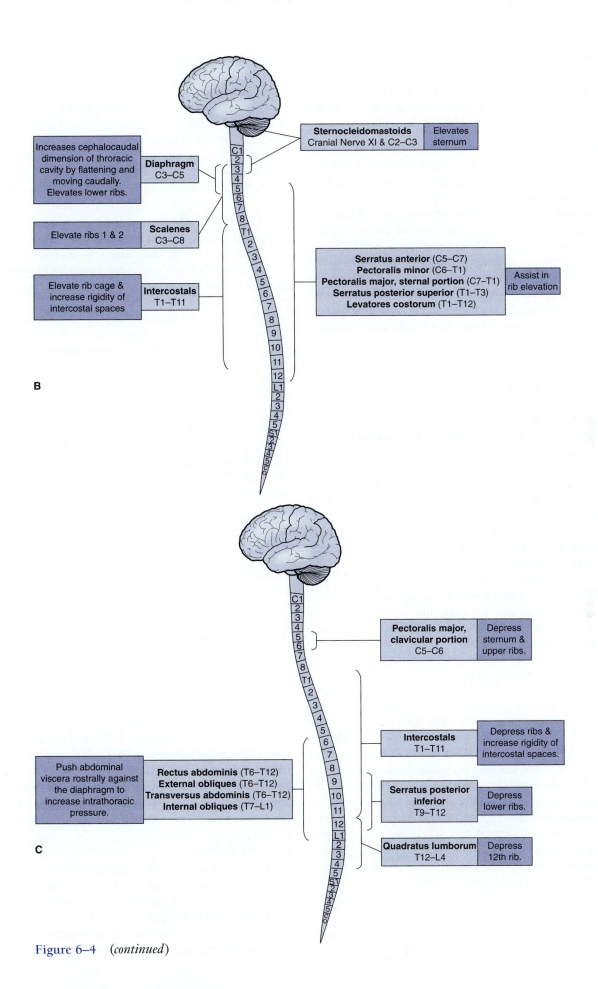

Figure 6-4 (continued)

The following descriptions of ventilatory function after spinal cord injury refer to complete lesions. Breathing and coughing ability after an incomplete lesion will depend upon the degree to which motor sparing occurs in the ventilatory muscles innervated below the lesion.

C1 and C2

An individual with a C1 or C2 neurological level of injury retains partial innervation of her sternocleidomastoid, trapezius, and erector spinae but loses the use of her diaphragm and all other muscles of ventilation. Using the innervated accessory muscles, she may be able to inhale a minimal amount of air.[17] This air movement will be inadequate for survival. Because she lacks a functioning diaphragm, the person with C1 or C2 tetraplegia will require[d] ventilatory support.[21,31] Additionally, forced expiration will not be possible; exhalation will occur as a result of passive recoil of the lungs and rib cage. As a result, she will require assistance for airway clearance.

C3

At this level, the diaphragm and scalenes retain partial innervation. The accessory muscles are more functional than with higher lesions because of full innervation of the sternocleidomastoid and partial innervation of the levator scapulae. The weakly functioning diaphragm, scalenes, and accessory muscles may be able to create sufficient motions of the thoracic cavity to allow for independent breathing. These muscles are likely to fatigue quickly, however, resulting in ventilatory failure.[17,32] For this reason, the person with C3 tetraplegia will require ventilatory support, at least during the acute stage after injury. Fortunately, weaning from the ventilator is frequently possible.[31,33–35]

Forced expiration will not be possible for a person with C3 tetraplegia; exhalation will occur as a result of passive recoil of the lungs and rib cage and cephalad pressure from the abdominal contents. The individual will require assistance for airway clearance.

C4

A person with C4 tetraplegia retains almost full innervation of her diaphragm, the primary muscle of inspiration. Paralysis of her abdominal muscles, however, will interfere with the diaphragm's functioning. Because her abdominal muscles are unable to support her viscera, her diaphragm will descend and flatten when she sits with her torso elevated above horizontal. This mechanically disadvantageous position of the diaphragm will compromise her ability to inhale. Inhalation will be further impaired by the intercostals' lack of function.

Soon after an injury at this level, the average vital capacity is approximately 24% of normal. Although many people with C4 tetraplegia require mechanical ventilation during the acute phase following injury, most are able to develop the capacity for independent breathing without mechanical support.[31,35,36]

Although those with C4 tetraplegia are likely to retain or develop the ability to breathe independently, they will be unable to cough effectively. Because they lack innervation of the abdominals and intercostals, they will be unable to perform the forceful exhalation involved in coughing. As a result, they will require assistance for airway clearance.

C5 Through C8

People with neurological levels of injury from C5 through C8 retain full use of their diaphragms, partial to full innervation of their scalenes, and nearly full innervation in their accessory muscles. For this reason, their capacity for independent breathing is stronger than that exhibited by people with higher lesions. Ventilatory failure occurs less frequently and resolves more rapidly than it does in patients with higher lesions.[37] Because innervation in the intercostal and abdominal musculature is lacking, however, inhalation and forced exhalation remain impaired.[17] Vital capacity soon after the onset of C5 or lower tetraplegia averages approximately 30% of normal.[36]

Although forced exhalation is impaired at these levels of tetraplegia, some capacity for cough is retained. The clavicular portion of the pectoralis major, which receives C5 and C6 innervation, can depress the sternum and upper ribs during coughing.[15,38]

T1 Through T5

Spinal cord injuries at T1 through T5 differ from higher injuries in that intercostal function is preserved at and above the neurological level of injury. This preserved motor function may slightly enhance a person's capacity for both inhalation and forced exhalation. Because the abdominals and the majority of the intercostals remain nonfunctional, the ability to inhale is slightly below normal and coughing is severely impaired.[17,31]

T6 Through T12

People with T6 through T12 paraplegia retain the use of those abdominal and intercostal muscles that are innervated above their lesions. Because of this additional motor function, their ability to perform both inhalation and forced exhalation (including coughing) is superior to that exhibited by individuals with higher lesions. The ability to breathe and cough remain lower than normal, however.[31] This impairment decreases with successively caudal lesions.

L1 and Below

Spinal cord damage with a neurological level of injury at or below L1 leaves intact all of the muscles of ventilation (except the quadratus lumborum) and thus does not have a significant effect on a person's ability to breathe or cough. Respiratory dysfunction may occur, however, as a result of other problems, such as prolonged bed rest.

---

[d] With training, many can learn to breathe for limited periods of time using their neck accessory musculature (neck breathing) or using mouth, throat, and pharynx musculature (glossopharyngeal breathing).[31,61,75,87,92,109–111,133]

Airway Caliber

In addition to disrupting the innervation of respiratory muscles, spinal cord injury can affect the reactivity of the airways. Cervical lesions are associated with elevated resting bronchomotor tone, which causes reduced airway caliber and therefore increased resistance to airflow. Bronchomotor hyperactivity may result from any or all of the following: an interruption of the lungs' sympathetic innervation (leaving parasympathetic activity unopposed), low circulating epinephrine levels due to interruption of the sympathetic innervation of the adrenal glands, and reduced inspiratory forces, leading to inadequate stretching of the smooth muscle in the airways.[39–41]

Positional Influences

Following spinal cord injury, a person who lacks innervation of the abdominal musculature typically breathes most easily in supine. In upright positions such as sitting, the abdominal viscera are allowed to descend and protrude because of a lack of muscular support from the abdominal wall. As a result, the diaphragm descends and flattens to a lower resting position, which places it in a mechanically disadvantageous position and thus impairs inspiration. In contrast, in the supine position, gravity exerts force on the abdominal contents, pushing them inward and rostrally so that they support the diaphragm in its normal resting position.[22,42-44] This position both reduces residual volume[45] and optimizes the functioning of the diaphragm because of the length–tension relationship.[17, 20]

Paradoxical Breathing Pattern

When rib stabilization by the intercostals and scalenes is lacking, as occurs to varying degrees with cervical and high thoracic spinal cord injuries, abnormal rib motions occur during breathing. When the diaphragm contracts and descends during inhalation, the resulting decrease in intrathoracic pressure pulls the unstabilized ribs caudally and inward. Instead of expanding in its anteroposterior and lateral dimensions during inspiration, the chest decreases in diameter.[7,22] This motion, called a paradoxical breathing pattern, causes a reduction in the volume of air inspired.[42] Breathing is less efficient; more work is required to move air, and thus respiratory muscle fatigue is more likely to occur.[21] Paradoxical rib motions become less pronounced as time passes, because of increased tone in the intercostal muscles.[46]

Changes Over Time

Early After Injury

Breathing is most impaired during the early phase after a spinal cord injury. Among patients with cervical lesions, deterioration in breathing ability is common during this time[47]; ventilatory failure is most likely to develop during the first week after injury.[48]

Respiratory function begins to improve within a few weeks of injury, with rapid gains typically seen in the first 5 weeks and continued improvement during the first few months after injury. Vital capacity is likely to double[e] during this time.[17,36] Additional gains in vital capacity may continue to occur for several years after the injury.[49]

A number of factors may contribute to the improvement of respiratory status during the early months after spinal cord injury. Possible contributing factors include motor return, increasing strength in the accessory muscles and diaphragm, return of tone in the intercostals and abdominals with the resolution of spinal shock, and stiffening of the joints of the rib cage.[17,21,31,36,50]

Effect of Aging

Although respiratory function typically improves for a period of time after spinal cord injury, it eventually declines over the years.[22,39,51,52] During sleep, blood oxygenation may decrease and hypercapnia increase despite improvement in measurements of vital capacity in the sitting and supine positions when the patient is awake. These findings, evidence of chronic alveolar hypoventilation, may be caused by normal aging, increased obesity and inactivity, or reduced compliance of the lungs and chest wall with chronic spinal cord injury.[49] Chronic alveolar hypoventilation may cause problems similar to those caused by sleep apnea, described in the following section.[34]

Sleep Apnea

Sleep apnea, characterized by multiple interruptions of breathing during sleep, is common following spinal cord injury. Most estimates of the prevalence of sleep apnea in individuals with spinal cord injury range from 25% to 45%.[34] This compares with an estimated prevalence of 10% or less in the general population.[53–56] Sleep apnea is thought to be under-diagnosed, both in patients with spinal cord injuries[57,58] and in the general population.[53,55,56]

Sleep apnea is more common in people with tetraplegia as opposed to paraplegia, with the highest prevalence associated with C4 and C5[f] motor levels.[58] Completeness of injury is not a significant risk factor.[58–60] Age and time since injury may[60] or may not[58,59] be related to sleep apnea. As is true in the general population, sleep apnea following spinal cord injury is associated with obesity,[g,58,59] higher body-mass index,[58–60] larger neck and abdominal girth,[57,59,60] and male gender.[60]

---

[e] Other studies have shown that pulmonary function improves as time passes after spinal cord injury but have found more variability in the timing and magnitude of these gains.[57,134]

[f] Two small studies of subjects with tetraplegia found no significant association between sleep apnea and lesion level.[59,60]

[g] Obesity is strongly associated with sleep apnea in noninjured individuals and in those with paraplegia, but the association appears to be weaker in individuals with tetraplegia.[58]

Most sleep apnea following spinal cord injury is classified as obstructive: respiratory effort is not interrupted but airflow is blocked by closure of the upper airways.[60] Although the mechanism of sleep apnea after spinal cord injury is unknown, it is likely that it results from a combination of factors. Possible contributing factors related to spinal cord injury include weakness in respiratory muscles, impaired sensory feedback from the chest wall, prevalence of the supine sleep posture, medications, neck muscle hypertrophy, and elevated resistance in the upper airways due to airway hyperreactivity.[57,58,60]

Problems associated with obstructive sleep apnea include sleepiness during the day, cognitive dysfunction, increased sympathetic activity, pulmonary and systemic hypertension, cardiovascular disease, stroke, cardiac arrhythmias, hyperlipidemia, abnormal glucose metabolism, and increased appetite with resulting weight gain.[12,34,53-56,58-60] Sleep apnea may also contribute to the development of atelectasis.[34]

Phonation

After spinal cord injury, speech may be impaired because of inadequate breath support. Breath support for speech requires adequate inspiration, followed by controlled exhalation involving eccentric contraction of the muscles of inhalation.[61] Individuals with midcervical or higher lesions are most likely to experience impairments in phonation. As respiratory status improves with time after injury, phonation should improve.

RESPIRATORY COMPLICATIONS

Respiratory complications are extremely common after spinal cord injury. Factors associated with greater risk of respiratory complications include higher lesion level, advanced age, concomitant thoracic trauma, and a prior history of respiratory disease, aspiration, or smoking.[62-64]

One large study found that the incidence of respiratory complications during the initial acute and rehabilitation hospitalizations was 84% among people with neurological levels of injury between C1 and C4, 60% among those with levels between C5 and C8, and 65% among those with thoracic levels. Pneumonia, ventilatory failure, and atelectasis were the most common respiratory complications among people with neurological levels of injury in the cervical region. Pleural effusion, atelectasis, and pneumothorax or hemothorax were the most prevalent respiratory complications developed by people with thoracic neurological levels of injury.[37]

Most of the respiratory complications associated with spinal cord injury are the result of impaired functioning in the muscles of ventilation.[h] Figure 6–5 illustrates how weakness in the muscles of inspiration and expiration can lead to atelectasis and respiratory failure. Inspiratory muscle weakness results in a reduction in the force of inspiration. Because inspiratory forces are important for maintaining open airways, this reduction in inspiratory force can cause airway closure and atelectasis. Atelectasis causes a loss of surfactant and reduces lung compliance, which results in an increase in the difficulty of breathing. This increased difficulty, combined with weakness in the muscles of inspiration, can lead to respiratory failure.[34] Inadequate strength in the expiratory muscles[i] impairs coughing ability, allowing secretions to accumulate and block the airways. Atelectasis, pneumonia, and respiratory failure can result.[34]

Another factor that can lead to respiratory complications following spinal cord injury is aspiration, which can be caused by gastric reflux or regurgitation combined with positioning (supine) or motor impairments that impede clearance of the airways. Gastrointestinal ileus or slowing, either as a direct result of the neurological injury or due to medications, increase the risk of aspiration.[34,65] Aspiration can also be caused by dysphagia, which is common[j] in

---

[h] Exceptions include pulmonary thromboembolism (discussed in Chapters 2 and 3), pulmonary edema, and complications from chest trauma such as pleural effusion, pneumothorax, and hemothorax.

[i] Inspiratory muscle weakness also impairs coughing ability,[79] because the first stage of an effective cough is the inhalation of a large volume of air.

[j] The reported incidence ranges from 16.6% [69] to 55%.[66]

Problem-Solving Exercise 6–1

Your patient was recently injured in an automobile accident, sustaining a spinal cord injury resulting in complete (ASIA A) C8 tetraplegia.

- List the muscles of inhalation that you would expect to remain fully innervated, partially innervated, and lacking innervation.
- List the muscles used for forced exhalation that you would expect to remain fully innervated, partially innervated, and lacking innervation.

- When the patient lies in a horizontal position, he breathes without any apparent difficulty. When the head of the bed is elevated, his respiratory rate increases and he complains of shortness of breath. Explain the most likely cause of the patient's dyspnea.

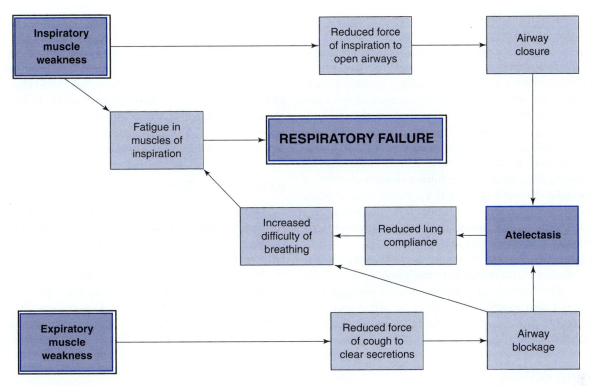

Figure 6–5   Schematic representation of weakness in the muscles of inspiration and expiration leading to atelectasis and respiratory failure.

the acute phase after cervical injury.[66–68] Risk factors for dysphagia include tracheostomy, mechanical ventilation, anterior-approach cervical spine surgery, older age, higher lesion level, and concomitant brain injury.[34,66,67,69] Dysphagia and aspiration can cause atelectasis, pneumonia, mechanical obstruction, and bronchospasm.[34]

Although respiratory complications occur most frequently during the initial postinjury phase,[70] they are not limited to the early weeks or months after injury. Both during the acute phase and in subsequent years, respiratory complications are the most common cause of death among people with spinal cord injuries. Pneumonia in particular is the most prevalent cause of death and causes fatality with greatest frequency when the patient is elderly or has a cervical neurological level of injury.[2,71–73]

EXAMINATION OF RESPIRATORY FUNCTION

A thorough respiratory examination should be performed as soon as feasible after injury. This early examination will make it possible to formulate an appropriate plan of care and establish a baseline against which to compare future findings. The examination should include assessment of strength in the muscles of ventilation, pattern of chest and abdominal motions during breathing, chest excursion, respiratory rate, coughing ability, ability to move air during breathing (pulmonary function testing), posture, and adequacy of breath support for speech. It should also

investigate the presence of respiratory complaints and complicating conditions such as chest injury, a history of smoking, or preexisting pulmonary disease. Additional examination procedures may be indicated during the acute phase after injury or in patients who are at high risk for pulmonary complications.[34]

Respiratory examinations should be repeated periodically during the acute and rehabilitation phases of care and during postdischarge follow-up visits. These examinations will enable the rehabilitation team to monitor progress or deterioration in respiratory status and to respond appropriately.

Strength in the Muscles of Ventilation

Innervation of the ventilatory muscles is the most significant determinant of breathing and coughing ability after spinal cord injury. It follows that an assessment of the strength in these muscles is an important component of the respiratory examination. The results of muscle testing can be used to predict the individual's potential for independent breathing and coughing. The findings of the muscle test will also indicate areas of weakness that should be addressed in a strengthening program.

If the patient's spine is stable, the physical therapist can examine the strength of the accessory muscles and abdominals using standard muscle testing procedures, adapted as indicated. If the spine is not yet stable, the therapist should avoid muscle testing procedures that could cause motion at or create a muscular pull on the affected vertebral area.

Chapter 7 presents additional considerations for manual muscle testing of patients with spinal cord injuries.

The respiratory examination should include an assessment of diaphragmatic function. Although the strength of the diaphragm cannot be examined using a manual muscle test, the therapist can gain some understanding of this muscle's functioning by observing the motion of the patient's abdomen during breathing.[74] With the patient supine, the therapist should watch for protrusion of the abdomen during inhalation. If the diaphragm contracts through its full excursion, the patient will exhibit a normal amount of epigastric rise. Limited or absent epigastric rise indicate impairment in diaphragm functioning. If the patient is on a ventilator, the therapist can disconnect the ventilator briefly to assess epigastric rise during inhalation.[42]

In addition to testing the muscles of ventilation, the therapist should assess strength in the musculature of the trunk and upper extremities. These muscles provide postural support and enable the patient to self-cough and perform trunk and shoulder girdle motions to optimize her ventilatory capacity.

Breathing Pattern

Motions of the abdomen and chest, and visible contractions of the neck accessory muscles, provide information on the patient's breathing ability. Normal epigastric motions indicate good diaphragmatic function. Chest expansion during inhalation gives evidence of intercostal functioning; a paradoxical breathing pattern indicates an absence of intercostal innervation. Visible contraction of the sternocleidomastoids and scalenes during inhalation when the patient is at rest is an indication of diaphragmatic weakness.[42,75]

The therapist can assess the patient's breathing pattern by observing and palpating the patient's abdomen, chest, and neck accessory muscles during breathing. This assessment should be performed with the patient in both the supine and sitting positions, since upright postures alter diaphragmatic functioning when the abdominals are not innervated. The therapist should also note any changes in breathing pattern that occur as a result of increased activity.[42,75]

Chest Excursion

Motions of the rib cage during breathing are a reflection of both ventilatory muscle functioning and chest wall mobility. Chest motions can be assessed using a tape measure with the patient supine. The therapist should measure the chest's diameter at the end of maximal exhalation and at the end of maximal inhalation. The measurements should be taken at the levels of the axilla and the xiphoid process to assess motions of the upper and lower chest, respectively.[42,75] An increase in chest diameter during inhalation is an indication of functioning intercostals. A decrease in chest diameter during inhalation (paradoxical breathing pattern) indicates that intercostal functioning is absent.

In addition to measuring chest diameter before and after inhalation, the therapist can measure the patient's chest after an airshift maneuver is performed. In this maneuver, the patient inhales maximally, closes her glottis, and relaxes her diaphragm while maintaining closure of the glottis. This causes a redistribution of air from the lower chest to the upper chest, with a resulting expansion of the upper chest.[42,76] Using an airshift maneuver, a patient who lacks intercostal innervation can achieve such expansion.

Respiratory Rate

Respiratory rate can be a reflection of the patient's overall respiratory status. In adults, the normal rate of respiration ranges from 12 to 16 breaths per minute.[75,76] Rapid breathing can be an indication that the individual's ventilatory efforts are not adequate to sustain good oxygenation.

People tend to alter their breathing rate if they realize that it is being observed. For this reason, the therapist should assess respiratory rate without the patient's awareness.[42,75] One way to do this is to count the patient's breaths while appearing to take her pulse.

Cough

Coughing ability is crucial to survival; a person who cannot cough effectively will be unable to clear her airways of respiratory secretions or foreign substances that she inadvertently inhales. The therapist should observe as the patient attempts to cough, and note the quality of cough that is produced (Table 6–4). If the patient is unable to generate an effective cough, the therapist should note her performance in each of the stages of cough. The patient may have difficulty with any of the following: inhaling an adequate volume of air, exhaling with adequate force, or opening and closing the glottis with appropriate timing during the cough.[26]

Pulmonary Function Tests

Pulmonary function testing can include a variety of measurements of ventilatory ability (Table 6–1). They can provide objective data to assist in both treatment planning and documentation of progress.

Vital capacity should be assessed every 6[48] to 8[31] hours during the first few days after injury, as the ventilatory status may deteriorate during this time. This test provides a good measure of ventilatory function in people with spinal cord injuries because it correlates significantly with most[k] other

---

[k] Roth et al.[77] performed pulmonary function tests on 52 patients with recent spinal cord injuries (C4 through T6) and found that vital capacity correlated significantly with forced expiratory volume in 1 second, inspiratory capacity, expiratory reserve volume, functional residual capacity, residual volume, total lung capacity, and the residual volume/total lung capacity ratio. Vital capacity did not correlate significantly with maximum positive expiratory pressure or maximum negative inspiratory pressure.

TABLE 6–4   Quality of Cough

Cough Quality	Sound	Number of Coughs Possible per Exhalation	Functional Significance
Functional cough	Loud and forceful	Two or more	Independent in respiratory secretion clearance.
Weak functional cough	Soft, less forceful	One per exhalation	Independent for clearing throat and small amount of secretions. Assistance needed for clearing large amounts of secretions.
Nonfunctional cough	Sigh or throat clearing	No true coughs; cough attempt has no expulsive force	Assistance needed for airway clearance.

Sources: references 42, 75, and 76.

pulmonary function tests.[77] Moreover, assessment of vital capacity is a practical means of examining ventilatory function in today's health care environment because it can be performed using a handheld spirometer, which is portable and inexpensive. If the patient has begun sitting, measurements should be taken in both the supine and sitting positions, as breathing ability is likely to differ between the two.

In addition to assessing vital capacity, the Consortium for Spinal Cord Medicine recommends periodically testing maximal negative inspiratory pressure, and forced expiratory volume in 1 second or peak cough flow.[34] Maximal negative inspiratory pressure can be predictive of ventilatory failure.[17] For individuals using mechanical ventilators, it can provide information on the potential for ventilator weaning.[78] Forced expiratory volume in 1second and peak cough flow provide information about the patient's capacity to cough effectively.[79]

Posture

The respiratory examination should include a postural assessment. The therapist should note any deformities such as thoracic kyphosis or scoliosis that might interfere with chest motion. The therapist should also assess the patient's sitting posture in a wheelchair, investigating whether her body's alignment will enhance or impede the activity of her respiratory muscles and motions of her thorax and abdomen. Any of the following postures can make breathing more difficult: posterior pelvic tilt, thoracic kyphosis, forward shoulders, or forward head.[24]

Breath Support for Speech

The respiratory examination should include an assessment of the patient's breath support for speech. The therapist can ask the patient to inhale maximally and then either count out loud or say "ah" or "oh" for as long as possible in one breath. The therapist can measure this performance by noting the number that the patient can count to, or by timing the phonation. Patients who have better inspiratory capacity

and better eccentric control of their inspiratory muscles will be able to phonate for a longer time with a single breath.[61]

Additional Examination Procedures

The respiratory examination may include additional assessments, particularly during the acute phase following injury and with patients who have severely compromised respiratory systems. Patients can be screened for atelectasis, pneumonia, and pneumothorax by chest x-ray.[31] Fluoroscopy can be used to evaluate diaphragmatic function. Arterial blood gases can be measured to detect levels of oxygen and carbon dioxide in the blood. Noninvasive pulse oximetry can provide ongoing information on the oxygenation of the patient's blood, both at rest and during activity.[17,34,80] Monitoring of the end-tidal pressure of carbon dioxide (Pco_2), also noninvasive, can be used to detect hypercapnia, or an elevated level of carbon dioxide in the blood.[34,49] Monitoring with pulse oximetry and end-tidal Pco_2 can reduce the frequency of arterial blood gas testing needed.[31]

Patients in the acute phase after injury should be screened for risk factors of dysphagia and aspiration.[34] Individuals found to be at risk should be assessed through a clinical evaluation of swallowing, followed by flexible endoscopic evaluation of swallowing (FEES) or a videofluoroscopic swallow study (VFSS) if indicated.[67,68]

Individuals with chronic spinal cord injury who show signs or symptoms of possible sleep-disordered breathing should undergo a polysomnographic evaluation of their breathing during sleep. Indications for evaluation include excessive daytime sleepiness that cannot be explained by other causes, severe snoring, hypertension not responsive to pharmacologic treatment, and persistent nocturnal bradycardia.[34]

*T*HERAPEUTIC INTERVENTIONS

Respiratory function is a critical focus of medical and rehabilitative care after spinal cord injury. This focus should begin soon after injury and continue throughout acute and postacute rehabilitation and postdischarge follow-up.

The respiratory component of a comprehensive rehabilitation program is directed toward the maximization of ventilatory ability and the prevention of pulmonary complications. It includes interventions to ensure adequate ventilation, enhance breathing and coughing ability, mobilize secretions, and provide the patient with the knowledge and skills required to avoid complications after discharge. The specific focus and design of each individual's program will depend on the results of her respiratory evaluation.

Ensuring Adequate Ventilation

The most basic focus of respiratory care after spinal cord injury is ensuring that the patient has adequate motion of air in and out of her lungs. A person who is unable to breathe, or whose breathing ability is inadequate to maintain alveolar ventilation and meet her metabolic needs, will require assistance in ventilation.

A high cervical lesion that results in seriously impaired breathing ability may make it necessary to initiate mechanical ventilation during the emergency phase of management. Mechanical ventilation may also be required in the presence of lower lesions, particularly if concomitant injuries, preexisting respiratory conditions, or advanced age compromise the patient's pulmonary function.

Even if unassisted ventilation is adequate initially, ventilatory ability can deteriorate in the first few days after a spinal cord injury. This decline in ventilatory function can occur as a result of an ascending lesion, atelectasis, accumulation of pulmonary secretions, pneumonia, or fatigue in the muscles of ventilation.[34,81,82] Because of the potential for deterioration, respiratory status should be monitored closely during the initial phase following injury. Repeated checks of arterial blood gases, vital capacity, and chest radiographs will provide information on the patient's status and allow a prompt response if needed. The Consortium for Spinal Cord Medicine recommends seriously considering mechanical ventilation if vital capacity is decreasing and less than 10 to 15 mL/kg of ideal body weight. Arterial blood gas testing (with the patient on room air) showing Po_2 under 50 or Pco_2 over 50 indicates respiratory failure and necessitates mechanical ventilation.[34] Warning signs of impending ventilatory failure include rapid shallow breathing, a drop in maximal negative inspiratory pressure to under 20 cm H_2O,[17] or a tidal volume of 6 mL/kg or less.[22] The patient may experience shortness of breath, increased anxiety, or reduced alertness.[34]

Some individuals with spinal cord injury develop ventilatory insufficiency after years of breathing without mechanical assistance. Late-onset chronic alveolar hypoventilation (CAH) may be due to a decline in vital capacity as a result of aging, obesity, inactivity, or reduced compliance of the lungs and chest walls. Individuals with CAH may exhibit hypersomnolence, frequent sleep arousals, dyspnea, fatigue, sleep-disordered breathing, morning headache, and more frequent respiratory infections. Acute respiratory failure can result.[49,83]

Positive-Pressure Ventilators

Most assisted breathing is achieved using intermittent positive-pressure ventilators (IPPVs). This type of ventilator causes inhalation either by delivering a set volume of air (volume-regulated ventilation) or delivering a set pressure (pressure-regulated ventilation) during inspiration.[32,84] Exhalation occurs as a result of passive recoil of the lungs and chest wall.

Positive-pressure ventilators can work through a variety of modes. These modes differ in the manner in which they support ventilation and in the degree to which they allow for spontaneous breathing (Table 6–5). Ventilation at high volumes may help to prevent or treat atelectasis and pneumonia, and enhance weaning from the ventilator.[31,34,85]

Positive-pressure ventilators are available in both stationary and portable models. With a portable ventilator, the person can be mobile at home and in the community using a power wheelchair.

Both portable and stationary PPVs typically interface with the patient through a tracheostomy tube.[86] Over the past few years, there has been increased focus on noninvasive alternative interfaces for ventilators. This is in part because of the high incidence of complications associated with tracheostomies.[1] Noninvasive positive-pressure ventilation (NPPV) can be provided using oral, nasal, oronasal, or total-face interfaces. During the day, a mouthpiece can be placed close to the user's face so that she can access it for assisted inspirations as needed. At night, a mouthpiece with a lip seal retention system reduces leakage from the mouth and makes it possible for the ventilator to deliver breaths while the user sleeps.[87–90] In general, people who have utilized intermittent positive-pressure ventilation via both tracheostomy and noninvasive alternatives find the noninvasive methods of ventilation preferable in terms of comfort, convenience, appearance, and impact on speaking, swallowing, and glossopharyngeal breathing.[91] Because noninvasive methods of ventilation require specialized skills, ventilation with intubation is recommended for patients in facilities where the staff does not have adequate experience with these techniques.[34]

Alternative Means of Providing Assistance to Ventilation

There are several alternatives to standard positive-pressure ventilators. These alternatives include intermittent abdominal pressure ventilators, negative-pressure body ventilators, biphasic cuirass ventilators, and phrenic nerve stimulators.

Intermittent abdominal pressure ventilators (IAPVs) work by applying intermittent pressure externally to the abdomen. This type of ventilator interfaces with the patient through an inflatable bladder built into an abdominal corset or belt. The corset or belt is worn with the inflatable

---

[1] Numerous severe complications are associated with tracheostomies. These complications result from infections, trauma to the trachea, and impairment of swallowing and airway clearance.[89,92,110]

TABLE 6–5   Modes of Mechanical Ventilation

Mode	Description	Patient's Involvement in Ventilation
Control	The rate and tidal volume are set to deliver a given minute ventilation.	The patient's spontaneous breathing efforts are ignored.
Assist control (AC)	The rate and tidal volume are set to deliver a minimum minute ventilation. If the patient has any spontaneous breathing efforts, these efforts trigger the ventilator to deliver the set tidal volume.	The patient can increase the respiratory rate and minute ventilation by triggering more than the set minimum number of breaths. If the patient has no spontaneous breaths, the ventilator will deliver the preset minimum minute ventilation.
Synchronized intermittent mandatory ventilation (SIMV)	The rate and tidal volume are set to deliver a minimum minute ventilation.	The patient can breathe spontaneously between the breaths delivered by the ventilator.
Pressure-control ventilation (PCV)	The rate and pressure to be delivered during inspiration are set. If the patient has any spontaneous breathing efforts, these efforts trigger the ventilator to deliver the set pressure for inhalation.	The patient can increase the respiratory rate and minute ventilation by triggering more than the set minimum number of breaths. If the patient has no spontaneous breaths, the ventilator will deliver the preset number of breaths.
Pressure-support ventilation (PSV)	The ventilator delivers a set pressure only when triggered by the patient's spontaneous breathing effort.	The patient controls the respiratory rate, tidal volume, timing of inhalation and exhalation, and minute ventilation.
Continuous positive airway pressure (CPAP)	The ventilator delivers positive pressure at the end of exhalation to prevent alveolar collapse.	The patient breathes spontaneously, performing the work of ventilation without assistance from the ventilator.

Source: reference 84.

bladder positioned against the wearer's abdomen. When the positive-pressure ventilator inflates the bladder, it compresses the abdominal contents. This compression causes the abdominal contents to push up against the diaphragm, resulting in exhalation. When the ventilator releases this pressure, gravity pulls the abdominal contents caudally, causing the diaphragm to descend, with resulting inhalation. Because this method of ventilation depends on the force of gravity, an IAPV is effective only when the wearer sits with her trunk elevated at least 30 degrees[m] above horizontal.[90] These ventilators are portable and do not require the presence of artificial airways. They can be used to provide ventilation to people who have no measurable vital capacity or to supplement the breathing efforts of people who are able to breathe to a limited degree on their own.[87,88,92,93]

Negative-pressure body ventilators encompass the torso and cause inhalation by creating a negative pressure on the thorax and abdomen. This results in expansion of the thoracic cavity, causing air to be drawn into the lungs. Examples of this type of ventilator include iron lungs, chest shell (cuirass) negative-pressure ventilators, and wrap-style ventilators.[87,92] The cuirass is the only one of these that can be used in a sitting position.[34] Negative-pressure ventilators are not in common use.[90]

Biphasic cuirass ventilators include a cuirass strapped to the chest anteriorly, and a ventilator that delivers negative pressure to cause inhalation and positive pressure to cause exhalation. Biphasic cuirass ventilators can be used to provide the same patterns of ventilation as positive-pressure ventilators, including synchronized intermittent mandatory ventilation and continuous negative pressure. The latter is analogous to continuous positive airway pressure.[94]

Phrenic nerve stimulators—also called phrenic nerve pacers, diaphragmatic pacemakers, or electrophrenic stimulators—are an alternative to mechanical ventilation for people who have been injured for over a year and have permanently paralyzed diaphragms. Intact phrenic nerves, diaphragm, lungs, and airway are required. Breathing is accomplished through the use of surgically implanted electrodes that stimulate the phrenic nerves.[n] The system includes an external power supply, transmitter and antennas,

---

[m] Intermittent abdominal pressure ventilators work *optimally* when the trunk is 70 to 80 degrees above horizontal.[87]

[n] Alternative approaches under development include stimulation of the diaphragm itself or combined pacing of the diaphragm and intercostals. The latter can be utilized for individuals with only one intact phrenic nerve.[95]

and an implanted receiver and electrodes (Figure 6–6). Typically, a program of diaphragmatic reconditioning is initiated approximately 2 weeks after the receiver and electrodes are implanted. The reconditioning program develops strength and endurance in the diaphragm by pacing for brief periods each hour throughout the day, with the duration of pacing gradually increasing as the patient tolerates.[95]

Diaphragmatic pacing can free the individual from a mechanical ventilator, achieve superior oxygenation, increase comfort, allow more normal speech and breathing patterns, and lower health care costs.[21,95–99] Disadvantages include the risk of phrenic nerve damage, as well as the need for continued use of a tracheostomy in most cases due to the potential for upper airway collapse during sleep.[21,95] Because of the potential for failure of the system, a backup ventilator is generally recommended for the home.[99]

Enhancing Breathing Ability

One of the most important outcomes of respiratory rehabilitation following spinal cord injury is maximization of the patient's ability to breathe. This task is accomplished by teaching the patient an efficient breathing pattern, strengthening the ventilatory musculature, preserving the mobility of the thoracic cage, optimizing posture, and providing abdominal support when needed.

Breathing Pattern

The patient should be encouraged to use a diaphragmatic breathing pattern during quiet breathing, as this pattern is more normal and efficient than an upper chest breathing pattern. To encourage diaphragmatic breathing, the therapist can use verbal and visual cues. If the patient is supine, visual feedback can be provided by placing a large light object, such as a box of tissues, on the abdomen so that the patient can observe its motions as she breathes.

In addition to providing verbal and visual cues, the therapist can provide a quick stretch to facilitate diaphragm contraction. Quick stretch to the diaphragm is performed by pushing the epigastric area in and rostrally immediately prior to asking for the inspiratory effort. Instructing the patient to sniff may also elicit a diaphragmatic response.[61]

Upper chest breathing occurs when the accessory muscles are used for ventilation. Upper chest expansion can be used to increase the volume of inspired air to enhance coughing, improve breath support for speech, or to meet the ventilatory requirements of increased activity. To develop upper chest expansion, the therapist can place her hands against the patient's upper chest and ask her to push against them while breathing in deeply. To facilitate this motion, the therapist can provide a quick stretch to the pectoralis major, sternocleidomastoids, and scalenes by pushing the upper chest in and caudally just before asking for the patient's inspiratory effort.[61]

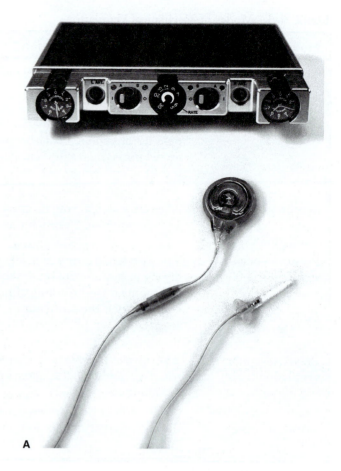

A

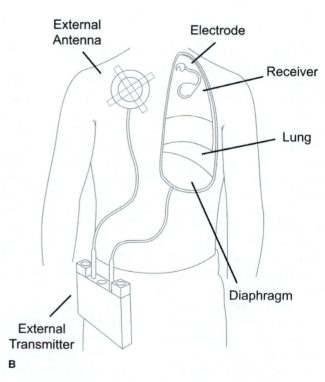

B

Figure 6–6 Phrenic nerve stimulator. (A) Stimulator. (B) Diagram showing stimulator in place. (Reproduced with permission from Avery Biomedical Devices, Inc., Commack, NY.)

Strength and Endurance

In both acute and chronic spinal cord injury, resisted exercises of the muscles of ventilation may[o] increase the strength and endurance of innervated respiratory musculature, improve performance on pulmonary function tests, and reduce the perceived difficulty of breathing.[21,100–104]

Because the diaphragm is the principal muscle of normal inspiration, and because diaphragmatic breathing is more efficient than breathing with the neck muscles,[42] diaphragmatic strengthening is an important component of the exercise program. During initial exercises, the therapist should work with the patient to develop a diaphragmatic breathing pattern. Strategies for teaching diaphragmatic breathing are presented above.

One approach to inspiratory muscle strengthening, resisting the patient's abdominal motion while she breathes, differentially promotes diaphragmatic contraction.[105] The patient can practice breathing deeply while the therapist applies manual resistance to her epigastric area and progress to breathing with weights placed on her abdomen. The weights should allow full epigastric rise during inspiration; a reduced rise during inhalation with the weights in place indicates that the resistance is excessive for the patient. To avoid overfatiguing the diaphragm, the therapist should observe the patient's breathing pattern and stop the exercises or reduce the resistance if the patient begins using her neck accessory muscles for inspiration.[42,75,76,106]

Resistive inspiratory muscle trainers (Figure 6–7) can be a useful alternative to abdominal weight training. Using one of these devices, the patient inhales against resistance. The resistance can be adjusted to accommodate the individual's inspiratory ability, with increasing resistance provided as her ability improves. Use of inspiratory muscle trainers can result in improved strength and endurance in the muscles of ventilation, improved performance on pulmonary function tests,[100–104] slower and deeper breathing both during the training sessions and at rest,[107] reduced use of the neck accessory muscles for inhalation, and increased tolerance for physical activity.[103] Because resistive inspiratory muscle trainers are small and can be self-administered, they can be useful tools for continued respiratory exercise after discharge.[101]

In addition to a strengthening program for the inspiratory muscles, the patient may benefit from exercises that develop strength in her trunk and upper extremities. These muscles provide postural support and enable the patient to perform trunk and shoulder girdle motions to optimize ventilatory capacity.

Once the patient is medically able to participate in aerobic activities, aerobic training may be another beneficial component of the respiratory rehabilitation program. Arm cranking exercises have been shown to improve ventilatory

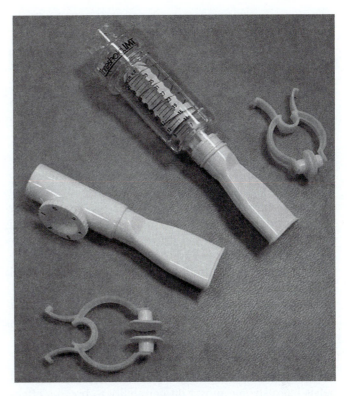

Figure 6–7   Resistive inspiratory muscle trainers, shown with nose clips.

muscle endurance in subjects with long-standing thoracic spinal cord injuries.[108]

Eccentric Control of Exhalation

Patients who have impaired eccentric control of exhalation may benefit from exercises directed at developing this control. Eccentric control of exhalation is required for normal speech production.

To develop eccentric control of exhalation, the patient can practice inhaling maximally and counting or saying "ah" or "oh" for as long as possible before taking another breath. If she can develop the ability to phonate for 10 to 12 seconds, she may be better able to speak normally.[61] The therapist can promote the development of eccentric control by applying manual vibration or resistance to the patient's chest wall during the exhalation.[61]

Glossopharyngeal breathing

Many people whose ability to breathe is severely limited can learn to use glossopharyngeal breathing to increase the volume of air that they can inhale. This technique involves using the tongue and pharyngeal musculature to force air into the lungs in a series of "gulps." This added volume of inspired air can assist with breath support for speech or coughing, improve oxygenation to allow more physical activity, and expand the lungs to enhance chest mobility. Glossopharyngeal breathing can also make it possible for people with high cervical lesions and no diaphragmatic function to breathe on their own for limited periods of time (in some cases for hours[92,109,110]) in the event that their ventilators are

---

[o] Because of a lack of randomized controlled trials and inconsistency in research findings, further study is required to determine the efficacy of inspiratory muscle training following spinal cord injury.[135,136]

disconnected or cease to function.[31,61,75,87,92,111] If the individual has a tracheostomy, it must be plugged or have a one-way speaking valve in place for effective glossopharyngeal breathing to occur.[111]

Teaching glossopharyngeal breathing is a highly specialized skill. Therapists who have not undergone training in this area should refer appropriate patients to therapists who are capable of teaching glossopharyngeal breathing.

Chest Wall Mobility

Chest wall mobility is an important focus of respiratory rehabilitation following spinal cord injury. When the muscles of inhalation are impaired, the rib cage does not move through its normal excursions as the individual breathes, and the chest wall stiffens as a result. Lung compliance is also reduced. Both of these factors increase the work of breathing.[103] Range of motion in the chest wall can be preserved or improved through deep-breathing exercises, passive stretching, joint mobilization, intermittent positive-pressure breathing, glossopharyngeal breathing, and air-shift maneuvers.[42,75,76,106,112]

Posture

The alignment of a person's spine, shoulder girdle, and pelvis has a strong impact on her ability to breathe effectively. Sitting posture is particularly important after spinal cord injury because of the amount of time that the individual is likely to spend in sitting. Sitting with an anteriorly tilted pelvis, erect trunk, adducted scapulae, and neutral head and neck alignment will enhance breathing by placing the ribs and accessory muscles in mechanically advantageous positions.[113] During rehabilitation after spinal cord injury, posture should be optimized through exercise, functional training, and the acquisition of appropriate seating equipment.

Abdominal Support

As described earlier in this chapter, patients with paralysis of the abdominal musculature breathe less effectively in sitting than in the supine position. To address this problem, an abdominal binder or corset can be used during out-of-bed activities to contain the abdominal contents and position the diaphragm for more effective function. These devices have been shown to improve a variety of measurements in sitting, including vital capacity, tidal volume, maximal expiratory pressure, and blood oxygenation.[22,31,34,36,75,106,112,114,115]

In most cases, abdominal binders or corsets can be used as a temporary measure to ease the transition to upright activities. As a person's breathing capacity improves, the binder or corset can be loosened gradually over a period of days, and finally discontinued as the patient accommodates to breathing without it.

Weaning From the Ventilator

Many people with spinal cord injuries, particularly those who have cervical lesions, require mechanical ventilators during the acute phase after injury. Most who have a neurological level of injury at C3 or lower are able to regain the capacity to breathe independently.[33,35] Factors that can reduce a person's potential to wean from a ventilator include respiratory or other medical complications, preexisting respiratory conditions, age over 50 years, a vital capacity under 1000, maximal negative inspiratory pressure less than 30 cm H_2O, and a history of smoking.[15,78,82]

When a ventilator is used during the acute or rehabilitation phase of hospitalization after injury, the therapeutic program should work toward developing the capacity to breathe without this mechanical assistance. Even when a patient lacks the potential to develop complete independence from mechanical ventilation, a ventilator weaning program may enable her to gain the capacity to breathe independently for brief periods. This ability may enhance her survival potential in the event of power failure, ventilator failure, or accidental disconnection.[33,34,82] It may also allow her to be off of the ventilator for brief periods during activities such as transfers, bathing, or tracheostomy care, or for longer periods for various other activities during the day.[34]

Ventilator weaning involves gradually reducing the patient's dependence on a ventilator. Although there are several approaches to ventilator weaning, one method has been used most successfully for people with spinal cord injuries and others who have difficulty developing independence from a ventilator. This approach to weaning, progressive ventilator-free breathing (PVFB), involves disconnecting the patient from the ventilator for increasing lengths of time. This process can start with the patient breathing independently for as little as 1 or 2 minutes at a time. Between sessions she continues to use a ventilator. As her breathing ability develops, the duration and frequency of ventilator-free breathing sessions can be increased.[17,33,78,86,116] Initial independent breathing sessions should take place with the patient supine,[P] as unassisted breathing will be easier in this position.[15,31,35,82,86]

[P] Patients with central cord syndrome who have intact intercostals but paralyzed diaphragms may breathe easier with their heads elevated rather than in the supine position.[31]

Problem-Solving Exercise 6–2

Your patient with complete (ASIA A) C4 tetraplegia exhibits visible contraction of her neck accessory muscles during quiet breathing. Design a treatment program that will decrease her reliance on her accessory muscles for breathing.

The patient is more likely to develop ventilator independence if the respiratory program includes inspiratory muscle training[15,117,118] and other measures to enhance breathing capacity, as described earlier in this chapter. The management of secretions is also critical for ventilator weaning,[78,118] as the accumulation of secretions will increase the work of breathing and lead to the development of respiratory complications.

Clearing Secretions

An inability to cough effectively leads to the accumulation of secretions within the lungs. Enforced recumbency after spinal cord injury compounds the problem. Retention of secretions can lead to atelectasis, pneumonia, and respiratory insufficiency. These complications can be avoided with appropriate management. Acutely following injury, patients with impaired respiratory ability are treated prophylactically with postural drainage and percussion and vibration of the chest.[17,31,81] Some specialty beds can provide positioning and vibration to enhance the clearance of secretions.[31] Intermittent positive-pressure breathing (IPPB) may also be used prophylactically or as an adjunct to these treatments when patients exhibit retention of secretions and atelectasis.[17,35] Tracheal and bronchial suctioning may be required to clear secretions, especially when the patient has a tracheostomy or a respiratory tract infection.

Postural drainage, percussion, vibration, IPPB, and suctioning are standard techniques used by respiratory and physical therapists. These techniques can be adapted as indicated to accommodate each individual's medical and orthopedic needs. Additional strategies utilized to enhance the clearance of secretions following spinal cord injury include manually assisted coughing, mechanical insufflation–exsufflation, self-coughing, positional changes, and muscle strengthening.[q]

Manually Assisted Coughing

Manually assisted coughing is an effective means of helping people who lack abdominal musculature clear their respiratory secretions by achieving forceful expiration while coughing.[119–121] To assist in a cough, the person providing the assistance applies force to the patient's abdomen or chest to push air out of the lungs. This maneuver should be coordinated with the patient's voluntary efforts at coughing after maximal inhalation.

There are several approaches to providing a manually assisted cough.[26,31,42,75,122] Probably the simplest technique involves a Heimlich-like maneuver (abdominal thrust). Using this technique, the helper pushes up and in on the patient's epigastric area, taking care to avoid applying force over the xiphoid process (Figure 6–8). An alternative technique involves applying inward and caudally directed forces to the lower lateral ribs. Either of these cough-assist techniques can be administered with the patient in the supine or side-lying position or sitting in a wheelchair. In a third technique, which can be applied with the patient in the supine, semisupine, or side-lying position, the therapist applies force to the patient's upper chest and lower chest or abdomen. A final technique, which involves applying rotational forces to the patient's trunk, is provided in the side-lying position only. The appropriate choice of assisted coughing technique will depend on such factors as medical or orthopedic restrictions,[r] the position of the patient when she needs to cough, effectiveness of cough production with each method, and the preferences of both the person coughing and the person providing assistance.

Regardless of the technique employed for cough assistance, the patient can enhance the cough's effectiveness by participating in all phases of the cough. Instruction in cough assistance should include the steps of cough and the actions that the patient and helper will perform during the assisted cough (Table 6–6). Both patient and helper are likely to require practice to develop optimal timing.

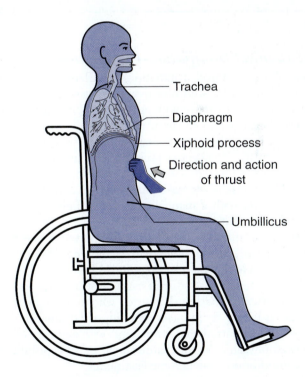

Figure 6–8 Assisted cough, using a Heimlich-like maneuver.

---

[q] Cough can also be elicited by activating the abdominal musculature using surface electrical stimulation, spinal cord stimulation, or functional magnetic stimulation.[28,29,120,121,137–139] These methods remain experimental.

[r] Precautions include any conditions that could make application of force to the thorax or abdomen hazardous. Examples are abdominal surgery, osteoporosis or fractures of the ribs,[119] an abdominal aortic aneurysm,[21] and the presence of a new inferior vena cava filter.[31]

TABLE 6–6 Instructions to Patient for Manually Assisted Coughing

Instructions to the Patient	Strategies to Enhance Performance	Purpose
1. Breathe as deeply as possible.	• If possible, combine inhalation with trunk and neck extension as well as shoulder flexion or scapular adduction. • If needed, the patient can use glossopharyngeal breathing to augment inhalation. If the patient is unable to inhale adequately unassisted, the helper may provide a deep breath using a ventilator, manual ventilation bag, positive-pressure blower, or IPPB machine.	• The positional changes listed will help maximize the volume of inspired air, which in turn will make it possible to generate a more effective cough. • The patient must inhale an adequate volume of air in order to cough effectively.
2. Hold breath briefly.	• Allow adequate time for inspiration prior to the "hold" phase of the cough.	• Closure of the glottis is required to allow a buildup of intrathoracic pressure for the expulsion phase of the cough.
3. Cough.	• If possible, combine forced exhalation with trunk and neck flexion, and shoulder extension or scapular abduction. • The helper should apply the cough-assist forces just prior to the opening of the patient's glottis, and continue applying force as the patient coughs.	• The positional changes listed will help maximize the force and velocity of the exhalation, which in turn will make it possible to generate a more effective cough. • Application of force prior to and after opening of the glottis will maximize the velocity and force of the expired air.

Sources: References 28, 42, 75, 89, 113, and 122.

Mechanical Insufflation–Exsufflation

Use of a mechanical insufflation–exsufflation (MI-E) device (Figure 6–9) is an effective alternative to suctioning or manually assisted coughing.[31,123,124] This device provides a deep breath to the patient through positive pressure, followed by forced exsufflation ("sucking the air out"[34]) created by negative pressure. The treatment can be administered through a face mask, mouthpiece, or endotracheal or tracheostomy tube. An MI-E may be used in combination with a manually-assisted cough when there are no contraindications to the latter.[27,31,34,92,119,123,125] Mechanical insufflation-exsufflation is reported to be more effective and comfortable than suctioning.[31,123,124,126] It can be used in inpatient settings and at home.[123,124]

MI-E should be used with caution in patients with recent cervical spinal cord injuries who remain in spinal shock, as it may result in severe bradyarrhythmias in these cases.[92] It is contradicted for patients with a history of bullous emphysema, recent barotrauma, or susceptibility to pneumothorax or pneumomediastinum.[31,123]

Self-Cough

One disadvantage of both manually assisted coughing and mechanical insufflation-exsufflation is that they require the presence of a helper. A person who cannot cough effectively without assistance may not cough as frequently as needed, since a helper will not always be available. As a result, respiratory complications will be more likely to develop.[11,120]

Most people with C5 or lower spinal cord injuries are able to learn self-cough techniques to "assist" their own coughs.[26,122] This capability is an important survival skill, as it makes it possible to clear secretions independently.

Self-coughing can be performed using a Heimlich-like maneuver by pushing up and in on the epigastric area

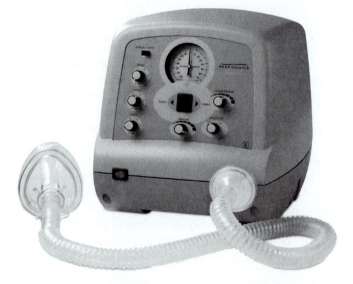

Figure 6–9 CoughAssist® mechanical insufflation–exsufflation device. (Used with permission of Philips Respironics, Inc., Murrysville, PA.)

while coughing. The strategies presented in Table 6–6 for maximizing cough effectiveness can be utilized during a self-cough. For example, a person who cannot generate adequate cough force using her upper extremities may be able to enhance her cough by falling forward from a sitting position while coughing. By flexing her trunk and neck while falling forward and pushing on her epigastric area, she may be able to expel air more forcefully.[75,22]

Positional Changes

Frequent changes in position are also helpful in mobilizing secretions.[82] When a person lies in bed in one position for prolonged periods, fluid accumulates in the dependent portions of her lungs. Regular changes in position help to alleviate this problem by preventing each area of the lung from being dependent too long.[76,127,128] As an alternative to regular turning on standard hospital beds, patients can be placed on rotating beds that keep them in constant motion (Figures 3–3 and 6–10). These beds may prevent the buildup of secretions within the lungs and reduce the incidence of pulmonary complications.[17,70] Additionally, early activity out of bed can help to mobilize secretions. As soon as it is medically and orthopedically feasible, patients should begin participating in out-of-bed activities.

Strengthening

Strengthening the muscles of exhalation may result in improved cough ability. Patients with innervated abdominal musculature can perform standard strengthening exercises of these muscles, adapted as needed to accommodate profound weakness or orthopedic restrictions. Individuals who lack abdominal musculature but have function in the clavicular portions of the pectoralis majors (C5 and 6 innervation) can use these muscles for forced exhalation. Strengthening of these muscles can lead to an improved capacity for forced exhalation, as evidenced by an increase in expiratory reserve volume.[38]

Strengthening the inspiratory muscles can also enhance cough ability, since efficient coughing requires inhalation of an adequate volume of air. A small study of patients with cervical injuries found that maximum negative inspiratory pressure correlated with peak cough flow in both unassisted and assisted coughing.[79]

Finally, patients may benefit from exercises that develop strength in innervated muscles of the back, shoulder girdle, and upper extremities. These muscles provide postural support and enable the patient to perform trunk and shoulder girdle motions to optimize the capacity for inhalation and forced exhalation.

Treatment of Sleep Apnea

The most common treatment for sleep apnea is continuous positive airway pressure (CPAP) therapy. CPAP delivers pressurized air through a nasal or oral/nasal mask while the individual sleeps, preventing airway collapse. Acceptance of CPAP therapy may be relatively low because of mask discomfort, interference with sleep, and claustrophobia. Alternative treatments for sleep apnea can be tried but have not been studied in patients with spinal cord injury. These treatments include enhancing airway patency during sleep using bilevel positive airway pressure (BiPAP),[s] upper airway surgery, or dental appliances.[34,129] Tracheostomies can also be used in severe cases.[34]

Education and Training

Respiratory complications pose a very real threat to the health and survival of a person with a spinal cord injury. Before patients are discharged from the inpatient phase of their rehabilitation programs, they should obtain the knowledge and skills that will be necessary to avoid these complications. If family members or others will be assisting in care after discharge, they too should be included in the education and training. Areas of knowledge to develop include potential respiratory complications, their prevention and early signs, and appropriate measures to take if complications occur. Skills to develop include techniques for secretion clearance and a home program of respiratory exercises for strength, endurance, and chest wall mobility. If a mechanical ventilator or electrophrenic stimulator is used, patients and those involved in their care must learn how to operate these devices.[t] They must also learn techniques for

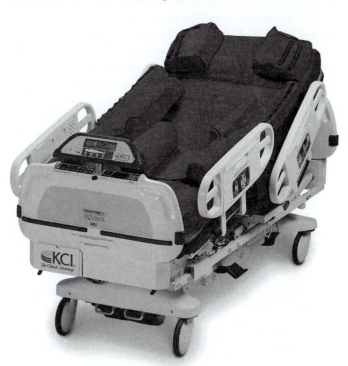

Figure 6–10   Bed providing rotation to enhance pulmonary health. (Courtesy of KCI Licensing, Inc. 2009.)

---

s BiPAP is a variation of CPAP that delivers different pressures during inspiration and expiration.[129]

t Even if the individual using the ventilator lacks the physical ability to operate it, she should be able to instruct others.

Problem-Solving Exercise 6–3

Your patient has incomplete C6 tetraplegia, ASIA C. He is unable to cough effectively without assistance.

- What examination procedures would you perform?

- Design a treatment program that would enhance the patient's independence in effective coughing.

---

providing adequate ventilation in the event of mechanical failure.

Most people with high tetraplegia return to home environments after discharge, and most utilize attendant care. This care is most frequently provided by aides rather than nurses, and the patient is likely to be the one who trains the attendant.[130] Although the rehabilitation team may be able to provide education and training to attendants who will be involved in the patient's care immediately after discharge, this task will fall on the patient or family in the years that follow. For this reason, both patients and their families should learn how to instruct others regarding respiratory care.

In addition to the education and training described in the preceding paragraphs, smoking cessation programs should be available to patients who smoke.[131] Smoking further compromises the functioning of an already impaired respiratory system[39] and increases the risk of mortality following spinal cord injury.[132] Finally, patients should be encouraged to receive influenza (yearly) and pneumococcal (every 5 years) vaccinations to help prevent respiratory infections.[71,131]

Summary

- Breathing is accomplished through cyclic changes of the volume within the thoracic cavity; increases and decreases in the space within this cavity cause inhalation and exhalation, respectively. The motions involved in breathing occur as a result of the coordinated action of the diaphragm, scalenes, accessory muscles, intercostals, and abdominal musculature.

- Coughing involves the following sequence of actions: maximal inhalation, glottis closure, contraction of the muscles of forced exhalation with the glottis closed, and continued forced exhalation with the glottis open.

- Spinal cord injury that results in paralysis of any of the muscles of ventilation will interfere with normal breathing and coughing. This can occur when the neurological level of injury is T12 or higher. With complete lesions, the level of injury determines the extent to which breathing and coughing are impaired. Higher lesions result in impairment of both inhalation and exhalation. Lower lesions interfere less with inhalation, but coughing remains impaired. The extent to which incomplete lesions interfere with breathing and coughing depends on both the level of injury and the amount of motor sparing below the lesion.

- Because spinal cord injury impairs breathing and coughing, respiratory complications are common and pose a significant threat to the individual's health and survival.

- The respiratory component of a rehabilitation program after spinal cord injury should begin soon after injury and continue through postdischarge follow-up. The program is directed at maximizing breathing and coughing ability and minimizing the potential for respiratory complications.

Suggested Resources

ORGANIZATIONS

American Association for Respiratory Care: *www.aarc.org*
International Ventilator Users Network: *www.ventusers.org*

PUBLICATIONS

Clinical practice guidelines published by Paralyzed Veterans of America, available for free download from *www.pva.org*:

- *Respiratory Management Following Spinal Cord Injury: A Clinical Practice Guideline for Health-Care Professionals,* 2005.

Frownfelter D, Dean E, eds. *Cardiovascular and Pulmonary Physical Therapy: Evidence and Practice,* 4th ed. St. Louis: Mosby Elsevier, 2006.

7

Physical Therapy Examination, Evaluation, and Goal Setting

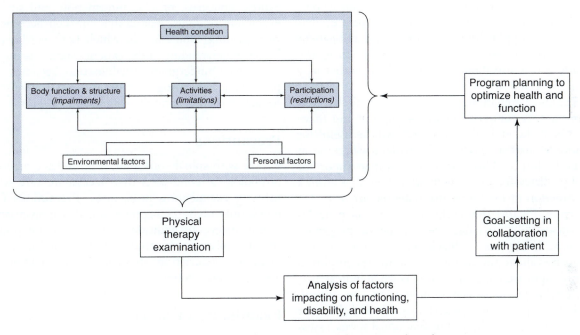

Chapter 7 presents information on physical therapy examination, evaluation and goal setting.

The purpose of rehabilitation is to enhance health and function. Appropriate intervention must be based on a careful analysis of the factors that may affect the patient's current and future health as well as those that contribute to his activity limitations and participation restrictions. This analysis starts with an examination of the patient's physical and functional status, as well as other areas relevant to health and function. After identifying the individual's impairments and activity limitations (functional limitations), the therapist makes an estimation of the patient's potential for functional gains. The findings of this assessment are then considered in the context of the patient's priorities, role requirements, social support systems, physical environment, and resources. Together the patient and therapist establish goals aimed at optimizing health, activities, and social participation.

EXAMINATION AND EVALUATION

Examination and evaluation are the foundations of any physical therapy program.[a] The physical therapist requires a thorough and accurate understanding of the patient's status in order to identify areas of strength and weakness, and

---

[a] The American Physical Therapy Association makes a distinction between examination, which involves gathering data, and evaluation, which involves making clinical judgments based on the examination results.[48]

potential roadblocks to progress. The therapist's evaluation of this data provides the basis for the development of goals and a plan of action tailored to the individual involved.

In addition to providing the information required for setting goals and planning treatment, the therapist's examination establishes a baseline. Documentation of the patient's initial status is needed for later comparison, facilitating the detection of any improvement or deterioration in the patient's condition.

The evaluation process should continue throughout the program. This is not to say that complete, formal evaluations should be performed continually. Rather, the therapist should remain aware of the patient's changing status. By monitoring any significant changes in physical and functional status, the therapist obtains feedback on the program's effectiveness. This feedback allows for adjustments to be made as appropriate.

Periodically, the therapist should perform a more complete reexamination and evaluation. These repeat evaluations provide the opportunity for the therapist and patient to assess progress, reassess goals, and update the program. Reevaluations can also direct attention to areas that may have been neglected inadvertently.

A thorough examination and evaluation at discharge is also important. A complete record of physical and functional status at the end of the program will be useful for health professionals with whom the patient will come in contact in the future. This evaluation is also an important source of feedback for the patient, who should be given a clear explanation of his status and potential areas for future progress. Finally, the discharge evaluation provides another opportunity to judge the therapeutic program's effectiveness. With this feedback on the program, the clinician can evaluate the therapeutic strategies employed and alter his approach to future patients when indicated.

After discharge, follow-up examinations are critical. During follow-up examinations, the patient and therapist can identify changes in physical or functional status, assess the patient's level of community reintegration, and determine whether additional services are indicated. They can also identify and address equipment needs during these visits. Perhaps the most efficient and effective approach to follow-up examinations is a clinic in which multiple members of the rehabilitation team are present. Individuals attending the clinic can then undergo a comprehensive multidisciplinary examination that addresses their various medical, orthopedic, psychosocial, and functional needs.

Cooperative Approach

The initial examination often constitutes the first contact between a health professional and a patient, and thus sets the stage for future interactions. Unfortunately this examination sometimes involves the pokings and proddings of an "expert" who approaches the patient as an object rather than as another person who happens to be a patient at the moment. When this occurs, the health professional dominates

the interaction, issuing commands and noting responses. Another unfortunate thing that can occur during evaluations is health professionals "protecting" their patients from evaluation results, filtering or sugar-coating their findings. This practice may stem from a belief that the information will somehow damage the patient. It may also be due to health professionals' own discomfort regarding communicating bad news to patients.

Whatever the reason behind these approaches to evaluation, they can have a negative impact. By assuming total command of the situation, by treating the person with a spinal cord injury as less than equal, and by withholding information, the health professional communicates to the patient that he is helpless and should assume a passive role.

To provide a more constructive experience, the therapist should include the patient as an active participant in the evaluation. This involves encouraging the patient to express concerns, provide information, and share in any evaluation findings. The evaluation then becomes a positive learning experience in which both parties achieve a better understanding of the patient's status. As importantly, the person undergoing rehabilitation becomes an active participant in his program from the outset. The stage is set for active participation throughout the program.

Precautions

People with spinal cord injuries often have orthopedic or physiological conditions that necessitate care when performing examination procedures. Precautions for treatment, presented in Chapter 8, are also appropriate during examinations. In addition to these general precautions, the therapist should note and abide by any medical or orthopedic restrictions that have been placed on the individual patient's activities.

Examination Content

Any complete physical therapy examination includes subjective statements and a history. The examination of someone who has had a spinal cord injury should also include an assessment of the areas of physical functioning that are directly affected by damage to the cord, as well as the areas in which secondary conditions are likely to occur. The physical therapist should also investigate the patient's functional capabilities, equipment needs, and home environment. Examinations performed after discharge from inpatient rehabilitation may include measures of participation.

History and Subjective Statements
Information for the history can be gathered by reading the medical record and interviewing the patient, family members, and others close to the patient. The history should contain any information relevant to the individual's physical or psychosocial status, prognosis, preinjury functional status, and discharge plans. This information will affect

goal setting and the therapeutic strategies employed during rehabilitation.

The therapist should document any relevant statements made by the patient or others that provide information on such matters as the patient's emotional state, concerns, or understanding of the injury. The patient's stated goals should also be included, as they give insight into his priorities.

A history should include the date, level, extent, and etiology of the damage to the spinal cord, any complications or additional injuries sustained at or since the time of the cord injury, and a brief summary of the medical and surgical management received since the injury. It should also note any changes in neurological status that have occurred since the injury. Any preexisting medical conditions that could impact on the person's health or functional status should also be documented. In addition, the history should include a brief summary of any rehabilitation that the patient has undergone since the time of the injury, and a description of his functioning since the injury.

In addition to obtaining information on the patient's medical history, the therapist should investigate social issues, getting a sense of the patient's social environment as well as his roles and participation in life situations prior to and since the injury. Pertinent areas to investigate include vocation and avocations, living arrangements prior to the injury, expected discharge destination, social support available, and the patient's accustomed roles within the various social arenas such as home, work, school, and the community at large.

Voluntary Motor Function

Motor function is one of the most important factors that affect a person's abilities following spinal cord injury; his ultimate potential for physical activities is largely dependent upon the musculature that remains innervated. The results of the manual muscle test[b] are used to predict the level of functional independence that an individual can expect to achieve, and to identify areas of weakness that should be addressed in a strengthening program.

Motor function is also significant in that it is a reflection of neurological status. The neurological level of injury is in part defined by the strength that the patient exhibits in the key muscles representative of each cord segment.[c] These key muscles, described by the American Spinal Injury Association (ASIA),[1] are shown in Figure 7–1. An accurate and complete baseline muscle test will allow comparison to future findings. This is especially important when the cord injury has occurred very recently, because at this stage, it is not unusual for improvement or deterioration of neurological function to occur.

---

[b] Manual muscle testing is the most frequently used method of assessing muscle strength in clinical settings, and is recommended by the American Spinal Injury Association. Alternative strategies include handheld and isokinetic dynamometry.[83,84]

[c] The ASIA classification system is explained in Chapter 2.

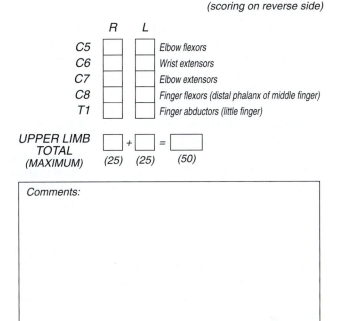

Figure 7–1 Motor portion of the scoring form for the International Standards for Neurological Classification of Spinal Cord Injury. (Reproduced with permission from the American Spinal Injury Association.)

In addition to providing information on the patient's current neurological status, motor function below the lesion during the acute phase after injury can be an indicator of possible future motor return.[2–7] Thus, the results of early muscle tests are important for patient education as well as for making predictions regarding future motor recovery and functional potentials.

Muscles to Be Tested

A specific manual muscle test is required for accurate assessment of motor function following spinal cord injury. The therapist should test all key muscles on both sides of the body.[d] After testing these muscles, the therapist can calculate the patient's upper- and lower-limb motor scores by adding the scores for all of the key muscles in the upper and lower extremities, respectively (Figure 7–1). These scores may be useful for documentation of changes in motor function.[8] When performing a muscle test, the therapist should never assume that all musculature above the diagnosed level of lesion is functioning normally. A therapist who makes this assumption will miss any pre-existing weakness or previously undetected signs of neurological damage. To avoid this oversight, all key muscles innervated above the lesion should be tested.

In like manner, the therapist should not assume that motor function is absent below the lesion. When examining an extremity that appears to lack any motor function, it can be tempting to check only a muscle or two, or even to forgo the muscle test altogether. This can lead to inaccurate results, with spared motor function going undetected. To avoid this problem, the therapist should test all key muscles at and below the neurological level of injury.

Certain muscles are functionally relevant but not identified as key muscles. This group includes the deltoids; serratus anterior; latissimus dorsi; trunk musculature; hip extensors, abductors, and adductors; and hamstrings. In extremities where voluntary motor function is found in the key muscles, the therapist should test the strength in other functionally relevant muscles. Additional musculature can be tested as indicated and as time allows.

Substitution

People with spinal cord injuries quickly learn to use functioning musculature to perform the actions of muscles that are weakened or absent. For example, the anterior deltoid can be used to extend the elbow in the absence of triceps function, and the radial wrist extensors can be used to flex the fingers in the absence of any functioning finger flexors (tenodesis grasp). These compensations can give the appearance of normal or partial functioning in musculature that is paralyzed. To prevent substitution during a muscle test,

---

[d] For the purpose of ASIA classification, muscles are scored without using + or − grades. Figure 2–11 in Chapter 2 presents the complete worksheet and definitions of muscle grades.

the therapist should eliminate motions at other joints and carefully palpate the muscle being tested to verify that it is contracting.

Stabilization

Musculature normally used for stabilization during manual muscle testing may be weak or absent. Failure to accommodate for this impaired ability to stabilize can make muscles appear to be weaker than they are. For example, someone with normal (5/5) deltoids and a weak serratus anterior may give the appearance of having weak deltoids during a manual muscle test. He may be able to perform the test motion without resistance, but scapular instability will enable the therapist to "break" the position with less than 5/5 force.

A person's ability to stabilize his entire body must also be taken into account during muscle testing. For example, someone who has recently sustained a cervical or thoracic injury may not have learned how to stabilize his trunk while sitting upright in a wheelchair. During manual muscle testing of his deltoids, he will be unable to maintain the test position against 5/5 force; his inability to stabilize his trunk will make his deltoids appear weak. Thus, if a therapist does not provide the needed trunk stabilization during muscle testing, the test results will be inaccurate.

To obtain accurate results, the therapist must stabilize the patient appropriately. Whenever stabilizing musculature is weak or absent, the therapist must provide the needed stability.

Muscle Tone Considerations During Muscle Testing

Involuntary contraction can occur when a muscle is being tested, making the muscle appear to be stronger than it actually is. Since abnormal tone can affect muscle test results, its presence should be noted when muscle strength is documented. In addition, the therapist must distinguish between voluntary and involuntary motor function. To make this distinction, the therapist should ask the patient to contract and relax the muscle on command.

Limiting Conditions

Orthoses and orthopedic restrictions often interfere with standard positioning for manual muscle testing. When this is the case, the therapist should simply adapt the tests by performing them in the best positions possible within

---

Problem-Solving Exercise 7–1

According to the medical record, your patient has complete (ASIA A) C6 tetraplegia. You are performing her initial examination.

- What muscles should you test for strength?

When you are testing for strength in her finger flexors, she is able to flex her fingers through about half of the available range.

- What should you do to determine whether the patient performs this motion by contracting her finger flexors or through muscle substitution?

Problem-Solving Exercise 7–2

You are performing a manual muscle test on your patient's anterior deltoid while he sits in a wheelchair. He is able to flex his shoulder to 90 degrees, but he is unable to maintain that position when you apply downward force on his arm.

- How can you determine whether he is exhibiting weak deltoids, weak serratus anterior, or both?
- Describe how you could muscle test the anterior deltoid and serratus anterior separately.

---

the limitations. The adaptations in muscle test procedure should be documented.

Precautions

If the spine is not yet stable, the therapist should exercise caution when testing musculature. Strong contraction of muscles that may exert a pull on the affected vertebral area should be avoided. For example, it is prudent to avoid resistance to the hip flexors if the patient has an unstable lumbar fracture.

Trunk Musculature

Testing trunk musculature presents a unique problem. The standard tests for the abdominals and back extensors assume that the musculature is functioning along its entire length. This is often not the case after a spinal cord injury. For example, a patient may have strong contraction of the rectus abdominis from the ribs to the umbilicus and no contraction below this level. What grade can be assigned to this muscle? Instead of trying to assign a grade to the musculature in such instances, it may be more meaningful to focus on identifying the approximate myotome levels in which the musculature functions.

The position of the umbilicus during muscle testing can be used as an indicator of function in the abdominal musculature. If it remains central during testing, this indicates that there is a uniform pull in the abdominals; abdominal musculature functions uniformly above, below, and to either side of the umbilicus. For this condition to exist, the abdominals are either absent or functioning uniformly along their entire length; the level of motor paralysis must be either above T5 or below T12. The therapist should palpate to determine which of these is the case. If the umbilicus moves cephalad during testing (Beevor's sign), the muscular pull is greater above the umbilicus than below; the lesion lies between T5 and T12. If the umbilicus moves to the side, the musculature is stronger on the side toward which it moves.

As is true with abdominal musculature, standard manual muscle testing for the back extensors is not appropriate when this musculature is not innervated along its entire length. When testing the back extensors, the therapist can palpate the paraspinals while the patient attempts back extension.

Sensation

Like voluntary motor function, sensation is directly affected by spinal cord injury and is a reflection of neurological status. Pin prick and light touch sensation at key points in each dermatome are used along with motor function to determine the patient's neurological level of injury.[1] Improvement or deterioration in neurological function can be evidenced by a change in sensation. Moreover, spared sensation below the lesion, particularly spared pin prick, during the acute phase after injury can be an indicator of possible future motor return.[3,5,7]

Sensation also has an impact on the capacity to perform functional skills, though to a smaller degree than does strength. A person who has intact proprioception and touch sensation in an extremity will find it easier to learn to use that extremity. For example, learning to propel a wheelchair will be easier if some touch sensation is present in the hands, and intact proprioception in the lower extremities will make it easier to control the legs during ambulation.

Pain sensation is particularly important because it serves to protect the skin. The normal reaction to pain is to withdraw from the stimulus, thus avoiding or reducing damage to the skin. Without this protection, an area that lacks pain sensitivity is more vulnerable to trauma. People who lack protective sensation need to know about this vulnerability and must take measures to avoid trauma to insensate areas.

Sensation to Be Tested

The therapist should test sensitivity to both pin prick and light touch in all of the key sensory points on both sides of the body. As is true with motor testing, sensory testing should be performed at all key points regardless of whether they fall above, at, or below the level of injury.[1] Figure 7–2 contains the American Spinal Injury Association (ASIA) key sensory points, as well as the form for recording sensory examination results. After testing sensation in all of the key points bilaterally, the therapist can calculate the patient's pin prick and light touch scores by adding the scores for all of the key sensory points. These scores can be useful for documenting changes in sensory function.

ASIA also recommends testing the patient's awareness of deep pressure/pain and position sense in one joint for each extremity.[1] The therapist may find it useful to test movement and position sense in all major joints of the affected extremities, as this sensation can influence the performance of functional skills.

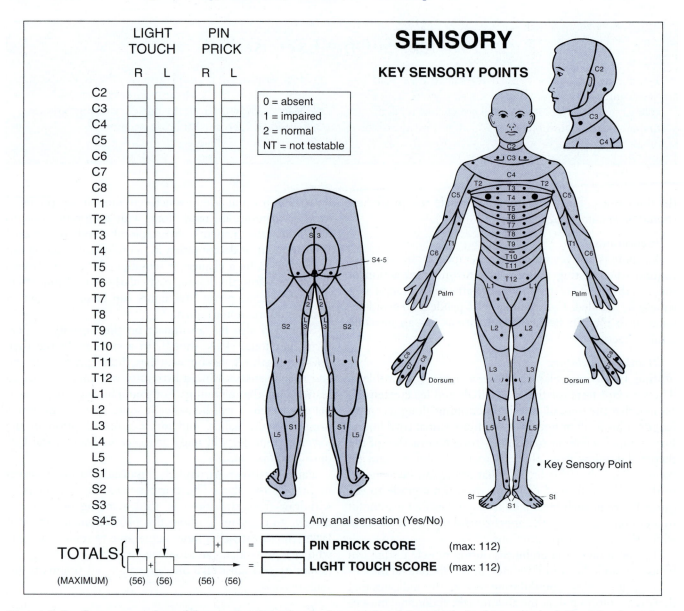

Figure 7–2   Sensory portion of the scoring form for the International Standards for Neurological Classification of Spinal Cord Injury. (Reproduced with permission from the American Spinal Injury Association.)

Sensory Substitution

When performing sensory tests, it is important for the therapist to prevent substitution from other senses. Various senses can be used for sensory substitution. The patient can watch the therapist performing the test. The therapist's voice intonation and choice of words can also provide hints. A patient who lacks proprioception in a joint can often detect movement through other sensory cues. For example, someone who is lying in bed may feel his body being pushed toward the head of the bed when his hip is flexed passively. To increase the accuracy of sensory testing, the therapist should take measures to eliminate these supplemental sensory cues.

Muscle Tone

Abnormal muscle tone is another consequence of spinal cord injury that can have a negative impact on health and function. Elevated muscle tone can cause pain, joint contractures, and skin breakdown. When severe, it can interfere with functional activities [9,10] and quality of life.[11] On the other hand, some individuals can use abnormal muscle tone to their advantage.[11] For example, some people with incomplete lesions depend upon their elevated muscle tone to augment their voluntary quadriceps function when standing or walking.

A patient's muscle tone can also provide information regarding his medical status. Following spinal cord injury,

TABLE 7–1 Modified Ashworth Scale for Grading Spasticity*

0	No increase in muscle tone.
1	Slight increase in muscle tone, manifested by a catch and release or by minimal resistance at the end of the range of motion (ROM) when the affected part(s) is moved in flexion or extension.
1+	Slight increase in muscle tone, manifested by a catch, followed by minimal resistance throughout the remainder (less than half) of the ROM.
2	More marked increase in muscle tone through most of the ROM, but affected part(s) easily moved.
3	Considerable increase in muscle tone, passive movement difficult.
4	Affected part(s) rigid in flexion or extension.

*During testing, the clinician asks the patient to relax and moves the patient's extremities passively through the available range of motion.[14]

Source: Bohannon R, Smith M. Interrater reliability of a modified Ashworth scale of muscle spasticity. *Physical Therapy.* 1987, 67(2): 207. Reproduced with permission from the American Physical Therapy Association.

an increase in muscle tone can be a sign that something is wrong physically, because a noxious stimulus below the lesion can cause an increase in tone. For example, sometimes an increase in spasticity is an early indication of a urinary tract infection.

When testing muscle tone, the therapist should check for spasticity, which is a velocity-dependent involuntary response to passive stretch.[12,13] If spasticity is present, the therapist should rate its severity and determine whether it interferes with function. Table 7–1 presents the Modified Ashworth Scale for grading spasticity.

The patient with elevated muscle tone may exhibit spasms in addition to spasticity. Spasms are involuntary muscle contractions that appear to occur spontaneously or are elicited by stimuli such as tactile stimulation.[15] If the patient exhibits spasms, the therapist should note their frequency and severity, and whether they cause pain or interfere with function.

While examining a patient's spasticity and spasms, the therapist should note whether they are constant or fluctuating and whether certain conditions, stimuli, or bodily motions influence the patient's muscle tone. This information can be useful to the patient and therapist, who may find ways to utilize these involuntary motor responses to enhance the performance of functional tasks.[16] For example, a patient who exhibits lateral trunk flexion on tactile stimulation of his thigh may be able to use this motor response for righting his trunk in a wheelchair. An understanding of the factors that influence a patient's tone can also be helpful to the patient and therapist as they seek ways to avoid involuntary motor responses that interfere with function. For example, a patient who exhibits trunk and extremity spasms when he uses a power recline to perform pressure reliefs in a wheelchair may be able to avoid those spasms by using a power tilt system instead.

The Patient Reported Impact of Spasticity Measure (PRISM) is a new self-report instrument that assesses the impact of abnormal muscle tone on quality of life. Its subscales measure this impact on social avoidance/anxiety, psychological agitation, daily activities, need for assistance/positioning, need for intervention, and social embarrassment. A unique feature of the PRISM is that it also measures the positive impact of abnormal muscle tone.[11]

Passive Range of Motion

Range of motion[e] can have a profound impact on functional ability after spinal cord injury. Even mild restrictions in motion at crucial joints such as the elbows or shoulders can severely limit a person's functional potential. The therapist should check passive range of motion of all major joints, starting with a gross test and specifically examining any areas where functionally relevant limitations exist.[f]

The examination should include measurement of hamstring flexibility, due to its impact on functional capabilities. Hamstring flexibility should be tested in supine with the pelvis stabilized. Having a person with a spinal cord injury long-sit and reach for his toes is not an appropriate technique for performing this assessment, as excessive back flexibility can mask hamstring tightness. In addition to checking hamstring length, the therapist may examine flexibility of the biceps brachii, pectoralis major, long finger flexors and extensors, rectus femoris, and gastrocnemius if motion restrictions or functional limitations indicate possible problems in these muscles.

When testing the joint range of motion or muscle flexibility of someone with a recent spinal injury, the therapist should avoid stress to areas of vertebral instability. For example, if a patient with an unstable lumbar fracture has limited hip range of motion, the hip should not be moved beyond the point at which resistance to motion occurs. Even when range does not appear to be limited, it may be

---

[e] The phrase *range of motion* in this section is used to refer to both joint range of motion and the flexibility of two-joint musculature such as the hamstrings or the biceps brachii.
[f] Table 8–2 in Chapter 8 presents range of motion requirements for function.

prudent to avoid hip flexion past 90 degrees or straight leg raising past 60 degrees in the presence of an unstable lumbar fracture. In like manner, an unstable cervical spine necessitates caution when moving the shoulders.

Functional Abilities

A functional examination investigates what a person is capable of doing, how much assistance he needs, and what equipment he requires to perform various activities. Because the major thrust of the physical therapy component of rehabilitation is to increase functional capability, this part of the examination is very important. The initial functional evaluation provides a starting point for goal setting and program development.

The functional examination performed on completion of the therapeutic program is also critical, as it provides a measure of the program's success. A physical rehabilitation program usually results in improvements in other areas, such as strength and range of motion, but these gains are significant only if they contribute to an increase in functional abilities. If the patient is no more independent at discharge than he was initially, the functional training program has failed.[g]

Examination and documentation of functional skills should be specific enough to provide a complete picture of the patient's abilities. Blanket statements about areas of functioning do not provide adequate information, as these statements can be interpreted differently by various readers. For example, a statement that an individual is "independent in wheelchair propulsion" does not provide enough information. Does this refer to even surfaces only? To 100 feet or 10 miles? How long does it take for the patient to propel over a given distance? Can he negotiate stairs with the wheelchair? Are specific wheelchair accessories such as handrim projections required? To effectively communicate about the patient's functional status, the therapist should specify the environmental conditions under which the various functional skills can be performed,[h] the equipment required, the patient's level of safety, and other measures relevant to each task, such as distance negotiated or time required.

The therapist should also be specific when documenting the amount of assistance that the patient needs to perform each task. Merely noting that a person "needs assistance" does not provide adequate information. For example, the statement that a patient "requires assistance in level transfers" could be true with an individual who is totally dependent, someone who requires only standby guarding, or anyone who falls between the two extremes. The terminology used in the Functional Independence Measure (FIM) can be useful for describing the level of assistance needed. This terminology defines terms according to the patient's contribution to the total effort required to accomplish the task. These terms, and the corresponding percentage of the effort that the patient contributes to the task, are as follows: total assistance ($<25\%$), maximal assistance (25 to $<50\%$), moderate assistance (50% to $<75\%$), minimal contact assistance ($\geq75\%$), supervision or setup (the patient requires only standby assistance or help with preparatory activities such as application of orthoses), modified independence (the patient provides 100% of the effort but takes excessive time, is unsafe, or requires an assistive device), and complete independence (100% of the effort and safe, without excessive time or assistive devices.)[17]

In addition to being specific and thorough, documentation of functional abilities must be as accurate as all other areas of the examination. It can be tempting to "give the patient the benefit of the doubt," calling him independent in an activity when he actually falls slightly short of the mark. For example, a therapist may report that an individual is independent in level transfers, even though he requires guarding because he occasionally loses his balance and falls. A patient should not be called independent in an activity unless he is capable of performing the task alone, without anyone in the area to provide setup or supervision.

To ensure accuracy in the functional examination, the therapist must observe the patient performing the activity; he should not take the patient's (or anyone else's) word on his capabilities.[i] An inexperienced person may feel that he is safe in a given activity when in fact he is not. For example, the author once had a patient report that he could negotiate ramps safely in a wheelchair. When asked to demonstrate, he careened down the ramp at a high speed, stopping only when he struck a glass door (fortunately, a sturdy one) about 20 feet beyond the bottom of the ramp. Following this hair-raising display, the patient still maintained that his technique was safe.[j]

Functional Skills to Examine

Mat and Bed Skills: The therapist should examine the patient's capabilities in rolling, coming to sitting, gross mobility (moving to the side, forward, or backward), and leg management. For the sake of convenience, these skills are frequently assessed on an exercise mat in a physical therapy gym. Exercise mats are typically firmer than beds, however, and are therefore easier surfaces on which to

---

[g] This is not meant to imply that functional gains are the only relevant outcomes of a comprehensive rehabilitation program. Certainly gains made in other areas such as breathing ability, skin integrity, psychosocial adaptation, patient and family education, bowel and bladder regulation, equipment procurement, and home modification are also extremely important.

[h] Environmental conditions include the surfaces on which mat skills and transfers are performed (mat versus bed, for example) as well as the surfaces over which the individual can walk or propel a wheelchair (linoleum versus sidewalk versus grass, for example).

---

[i] If direct observation of the skill is not indicated, the documentation should make it clear that it is the patient's judgment of independence, not the clinician's, that is being reported.

[j] This example illustrates both the need to observe a patient's performance of functional activities and the need to guard him while doing so!

function. A patient who functions independently on a mat may not perform as well on a bed. For this reason, mat and bed skills should be examined with the patient on a bed before he is judged to be independent.

Transfers: The evaluation should address even and uneven transfers, also called level and unlevel transfers. Even transfers involve moving between the wheelchair and a surface that is level with the wheelchair seat.[k] An uneven transfer involves moving between the wheelchair and a higher or lower surface such as a bathtub, toilet, couch, truck, car, plinth, or the floor. Transfers between a wheelchair and a bed may be even or uneven, depending on the relative heights of the wheelchair and bed.

An independent transfer involves more than merely moving the buttocks from one surface to another. To be independent in a transfer from a wheelchair, a person must be able to set up for the transfer: position the wheelchair, lock the brakes, remove or reposition an armrest, position the feet and footrests, and position the transfer board, if one is used. The person must be able to move his entire body onto the surface, including his legs. To be independent in a transfer to the wheelchair, he must be able to prepare to leave the area following the transfer: position his buttocks appropriately on the wheelchair seat, place his trunk in an upright position, remove the transfer board (if used), position the wheelchair's footrests and armrests, place his feet on the footrests, and unlock the brakes.

To transfer safely, a person with a spinal cord injury must move from one surface to another without falling and without traumatizing his skin. Someone who scrapes his buttocks across the wheelchair's tire while transferring has not performed the transfer safely.

Wheelchair Skills: If a patient will require a wheelchair, these skills should be included in the functional examination. Because wheelchair characteristics significantly influence functional performance, this portion of the examination investigates both the patient's abilities and the suitability of the equipment. The evaluation report should include a description of the wheelchair, including the type of chair, alignment, and relevant components such as handrim projections.

The therapist should check the patient's capabilities in propulsion over even surfaces, including the distance that he is able to travel, the time required to propel this distance, and the propulsion pattern used.[l] Obstacle negotiation should also be addressed, including maneuvering over uneven terrain (grass, dirt, gravel, sidewalk), curbs

(the therapist should specify the height), inclined surfaces, doorways, carpet, and stairs. If the patient negotiates obstacles by performing wheelies, the functional assessment should also address his ability to fall safely and right the wheelchair after a fall.

Another important skill to assess is the performance of pressure reliefs, as this skill is critical for health and survival. The examination should determine both whether the person is capable of performing pressure reliefs and whether he assumes the responsibility to get the relief at appropriate intervals.

Numerous wheelchair skills assessment tools have been developed.[18-22] Perhaps the most comprehensive of these is the Wheelchair Skills Test.[21,23] (Figure 7–3)

Ambulation: If a patient is ambulatory, the therapist should determine how far he can walk, the time required to walk this distance, the gait pattern and equipment used, and the level of assistance required. Capabilities in obstacle negotiation (obstacles listed above in wheelchair skills section) should also be assessed. Additional ambulatory skills that should be addressed include donning and doffing the orthoses (if used), walking backward and to the side, safe falling techniques, coming to stand from the floor, coming to stand from sitting, and returning to sitting from a standing position.

In addition to investigating the patient's ambulatory ability as it relates to level of functional independence, the therapist should perform a gait analysis. This analysis will assist in program planning and equipment selection as the therapist and patient work together to optimize gait.

Several standardized assessment tools are valid and reliable for measuring walking performance in individuals with spinal cord injury. The 6-minute walk test (6MWT), 10-meter walk test (10MWT), and Timed Up and Go[m] are relatively simple tests that can be used to measure progress and outcomes.[24] The 6MWT and 10MWT may be particularly useful in detecting change in the walking capacity of high-functioning individuals with incomplete lesions.[25] The Walking Index for Spinal Cord Injury (WISCI II) rates performance on a scale of 0 to 20 based on the assistive devices, orthoses, and assistance that a patient requires to walk 10 meters.[24,26,27] The Spinal Cord Injury Functional Ambulation Inventory (SCI-FAI) rates performance in three areas: gait pattern, equipment required, and measures of speed and walking performance in the home and community.[28] (See Figure 7–4.)

Instruction of Others: The therapist should determine whether the patient is able to instruct others in safe techniques to assist him with activities in which he is dependent.

---

[k] An even transfer is actually between the wheelchair and a surface that is level with the sitting surface. If a wheelchair cushion is used, its top is the sitting surface.

[l] The pattern of upper extremity motions used to propel a manual wheelchair influences the efficiency of propulsion and the potential for upper extremity overuse syndromes. Additional information is presented in Chapter 11.

[m] The 6-minute walk test measures the distance that a patient can walk in 6 minutes, the 10-meter walk test measures the time required to walk 10 meters, and the Timed Up and Go measures the time required to stand from an armchair, walk 3 meters, return to the chair, and sit down.[24]

Wheelchair Skills Test 4.1
Manual Wheelchair - Wheelchair User

Name: ______________________

Date: ____________ Time start: ____________

Tester: ____________ Time finish: ____________

Scoring Guide (see over for details)
✔ = pass, safe
✗ = fail, unsafe
NP = no part (only for indicated skills)
TE = testing error
NT = not tested (safety only)

	Individual Skills	Performance	Safety	**Comments**
1.	Rolls forward 10m			
2.	Rolls forward 10m in 30s			
3.	Rolls backward 5m			
4.	Turns 90° while moving forward[L&R]			
5.	Turns 90° while moving backward[L&R]			
6.	Turns 180° in place[L&R]			
7.	Maneuvers sideways[L&R]			
8.	Gets through hinged door in both directions			
9.	Reaches 1.5m high object			
10.	Picks object from floor			
11.	Relieves weight from buttocks			
12.	Transfers from WC to bench and back			
13.	Folds and unfolds wheelchair			No Part?
14.	Rolls 100m			
15.	Avoids moving obstacles[L&R]			
16.	Ascends 5° incline			
17.	Descends 5° incline			
18.	Ascends 10° incline			
19.	Descends 10° incline			
20.	Rolls 2m across 5° side-slope[L&R]			
21.	Rolls 2m on soft surface			
22.	Gets over 15cm pot-hole			
23.	Gets over 2cm threshold			
24.	Ascends 5cm level change			
25.	Descends 5cm level change			
26.	Ascends 15cm curb			
27.	Descends 15cm curb			
28.	Performs 30s stationary wheelie			
29.	Turns 180° in place in wheelie position[L&R]			
30.	Gets from ground into wheelchair			
31.	Ascends stairs			
32.	Descends stairs			
	Total Percentage Scores			(Please see over for scoring formulae)

Additional comments: ______________________

Data Collection Form FORM WST_M_WCU 4.1.9 Aug 5 2008

Figure 7–3 Wheelchair Skills Test. Forms for assessing power wheelchair skills and caregiver skills are also available. (Reproduced with permission from Dalhousie University. Forms and instructions are available on www.wheelchairskillsprogram.ca.)

TIPS FOR SCORING

General
- The WST 4.1 Manual should be consulted for details (www.wheelchairskillsprogram.ca)
- Each skill should be scored for both Performance and Safety, unless there is "No Part"
- **Left and Right:** (L&R): For skills with a left and right component, the participant needs to pass the skill on both sides to receive a pass. If the participant is successful on only one side, a fail is awarded and a note should be made in the comment section.
- **Comments section:** Document anything requiring action (e.g. wheelchair part malfunction, dangerous behaviour, training needs).

Scale for Scoring Skill Performance

Pass: (record "P" or ✔)
- Task independently and safely accomplished. Unless otherwise specified in the manual, the skill may be performed in any manner. The focus is on the task requirements, not the method used. Aids may be used if carried or available in the subject's environment.
- A pass may be awarded if the subject passed a more difficult version of the same skill (e.g. if a subject successfully ascends a 15cm curb, a pass may be awarded on the 5cm level change without the subject needing to actually perform the latter).

Fail: (record "F" or ✘)
- Task incomplete.
- Unsafe performance (defined opposite).
- Likely to be unsafe in the opinion of the clinician or tester (e.g. on the basis of the subject's description of how a task will be attempted).
- Unwilling to try.
- Has failed an easier version of the same skill (e.g. if the subject cannot roll forward 10m, he/she need not be asked to roll 100m).
- If a caregiver is the subject of testing, he/she may not ask the wheelchair occupant for advice or physical assistance in the performance of the skill unless specifically permitted in the caregiver section of the individual skill descriptions.
- Wheelchair part malfunction.

Scale for Scoring Skill Safety

Safe: (record "S" or ✔)
- None of the unsafe criteria were met.
- Although a failing performance score will be awarded in such circumstances, a safe score can be awarded to a person who states that he/she cannot do and will not attempt a skill.

Unsafe: (record "US" or ✘)
- Subject requires appropriate, significant spotter intervention to prevent acute injury to the subject or others. Performing a skill quickly is not, in and of itself, unsafe. A significant intervention is one that affects performance of the skill.
- A significant acute injury occurred. This may include sprains, strains, fractures or head injury, but does not include minor blisters, abrasions or superficial lacerations. Poor technique that may or may not lead to overuse injury at a later time should be noted in the comments section, but does not warrant awarding an unsafe score.
- During screening questions, the subject describes a method of performing a skill that the tester considers dangerous.
- If a caregiver creates more than minimal discomfort or potential harm (e.g. using excessive force with the knee against a flexible backrest of the wheelchair to help push the wheelchair through gravel).
- Specific risks as listed in the Manual.

Not Tested: (record "NT")
If an easier version of the skill has been failed, the skill under consideration is not tested, so it is not possible to determine whether the attempt would have been safe or unsafe.

Scale for both Scoring Skill Performance and Safety

Testing Error: (record "TE")
If testing of the skill was appropriate, but was not sufficiently well observed to provide a score (e.g. if the tester failed to test the skill fully or if the skill was being scored from videotape and the entire skill could not be viewed).

No Part: (record "NP")
The Wheelchair does not have the component. This score should only be used if both left and right parts are missing.

Total Performance Score = # passed skills _____ / (32 - #NP - #TE) × 100% = _____
Total Safety Score = # safe skills _____ / (32 - #NP - #TE - #NT) × 100% = _____

Data Collection Form

FORM WST_M_WCU 4.1.9 Aug 5 2008

Figure 7–3 *(Continued)*

SCI Functional Ambulation Inventory (SCI-FAI)

Name: Session: Date:

PARAMETER	CRITERION	L	R
A. Weight shift	shifts weight to stance limb	1	1
	weight shift absent or only onto assistive device	0	0
B. Step width	swing foot clears stance foot on limb advancement	1	1
	stance foot obstructs swing foot on limb advancement	0	0
	final foot placement does not obstruct swing limb	1	1
	final foot placement obstructs swing limb	0	0
C. Step rhythm	at heel strike of stance limb, the swing limb:		
(relative time needed	begins to advance in <1 second *or*	2	2
to advance swing limb)	requires 1–3 seconds to begin advancing *or*	1	1
	requires >3 seconds to begin advancing	0	0
D. Step height	toe clears floor throughout swing phase *or*	2	2
	toe drags at initiation of swing phase only *or*	1	1
	toe drags throughout swing phase	0	0
E. Foot contact	heel contacts floor before forefoot *or*	1	1
	forefoot or foot flat first contact with floor	0	0
F. Step length	swing heel placed forward of stance toe *or*	2	2
	swing toe placed forward of stance toe *or*	1	1
	swing toe placed rearward of stance toe	0	0
	Parameter total		Sum /20

ASSISTIVE DEVICES		L	R	
Upper extremity	None	4	4	
balance/weightbearing	Cane(s)	3	3	
devices	Quad cane(s), Crutch(es) (forearm/axillary)	2	2	
	Walker		2	
	Parallel bars		0	
Lower extremity assistive devices	None	3	3	
	AFO	2	2	
	KAFO	1	1	
	RGO	0	0	
	Assistive device total		Sum /14	

TEMPORAL/DISTANCE MEASURES			
Walking mobility	Walks …		
(typical walking practice	regularly in community (rarely/never use W/C)	5	
as opposed to W/C use)	regularly in home/occasionally in community	4	
	occasionally in home/rarely in community	3	
	rarely in home/never in community	2	
	for exercise only	1	
	does not walk	0	
	Walking mobility score		Sum /5
Two-minute walk test	Distance walked in 2 minutes = ...	feet/minute	meters/ minute
(distance walked in 2 minutes)			

AFO: ankle-foot orthosis; KAFO: knee-ankle-foot orthosis.

Figure 7–4   Spinal Cord Injury Functional Ambulation Inventory. (Reproduced with permission from Taylor & Francis. Field-Fote, EC, GG Fluet, et al 2001. The Spinal Cord Injury Functional Ambulation Inventory (SCI-FAI) *J Rehabil Med* 33(4): 177–81)

Global Functional Assessment Tools

Standardized functional assessment tools are frequently utilized as a component of a functional evaluation. They provide quantified data that can be useful for clinical research, and for communication with insurance providers about an individual's functional gains. Data gained using a standardized assessment tool can also be used as a measure of a facility's effectiveness, as patients' performance can be compared to the outcomes achieved at other facilities. This information on programmatic effectiveness may be used internally for program development, or externally for accreditation or communication with insurance providers.[29]

The Functional Independence Measure (FIM) is widely used both in the United States and abroad. Designed to assess burden of care, this 18-item instrument addresses performance in self-care, sphincter control, transfers, locomotion (walking or using a wheelchair), communication, and social cognition.[17] The FIM has been investigated extensively and has been demonstrated to be reliable and valid in general, but may lack the sensitivity to detect some functionally relevant changes among people with spinal cord injury.[30–33] For example, a person who uses a cane to walk 150 feet would receive the same rating for locomotion as a person who requires a power wheelchair to travel the same distance.

The Spinal Cord Independence Measure (SCIM III) is a comprehensive functional assessment tool designed specifically for individuals with spinal cord lesions (Figure 7–5). This 17-item instrument addresses performance in self-care (feeding, bathing, dressing, grooming, toileting), breathing and coughing, bowel and bladder management, bed mobility and pressure reliefs, transfers (between wheelchair and bed, toilet, tub, car, ground), mobility (walking or wheelchair), and stair negotiation.[34] The SCIM has been shown to be valid and reliable, and more sensitive than the FIM to functional changes in this population.[32–38]

Alternative standardized tools include the Quadriplegia Index of Function,[39–41] which is relatively limited in scope, and the Barthel Index,[39,42] which is less sensitive to change than the SCIM.[36] The Modified Barthel Index[43] is no more sensitive to change than the Barthel Index.[44]

Participation

Examinations performed after discharge from inpatient rehabilitation (outpatient or follow-up examinations, for example) should include a measure of participation. This investigation may help identify problems in community reintegration that can be addressed through physical therapy or referral to other rehabilitation professionals. Standardized tools related to participation include the Craig Handicap Assessment and Reporting Technique, the Community Integration Questionnaire, the Assessment of Life Habits, the Impact on Participation and Autonomy Questionnaire, and the Craig Hospital Inventory of Environmental Factors.[31,45]

Skin Integrity

Skin breakdown is a complication of spinal cord injury that can lead to severe medical problems, even death. During the initial examination, the therapist should note any pressure ulcers or early signs of skin breakdown.[n] If a problem is found, pressure over the area must be relieved and the therapeutic program must be modified to avoid any further trauma to the area. The therapist should also notify other members of the team if they are not already aware of the breakdown.

Areas of scarring from healed pressure ulcers should also be noted in the examination. Because scar tissue is more susceptible than normal skin to breakdown, care must be taken to minimize trauma to scarred areas. Areas of scarring are also important to note because they provide a history of past skin problems. The presence of healed pressure ulcers may indicate that the patient has neglected skin care in the past and needs to learn better habits in this area. These scars may also be the legacy of poor medical care.

Breathing and Coughing

Most spinal cord injuries result in at least partial impairment of breathing and coughing ability. As a result, respiratory complications are a significant source of mortality among people with spinal cord injuries. The respiratory evaluation investigates the patient's ability to breathe and clear secretions from his lungs.[o]

Pain

Because pain is a common problem during all time frames following spinal cord injury, it should be addressed in all physical therapy examinations. If a patient reports experiencing pain, the examination should investigate the history (onset, intermittent versus constant, factors that aggravate or relieve it, past interventions if chronic), quality, location, and severity of the pain. Additional examination procedures by the therapist or other health professionals may be indicated to determine the cause of the pain (musculoskeletal, visceral, or neuropathic), and contributing factors.[46,47]

Equipment

Equipment has a significant impact on function, disability, and health. Someone who lacks needed equipment, or has equipment that is inappropriate or in disrepair, is likely to experience activity limitations and participation restrictions as a result. He may also develop secondary pathologies that could have been prevented with appropriate equipment.

An equipment check during the initial examination helps to focus attention early on this important area. As soon as a patient's equipment needs have been identified, the process

---

[n] Skin care and assessment are presented in greater depth in Chapter 5.
[o] Chapter 6 addresses respiratory examination and interventions.

LOEWENSTEIN HOSPITAL REHABILITATION CENTER

Affiliated with the Sackler Faculty of Medicine, Tel-Aviv University

Department IV, Medical Director: Dr. Amiram Catz   **Tel:** 972-9-7709090   **Fax:** 972-9-7709986   **e-mail: amiramc@clalit.org.il**

Patient Name: _____   ID: _____   Examiner Name: _____

(Enter the score for each function in the adjacent square, below the date. The form may be used for up to 6 examinations.)

SCIM-SPINAL CORD INDEPENDENCE MEASURE

Version III, Sept 14, 2002

Self-Care   DATE

EXam 1 2 3 4 5 6

1. Feeding (cutting, opening containers, pouring, bringing food to mouth, holding cup with fluid)
0. Needs parenteral, gastrostomy, or fully assisted oral feeding
1. Needs partial assistance for eating and/or drinking, or for wearing adaptive devices
2. Eats independently; needs adaptive devices or assistance only for cutting food and/or pouring and/or opening containers
3. Eats and drinks independently; does not require assistance or adaptive devices

2. Bathing (soaping, washing, drying body and head, manipulating water tap). **A-upper body; B-lower body**
A. 0. Requires total assistance
   1. Requires partial assistance
   2. Washes independently with adaptive devices or in a specific setting (e.g., bars, chair)
   3. Washes independently; does not require adaptive devices or specific setting (not customary for healthy people) (adss)
B. 0. Requires total assistance
   1. Requires partial assistance
   2. Washes independently with adaptive devices or in a specific setting (adss)
   3. Washes independently; does not require adaptive devices (adss) or specific setting

3. Dressing (clothes, shoes, permanent orthoses: dressing, wearing, undressing). **A-upper body; B-lower body**
A. 0. Requires total assistance
   1. Requires partial assistance with clothes without buttons, zippers or laces (cwobzl)
   2. Independent with cwobzl; requires adaptive devices and/or specific settings (adss)
   3. Independent with cwobzl; does not require adss; needs assistance or adss only for bzl
   4. Dresses (any cloth) independently; does not require adaptive devices or specific setting
B. 0. Requires total assistance
   1. Requires partial assistance with clothes without buttons, zipps or laces (cwobzl)
   2. Independent with cwobzl; requires adaptive devices and/or specific settings (adss)
   3. Independent with cwobzl without adss; needs assistance or adss only for bzl
   4. Dresses (any cloth) independently; does not require adaptive devices or specific setting

4. Grooming (washing hands and face, brushing teeth, combing hair, shaving, applying makeup)
0. Requires total assistance
1. Requires partial assistance
2. Grooms independently with adaptive devices
3. Grooms independently without adaptive devices

SUBTOTAL (0–20)

Respiration and Sphincter Management

5. Respiration
0. Requires tracheal tube (TT) and permanent or intermittent assisted ventilation (IAV)
2. Breathes independently with TT; requires oxygen, much assistance in coughing or TT management
4. Breathes independently with TT; requires little assistance in coughing or TT management
6. Breathes independently without TT; requires oxygen, much assistance in coughing, a mask (e.g., peep) or IAV (bipap)
8. Breathes independently without TT; requires little assistance or stimulation for coughing
10. Breathes independently without assistance or device

6. Sphincter Management - Bladder
0. Indwelling catheter
3. Residual urine volume (RUV) > 100cc; no regular catheterization or assisted intermittent catheterization
6. RUV <100cc or intermittent self-catheterization; needs assistance for applying drainage instrument
9. Intermittent self-catheterization; uses external drainage instrument; does not need assistance for applying
11. Intermittent self-catheterization; continent between catheterizations; does not use external drainage instrument
13. RUV <100cc; needs only external urine drainage; no assistance is required for drainage
15. RUV <100cc; continent; does not use external drainage instrument

7. Sphincter Management-Bowel
0. Irregular timing or very low frequency (less than once in 3 days) of bowel movements
5. Regular timing, but requires assistance (e.g., for applying suppository); rare accidents (less than twice a month)
8. Regular bowel movements, without assistance; rare accidents (less than twice a month)
10. Regular bowel movements, without assistance; no accidents

8. Use of Toilet (perineal hygiene, adjustment of clothes before/after, use of napkins or diapers).
0. Requires total assistance
1. Requires partial assistance; does not clean self

Figure 7–5   Spinal Cord Independence Measure, version III. (Itzkovich et al. 2007. The Spinal Cord Independence Measure [SCIM] version III: Reliability and validity in a multi-center international study. Disability and Rehabilitation, 29[24]: 1926–1933.)

2. Requires partial assistance; cleans self independently
4. Uses toilet independently in all tasks but needs adaptive devices or special setting (e.g., bars)
5. Uses toilet independently; does not require adaptive devices or special setting)

SUBTOTAL (0-40)

DATE

Mobility (room and toilet)

9. Mobility in Bed and Action to Prevent Pressure Sores
   0. Needs assistance in all activities: turning upper body in bed, turning lower body in bed, sitting up in bed, doing push-ups in wheelchair, with or without adaptive devices, but not with electric aids
   2. Performs one of the activities without assistance
   4. Performs two or three of the activities without assistance
   6. Performs all the bed mobility and pressure release activities independently

10. Transfers: bed-wheelchair (locking wheelchair, lifting footrests, removing and adjusting arm rests, transferring, lifting feet).
   0. Requires total assistance
   1. Needs partial assistance and/or supervision, and/or adaptive devices (e.g., sliding board)
   2. Independent (or does not require wheelchair)

11. Transfers: wheelchair-toilet-tub (if uses toilet wheelchair: transfers to and from; if uses regular wheelchair: locking wheelchair, lifting footrests, removing and adjusting armrests, transferring, lifting feet)
   0. Requires total assistance
   1. Needs partial assistance and/or supervision, and/or adaptive devices (e.g., grab-bars)
   2. Independent (or does not require wheelchair)

Mobility (indoors and outdoors, on even surface)

12. Mobility Indoors
   0. Requires total assistance
   1. Needs electric wheelchair or partial assistance to operate manual wheelchair
   2. Moves independently in manual wheelchair
   3. Requires supervision while walking (with or without devices)
   4. Walks with a walking frame or crutches (swing)
   5. Walks with crutches or two canes (reciprocal walking)
   6. Walks with one cane
   7. Needs leg orthosis only
   8. Walks without walking aids

13. Mobility for Moderate Distances (10–100 meters)
   0. Requires total assistance
   1. Needs electric wheelchair or partial assistance to operate manual wheelchair
   2. Moves independently in manual wheelchair
   3. Requires supervision while walking (with or without devices)
   4. Walks with a walking frame or crutches (swing)
   5. Walks with crutches or two canes (reciprocal walking)
   6. Walks with one cane
   7. Needs leg orthosis only
   8. Walks without walking aids

14. Mobility Outdoors (more than 100 meters)
   0. Requires total assistance
   1. Needs electric wheelchair or partial assistance to operate manual wheelchair
   2. Moves independently in manual wheelchair
   3. Requires supervision while walking (with or without devices)
   4. Walks with a walking frame or crutches (swing)
   5. Walks with crutches or two canes (reciprocal waking)
   6. Walks with one cane
   7. Needs leg orthosis only
   8. Walks without walking aids

15. Stair Management
   0. Unable to ascend or descend stairs
   1. Ascends and descends at least 3 steps with support or supervision of another person
   2. Ascends and descends at least 3 steps with support of handrail and/or crutch or cane
   3. Ascends and descends at least 3 steps without any support or supervision

16. Transfers: wheelchair-car (approaching car, locking wheelchair, removing arm- and footrests, transferring to and from car, bringing wheelchair into and out of car)
   0. Requires total assistance
   1. Needs partial assistance and/or supervision and/or adaptive devices
   2. Transfers independent; does not require adaptive devices (or does not require wheelchair)

17. Transfers: ground-wheelchair
   0. Requires assistance
   1. Transfers independent with or without adaptive devices (or does not require wheelchair)

SUBTOTAL (0–40)

TOTAL SCIM SCORE (0–100)

EXam   1   2   3   4   5   6

Figure 7–5   (*Continued*)

of meeting those needs should be started. If arrangements for equipment purchase or repair are initiated early, the results are likely to be more satisfactory than if equipment procurement is attempted in a rush just prior to discharge.

The therapist should record any orthoses, wheelchairs, or other equipment in the patient's possession and note whether it is rented, on loan, or owned by the patient. The fit, function, and condition of the equipment should be evaluated.[p]

Home Environment

One important task during rehabilitation is preparing the person to function in his home. This preparation involves a combination of developing functional skills and adapting the home environment as necessary.

During the initial evaluation, the therapist should find out what environment the patient intends to return to on completion of rehabilitation, and whether the home has architectural barriers such as stairs or small bathrooms. A more detailed assessment of the home should follow.[q]

Other

The physical therapy examination should cover any other areas that may require intervention, impact on prognosis, or influence goals or treatment strategies. Possible additional areas of examination that may be indicated include edema, aerobic capacity and endurance, balance, posture, deep tendon reflexes, and environmental barriers in the community.[48]

FUNCTIONAL POTENTIALS

After completing the initial examination, the physical therapist makes an informed estimate of the patient's potential for functional gains. This estimate, or prognosis, is needed for patient and family education as well as for goal setting.[r] Table 7–2 presents descriptions of typical functional outcomes of people with *complete* traumatic spinal cord injuries. The functional potentials presented here are meant to be used as general "ballpark" guides rather than as rigid guidelines for goal setting. A given individual may either exceed or fall short of the outcomes presented.

Factors Affecting Functional Outcomes

Following spinal cord injury, an individual's potential for physical activity is determined largely by his motor function. As a rule, people with more innervated musculature have a greater capacity for independence.[50–56] The level and extent of a cord lesion determine the motor function that remains after the injury: lower lesions and incomplete lesions leave more of the body's musculature innervated.

If all other factors are equal, a person with a low complete spinal cord lesion can be expected to achieve independence in more advanced activities than would be possible for someone with a higher complete lesion. Even the degree of motor sparing within a level can have an impact. For example, someone with only 3/5 strength in the muscles of the myotome at his neurological level of injury may not achieve the same level of independence as another person with the same neurological level of injury who has greater strength in the same musculature. In like manner, preserved motor function in the zone of partial preservation can result in greater functional independence.[s]

Whereas the neurological level of injury is the best predictor of functional gains after a complete injury, it is not a good predictor following incomplete spinal cord injury. When a lesion is incomplete, the degree of completeness and neurological recovery have more relevance to functional potential.[57] People with significant voluntary motor function below their lesions (ASIA D) tend to achieve greater functional independence than do people with more complete (ASIA A, B, or C) lesions.[58]

Although voluntary motor function has a major impact upon a person's functional capacity, it is not the sole determinant. Research has shown that the following factors are associated with lower functional outcomes: advanced age, pressure ulcers, spasticity, pain, limitations in range of motion, and concurrent head injury.[9,51,59–64] Clinical experience[65–67] points to several additional factors that can limit progress in functional training. These include obesity, disadvantageous body build (short arms, for example), sensory impairments, impaired mental functioning, inadequate psychological adjustment to the spinal cord injury, poor motivation, fear, medical complications, low endurance, limited equipment options, and poor premorbid athletic ability. Unfortunately, the rehabilitation that is available to an individual can also be a limiting factor. If not enough time is allotted to rehabilitation, functional gains may be limited. Such gains can also be constrained if the person undergoes rehabilitation in a setting that is not oriented toward the aggressive pursuit of independence.

---

[p] Evaluation of cushions, wheelchairs, and lower limb orthoses is addressed in Chapters 5, 11 and 12.

[q] Chapter 15 addresses architectural design.

[r] The *Guide to Physical Therapist Practice*[48] published by the American Physical Therapy Association distinguishes between goals and outcomes. The term *goals* refers to intended accomplishments related to impairments, and *outcomes* refers to intended accomplishments related to functional limitations and health status. In the portion of that publication which discusses practice patterns, however, both types of intended accomplishments are referred to as goals. This text follows that lead: it uses the term *goals* in reference to intended accomplishments in all areas rather than limiting it to those relating to impairments.

---

[s] The zone of partial preservation consists of the myotomes and dermatomes below the neurological level of injury that remain partially innervated after a complete spinal cord injury.[1]

TABLE 7–2 Typical Functional Outcomes Following Complete Spinal Cord Injury*

Neurological Level of Injury	Bed Skills	Transfers	Wheelchair (W/C) Skills	Ambulation
C1–C4	Total assist	Total assist	**Power W/C:** Independent driving using head, chin, mouth, or breath control. Independent in pressure reliefs using power tilt and/or recline. **Manual W/C:** Total assist.	No functional ambulation
C5	Some assist	Total assist	**Power W/C:** Independent driving using hand-control. Independent in pressure reliefs using power tilt and/or recline. **Manual W/C:** Independent to some assist indoors on uncarpeted level floors. Some to total assist outdoors.	No functional ambulation
C6	Some assist	**Even:** Some assist to independent **Uneven:** Some to total assist	**Power W/C:** Independent driving using hand-control. Independent in pressure reliefs either without specialty seating system or using power tilt and/or recline. **Manual W/C:** Independent indoors, some to total assist outdoors.	No functional ambulation
C7–C8	Independent to some assist	**Even:** Independent **Uneven:** Independent to some assist	**Manual W/C:** Independent indoors and outdoors on level terrain. Some assist with unlevel terrain.	No functional ambulation
T1–T9	Independent	**Even:** Independent **Uneven:** Independent	**Manual W/C:** Independent indoors and outdoors on level and unlevel terrain.	Functional ambulation not typical
T10–L1	Independent	**Even:** Independent **Uneven:** Independent	**Manual W/C:** Independent indoors and outdoors on level and unlevel terrain.	Some assist to independent in functional ambulation using knee-ankle-foot orthoses (KAFOs) and forearm crutches or walker
L2–S5	Independent	**Even:** Independent **Uneven:** Independent	**Manual W/C:** Independent indoors and outdoors on level and unlevel terrain.	Some assist to independent in functional ambulation using KAFOs or ankle-foot orthoses (AFOs) and forearm crutches or cane(s)

*This table is consistent with the outcomes published by the Consortium for Spinal Cord Medicine.[49] More detailed information on functional potentials is presented in Chapters 9 to 12.

Exceptional Cases

When youth, health, advantageous body build, a high degree of motivation, good funding, and access to good medical and rehabilitative care combine, the patient may acquire more advanced skills than are typical for his level of injury. Table 7–3 presents outcomes that are possible in exceptional cases.[t]

The information in Tables 7–2 and 7–3 should not be used to set strict upper limits in establishing goals. Therapists who impose inflexible ceilings on patients' goals can limit their functional gains. Greater independence may be achieved if rehabilitation professionals and people with spinal cord injuries attempt to accomplish higher goals, stretching past previous limits.

Incomplete Spinal Cord Injuries

The functional potential of an individual with an incomplete lesion depends largely on the degree of motor sparing or *return* that he experiences. When sparing is sensory only (ASIA B) or when voluntary motor function below the lesion is minimal (ASIA C), the functional capacity is essentially the same as if the individual had a complete lesion (ASIA A) at the same spinal cord level. When significant motor sparing or *return* occurs in the trunk and extremities (ASIA D and E), a higher degree of functional independence can be achieved. In predicting the potential for functional gains, the therapist should take into account the individual's potential for neurological return.[u]

---

[t] Table 7–3 presents exceptional outcomes for individuals with C8 or higher neurological levels of injury. Functional potentials for people with lower levels "max out" in Table 7–2, as these individuals typically achieve independent functioning.

[u] A patient who presents soon after injury with ASIA C, for example, may progress to ASIA D. This neurological return would bring the potential for greater functional independence. Chapter 2 includes information on predictors of neurological return.

As is true with complete injuries, voluntary motor function is not the sole determinant of functional outcomes after incomplete spinal cord injuries. Muscle tone is a particularly important consideration when predicting functional potential following incomplete spinal cord injury. Incomplete lesions tend to result in more spasticity than do complete lesions,[68,69] and severe spasticity can greatly impede progress. Sensory sparing and return can also impact on function after an incomplete spinal cord injury. Because somatosensory feedback is required for normal motor control, sensory impairments can prevent optimal utilization of musculature that remains or returns after a spinal cord injury. Additional factors that affect functional outcomes are presented above.

Functional Gains After Discharge

Many people with spinal cord injuries experience significant functional gains after they leave rehabilitation.[56,70–72] This improvement is due at least in part to the development of skill through practice. In addition, the strength gains that typically occur during the first year or more after cord injury[5–7,73–77] may lead to functional improvements.

GOAL SETTING

Goal setting is a critical component of a physical therapy evaluation because goals give direction in the development of therapeutic programs. They also provide a measure with which the therapist and patient can judge the program's effectiveness.

Setting therapeutic goals involves an analysis of the examination results as they relate to health and function. The therapist and patient together consider the impairments, activity limitations, and other factors that could affect the patient's future health and participation in life situations.

TABLE 7–3 Exceptional Functional Outcomes Following Complete Spinal Cord Injury

Neurological Level of Injury	Bed Skills	Transfers	Wheelchair (W/C) Skills
C4	—	—	**Power W/C:** Independent driving using hand control.
C5	Independent; may require equipment	**Even:** Independent; usually require transfer board, may require overhead frame with loops	**Power W/C:** Independent in pressure reliefs without specialty seating system.
C6	Independent	**Uneven:** Independent in slightly uneven transfers; may require transfer board	**Manual W/C:** Independent in negotiation of mild obstacles such as 1:12 grade ramps, slightly uneven (outdoor) terrain, 2- to 4-inch curbs.
C7–8	—	**Uneven:** Independent in uneven transfers, including floor-to-wheelchair	**Manual W/C:** Independent in negotiation of mild obstacles such as ramps with steeper than 1:12 grade, slightly uneven (outdoor) terrain, 4-inch curbs.

Problem-Solving Exercise 7–3

Your patient is a 52-year-old male with complete (ASIA A) C7 tetraplegia. His innervated musculature is strong, his passive range of motion is normal in all extremities, and he exhibits 1+ spasticity in both lower extremities. He has no medical problems other than the tetraplegia. Prior to his accident he had a sedentary lifestyle. He cooperates in therapy but does not show much drive or initiative.

Another patient is a 19-year-old otherwise healthy male with C7 tetraplegia who, remarkably, has identical strength, passive range of motion, and muscle tone as the 52-year-old. This patient was a star athlete prior to his accident and shows a very high level of motivation in therapy.

- What functional outcomes might be reasonable to expect for the 52-year-old patient?
- What functional outcomes might be reasonable to expect for the 19-year-old patient?

The therapist and patient then set goals directed toward minimizing disability, returning the patient to as healthy, independent, and active a lifestyle as possible.[v]

Patient Involvement

For the rehabilitation process to be successful, patients must be involved in establishing their own goals. A patient's participation in goal setting ensures that the program is directed toward mastering skills that he values. It also gives him some control over his program, thus promoting independence.

Setting Meaningful Goals

The only way to ensure that a program's goals are meaningful to the patient is to involve him in establishing them. The therapist cannot assume that what he wants a patient to achieve will coincide with what that individual wants to learn. A health professional who sets goals without the patient's input runs the risk of establishing goals that he does not value, and may neglect areas of functioning that the patient wants to address.

The therapist and patient should identify goals that reflect the patient's priorities, participation and role requirements, and environments in which he will function after discharge.[78] Doing so will ensure that the therapeutic program is directed toward outcomes that will be meaningful to the patient. This may result in better motivation to work in therapy, which in turn will enable the patient to achieve a higher level of independence.[78] It will also increase the likelihood that he will use his newly acquired skills following discharge. A program that focuses on gaining abilities that the patient has no wish to use will only waste time, effort, and money.

Program Control

A health professional who dictates a patient's goals places him in a position of dependence. The messages given to the patient are: "We are in control. We know what is best for you. You need us to make these decisions for you. Do as you are told." In contrast, having a patient set his own goals affirms his autonomy, giving him the responsibility of identifying what he wants to achieve. It emphasizes that he is still in control of his life, despite his spinal cord injury. Having responsibility for the goals may also encourage a feeling of greater involvement in the rehabilitation process, and enhance motivation.

The Collaborative Process

Having a patient set his goals does not mean that the therapist cannot provide suggestions and guidance. Goal setting involves a collaborative process in which the patient and therapist come to an agreement about the intended outcomes of the therapeutic program. The therapist brings to the process an estimation of the patient's functional potential based on the results of the physical therapy examination. The patient brings to the process his perspective, priorities, and understanding of the social and physical environments in which he is accustomed to living.

Soon After Injury

A person who participates in setting his therapeutic goals experiences control in at least one area of his life. This is particularly important for a recently injured person. In the bulk of his experiences since the injury, it is likely that health professionals, family, and even friends have been in charge. By giving the newly injured person some control over his program, the therapist supports his autonomy.

Although it is important to involve patients in setting their goals, a recently injured person cannot be expected to come up with a complete list of rehabilitation goals without any guidance. He is likely to have no idea of his functional potential or of the skills that he will require to

<hr/>

[v] In the United States, valuing personal independence is a cultural norm. Health professionals should be aware and respectful, however, of differing beliefs and values related to functional independence based on cultural background or other personal factors.

function and stay healthy. The day before or perhaps a week earlier, the recently injured person was probably oriented toward such achievements as paying off a loan, completing college, getting a promotion, or finding a date for the senior prom. The idea of therapeutic goals such as independent transfers or wheelchair mobility is likely to be completely foreign.

To prepare a recently injured person to set his rehabilitation goals, the therapist should share the initial examination results with him and provide an estimate of his functional potential. The therapist should explain what skills are possible to acquire and then ask the patient whether he is interested in learning to perform these activities. The patient should also be given the opportunity to identify any other goals that he might want to pursue.

When discussing goals with an acutely injured person, it is a challenge for the therapist to be forthright and yet tactful. It is important to remember that the patient has not had time to adjust to his injury or even to comprehend its impact. The therapist must also understand that the patient may not be overly thrilled with the list of functional skills presented as possible goals. Rehabilitation is not an appealing option compared with recovery.

"Rehabilitation's job is to take your body *as it is* and to maximize your capabilities within recognized limitations. This is a difficult acknowledgment. Rehabilitation seems only second best, which is exactly what it is. To fully accept rehabilitation, for most of us, is to effectively abandon recovery. Rehabilitation can give you strength, reeducation, skills and real improvement, but no cure. Many people find this an easy bridge to cross, and a few find it so upsetting that they temporarily want out of the game."

Barry Corbet[79]
author, filmmaker, father,
T12/L1 SCI survivor

Further Down the Road

A person who sustained a spinal cord injury months or years earlier is likely to have a good understanding of the impact of his injury and should be able to identify specific goals to pursue when he comes for rehabilitation. In these cases, the therapist should start the process of goal setting by asking the patient what he wants to achieve in therapy.

The therapist may know of additional functional abilities that the individual has the potential to achieve. These skills may well interest the patient even though they were not in his list of goals; it may not have occurred to him that these activities were possible. For example, few people would spontaneously come up with the idea of negotiating stairs in a wheelchair. To give the patient a chance to maximize his functional potential, the therapist should let him know what additional skills he has the potential to achieve and allow him to decide whether he wishes to develop these skills.

Prioritization of Goals

In today's health care environment, funding sources frequently limit the time that a patient can spend in the acute and postacute inpatient phases of rehabilitation.[80,81] Much rehabilitation now occurs in alternative settings[82] such as extended care facilities, day rehabilitation programs, outpatient clinics, and patients' homes. Rehabilitation may occur in stages at a series of settings, with the program in each setting reinforcing and building on the patient's prior accomplishments. (Figure 7–6) Because of time constraints, there is typically a limitation in the goals that an individual can achieve during each phase of rehabilitation.

When the time available in a given phase of rehabilitation is limited, the therapist and patient must identify the goals that are most critical to achieve at that point. Factors to consider when prioritizing goals include discharge destination, assistance available after discharge, availability of therapy following discharge, current medical or orthopedic restrictions on activity, likelihood of significant neurological return, functional potential, financial resources, and the patient's home and community environments.

When funding sources seriously limit the services, equipment, and time in rehabilitation that are available to patients with spinal cord injuries, rehabilitation professionals may

---

Problem-Solving Exercise 7–4

Your patient is a 22-year-old female with complete (ASIA A) C5 tetraplegia sustained in an automobile accident 3 weeks ago. When you ask her about the goals that she would like to achieve during rehabilitation, she tells you that she wants to walk.

- Is this a reasonable goal to set, given her current motor function?
- How should you respond to this patient?

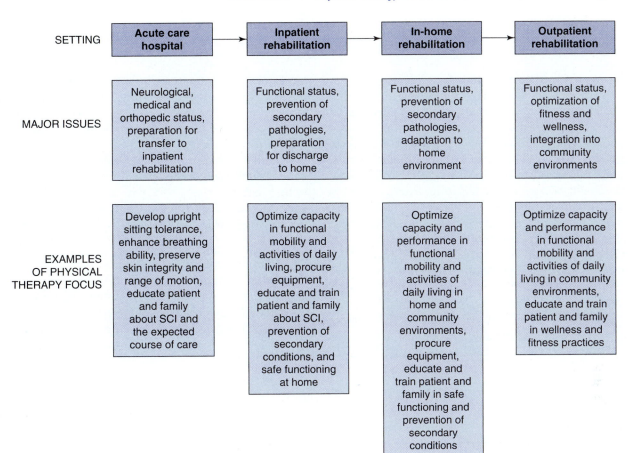

SETTING	Acute care hospital	→	Inpatient rehabilitation	→	In-home rehabilitation	→	Outpatient rehabilitation

MAJOR ISSUES	Neurological, medical and orthopedic status, preparation for transfer to inpatient rehabilitation	Functional status, prevention of secondary pathologies, preparation for discharge to home	Functional status, prevention of secondary pathologies, adaptation to home environment	Functional status, optimization of fitness and wellness, integration into community environments

EXAMPLES OF PHYSICAL THERAPY FOCUS	Develop upright sitting tolerance, enhance breathing ability, preserve skin integrity and range of motion, educate patient and family about SCI and the expected course of care	Optimize capacity in functional mobility and activities of daily living, procure equipment, educate and train patient and family about SCI, prevention of secondary conditions, and safe functioning at home	Optimize capacity and performance in functional mobility and activities of daily living in home and community environments, procure equipment, educate and train patient and family in safe functioning and prevention of secondary conditions	Optimize capacity and performance in functional mobility and activities of daily living in community environments, educate and train patient and family in wellness and fitness practices

Figure 7–6   Example of progression of rehabilitation in a series of settings. Note that this is a simplified example; it is not intended to provide a comprehensive summary of rehabilitative care in all environments.

have to settle for "adequate outcomes"[w] rather than striving for "optimal outcomes."[81] In these cases, highest priority should be given to goals related to basic survival, such as obtaining an appropriate seating system and developing skill in performing pressure reliefs. When setting goals related to functional skills, the therapist and patient may have to accept lower levels of independence, with greater reliance on equipment and assistance. Emphasis must then be placed on the education and training of the caregivers and on teaching the patient how to direct his assistance. The patient and therapist can also establish goals related to activities and a home exercise program that will enable the patient to continue progressing after discharge.

Writing the Goals

Therapeutic goals should focus on functional outcomes rather than impairments, as this focus is more pertinent to the patient's ability to fulfill role expectations and participate in life. The list of goals should specify exactly what functional skills will be pursued in therapy. It should also address the equipment procurement, architectural adaptation, and educational outcomes required for optimal functioning and health after discharge.

Goals provide direction, focus, and structure for therapeutic programs. Their wording should be specific, with measurable endpoints. In addition to providing better direction for program planning, this specificity will enhance communication with other health professionals and third-party payers regarding the purpose of the therapeutic program. A well-written functional goal should specify exactly what the patient will be able to do (ascend and descend 4-inch curbs in a manual wheelchair, for example), including the conditions under which he will perform the activity (cement curb, for example) and how much if any assistance he will require to perform it safely. Finally, goals should state a target date for achievement.

---

[w] This is not to say that the rehabilitation team should "go down without a fight." When faced with funding constraints limiting optimal outcomes, health professionals should utilize the appeals process, seek alternate sources of funding, or both. When these attempts are unsuccessful, the therapist and patient may be forced to settle for adequate rather than optimal outcomes.

Problem-Solving Exercise 7–5

Your patient was in an automobile accident a week ago. She sustained an incomplete spinal cord injury with T10 neurological level of injury, plus multiple extremity fractures. She was transferred to your facility today for inpatient rehabilitation. The following orthopedic restrictions are listed in her chart: (1) thoraco-lumbo-sacral orthosis (TLSO) to be worn at all times. (2) Strict non–weight bearing on the left lower extremity and bilateral upper extremities. You speak with the patient's surgeon about the restrictions and find that she should not push or pull with the upper extremities or bear any weight through either the hands or the forearms. The left lower extremity may be allowed to rest on the floor or on a wheelchair footrest, but the patient is not to bear any additional weight on it.

The TLSO will be worn for approximately 3 months. From your past experience, you do not expect it to hamper the patient's progress in rehabilitation to a large degree. The non–weight-bearing restrictions are to be in force for at least 6 weeks. While these restrictions are in place, you do not foresee any significant progress in her functional abilities.

Your facility's case manager informs you that the patient's insurance company will fund 5 weeks of inpatient rehabilitation. From past experience with this company, the case manager feels that it may be possible to extend the inpatient stay by a week or two at the most.

- What solution can you think of that would maximize the patient's benefit from therapy? To implement this plan, what will the case manager, nursing staff, and therapists need to do?
- What therapeutic goals would you set at this time?

Summary

- Physical therapy examination and evaluation involve an assessment of the patient's impairments, activity limitations, and other factors that impact on health and function. The data gathered in the examination establishes a baseline and provides the basis for program planning.

- The examination and evaluation should be a collaborative effort between the therapist and patient. Inclusion of the patient as an active participant in the process serves to reinforce his autonomy and ensures that the therapeutic goals established are meaningful to him.

- Following spinal cord injury, a physical therapy examination should include the patient's history and subjective statements, voluntary motor function, sensation, muscle tone, passive range of motion, functional abilities, pain, skin integrity, ability to breathe and clear secretions, equipment, and home environment.

- After the initial examination is completed, the therapist makes an informed estimate of the patient's potential for functional gains. This estimation is largely influenced by the patient's voluntary motor function. Additional factors to be considered include passive range of motion, spasticity, age, secondary or preexisting medical conditions, body build, sensation, cognitive and

emotional status, and funding for equipment and rehabilitation services.

- Goals are set in a collaborative process in which the patient and therapist come to an agreement about the intended outcomes of the therapeutic program. The patient and therapist must take into account the examination results, the estimated potential for functional gains, the patient's priorities, the social and physical environment in which the patient will function after discharge, and the resources available for rehabilitation.

- When funding sources limit the rehabilitation services available to the patient, goals must be prioritized. Factors to consider when prioritizing goals include discharge destination, assistance available after discharge, availability of therapy following discharge, current medical or orthopedic restrictions on activity, likelihood of significant neurological return, functional potential, financial resources, and the patient's home and community environments.

- Goals are established with an emphasis on increasing functional independence and reducing disability. All goals should be written with specified, measurable endpoints.

Suggested Resources

PUBLICATIONS

ASIA Standards Teaching Package: available for purchase at *www.asia-spinalinjury.org/publications/store.php*

Community Integration Questionnaire (CIQ): available free at *www.tbims.org/combi/ciq/index.html*

Craig Handicap Assessment & Reporting Technique (CHART): available free at *www.craighospital.org/research/CHART.asp*

Craig Hospital Inventory of Environmental Factors (CHIEF): available free at *www.craighospital.org/research/CHIEF.asp*

Functional Independence Measure (FIM): *www.udsmr.org*

Kendall FP et al. *Muscles: Testing and Function, with Posture and Pain*, 5th ed. Lippincott Williams & Wilkins.

PRISM (Patient Reported Impact of Spasticity Measure): available free at *http://uwcorr.washington.edu/prism.htm*

SCIM III (Spinal Cord Independence Measure, Version III): available free at *www.rehab.research.va.gov/jour/07/44/1/pdf/catzappend.pdf*

Standards for Neurological Classification of SCI Worksheet (Dermatomes Chart): available free at *www.asia-spinalinjury.org/publications/2006_Classif_worksheet.pdf*

Walking Index for Spinal Cord Injury (WISCI II): available free at *www.spinalcordcenter.org/research/wisci/resources/index.html*

Wheelchair Skills Test (versions available for manual and power wheelchairs, wheelchair user and caregiver): available free at *www.wheelchairskillsprogram.ca*

8

Strategies for Functional Rehabilitation

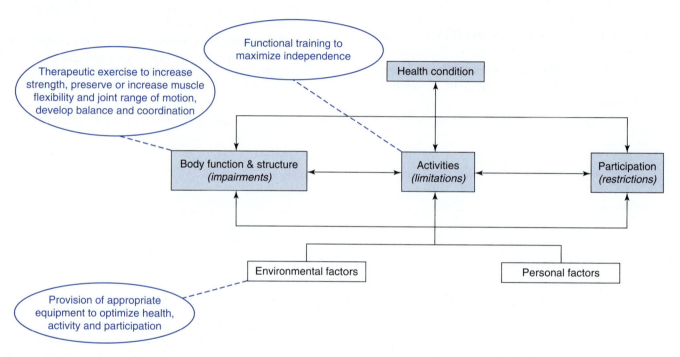

Chapter 8 presents strategies for functional rehabilitation after spinal cord injury, including compensation versus restoration, therapeutic exercise, functional training, and selection of equipment.

Function is a major focus of rehabilitation; the aim of functional rehabilitation is to optimize the individual's ability to perform activities and participate in life situations. Each activity involves the performance of a set of skills, and requires adequate strength, joint range of motion, and muscle flexibility (physical prerequisites) to carry out the actions involved. During rehabilitation, the patient develops the needed skills and physical prerequisites, and obtains the equipment that she will require for safe and independent functioning.

COMPENSATION VERSUS RESTORATION

Functional gains can be achieved through compensation, restoration of more normal movement capabilities, or a combination of the two. The strategies used depend largely on the individual's voluntary motor function below the lesion (Figure 8–1).

When voluntary motor function is absent below the lesion (ASIA A or B), functional independence is optimized through compensation. Rehabilitation emphasizes the acquisition of new motor skills (compensatory movement strategies) used to perform activities using innervated musculature; development of the strength and flexibility needed to perform these skills; provision of equipment such as ambulatory assistive devices, orthoses, wheelchairs, and adaptive devices for activities of daily living (ADL); and adaptation of the environment.

In contrast, individuals who have voluntary motor function that is preserved or returns after injury (ASIA C or D) have the potential to relearn more normal movement

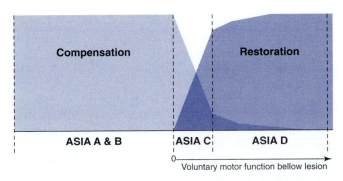

Figure 8–1   Compensation and restoration in functional rehabilitation following spinal cord injury. Schematic diagram shows compensation with motor complete injuries (ASIA A and B), and a shift from compensation to restoration with greater amounts of voluntary motor function below the lesion in motor incomplete injuries (ASIA C and D).

patterns. Rehabilitation emphasizes restoration of normal movement capacities and minimization of compensation to the extent possible. In recent years, an emerging understanding of the central nervous system's potential for adaptation after spinal cord injury has given rise to interventions designed to target this neuroplasticity.

Movement Strategies Following Spinal Cord Injury

Normal movement involves the coordinated action of an array of skeletal muscles functioning in concert to move the trunk and extremities. Damage to the spinal cord disrupts this normal pattern of motion. The extent of this disruption depends on the completeness and pattern of neurological damage. The manner in which an individual can move after a spinal cord injury will be influenced by the motor and sensory function that returns or is preserved following the injury.

Complete Injuries

After sustaining a complete spinal cord injury, a person who wishes to regain functional independence must learn to use the muscles that remain to perform the tasks of now absent musculature. With fewer muscles functioning, she must find new ways to move. Three compensatory movement strategies are available to enable a person with complete spinal cord injury to make the most of what musculature remains functional: muscle substitution, momentum, and the head–hips relationship.

Muscle Substitution

Muscle substitution can be used when the musculature normally causing a motion is weak or absent. In one method of substitution, agonistic musculature compensates

for a strength deficit. For example, the tensor fascia lata can substitute for a weak or absent gluteus medius in hip abduction. This and other substitutions by agonists should be familiar to all physical therapists, who monitor for them whenever they are performing manual muscle tests.[1,2]

Agonists are commonly used to substitute after spinal cord injury. Whenever the agonists of a weak or nonfunctioning muscle remain functional, they work to compensate for the motor deficit. In the paralysis that results from spinal cord injury, however, agonists often are not available for substitution. In these instances, other methods of substitution are used.

The substitutions used following spinal cord injury may seem mysterious to the uninitiated. (Muscles are used to move joints they do not even cross!) However, a muscle used to substitute does not do anything out of the ordinary. It simply contracts concentrically, eccentrically, or isometrically, pulling in the same direction that it always did. Unless a muscle is moved surgically, it cannot do otherwise. The key to muscle substitution after spinal cord injury is learning to use a muscle's pull differently.

In addition to substitution by agonists, there are three ways in which a muscle can be used to substitute. Muscle action can be combined with the effects of gravity, tension in passive structures, or fixation of the distal extremity to effect a desired motion.

Substitution Using Gravity

Functioning musculature can be used to reposition a part in such a way that gravity will effect the desired motion. For example, shoulder motion can be used to pronate the forearm. When a person is sitting upright, shoulder abduction and internal rotation can move the forearm to a position in which the palm faces downward slightly. Once the forearm is in this position, the downward pull of gravity will pronate the forearm.

When gravity is used in substitution, the movement's force will be very limited. Any significant resistance will prevent the motion.

Substitution Using Tension in Passive Structures

Tension in nonfunctioning musculature can also be used to effect motion. The tenodesis grasp is an example of this method of substitution. When a tenodesis grasp is used, the extensor carpi radialis longus and brevis are used to extend the wrist. The resulting increase in tension in the flexor digitorum profundus, flexor digitorum superficialis, and the flexor pollicis longus causes the fingers to flex and the thumb to approximate the fingers (Figure 8–2).[3]

This method of substitution can cause a more forceful motion than is possible in substitutions using gravity; the motion can be performed against some resistance. For this reason, a tenodesis grasp can be functionally useful in activities such as eating, dressing, and self-catheterization.

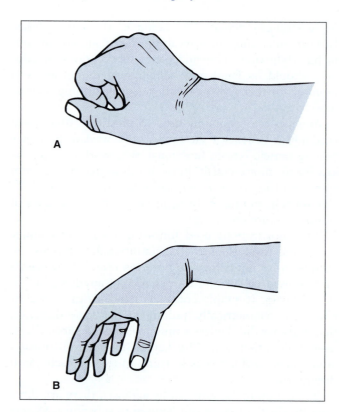

Figure 8–2   Tenodesis grasp used by people with C6 and C7 tetraplegia. (A) Fingers close upon wrist extension and (B) open upon wrist flexion. Gravity provides power for wrist flexion.

Substitution Using Fixation of the Distal Extremity

This method of muscle substitution involves fixing the distal end of an extremity by stabilizing it on an object and using proximal musculature to cause motion at an intermediate joint. The anterior deltoid and pectoralis major (clavicular portion) can be used to extend the elbow in this manner.[4–6] When a person with a spinal cord injury extends her elbow using her proximal musculature, she first stabilizes her hand. In this closed-chain position, she then uses her anterior deltoid and pectoralis major to adduct (Figure 8–3) or flex (Figure 8–4) the humerus. This motion pulls her elbow into extension.

Using this method of substitution, a fair amount of force can be generated. A patient who has adequate strength proximally will be able to extend her elbows forcefully enough to lift her trunk from a forward lean (Figure 8–4).

In a related maneuver, an individual who lacks functioning triceps can "lock" her elbows in extension during weight-bearing activities such as transfers. "Locking" the elbows involves placing the palms on the supporting surface (mat, wheelchair cushion, or bed) and positioning the arms with the shoulders externally rotated, the elbows and wrists extended, and the forearms supinated. Elbow extension is maintained during the weight-bearing activity through strong contraction of the anterior deltoids and external rotators.

Angular Momentum

Another compensatory movement strategy that is used following spinal cord injury involves the use of momentum. Momentum is the tendency of an object to continue moving once it has been set in motion. An object that is rotating about an axis has angular momentum, the tendency to continue its rotation.

Angular momentum can be used to augment motion at a given joint when musculature is weak. A patient who cannot complete an action when she "places" a body part, moving it slowly, may be able to complete the same action if she "throws" the part instead. An example would be someone with weak posterior deltoids who is sitting in a wheelchair and wishes to position her arm behind the wheelchair's push handle. She may find that she is unable to "place" her arm behind the push handle but can move her arm into position by throwing it.

In another use of angular momentum, innervated musculature causes motion, and the momentum of the moving part(s) results in movement in other areas of the body. This use of angular momentum is exemplified by a compensatory technique used to roll. A person who lacks innervated trunk and lower extremity musculature can roll by throwing her head and arms to the side. If the motion is forceful enough and timed correctly, the momentum of the head and arms will carry the trunk from supine.

The angular momentum of a large object (such as a person) is equal to the sum of the angular momenta of all of its parts. Each part's angular momentum is proportional to its velocity, mass, and the moment arm, or distance of the part from its axis of rotation. The effects of these characteristics of angular momentum are important to keep in mind during functional training. They are summarized in Table 8–1.

Head–Hips Relationship

The third compensatory movement strategy used to perform functional activities following complete spinal cord injury involves the head–hips relationship. When using this strategy, a person with a spinal cord injury moves her buttocks by moving her head in the opposite direction. To do so, she pivots on her shoulders, which act as a fulcrum in a first-class lever (Figure 8–5).

Transfers provide a good example of the use of the head–hips relationship. Someone with a complete injury who wishes to lift her buttocks up and to the left in a transfer does so by moving her head down and to the right while pivoting on her arms.

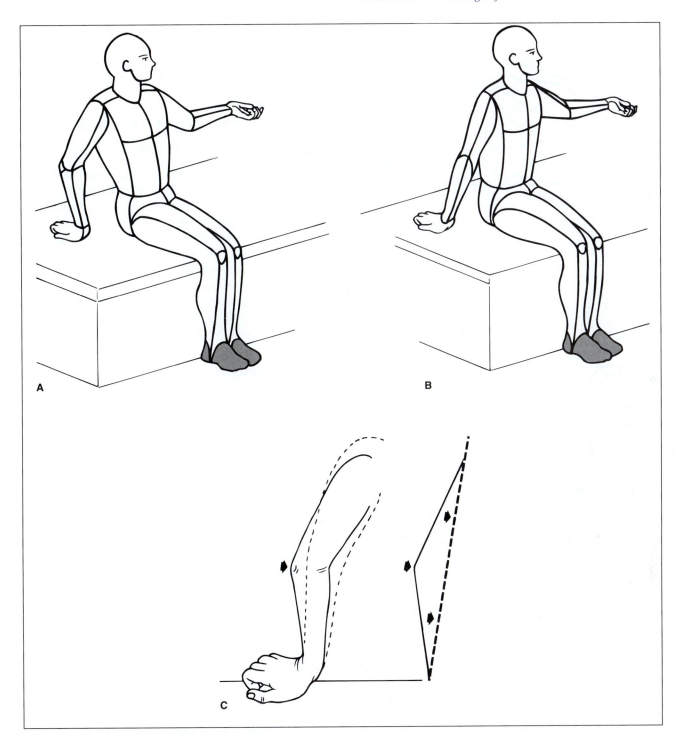

Figure 8–3   Substitution using fixation of the distal extremity. (A) An individual lacking triceps is sitting on a mat, leaning on one arm. The elbow is flexed and the hand is stabilized on the mat. (B) The elbow is extended by adducting the shoulder. (C) When the humerus is adducted, the proximal forearm also moves medially, resulting in elbow extension.

Incomplete Injuries

The motor and sensory function that remains or returns following incomplete spinal cord injury is highly variable. The movement strategies that an individual with an incomplete injury uses in order to function will depend on the extent and pattern of her neurological damage. A person who has sensory sparing but lacks any voluntary motor function below her lesion will utilize the same movement strategies as those used by people with complete spinal

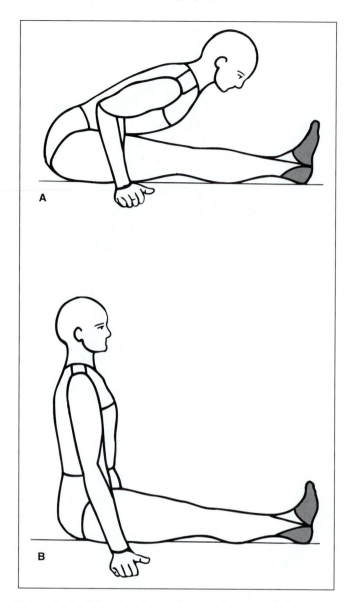

Figure 8–4   Muscle substitution used to extend the elbows and lift the trunk from a forward lean.

cord injuries: muscle substitution, momentum, and the head–hips relationship. Someone with minimal motor sparing is likely to use the same strategies, modified to incorporate the use of functioning musculature. For example, a person who retains or regains some use of her hip flexors could use these muscles while rolling, combining hip flexion with her head and arm motions.[a] In contrast, a person with significant voluntary motor function that remains or returns below her spinal cord lesion may be capable of more normal movement patterns; if adequate voluntary motor function is present below the lesion, she may be able to function without the use of muscle substitution,

momentum, or the head–hips relationship. Finally, a person who has an intermediate degree of motor return may utilize compensatory movement strategies for some activities, and more normal movement patterns for others.

PHYSICAL PREREQUISITES: STRENGTH AND RANGE OF MOTION

Whether an individual learns new movement strategies to compensate for lost musculature or relearns more normal movement patterns, she requires adequate muscle strength and range of motion to perform the motions involved.[b] During rehabilitation after spinal cord injury, appropriate measures must be taken to ensure that the individual will be prepared for the specific physical actions that she will eventually use to function. To accomplish this end, it is important for clinicians to keep in mind the manner in which the individual will ultimately function. (How will she transfer? How will she grasp objects?)

Muscle Strength

Strengthening exercises are an essential component of rehabilitation after spinal cord injury. The strengthening program should be designed to prepare the individual to function optimally using compensatory strategies, more normal movement patterns, or a combination of the two, depending on her motor function and potential.

After spinal cord injury, greater strength in upper extremity musculature is associated with higher levels of independence in a variety of functional tasks.[7–10] If the individual will be using compensatory strategies to function, the strengthening program should emphasize musculature that is used in elbow flexion and extension, shoulder flexion and horizontal adduction, and scapular protraction and depression, as these muscles are used for most functional activities.[c] Trunk and lower extremity musculature that remains innervated should also be strengthened to enhance function.

When compensatory movement strategies will be used to function, even musculature that exhibits normal (5/5) strength may need to be strengthened. In these cases, the muscles that remain innervated compensate for those that have been paralyzed. As a result, innervated muscles are often required to perform actions for which they are not ideally suited. An example is the use of the anterior deltoids to extend the elbows when the triceps are paralyzed. The anterior deltoids, which normally flex the glenohumeral joints, must extend the elbows during

---

[a] By flexing her hip while throwing her head and arms, she can add angular momentum in the direction of the roll. This technique is described in more detail in Chapter 9.

[b] Adequate cardiovascular endurance is also required for function. Cardiovascular fitness training is discussed in Chapter 3.
[c] The therapeutic exercise program should also be designed to preserve upper extremity function. Strategies for preventing upper extremity overuse injuries are discussed later in this chapter.

TABLE 8–1   Properties of Angular Momentum

Property	Impact on Momentum	Application	Clinical Example: Rolling
Summation of momenta	The angular momentum of a large object is equal to the sum of the angular momenta of all of its parts.	Following spinal cord injury, the motions of body parts that remain innervated are used to generate momentum to move parts that are paralyzed. Motions of relatively small body parts (head and upper extremities) are often used to cause larger parts (trunk and lower extremities) to move.	During rolling, momentum from head and arm motions is used to move the trunk and lower extremities. Isolated motions of the head or upper extremities may not create adequate momentum for rolling, but the combined momentum from the head and arms moving synchronously may generate adequate momentum to move the rest of the body.
Velocity	Angular momentum is proportional to the object's (or part's) velocity.	An extremity moving with higher velocity will have greater momentum than the same extremity moving at a slower speed. When a person uses momentum to perform a functional activity, his motions must be performed with adequate speed.	Someone who moves his arms and head too slowly while attempting to roll will not be able to work up enough momentum to move his trunk.
Mass	Angular momentum is proportional to the object's (or part's) mass.	If all other things are equal, an object with greater mass will have greater angular momentum. Because the arms are relatively small, it can be difficult at first to generate adequate momentum using arm motions to cause motion in the pelvis and lower extremities.	Rolling can be made easier by attaching a weight to a patient's forearm. This increases the angular momentum that the arm will have at a given speed, making rolling easier. Although adding a wrist weight to facilitate rolling is not practical as a permanent measure, it can be used to assist rolling during functional training.
Moment arm	Angular momentum is proportional to the object's (or part's) moment arm. A moment arm is the distance of the part from its axis of rotation.	For a given mass and velocity, an object with a longer moment arm will have greater angular momentum. When a person uses momentum from arm motions to move, he will be more successful if he moves his arms in an arc that is as distant as possible from the axis of rotation.	Rolling is easier when the elbows are held in extension and the shoulders are flexed to lift the arms above the trunk. Throwing the arms in this position keeps their mass further from the body, increasing their moment arms. This enables the patient to generate more angular momentum when he throws his arms.

transfers and maintain this extension while the person supports her weight on her arms. The stronger the anterior deltoids are, the more stable the arms will be during transfers.

Strengthening exercises should consist of active-assisted, active, or resisted motions, depending on the strength of the functioning musculature. To the degree possible within the constraints imposed by orthopedic precautions, the patient can be asked to contract her muscles maximally for short durations. This muscle activity should result in strengthening and hypertrophy of innervated musculature. Lower-intensity exercises of longer duration can also be included in the program to increase resistance to muscle fatigue.[11] The strengthening program may include any combination of the following: isometric exercises, progressive resistive exercises (concentric and eccentric), strengthening through functional activity, isokinetic exercise, proprioceptive neuromuscular facilitation (PNF) techniques, and electrical stimulation.[12–16] During strengthening exercises, care should be taken to avoid placing stress on unstable vertebral areas.

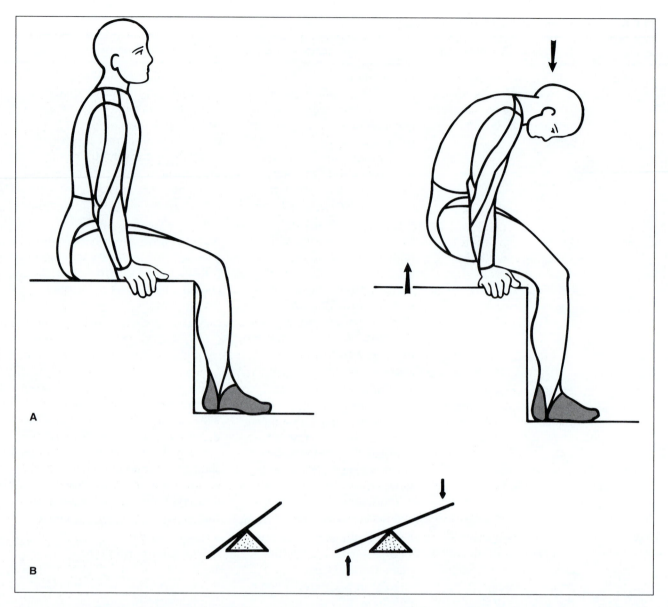

Figure 8–5   The head–hips relationship. (A) The person with a spinal cord injury pivots on his arms, moving his head down to lift his buttocks. (B) First-class lever.

Problem-Solving Exercise 8–1

Your patient has complete (ASIA A) T5 paraplegia. He is working toward the goal of independent floor-to-wheelchair transfers. He is sitting on the floor in front of his wheelchair, with his right hand on the wheelchair seat and his left hand on the floor.

- In what direction should the patient move his head in order to lift his buttocks up and to the right toward the wheelchair seat?

- Should he throw his head in a rapid motion, or should he place it using a slow and controlled motion?
- Will he need to use muscle substitution to maintain elbow extension on the left?

During rehabilitation, the patient with a spinal cord injury should be encouraged to use her functioning musculature as much as possible. While not in therapy, she can maximize her strength by performing isometric exercises, lifting weights, participating in her care, and propelling her wheelchair.

Range of Motion

Preservation or development of appropriate range of motion is critical during rehabilitation. At best, the development of contractures will slow the rehabilitation process. At worst, contractures will seriously limit the person's ultimate functional potential. To prevent the development of contractures, range-of-motion exercises should be initiated as soon as possible after spinal cord injury. When vertebral instability is present, care should be taken to avoid placing stress on the unstable segments of the spine.

Joint range of motion and muscle flexibility should be increased or maintained (as indicated) through positioning, splinting, and daily exercises during acute care and rehabilitation.[d] Passive and active range of motion exercises, PNF techniques, joint mobilization, prolonged static stretching, or a combination thereof may be employed.[15,17] To complement and eventually replace the exercise program provided by health professionals, the family can be instructed in range-of-motion exercises or the patient can be taught self–range of motion.

When range-of-motion limitations seriously impede functional progress, splints or casts may be used to help increase or maintain range between therapy sessions.[15,17] When these devices are used, however, the health care team must be aware of their potential hazards and take measures to avoid them.[e]

As a rule, normal joint range of motion and muscle flexibility will enhance function. After a motor complete spinal cord injury, however, greater than normal motion is required in some areas and mild tightness is desirable in others. Moreover, range and flexibility will have greater functional significance in some areas than in others. For example, limited elbow extension will have greater impact on function than will a comparable limitation in ankle plantar flexion. Table 8–2 summarizes the range-of-motion requirements of people with motor complete spinal cord injuries.

STRATEGIES FOR FUNCTIONAL TRAINING

A program limited to strengthening and range-of-motion exercises will not result in the development of functional skills. The most important component of a functional rehabilitation program is functional training. Through functional training, the individual with significant motor impairments learns the compensatory movement strategies that she will use to move her body, take care of herself, and manipulate her environment. The person with less severe motor deficits relearns more normal movement strategies for performing functional tasks.

The purpose of functional training is the acquisition of motor skills that can later be utilized in environments other than the therapy gym. By helping patients acquire functional skills that they can perform at home or in the community, therapists can enhance their capacity to return to their accustomed activities and participation in life situations. Theories of motor learning provide some concepts that can be useful in this process.[f] Table 8–3 presents some general suggestions for functional training that are consistent with these theories.

Functional training should be initiated as early as possible in the program rather than being postponed until strength and range have been maximized. Early functional training can have tremendous psychological benefit, enabling the newly injured person to do things for herself and experience tangible progress toward her goals. As the patient masters and uses more skills, her increased activity level also serves to further develop her strength and flexibility. A balanced program that addresses skill concurrently with strength, muscle flexibility, and joint range of motion will be most efficient in helping the patient progress toward independence.

The task of functional training may seem overwhelming when one is faced with a recently injured person who is unable to roll in bed or even to remain upright in a wheelchair. How on earth will this person achieve the lofty goals that she has identified? The answer is that functional goals can be achieved through the application of a few simple functional training strategies: building a foundation of movement skills, breaking down activities into their component parts, making tasks easier, and learning skills in reverse.

Building a Foundation of Movement Skills

Following spinal cord injury, an individual with significantly impaired or absent voluntary motor function below her level of injury has a limited number of innervated muscles with which to perform tasks that previously involved the coordinated action of the muscles of her entire body. To

---

[d] Studies of the effects of stretching following spinal cord injury have found no effect on hamstring flexibility[42] and little[43,44] or no[45] effect on ankle range of motion. Stretching remains a standard component of rehabilitation following spinal cord injury, however, as the clinical implications of these studies remain unclear.

[e] Splints and casts can impair circulation and cause skin breakdown and nerve damage. To avoid these complications, the health care team must ensure that the splints or casts have been fabricated correctly. These devices must also be evaluated regularly to ensure that they continue to fit and function appropriately.

---

[f] An in-depth discussion of motor learning is beyond the scope of this text. For more information on this topic, the reader is referred to the following references: 18, 20, 22, 23, and 27.

TABLE 8–2 Range of Motion Requirements Following MOTOR complete Spinal Cord Injury

	Ideal Range	**Functional Significance**
Neck	As normal as possible within orthopedic constraints and precautions.	Mat/bed activities, upper body dressing, self-care, and standing and sitting posture.
Low back	Mild tightness.	Transfers and mat/bed activities.
Shoulders	Normal range in all motions.	Mat/bed activities, upper body dressing, uneven transfers.
	In the absence of functioning triceps: greater than normal combined extension/external rotation with elbow extended.	Coming to sitting using certain methods. *Note: concerns regarding potential shoulder problems may direct the therapist and patient toward alternate methods of coming to sitting that do not require greater than normal shoulder range.*
Elbows	Full extension is essential.	Transfers, mat/bed activities, wheelchair skills, and ambulation.
	Normal or near normal flexion.	Self-care, eating, mat/bed activities, wheelchair skills, and floor-to-wheelchair transfers.
Forearms	Normal supination.	"Locking" elbows in the absence of functioning triceps.
	Normal pronation.	Manipulation of handheld joystick of power wheelchair.
Wrists	Normal extension.	"Locking" elbows in the absence of functioning triceps. Tenodesis grasp for the performance of ADLs.
	Normal flexion.	Release of tenodesis grasp for ADLs.
Fingers	In the absence of functioning finger flexors: normal metacarpophalangeal and interphalangeal motion, mild tightness in extrinsic finger and thumb flexors.	Tenodesis grasp and release for ADLs.
Hips	Full extension.	Ambulation.
	At least neutral extension.	Positioning and mat/bed activities in prone.
	Normal or near normal flexion.	Mat/bed activities, dressing, wheelchair skills, transfers, and coming to stand from the floor.
	Normal or near-normal external rotation.	Dressing.
Knees	Normal extension.	Ambulation.
Hamstrings	110 to 120 degrees of passive straight leg raise.	Long-sitting, dressing, mat mobility, floor-to-wheelchair transfers, and coming to stand from the floor.
Ankles	At least 10 degrees of dorsiflexion.	Ambulation.
	At least neutral dorsiflexion.	Prevention of skin breakdown due to excessive pressure over metatarsal heads and toes while sitting in a wheelchair.

compensate for lost musculature, she must learn to move in new ways, using muscle substitution, momentum, and the head–hips relationship to function. She must also learn to use her remaining musculature to maintain her balance in the various postures involved in functional activities. Physical therapy in this case involves the development of new motor skills used to move and maintain balance. The emphasis of treatment is on function rather than normalcy.

In contrast, a person who retains or regains adequate motor functioning below her spinal cord lesion may have the potential for more normal movement patterns. Coordinated motor function, however, will not necessarily appear spontaneously as neurological return occurs. For this reason, physical therapy should address the development of normalcy of motion in addition to functional status in instances where significant voluntary motor function remains or returns following spinal cord injury. Interventions designed to maximize the recovery of motor skills through neuroplasticity emphasize repetitive and intense practice of normal movement patterns.[g]

---

[g] To date, the most prominent of these approaches has been body weight–supported treadmill training (BWSTT). This topic is addressed in Chapter 12.

TABLE 8–3   Suggestions for Enhancing Motor Learning During Functional Training

Suggestion	Reasoning
Plan for successes as much as possible.	It can be frustrating and discouraging to attempt tasks that are too difficult to perform. In contrast, successful accomplishment of a task can be rewarding and motivating. A patient's motivation may be enhanced if her activities in therapy are structured so that she can experience success in many of the tasks that she is asked to perform.
Have the patient practice tasks that are difficult but doable.	If an activity can be performed too easily, practice will not lead to the development of new motor skills. Moreover, practice of a task that is too easy will not engage the patient as effectively in the active learning of the task. Functional training should include tasks that the patient can perform successfully but with effort.[18,19] Practice of these tasks will enable the patient to master new skills.
Encourage multiple repetitions of new skills.	Practice enhances motor learning.[20–23] A patient who successfully performs a new skill once may be unable to repeat the action in the future if she does not practice. If instead she repeats the maneuver multiple times, she is more likely to retain the ability to perform that task in the future.
Encourage patients to use their skills during nontherapy times.	Use of skills during nontherapy times (in addition to functional training sessions) will increase the time spent practicing, add variety to the conditions under which the skills are practiced, and encourage problem solving. All of these effects will enhance motor learning.[21]
Once a patient can perform a task, intersperse practice of this task with the practice of other tasks.	Except during early practice of a new motor pattern, retention of learned motor skills is enhanced when the task is interspersed with other tasks (random practice) instead of being practiced repetitively without interruption by practice of other tasks (blocked practice).[18,20,23]
During early practice of a skill, provide physical and verbal guidance to the patient. During subsequent practice, reduce guidance. To the extent possible while ensuring safety, allow the patient to make errors and discover her own solutions to movement problems.	Guidance during early practice can reduce the patient's fear, enhance safety, and guide the patient toward successful performance of the task. During later practice, allowing errors and encouraging the patient to "discover" movement strategies will enhance learning and retention.[20,22,23]
During early practice of a skill, provide frequent feedback regarding the patient's attempts at performing the task. During subsequent practice, reduce the frequency of the verbal feedback.	Feedback (knowledge of results) that is frequent during early practice and diminishes as the person continues to practice may promote the learning and retention of new skills. A possible explanation for this enhanced learning is that with reduced feedback, the person learns to detect errors in performance because she cannot rely so heavily on the feedback.[20]

Although motor function plays a critical role in movement, sensation is also important. Normal motor control involves input from the visual, vestibular, and somatosensory systems.[24] A person with sensory impairment following spinal cord injury may have limited or absent ability to sense her body's contact with the supporting surface, and may be unable to sense the positions and motions of her body parts relative to each other and relative to the environment. During rehabilitation, a person with significant sensory loss must learn to utilize remaining sensory cues (visual, vestibular, and somatosensory above the lesion) when performing motor tasks.

As a part of building a foundation of movement skills, the person with motor or sensory impairment needs to develop the ability to control her body in the various postures and different environments involved in functional activities. Concepts from theories of motor learning[18,20,22] as well as proprioceptive neuromuscular facilitation (PNF) techniques[15] can be applied to promote the development of coordinated movement in the trunk, neck, and extremities.

Progression of Postures

Motor control can be developed in a variety of postures. Typically, patients who have profound motor impairments following spinal cord injury first work in basic postures, such as side-lying and supine. Coordinated movement may be easier in these positions because of the low center of gravity and large base of support in these postures. Early work can also occur while sitting in a wheelchair. The support provided by a wheelchair can provide the postural stabilization that a recently injured person is likely to require in an upright posture.

As a patient's ability to stabilize herself and move within a basic posture develops, she can work in progressively more challenging positions. Depending on a patient's muscle function, she may progress to working in a variety of postures, such as prone on elbows, supine on elbows, long and short sitting with and without upper extremity support, kneeling, and standing. To develop a foundation of movement skills, the patient can work on the ability to stabilize and move within these and other postures.

"Stages of Motor Control"

The PNF approach involves progressing from more basic to more advanced motor abilities. The four "stages of motor control" conceptualized in PNF, progressing from most basic to most advanced, are mobility, stability, controlled mobility, and skill.[25] Before one can exhibit a given level of motor control in a particular posture, one must be capable of more basic levels of control in that posture.

Although the theoretical basis for PNF has been challenged,[26] it remains an approach that can be useful for planning interventions and developing movement skills.[15] For example, in planning interventions to develop transfer skills, an even transfer can be conceptualized as follows: transferring between a wheelchair and a bed by pivoting on the arms (skill) requires the ability to shift weight (controlled mobility, or dynamic postural control) in sitting with the hands on the supporting surfaces, which presupposes the ability to maintain a sitting posture (stability, or static postural control) with the hands on the supporting surfaces, which in turn requires adequate range of motion and the ability to initiate motion (mobility). In therapy, the patient can start by developing basic motor abilities (mobility, stability) if they are lacking, and then build on these abilities (progressing to controlled mobility and skill) as her control improves.

Breaking the Activity Down Into Its Component Parts

Following spinal cord injury, many functional activities are serial tasks, consisting of a sequence of discrete actions. A "simple" act such as coming to sitting, for example, can require a series of five or more separate steps. Each of these steps requires a different set of prerequisite skills. Rather than trying to tackle a complex multistep activity as a whole, it can be more productive to break it down and work toward mastery of each component. Once the patient masters the different steps, she can work on putting them together to perform the functional task (part-whole training).[20,21,23,27]

Making the Task Easier

Certain activities are exceedingly difficult initially, even when broken into separate steps. When working on such a challenging task, functional training may involve practicing an easier version of the task. Using this approach, the patient develops her skill by practicing a maneuver that involves the same technique as the activity in question but is easier to perform. As her skill improves, the maneuver that she practices should increase in difficulty, becoming more similar to the functional skill being addressed.

An example of a task that could be approached using this strategy is the side-approach transfer from the floor to a wheelchair. This activity includes a step in which the person lifts her buttocks all the way from the floor to the wheelchair seat. This maneuver requires great flexibility, strength, and finesse. A patient can develop her technique for floor-to-chair transfers by performing transfers between the floor and successively higher surfaces. She may begin by transferring between the floor and a surface 1 or 2 inches higher than the floor, and gradually increase the surface's height until she can transfer as high as the wheelchair seat.

Another example of this functional training strategy is the practice of bed skills on a mat. A mat, because it is a firmer surface than a bed, provides an environment in which it is easier to perform such tasks as coming to sitting or moving the legs while in a sitting position. It is often beneficial to develop these skills on a more stable surface (mat) during early practice, and progress to practice on a less stable surface (bed).

Learning the Skill in Reverse

Many activities are difficult to initiate and become easier as they approach completion. The task of assuming the prone-on-elbows position is an example of such an activity. It takes a good deal of strength for someone with C5 or C6 tetraplegia to lift her upper trunk off of a mat or bed from a sidelying or prone position. The task becomes easier as her upper trunk rises higher and her arms move into a more vertical position under her shoulders.

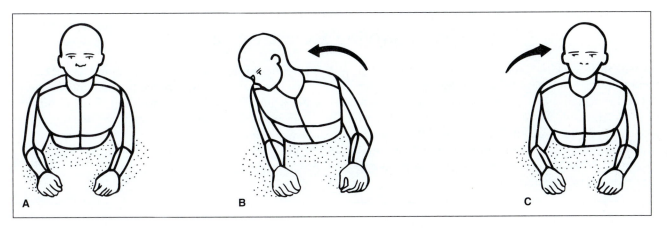

Figure 8–6   Learning a skill in reverse: assuming the prone-on-elbows position. (A) Begin in the end position (prone on elbows in this case). (B) Shift a short distance out of the position. (C) Return to the original position.

Working on the skill in reverse is a useful training strategy for this type of activity. Instead of starting at the beginning of the activity where the task is the most difficult, the patient starts at the endpoint and works backward. Emphasis should be placed on the patient controlling her motion as she works on the skill in reverse. For example, the individual learning to assume the prone-on-elbows position from sidelying can start in prone-on-elbows and practice moving toward sidelying. To develop her skill, she should move slightly toward sidelying in a controlled fashion and then actively return to prone-on-elbows (Figure 8–6). As her ability improves, she should work on moving progressively further from, and returning to, the prone-on-elbows position in a controlled fashion.

INDEPENDENT WORK

During rehabilitation, patients can learn to perform many therapeutic activities independently or with set-up assistance and distant supervision. Examples include strengthening exercises, self-stretching, and practice of newly or partially acquired motor skills. Independent work can enhance the individual's progress by maximizing the time spent exercising and practicing skills. Moreover, it may reinforce her sense of competence and control, and develop her capacity to continue progressing after discharge from rehabilitation.

PROGRAM DESIGN

The therapeutic program is designed to enable the patient to achieve all of her functional goals. The steps of program planning follow.

1. Identify the functional goals, based on the examination results.[h]

---
[h] Goal setting is addressed in Chapter 7.

2. Determine the methods that the patient will utilize to perform the activities identified in the goals. This determination will involve choosing the methods that provide the best match between the patient's characteristics (body build, impairments, potential for recovery of normal movement patterns, etc.) and the physical and skill requirements of the activities.
3. Consider the patient's impairments and activity limitations as they compare to the physical and skill requirements of the activities to be achieved.
4. Devise and implement a therapeutic program to develop the needed strength, range of motion, and motor skills.
5. Monitor the patient's status, and adapt the therapeutic program as appropriate.

For the purposes of program planning, it may be best for the therapist and patient first to consider each goal separately and devise a plan for achieving each goal. The different goals and their plans can then be considered together. Fortunately, there is much overlap of physical and skill prerequisites for the different functional activities. Thus a person working on rolling from supine is potentially progressing toward independence in rolling, assuming the prone-on-elbows position, and coming to sitting without equipment. Furthermore, work aimed at developing one ability can benefit other, seemingly unrelated, activities. For example, the strengthening and motor learning that results from practicing mat skills may benefit a patient's transfers or basic wheelchair skills.

PRECAUTIONS

Strengthening, range-of-motion exercises, and functional training are essential for maximizing functional capabilities following spinal cord injury. These interventions, however, can cause problems if they are applied improperly. Excessive shearing forces or blunt trauma can damage the skin over the buttocks during transfer training. Vigorous

Problem-Solving Exercise 8–2

Your patient is working toward the goal of rolling from supine to prone. You have instructed her to throw her head and arms (all moving in the same direction) back and forth from side to side in order to roll. From past experience, you know that rolling is most difficult while the patient is supine and the pelvis remains horizontal on the mat. Rolling becomes progressively easier as the pelvis rolls out of this position.

- The patient is unable to roll from supine. What can you do to enable her to practice this skill independently while you work with another patient? (Think of several things you could do to enable her to practice rolling.)
- As her skill develops, how will you progress the program?

---

strengthening or range-of-motion exercises can place undue stress on an unstable spine and compromise neurological status. Improper techniques in hand and wrist range of motion exercises can overstretch the long finger flexors and compromise the patient's functional grasp. To prevent these and other problems, the health practitioner must take appropriate precautions during all rehabilitative efforts.

Orthopedic Precautions

Following traumatic spinal cord injury, the injured segment of the spinal column is likely to be unstable for a period of time. The duration of spinal instability will vary with the type and severity of the bony and ligamentous injuries as well as the surgical and nonsurgical interventions applied. To avoid causing additional neurological injury, health professionals must remain cognizant of the status of the patient's spinal stability and precautions, and carefully avoid any activities that could put the unstable spine at risk. Until the patient has been cleared for unrestricted activity, the surgeon should be consulted about the patient's readiness for any new activities that could potentially place stress on the spinal column.

When the cervical spine is unstable, shoulder range-of-motion exercises should be performed cautiously, with the therapist performing the exercises gently to avoid stress to the cervical region. It may be advisable to avoid shoulder flexion or abduction past 90 degrees until the spine has been stabilized.[28] Strong contraction of the shoulder musculature should also be avoided while the cervical spine is unstable, as muscular contraction may place stress on this area of the spine.

When the lumbar spine is unstable, strong muscle contraction of the hip musculature should be avoided because it may cause motion of the lumbar vertebrae. Hip motions should also be restricted; the therapist should perform hip range-of-motion exercises gently, and may need to avoid flexion past 90 degrees. Passive straight-leg raise exercises should be limited to a range in which motions do not cause any tilting of the pelvis. The allowable range will vary depending on the patient's hamstring flexibility.

Spinal precautions are critical considerations in treatment planning and implementation during the acute and early rehabilitation stages following spinal cord injury. Another orthopedic concern that becomes important as time passes is osteoporosis. Bone mass is rapidly lost after the spinal cord is damaged, resulting in increased risk of fracture.[29] When severe osteoporosis is present, activities that place excessive stresses on the osteoporotic bones should be avoided.

Finally, measures should be taken to prevent overuse injuries of the upper extremities. Shoulder pain is a common problem among people with chronic spinal cord injury. It occurs more frequently in individuals with tetraplegia,[30,31] probably because of altered joint mechanics resulting from incomplete innervation of the upper extremities and shoulder girdle. The other upper extremity joints are also often painful, but the shoulders are most commonly affected.[32–34]

Abnormal stresses experienced repetitively during daily function are thought to be a significant source of overuse injuries after spinal cord injury. As a compensation for paralysis, the upper extremities are used for weight bearing during a variety of activities, as well as for wheelchair propulsion. To compound the potential damage arising from this daily function, muscle imbalances resulting from these activities may alter joint mechanics and further increase the risk of injury.

Strategies for preserving the upper extremities include exercises to develop endurance, balanced strength, and flexibility in the shoulder girdles (Table 8–4). These exercises may reduce damaging stresses by optimizing shoulder girdle mechanics. Additional strategies include minimizing damaging stresses on the upper extremities during daily function by providing appropriate equipment, adapting the physical environment, teaching functional techniques that minimize unnecessary stress on the upper extremities, and educating the patient about upper extremity preservation. Chapters 9 to 12 provide additional information.

Skin Precautions

Pressure ulcers are a common and preventable complication of spinal cord injury that can have serious effects on the person's health, activity, and participation in life situations. During functional training, care must be taken to

TABLE 8–4   Exercises Designed for Upper Extremity Preservation*

Exercises to develop strength and muscle endurance:

- Perform resisted exercises 2 to 3 days per week.
- Emphasize:
  - shoulder internal and external rotation: supraspinatus, infraspinatus and subscapularis
  - shoulder adduction: pectoralis major, latissimus dorsi
  - scapular retraction: middle trapezius and rhomboids
  - scapular upward rotation and stabilization: serratus anterior

Exercises to maintain normal flexibility:

- Perform flexibility exercises ≥2 to 3 times per week.
- Emphasize:
  - humeral external rotation
  - scapular retraction and upward rotation
  - cervical and upper trunk flexibility (prevent forward head posture and kyphosis)
- During stretching exercises for glenohumeral motions, include gentle distraction along the long axis of the humerus to avoid shoulder impingement.

*Exercises should be pain-free.
Sources: References 30, 35, and 36.

avoid prolonged pressure, blunt trauma, and excessive shear forces on the skin. The skin should also be monitored regularly for signs of breakdown. Special attention should be given to the areas of skin most likely to be damaged, based on the patient's activities and other contributing factors.[i]

Blood Pressure Precautions

Orthostatic hypotension, a drop in blood pressure that occurs when moving toward upright from a horizontal position, commonly occurs when sitting activities are initiated after spinal cord injury. Placing an abdominal binder and thigh-high elastic stockings on the patient can help prevent dizziness and loss of consciousness during initial upright activities. The patient should also be moved

gradually from supine to sitting with the legs placed in increasingly dependent positions.[j] When a patient experiences a drop in blood pressure during upright activities, the therapist can elevate the patient's legs, recline the trunk to a less upright position, or both (Figure 8–7).

Autonomic dysreflexia is a more serious problem that can occur in people who have cord lesions above T6, usually after 6 or more months have elapsed since the injury. It is caused by uncontrolled sympathetic discharge, brought on by a noxious stimulus (such as bladder distention or overly vigorous hamstring stretching) below the lesion. Signs and symptoms include elevated blood pressure, bradycardia, a pounding headache, and sweating and vasodilation above the lesion. When autonomic dysreflexia is suspected, the health professional should place the patient

[i] Strategies for protecting the skin during functional training are presented in Chapters 9 to 12.

[j] Chapter 2 presents additional information on orthostatic hypotension. Chapter 11 provides more in-depth information on accommodation to upright sitting.

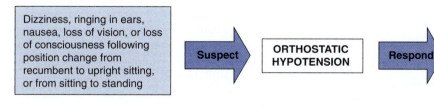

Figure 8–7   Orthostatic hypotension: symptoms and appropriate response.

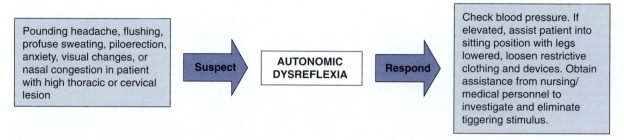

Figure 8–8   Autonomic dysreflexia: signs, symptoms and appropriate response.

in an upright sitting position with the legs dependent, and should remove the source of the problem (Figure 8–8).[k]

Preservation of Beneficial Tightness

The precautions just described are required for preventing medical complications and injuries. In contrast, the precautions presented in this section are aimed at preserving the patient's capacity to perform functional skills. Although these precautions may seem to be less important than those described previously, failure to adhere to them can lead to a profoundly diminished capacity for functional independence.

Tenodesis Grasp

People who lack active finger flexion but retain active wrist extension after spinal cord injury can learn to use a tenodesis grasp to hold and manipulate objects to perform functional tasks such as writing or self-catheterization. This grasp requires mild shortening of the long finger flexors. With the appropriate degree of tightness in these muscles, the fingers will close upon wrist extension and open fully when the wrist is flexed (Figure 8–2). Overstretching of the long finger flexors results in a loss of the functional tenodesis grasp. At the other extreme, excessive shortening of these muscles will inhibit release.

When the wrists and fingers are extended simultaneously, the long finger flexors are stretched and the tenodesis grasp can be damaged. To ensure the development of appropriate tension in these muscles, simultaneous wrist and finger extension must be avoided. Range-of-motion exercises should include finger extension to neutral (0 degrees in all joints) with the wrist fully flexed and full finger flexion with the wrist fully extended. Splints can also be used to encourage the development of appropriate tightness and flexibility for a tenodesis grasp and release.[3]

The tenodesis grasp is at risk during the performance of functional skills. Simultaneous wrist and finger extension can occur during transfers or functional mat activities when weight is borne on the palms. To avoid stretching the long finger flexors, an individual who uses a tenodesis

grasp (or may use this grasp in the future) should keep her interphalangeal joints flexed whenever she bears weight on her palms (Figure 8–9).

Preservation of mild tightness in the long finger flexors is particularly important because damage to the tenodesis mechanism may be permanent. Once the finger flexors become overstretched, it is difficult to get them to tighten. An overzealous but uninformed therapist can cause lasting problems by overstretching these muscles during the acute stage after injury. In like manner, an uninformed patient or family member may damage the tenodesis grasp mechanism. Many newly injured people and their families are eager to perform exercises on the paralyzed extremities in the hope that these exercises will bring about a return of function. Often, the hands are a focal point of these exercises. For this reason, the patient and her family should be educated regarding the importance of avoiding overstretching the long finger flexors.

To facilitate tenodesis grasp and release, appropriate shortening should be allowed to develop in the long finger flexors of people with C7 or higher tetraplegia. Although people with C5 and higher tetraplegia do not have the wrist extensors needed for a tenodesis grasp, their long finger flexors should be allowed to tighten. This tightness may make it possible to use the hand as a hook. Moreover, it is common for voluntary motor function to return in one or more levels caudal to the neurological level of injury during the months and years after injury.[37–40] Many people with C5 and a few with C4, tetraplegia (motor level) regain function in the C6 myotome during the first 8 months after their injuries.[41] Thus a person who initially lacks wrist extensor function can regain it and may then require finger flexor tightness for a tenodesis grasp.

In addition to requiring mild tightness in the long finger flexors, a tenodesis grasp requires adequate strength in the wrist extensors. During the early stages following spinal cord injury, care should also be taken to prevent overstretching of wrist extensors with less than fair (3/5) strength, as overstretching of weakened musculature can impair its functioning. Overstretching can occur when the wrists are allowed to remain positioned in flexion due to the effects of gravity. Positioning the wrists in extension with splints or hand rolls when at rest can prevent this problem.

---

[k] Chapters 2 and 3 address autonomic dysreflexia in greater depth.

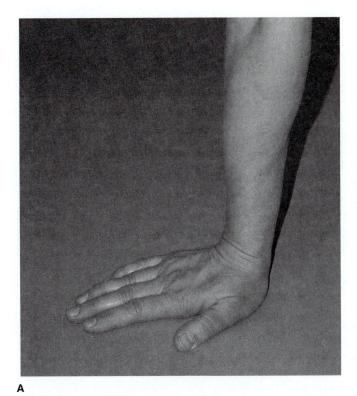
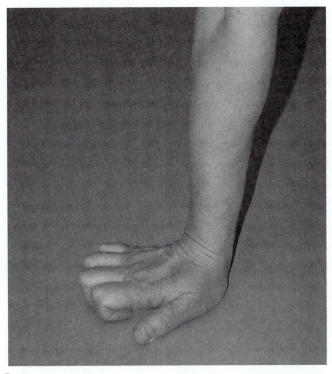

A   **B**

Figure 8–9   Preservation of tenodesis grasp. (A) Extension of wrist and interphalangeal joints in combination can impair potential for tenodesis grasp by overstretching long finger flexors. (B) Flexion of the interphalangeal joints when the wrist is extended preserves the tenodesis grasp.

Low Back

When spinal cord injury results in significant loss of motor function, many functional skills involve using motions of the arms, head, and upper trunk to move the pelvis and legs. Mild tightness in the low back can enhance the performance of functional skills by allowing head and shoulder motions to be transmitted to the lower body. Excessive flexibility in the low back can interfere with function by allowing disassociation between the upper and lower trunk, permitting the upper trunk to move without any motion occurring in the lower trunk or legs. For example, people with complete spinal cord injuries pivot on their arms and use head and scapular motions to move their buttocks during transfers. A person with an overstretched low back who attempts to lift her buttocks in this manner may find that her back elongates and her buttocks remain on the supporting surface when she attempts to pivot on her arms. To prevent this dissociation between motions of the upper and lower trunk, care should be taken to preserve mild tightness in the low back.

Perhaps the most important precautionary measure that can be taken to preserve beneficial tightness in the low back is the maintenance of proper positioning in a wheelchair: the buttocks should be positioned well back on the seat during prolonged sitting.[1] Additional strategies for preserving beneficial tightness in the low back include performing hamstring stretching in supine rather than in long-sitting, and avoiding long-sitting when the hamstrings are shortened.

SELECTION OF EQUIPMENT

Equipment selection is a critical component of functional rehabilitation following spinal cord injury. Regardless of the level or degree of completeness of an individual's spinal cord lesion, she is likely to require equipment in order to function optimally. The extent and level of the person's neurological damage will influence the type of equipment needed. At one extreme, an individual who has either a very low lesion or near-normal motor and sensory function below the lesion may need equipment as simple as a cane or an ankle–foot orthosis in order to function safely and independently. At the other extreme, a person who has a high cervical lesion with minimal or no motor function below her injury may require a power tilt-and-recline wheelchair with controls that interface with environmental control units.

In recent years there has been a virtual explosion in the adaptive equipment market. There is much variability in the quality and usefulness of available products; some are excellent, others have little value. Additionally, a given piece of equipment may be beneficial for some people and useless or even detrimental to others. To maximize functional

---

[1] Sitting posture in a wheelchair is addressed in greater depth in Chapter 11.

status, health, and satisfaction and gain the most for each equipment dollar, health professionals and people with disabilities should select equipment carefully.

Establishing Need

The first step in ordering equipment is establishing a need. A person's need for equipment may be functional, medical, or both.

Functional Need

Equipment such as wheelchairs, doorknob adapters, and lower extremity orthoses can meet functional needs. Equipment can make the life of a person with physical impairments easier, enable her to do things that she otherwise could not do, and conserve time and energy. Clinicians should be mindful, however, that equipment is a double-edged sword: it can also create dependence on itself, reducing the user's ability to function without it. A person who is dependent on a piece of equipment has to put up with its drawbacks (bulk, cosmesis, maintenance, etc.). She will also be unable to function in the event that the equipment is lost, broken, misplaced, or left behind.

One challenge in recommending equipment to improve function is determining whether equipment is truly needed. If someone cannot perform an activity satisfactorily without equipment, she may benefit from equipment designed to aid in the task. Alternatively, she may benefit from additional training to learn to function without the equipment. Therapists should be wary of equipment that at first appears to improve function but that the patient could learn to do without. Often, like training wheels on a bike, equipment can make a task easier while someone is first learning a skill. The problem is that therapists sometimes leave these "training wheels" on, thinking that the need remains. The result is that the need does remain and the person is left using unnecessary equipment.

Once it has been determined that someone cannot function well *without* a given piece of equipment, she and the therapist should ascertain whether she can function better *with* it. Through the years, much money has been wasted on equipment that turned out to be of limited or no benefit to the intended users. Prior functional training with and "test drives" of equipment prior to purchase can help to eliminate this problem.

Medical Need

A medical need exists if a piece of equipment is required for an individual to maintain or return to a healthy state. Wheelchairs, wheelchair cushions, and vertebral orthoses are examples of equipment that meets medical needs.

Some medical needs are temporary. For example, during the acute phase of rehabilitation, a person with a spinal cord injury may experience orthostatic hypotension as her body readjusts to upright sitting. During this adjustment period, she may require a wheelchair with a reclining back and elevating leg rests. Within a brief period

of time, however, she will most likely adjust to upright sitting and will not need these features in a wheelchair. With a temporary medical problem such as this, the needed equipment should be rented or borrowed rather than purchased.[m]

Regardless of whether a piece of equipment meets a temporary or permanent medical need, it should be chosen carefully. Ideally, the equipment will achieve the medically necessary outcome while allowing the patient to function as independently as possible. For example, the vertebral orthosis will stabilize the spine adequately without unnecessarily restricting the patient's extremity motions, or the wheelchair cushion will provide the needed pressure distribution without interfering unnecessarily with transfers.

Choosing Equipment

Once a functional or medical need has been established, the health professional and patient must determine which piece of equipment best meets this need. For most types of equipment, there is a large selection from which to choose. The various brands generally offer different options and vary in quality, price, durability, maintenance required, availability of replacement parts and qualified maintenance facilities, warranty specifications, and other characteristics. With the market constantly expanding, clinicians who are involved in prescribing and advising on equipment must keep current.

When deciding on a piece of equipment, it is best to keep in mind the fact that any equipment has both advantages and disadvantages. For example, pneumatic wheelchair tires are better than solid tires in the following respects: smoother ride and easier propulsion over uneven surfaces, easier negotiation of curbs, and greater traction. Pneumatic tires also have their drawbacks. They go flat if punctured, increase the overall width of the wheelchair, cost more than solid tires, track more dirt into buildings, and must be filled with air periodically. Like pneumatic tires, any equipment or component will have both positive and negative qualities. Clinicians involved in prescribing or advising on equipment should investigate the benefits and drawbacks of the available equipment options.

When possible, equipment (or an identical model) should be used for a trial period before it is purchased. Ideally, several different models will be made available for trials.[n] This practice increases the likelihood that the equipment chosen is really the best match for the individual concerned.

The decision about any piece of equipment should be based on its advantages and disadvantages, considering the needs and priorities of the prospective user. Ultimately,

---

[m] This is not possible with all types of equipment. Vertebral orthoses, for example, must be purchased.

[n] Vendors and company representatives are often accommodating when asked to provide equipment for trial.

the final choice between equipment options is based on values. When weighing the positives and negatives of different options, should ease of use take priority, or should greatest consideration be given to convenience, durability, maintenance requirements, price, or esthetics? Because equipment choice is a value-laden decision with no universal right and wrong answers, the person for whom the equipment is being ordered must be involved in the decision. Otherwise the piece of equipment chosen by the clinician may not be the one most suitable to the values and priorities of the user. Involving the prospective user in

equipment selection also promotes independence, and encourages personal responsibility and consumerism.°

° Involving patients in ordering equipment does not mean ordering everything that they want or everything that their funding sources are willing to purchase. An individual may want something that is not truly needed or that will be detrimental to her physical or functional status. In an instance such as this, the health professional would be doing the patient a disservice by ordering the requested equipment. The clinician also has a responsibility to third-party payers to recommend equipment only when it can be justified as meeting a true need.

Summary

- Functional rehabilitation after spinal cord injury is a challenging task. Depending on the voluntary motor function that an individual retains or regains after injury, she must either learn to use her muscles and move her body in new ways, or relearn more normal movement patterns as motor return occurs.

- An individual who has a complete injury learns to use compensatory movement strategies to perform functional tasks. These strategies include muscle substitution, angular momentum, and the head–hips relationship.

- A person who has an incomplete injury will learn to use compensatory movement strategies, more normal movement patterns, or a combination of the two, depending on her motor function.

- The individual with a spinal cord injury who wishes to optimize her functional capacity must develop an array of physical skills, and develop the muscle strength, joint range of motion, and muscle flexibility needed to perform these skills. The physical therapist assists in

this process by working with the patient to develop and implement a program of therapeutic exercise and functional training.

- Four basic strategies can be used in functional training after motor complete spinal cord injury: building a foundation of movement skills, breaking activities down into their component parts, making tasks easier, and learning skills in reverse. After motor incomplete injuries, interventions designed to maximize the recovery of motor skills through neuroplasticity emphasize repetitive and intense practice of normal movement patterns.

- During functional training and therapeutic exercise, health professionals must take appropriate precautions. These include a variety of orthopedic and medical precautions as well as measures to preserve beneficial tightness in the long finger flexors and the low back.

- The patient and therapist also work together to select appropriate equipment that will promote health and enhance function.

Suggested Resources

AUDIOVISUAL MATERIAL

Clinical Kinesiology Applied to Persons with Quadriplegia, Parts I and II (2002). (Videotapes by Donald Neumann and Michelle Lanouette, Marquette University, Milwaukee, WI.)

PUBLICATION

Preservation of Upper Limb Function Following Spinal Cord Injury: A Clinical Practice Guideline for Health-Care Professionals, 2005. Published by the Paralyzed Veterans of America. Available for free download from *www.pva.org*

WEB SITES

Physiotherapy Exercises for People with Spinal Cord Injuries and Other Neurological Conditions: www.physiotherapy exercises.com

Spinal Cord Injury Rehabilitation Evidence, Chapter 5, Upper Limb Rehabilitation Following Spinal Cord Injury: *www.icord.org/scire/chapters.php*

9

Functional Mat Skills

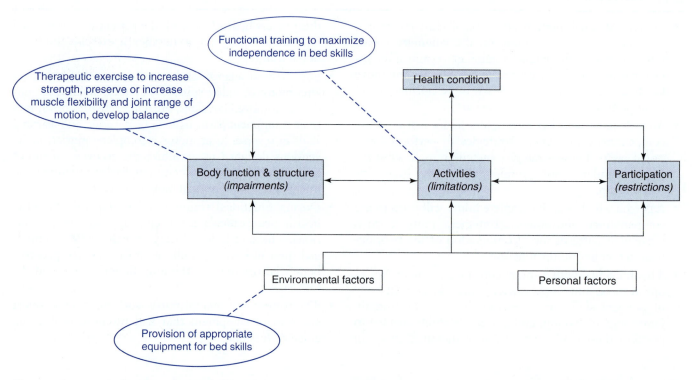

Chapter 9 presents functional mat skills and therapeutic strategies for increasing independence in these activities.

Functional mat skills include rolling, coming to sitting, gross mobility on a mat or bed (moving around on a mat or bed), maintenance of an unsupported sitting posture,[a] and leg management. These skills are required for independent mobility; before someone can get out of bed in the morning, he must first be able to sit up and move to the edge of the bed. These skills are also required for independent dressing.

This chapter presents a variety of functional mat techniques[b] as well as suggestions on how to teach them. The

descriptions of techniques and training should be used as a guide, not as a set of hard and fast rules. The exact motions used to perform any activity vary among people because of differences in body build, skill level, range of motion, muscle tone, patterns of strength and weakness, and presence or absence of additional impairments. During functional training, the therapist and patient should work together to find the techniques that best suit that particular individual.

PRECAUTIONS

Following spinal cord injuries, the activities involved in functional mat training can cause problems if appropriate precautions are not taken. Mat activities can result in excessive motion in unstable segments of the spine, skin damage, and overstretching of the low back and long finger flexors.

---

[a] Unsupported sitting balance is addressed in Chapter 10.
[b] This chapter does not attempt to present all possible functional mat techniques. An individual who is unable to master a skill described in this chapter may fare better with a variation of that technique or with an altogether different method.

TABLE 9–1   Precautions During Functional Mat Training

Potential Problems	Mat Activities That Place Patients at Risk	Precautions
Excessive motion at site of vertebral instability, potentially causing additional neurological and orthopedic damage	Any activity involving excessive motion or muscular action at or near the site of spinal instability. Examples: prone-on-elbows activities while the cervical spine remains unstable, long sitting while the lumbar spine remains unstable.	• Strictly adhere to orthopedic precautions. • Check fit of vertebral orthoses with patients in the different postures involved in mat training. • When the spine is unstable, avoid activities that may cause motion or strong muscular contraction at site of instability.
Skin abrasions and pressure ulcers	Any activities creating shearing forces on skin. Examples: dynamic activities while bearing weight on the elbows, practice moving the buttocks on a mat. Any activities causing prolonged pressure over areas vulnerable to skin damage. Examples: supine activities when there is a pressure ulcer over the sacrum, side-lying activities when there is scarring over the greater trochanters.	• Protective padding over the elbows or buttocks during prolonged practice of activities that create shear forces on skin. • Limited time spent in activities that cause shear forces to skin that is not protected by padding. • Bridge vulnerable areas during activities that would expose them to prolonged pressure: have the patient lie on cushions that are positioned proximal and distal to the wound or vulnerable skin but not in contact with it.
Impaired tenodesis grasp due to overstretching of the long finger flexors	Any activities involving simultaneous wrist and finger extension. Examples: weight bearing on the palms with the fingers extended while coming to sitting or propping in long sitting.	• With patients who may utilize a tenodesis grasp (people with C7 or higher tetraplegia), avoid simultaneous wrist and finger extension. • When bearing weight on the palms, maintain the interphalangeal joints in flexion.
Overstretched low back, resulting in diminished capacity for functional independence	Any activities involving simultaneous hip flexion with knee extension in patients with hamstring tightness, placing stress on the low back. Example: long sitting when the hamstrings are tight.	• Avoid long sitting in patients who lack a minimum of 90 degrees of passive straight leg raise. • Patients with hamstring tightness may sit safely with their knees flexed and hips externally rotated.
Overuse injuries of the upper extremities	Activities involving potentially injurious positions of the upper extremities, performed repetitively over time.	• Avoid positioning joints at extremes of motion or in potentially injurious positions, including internal rotation of the shoulder combined with abduction or flexion.[1]

Over time, activities that subject the joints of the upper extremities to damaging forces may also cause overuse injuries. Table 9–1 presents a summary of precautions for functional mat training.

FUNCTIONAL POTENTIALS

After a spinal cord injury, a person's potential for achieving independence in bed skills is determined largely by his voluntary motor function. Table 9–2 presents a summary of the level of independence in bed skills that can be achieved by people who have complete spinal cord injuries

at different motor levels (motor component of neurological level of injury). When predicting an individual's capacity to develop bed skills, the clinician should take into consideration the many other factors that also affect functional gains.[c] In addition, it is important to recall that these skills take time to develop. Functional gains are likely to continue during all phases of rehabilitation (inpatient, in home, outpatient), and may continue for months or years after discharge.

---

[c] Chapter 7 presents factors that can influence functional outcomes.

TABLE 9–2   Functional Potentials

Motor Level	Significance of Innervated Musculature	Potential for Independence in Bed Skills
C4 and higher	Inadequate voluntary motor function to contribute to bed skills.	Using hospital bed and input through mouth or voice control, independent in coming to a sitting position from supine. Dependent in all other bed skills.
C5	**Partial innervation of the deltoids** makes it possible to extend the elbows using muscle substitution. Deltoid function plus **partial innervation of the infraspinatus and teres minor** make it possible to "lock" the elbows in extension. **Partial innervation of the biceps brachii, brachialis, and brachioradialis** makes it possible to use elbow flexion to pull. Lack of triceps function makes rolling difficult because active elbow extension is lacking. Minimal serratus anterior function is inadequate to stabilize the scapulae against the thorax.	**Typical Functional Outcomes** **Rolling:** some assist, pulling on bed rail or loops **Coming to sitting:** some assist, either walking on elbows or pulling on loops. **Gross mobility in sitting:** dependent to some assist. **Leg management:** dependent to some assist. **Exceptional Functional Outcomes** Independent in bed skills. Likely to require bed rails or loops.
C6	**Fully innervated deltoids, infraspinatus, teres minor, and clavicular portion of the pectoralis major** allow for stronger elbow extension and "locking" using muscle substitution. **Fully innervated biceps brachii** allows for stronger pull using elbow flexion. **Partial innervation of the serratus anterior** makes it possible to stabilize the scapulae against the thorax. Scapular protraction allows greater lift of the buttocks. **Partial innervation of the latissimus dorsi** enhances shoulder girdle depression. Minimal innervation of the triceps brachii is inadequate to contribute significantly to bed skills.	**Typical Functional Outcomes** **Rolling:** some assist to independent, with or without equipment. **Coming to sitting:** some assist to independent, with or without loops. **Gross mobility in sitting:** some assist. **Leg management:** some assist. **Exceptional Functional Outcomes** Independent in all bed skills without equipment.
C7	**Partial innervation of the triceps brachii** allows for stronger elbow extension. **Full innervation of the serratus anterior** provides more stable scapulae as well as stronger protraction and upward rotation. **Partial innervation of the latissimus dorsi and sternocostal portion of pectoralis major** enhances shoulder girdle depression, allowing greater lift of the buttocks.	**Typical Functional Outcomes** Independent to some assist in bed skills without equipment. **Rolling:** independent. **Coming to sitting:** independent. **Gross mobility in sitting:** independent to some assist. **Leg management:** independent to some assist.

TABLE 9–2   *(Continued)*

Motor Level	Significance of Innervated Musculature	Potential for Independence in Bed Skills
C8	**Full innervation of the triceps brachii** provides normal strength in elbow extension. **Full innervation of the latissimus dorsi and nearly full innervation of pectoralis major** allow strong shoulder girdle depression. **Nearly full innervation of flexor digitorum superficialis and profundus and partial innervation of flexor pollicus longus and brevis** provide grasp without muscle substitution, making leg management easier.	**Typical Functional Outcomes** Independent to some assist in bed skills without equipment. **Rolling:** independent. **Coming to sitting:** independent. **Gross mobility in sitting:** independent to some assist. **Leg management:** independent to some assist.
T1 and below	**Fully innervated upper extremities** make all bed skills easier to achieve. (Innervation of musculature associated with lower levels of injury enhances performance.)	**Typical Functional Outcomes** Independent in all bed skills without equipment.

References for innervation: 2 to 6.

PHYSICAL AND SKILL PREREQUISITES

Each method of performing a functional activity involves a particular set of skills. Each activity also has strength, joint range of motion, and muscle flexibility requirements. A deficiency in any of these skill or physical prerequisites will impair a person's performance of the activity.

The descriptions of functional techniques presented in this chapter are accompanied by tables that summarize the skill and physical prerequisites. Exact values for the physical prerequisites are not given because the requirements vary among individuals. For example, when coming to sitting using a given method, someone who is strong and coordinated may require less range in shoulder hyperextension than another person who is weaker or less coordinated.

PRACTICE ON MAT AND BED

An exercise mat is a good surface on which to learn mat skills. It is firmer than a bed, making it an easier surface on which to practice. The goal, however, should be for the patient to function on a bed. This is the surface on which he will most often use these skills during daily life. Since a bed is a more difficult surface on which to function, ability developed on a mat will not automatically transfer to bed function. Thus after an individual has begun to develop some skills on a mat, he should practice them both on a mat and on a bed. This will increase the likelihood that the skills learned in therapy will be utilized outside of therapy.

MAT SKILLS FOLLOWING COMPLETE SPINAL CORD INJURY: FUNCTIONAL TECHNIQUES AND THERAPEUTIC STRATEGIES

Regardless of the level of injury, a person who sustains a complete spinal cord injury has a limited number of muscles with which to perform functional mat skills. To roll, come to sitting, or move about on a bed, he must utilize the muscles innervated above his lesion to move his entire body. During rehabilitation, the patient learns how to perform mat skills using a variety of compensatory strategies, including muscle substitution, momentum, and the head–hips relationship.[d]

General Therapeutic Strategies

To perform a functional mat activity, a person with a spinal cord injury must acquire the activity's physical and skill prerequisites. The therapeutic program should work toward developing all of the needed range of motion, strength, and skills.

Rolling, gross mat mobility, and leg management are relatively simple activities, with few skill prerequisites. As a result, planning a functional training program to develop one of these abilities is fairly straightforward. The patient

---

[d] These movement strategies are explained in Chapter 8.

should start by developing the most basic prerequisite skills and then build on these skills until he is able to perform the activity.

In contrast, each method of coming to sitting involves several steps. Many of the steps are unrelated; the skills required to perform one step are not needed to perform any other steps. As a result, decisions in functional training are less clear cut. When working toward coming to sitting using the method that involves rolling and throwing the arms, is it best to work first on assuming the prone-on-elbows position or on balancing on one extended arm? The two steps involve different skills, and neither step is required to practice the other.

In instances in which an individual has a number of unrelated skills to master, it may be best to work on several different skills during a treatment session. Doing so will add variety to the program. This variety will make it possible to change activities when a group of muscles becomes fatigued, enabling the patient to work in therapy for longer periods of time by distributing the demands on his musculature. Changing activities will also alter the stresses being placed on his joints and skin. Varying activities may also help to keep the patient's interest in the program.

Before asking a patient to attempt a new skill, the therapist should explain and demonstrate the technique.[e] The demonstration should provide a clear idea of the motions involved as well as the timing of these motions. The therapist should also demonstrate or explain how the new skill will be used in daily activities.

During functional training, the therapist should remember that every individual with a spinal cord injury will perform a particular activity differently. Each person has a unique combination of body build, coordination, strength, flexibility, and muscle tone, and these characteristics influence the manner in which he performs functional tasks. What works for one patient may be a total disaster for the next. The challenge of functional training is finding the timing and maneuvers that best suit the individual involved.

Basic Skills

Certain prerequisite skills are required to perform many different mat skills. These include positioning the elbows in extension, maintaining elbow extension while flexing the shoulder, and static and dynamic control while propping on the upper extremities. The following paragraphs include descriptions of these skills and therapeutic strategies for teaching them.

Position Elbows in Extension

People with complete C5 or C6 tetraplegia have innervated elbow flexors but lack extensors. As a result, a problem that they often experience when lying supine is that they cannot straighten their elbows once they become flexed. Because these individuals lack functioning triceps, they need to learn an alternate method for extending their elbows. In supine, momentum is used to accomplish this task.[f]

Commonly, an elbow is positioned in flexion with the shoulder internally rotated so that the forearm rests on the trunk. To extend his elbow when his arm is in this position, a patient can flex his shoulder and then strike his elbow into the mat by extending and externally rotating the shoulder abruptly. If he performs this maneuver with enough force *and if he relaxes his elbow flexors while doing so,* the forearm's momentum will carry it caudally and the elbow will extend.

If the shoulder is initially positioned in external rotation, the elbow can be extended by internally rotating the shoulder while striking the elbow into the mat. Alternatively, the patient can internally rotate the shoulder to position his forearm across his body and proceed from there as described above.

Therapeutic Strategies

Many people with spinal cord injuries discover these maneuvers on their own. Others require instruction and practice. Those who have difficulty learning to extend their elbows can practice the techniques starting with their elbows only slightly flexed. (Extending the elbows will be easiest from this position.) As they develop skill, they can practice from increasingly flexed positions. During early practice, the therapist can assist with the motion and provide verbal and tactile cueing. These inputs should be withdrawn as the patient's ability develops.

Maintain Elbow Extension While Flexing Shoulders

In the absence of functioning triceps, a person with C5 or C6 tetraplegia must use gravity to hold his elbows in extension when he flexes his shoulders. For gravity to hold the elbows in extension, appropriate positioning is required; the shoulders must be held in external rotation. Internal rotation of the shoulders will result in elbow flexion.

Maintaining elbow extension during shoulder flexion involves more than simply positioning the arms so that gravity extends the elbows. People who lack functioning triceps must also keep their elbow flexors relaxed while they flex their shoulders. After sustaining cervical spinal cord injuries, people often tend to perform shoulder and elbow flexion in combination. (This may be a result of

---

[e] This demonstration can also be provided by another person with a spinal cord injury, if someone is available who has similar impairments but a higher level of functional ability. Alternatively, the patient may watch a videotaped demonstration of the skill.

[f] Muscle substitution using the anterior deltoid is not generally feasible in supine because it requires the presence of an object on which to stabilize the hand.

recruitment in response to a partial loss of deltoid inner-vation.) To use their arms functionally, these individuals must learn to isolate these motions.

Therapeutic Strategies

Some patients learn without instruction how to maintain their elbows in extension while flexing their shoulders; however, many require instruction and practice. A therapist may assist by giving verbal and tactile cues as the patient learns to contract his shoulder flexors while keeping his elbow flexors relaxed. This assistance should be withdrawn as the patient's ability develops. A patient who has difficulty keeping his elbow flexors relaxed while flexing his shoulders should practice flexing his shoulders through only a few degrees of motion, and progress through larger arcs as his skill increases.

Static and Dynamic Control While Propping on the Upper Extremities

Many functional mat skills involve propping on one or both upper extremities, balancing in these positions, and changing positions without a loss of balance. During functional training, the person with a spinal cord injury develops his static and dynamic control in each of the postures involved in the functional skills that he is working to master, and practices moving between the postures. Early practice in a given position involves developing static stability, the ability to maintain the posture once in that position. After a patient gains static stability in a posture, he can begin to work on developing dynamic stability, first shifting weight in the posture and then progressing to more challenging tasks as his skill develops.

Therapeutic Strategies: Maintain Position (Static Stability)

Mat activities involve stabilizing in a variety of positions: prone on elbows, supine on elbows, supine supported on one elbow, supine supported on one elbow and one hand, forearm-supported side lying, and long sitting propped on one or two hands. The postures involved depend on the particular method used to perform the activity. For example, one method of coming to sitting involves positioning in prone on elbows, another method involves supine on elbows, and a third method involves both postures. During functional training, a patient with a spinal cord injury should work to develop the ability to stabilize in each of the positions involved in the particular functional techniques that he is working to master.

When propping on the upper extremities, the location of the hands or elbows on the mat or bed influences the difficulty of maintaining the posture. During early practice propping on one or two arms, the supporting elbows or hands should be located on the mat in positions that will make the task easiest. For example, the prone-on-elbows position is typically easiest to maintain when the elbows are on the mat directly beneath the shoulders. If the elbows are located in a different position, (lateral to the shoulders, for example), the patient will have to exert more effort to remain in position. When he begins working on stabilizing in the prone-on-elbows position, the patient should practice with his elbows directly beneath his shoulders. As his skill develops, he can progress to stabilizing with the elbows lateral, caudal, or rostral to this position.

The difficulty of propping on the upper extremities is also influenced by whether the person is using one or two extremities for support. Stabilizing on two upper extremities is less difficult because of the relatively large base of support. Moreover, with both upper extremities in closed-chain positions, the individual can use muscles in both extremities to resist motion out of the posture. (For example, a person propping on two elbows can use bilateral shoulder girdle musculature to maintain the position.) In contrast, a person propping on one upper extremity has a smaller base of support, and has only one upper extremity in a closed-chain position. In addition to using the musculature of his supporting arm to maintain stability in the position, he uses motions of his head and free (non–weight-bearing) arm keep his center of gravity over his base of support. When his trunk starts to fall, he moves his head and free arm in the direction opposite the fall.

Because of the difficulty of balancing with only one extremity for support, patients typically practice stabilizing on two elbows or hands before they practice propping on a single upper extremity. To help a patient develop the ability to maintain a given posture, the therapist can assist him into the position and ask him to hold himself there. At first, the therapist may need to help the patient stabilize by providing verbal cues and manual assistance. As the patient's ability improves, the therapist can withdraw this assistance and guard the patient as he holds the position. With further development of the patient's ability to stabilize, the therapist can apply resistance to his shoulders in various directions while the patient holds the posture.

Once a patient has learned to prop on two extremities, he can progress to maintaining his balance while propping on one.[g] After explaining and demonstrating how the patient can use motions of his head and free arm to help maintain his balance, the therapist can assist the patient into position and ask him to maintain the position. The therapist can provide assistance and verbal cueing at first, and withdraw this input as the patient's skill develops.

Practice of stability in sitting requires two capabilities that are not needed in other positions. First, before working on any sitting skills, individuals who experience orthostatic hypotension must develop tolerance to sitting.[h] A second requirement for propping on the upper extremities in sitting is the ability to hold the elbows in extension.

---

[g] Prior training in unsupported sitting balance may help prepare the patient for this maneuver. Strategies for developing unsupported sitting balance are presented in Chapter 10.

[h] Strategies for developing tolerance to upright sitting are presented in Chapter 11.

Patients who lack functioning triceps must learn to stabilize their elbows using muscle substitution.[i]

Therapeutic Strategies: Weight-Shift While Propped on Two Upper Extremities (Dynamic Stability)

Mat activities involve a variety of postures in which the individual supports his trunk by propping on two upper extremities: prone on elbows, supine on elbows, supine supported on one elbow and one hand, and sitting propped on two hands. Patients should practice shifting weight in each of the positions involved in the particular methods that they will use to function. Before practicing weight shifts in a particular posture, a person should first practice stabilizing in that position. Adequate static stability in the posture will make it possible to begin developing dynamic stability.

Weight shifts are likely to be easiest when the supporting extremities are symmetrical, with either two hands or two elbows on the mat. Shifting weight will also be easier when the hands or elbows are relatively close to midline and positioned in a way that places the shoulders level with each other. During early practice of weight shifts, it is probably best to develop skill in easier positions first. For example, practice in the supine-on-elbows position should precede practice shifting weight while in supine propped on one elbow and one hand.

During early practice of weight shifts in a given posture, the therapist can assist the patient into position and ask him to shift his weight laterally. If the patient has difficulty shifting his weight, the therapist can place a hand against one of the patient's shoulders and ask him to push against it. After the patient has shifted slightly, he can return to upright by pushing against a hand placed on the opposite shoulder. As the patient's skill develops, he can progress to practicing without any manual contact from the therapist.

The patient should practice leaning alternately to one side, then the other. He should start with small motions, shifting only as far as he is able to control the motion and return to the starting position. As his skill increases, he can increase the arcs of motion.

Therapeutic Strategies: Dynamic Shoulder Control (Pivot) Balancing on One Upper Extremity

Various functional mat activities involve this skill, performed in several different positions: supine supported on one elbow, forearm-supported side lying, and long sitting propped on one hand. To perform this maneuver, a person with a spinal cord injury pivots his trunk over one supporting shoulder. This involves maintaining balance while moving the supporting shoulder forward and back (see Figure 9–1 for examples). To do this, he pivots his trunk in the direction opposite the supporting shoulder's movements: as the supporting shoulder moves forward, his trunk rotates back. Motions of the head and free arm are used to augment balance.

Once a patient is able to maintain his balance while propping on one extremity, he is ready to practice dynamic shoulder control in that position. He should start by moving his supporting shoulder forward and back through small arcs of motion, pivoting his trunk in the opposite direction as he does so. The therapist may first move him passively to give him a feel for the motion involved. The patient should then perform the motions with assistance and guarding.

---

[i] Strategies for developing the ability to extend the elbows using muscle substitution, lock the elbows, and prop on extended arms in sitting are presented in Chapter 10.

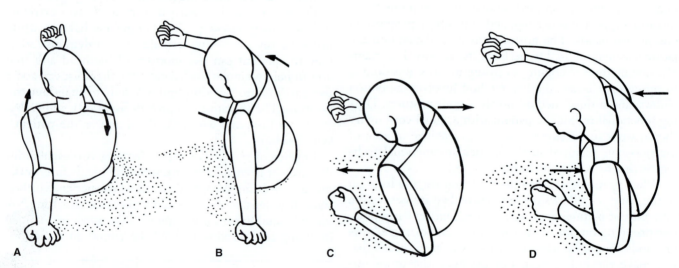

Figure 9–1   Dynamic shoulder control, balancing on one extremity. As the supporting shoulder moves forward, the trunk rotates back. As the supporting shoulder moves back, the trunk rotates forward. (A & B) Dynamic shoulder control in sitting, propped back on one hand. (C & D) Dynamic shoulder control in forearm-supported sidelying.

TABLE 9–3   Rolling—Physical Prerequisites

	Supine to Prone Without Equipment	Supine to Prone With Equipment	Prone to Supine
Strength			
Anterior deltoids	☑	☑	√
Middle deltoids	√	√	√
Posterior deltoids	☑	√	√
Biceps, brachialis, and/or brachioradialis		☑	
Infraspinatus and teres minor	√	√	√
Serratus anterior	•	•	•
Triceps brachii	•	•	•
Range of Motion			
Shoulder Flexion		√	√
External rotation	☑		
Horizontal adduction	√	√	
Horizontal abduction	√		
Elbow Extension	☑		√
Flexion		√	
Forearm Supination	√		√

√ Some strength is needed for this activity, or severe limitations in range will inhibit this activity.
☑ A large amount of strength or normal or greater range is needed for this activity.
• Not required but helpful.

As the patient's skill develops, he can increase the forward and back motions of his supporting shoulder until he is able to pivot through large arcs. He should practice moving through arcs that are large enough to be a challenge but small enough for him to retain control.

The patient should also practice abducting the scapula of his supporting shoulder when his trunk is rotated into a position vertically over this shoulder. This scapular abduction raises the trunk, increasing the distance between the free shoulder and the mat. This skill is important for functional tasks that involve throwing one upper extremity while balancing on the other.

Rolling

Rolling is an important skill for comfort, health, and function. A person who can roll in bed independently will be able to reposition himself during the night to remain comfortable (shift pressures on his shoulders, for example) and prevent pressure ulcers. Rolling is also a prerequisite skill for several methods of coming to sitting. Finally, independent dressing in bed also involves rolling.

The following paragraphs describe techniques for rolling from supine to prone with and without equipment, and for rolling from prone to supine. The physical prerequisites for these techniques are summarized in Table 9–3. Table 9–4 summarizes the prerequisite skills for rolling.

Supine to Prone Without Equipment

To roll from supine to prone without equipment, a person with a complete spinal cord injury turns his body using momentum from head and arm motions.

Some people with complete injuries who are very coordinated, strong, or have low lesions (or any combination thereof) are able to roll in a single maneuver. An individual with this capability simply throws his head and arms forcefully in the direction toward which he wants to roll. For most people with complete injuries, rolling requires more effort. Momentum for the roll is built by rocking back and forth. To roll in this manner, the person swings his head and arms forcefully to one side and then the other. His trunk rocks from supine with each swing, rolling partially in the direction of the throw. As his trunk falls back toward supine, he adds momentum to the motion by throwing his head and arms. By repeatedly throwing his head and arms left and right in coordination with the trunk's rocking motion, the person can build enough momentum to roll (Figure 9–2). The number of throws that an individual uses to roll will depend on several factors. Someone with greater strength and skill will be able

TABLE 9–4   Rolling—Skill Prerequisites

	Supine to Prone Without Equipment	Supine to Prone With Equipment	Prone to Supine
Position elbows in extension (p. 158)	√	√	
Maintain elbow extension while flexing shoulders (pp. 158–159)	√	√	
Throw arm(s) across body, elbow(s) extended (p. 164)	√	√	
Combined arm throw and head swing (pp. 164–165)	√	√	
Roll supine to prone using momentum (p. 165)	√		
Position arm to assist in rolling with equipment (p. 165)		√	
Roll toward prone by pulling on equipment (p. 165)		√	
Roll from prone by pushing with arm (p. 165)			√

√ This prerequisite skill is required to perform this activity.

to roll with fewer throws. Body build will also have an impact; obesity or wide hips will make rolling more difficult.

A good deal of momentum is required to move the large mass of the trunk and lower extremities. When the relatively small mass of the head and upper extremities is used to roll, their momentum must be maximized. Several things can be done to increase momentum. The elbows should be held in extension to maximize the moment arm. Protracting the scapula at the end of the swing will also increase the moment arm. Arm and head swings should be synchronized and performed forcefully, with maximal velocity.

People with innervated triceps can throw their arms in an arc that is perpendicular to the mat. This is not true for people with C5 or C6 tetraplegia, as they lack functioning triceps. In these cases, the elbows will flex when thrown in this manner, which can result in the person hitting himself in the face. To avoid this problem, an individual who lacks functioning triceps should swing his arms in an arc that is approximately 45 degrees above the plane of his body. (The shoulders are flexed to about 45 degrees.) This position, combined with shoulder external rotation and forearm supination, helps maintain the elbows in extension. It is, however, a less advantageous position for generating momentum for the roll because the arms' mass is positioned closer to the body's axis of rotation.[j] This disadvantageous

arm position, combined with absent or minimal pectoralis major innervation, makes rolling difficult for people with C5 or C6 tetraplegia.

Supine to Prone With Equipment
Weakness, contractures, obesity, spasticity, confusion, low motivation, or inadequate time funded for rehabilitation can keep someone from achieving independence in rolling without equipment. In these instances, many people can learn to roll by pulling on a looped strap, a bed rail, or a wheelchair parked next to the mat or bed. The use of a wheelchair is preferable to a looped strap or bed rail, as it does not require any special equipment.

To prepare to roll using equipment, a person who lacks hand function first positions the arm toward which he plans to roll, stabilizing his arm in a loop, under a bed rail, or under his wheelchair's armrest or wheel rim. The arm should be positioned with the shoulder abducted to about 90 degrees and the antecubital fossa facing the ceiling (Figure 9–3). The forearm should be supinated.

Pulling on the equipment using his biceps and anterior deltoid, the person rolls his trunk toward his stabilized arm. At the same time, he swings his head and free arm in the direction of the roll, adding momentum. In the absence of innervated triceps, the free arm should be swung in an arc that is about 45 degrees above the plane of the body.

The roll can be completed in one of two ways. At the end of the free arm's swing, this arm can be used to pull on the equipment. Alternatively, the person can reach or

---
[j] The properties of momentum are discussed in Chapter 8.

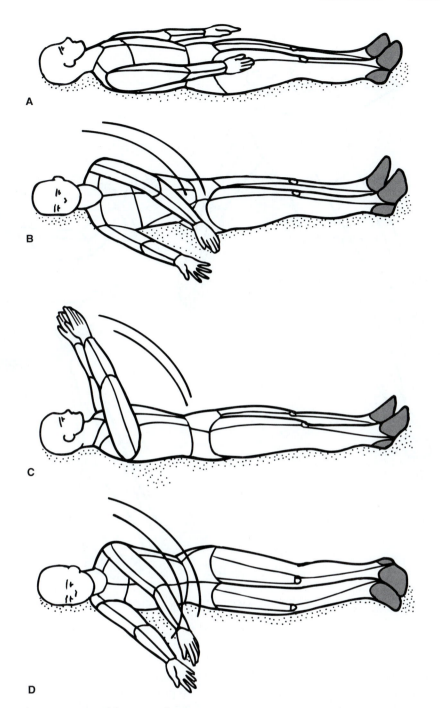

Figure 9–2 Rolling supine to prone without equipment.

punch with his free arm at the end of the swing, protract-ing his scapula to add momentum to the roll.

Prone to Supine

Rolling from prone to supine is far easier than rolling in the opposite direction. A person with a complete spinal cord injury simply pushes on the supporting surface, using the arm away from which he wants to roll. Once he reaches a side-lying position, he can throw his head and arm in the direction of the roll.

Rolling—Therapeutic Strategies

Some patients with intact upper extremity function can learn to roll with a brief period of practice. In contrast, people with tetraplegia or other limiting factors are likely to find the task more challenging. These individuals may benefit from prac-ticing the prerequisite skills appropriate to the method of rolling that they will use, and progress to rolling. Strategies for developing these prerequisite skills are described earlier in the chapter and in the following paragraphs.

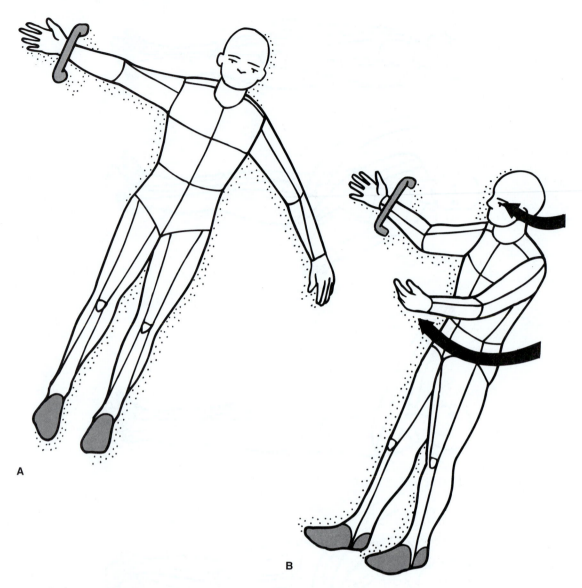

Figure 9–3   Rolling supine to prone with equipment, viewed from above.

Throw Arm(s) Across Body, Elbow(s) Extended

To practice this skill, a patient should be able to maintain his elbows in extension while flexing his shoulders. The position of the arms during this maneuver will depend on whether or not the individual's triceps are innervated. A person who lacks functioning triceps must use positioning to keep his elbows from flexing while he throws his arms across his body in supine, holding his shoulders in external rotation and flexing them only to about 45 degrees. Functioning triceps makes this positioning unnecessary; the person can throw his arms in whatever arcs of motion he finds most effective and comfortable.

A person with a spinal cord injury who wishes to use arm motions to roll must throw his arms forcefully. The therapist can help the patient get a feel for the position and velocity of the arm swings by assisting him through the motions. Once the patient gets a feel for the motion, he can practice on his own.

Some patients are able to throw their arms across their bodies without prior instruction, and do not need to practice this skill separately. These patients may proceed directly to practicing combined head and arm motions.

Combined Arm Throw and Head Swing

To practice this skill, a patient should be able to maintain his elbows in extension while throwing his arms across his body.

The patient should practice turning his head while throwing his arms across his body, turning his head in the direction of the arm throw. To build enough momentum to roll, he must perform the arm and head motions forcefully and simultaneously. The therapist can give the patient a feel for the velocity of the arm motions by moving him passively once or twice.

Roll Supine to Prone Using Momentum

Rolling toward prone can be practiced from side lying without the prior development of any skills. For practice rolling from supine, however, the patient must be able to throw his arms across his body while keeping his elbows extended, simultaneously throwing his head in the same direction.

It can be very difficult to learn to roll from supine to prone. To facilitate the acquisition of this skill, the therapist should make the task easier. One way to do so is to cross the patient's legs. During practice rolling to the left, the right leg should be crossed over the left.

Rolling is most difficult from supine and gets progressively easier as the individual approaches side lying. For this reason, practice should start in the side-lying position. The therapist should position the patient in side lying with his legs crossed, and instruct him to punch or reach his free arm forward. This motion will move his center of gravity forward, causing him to roll toward prone. Once the patient learns how to turn his body in this manner, the therapist can assist him to a slightly more supine position and have him practice rolling from there. As the patient's skill increases, he should practice rolling from progressively more supine positions. Throughout the practice, forceful head and arm motions should be encouraged.

A patient who is having difficulty learning to roll may benefit from having wrist weights placed on his arms. The added mass of the wrist weights adds to his arms' momentum, making it easier to roll. As a patient's skill increases, the weights should be removed.

The training strategies just described should be used judiciously. The patient should always start from a position as close to supine as possible,[k] and use as little weight as he can. Once he is able to roll from supine, he should practice with his legs uncrossed.

Position Arm to Assist in Rolling With Equipment

Before practicing this skill, a patient should be able to extend an elbow, using either triceps or momentum. If he can extend his elbow, positioning the arm to assist in rolling should take little practice.

The therapist should begin by showing the patient the appropriate arm position for rolling with equipment: the shoulder is abducted and in neutral rotation so that the antecubital fossa faces the ceiling. The forearm is supinated and stabilized in a loop or under either the bed rail or the armrest of a wheelchair (Figure 9–3).

Once shown the position, the patient should require little practice to learn this skill. An individual who lacks functioning triceps should first position his elbow in extension, then abduct his shoulder to place the arm.

Roll Toward Prone by Pulling on Equipment

Practice of this skill does not require the ability to position the arm. The therapist can assist the patient into position with one arm in a loop or stabilized against a bed rail or wheelchair, and then instruct the patient to roll his body by pulling on the equipment. If the patient is able, he should add momentum to the roll by swinging his head and free arm toward the equipment. Toward the end of the roll, he can use his free arm to assist by reaching or punching in the direction of the roll, by pulling on the equipment, or both.

The therapeutic strategies used to teach rolling with momentum can be used for rolling with equipment. To make the task easier, the therapist can have the patient practice initially from a side-lying position, with the legs crossed. A weight on the free arm may also be helpful during early practice. (A more complete description of strategies for teaching rolling is supplied above.)

Roll From Prone to Supine by Pushing With Arm

To practice this skill, a patient must be able to extend his elbow. He can do so using either triceps or muscle substitution with the anterior deltoid.[l]

Because rolling toward supine is most difficult from prone, practice can start in side lying. From this position, a small push will rotate the body slightly toward supine. Once the patient has moved out of side lying, gravity will complete the roll.

Once a patient is able to roll to supine from side lying, he should practice rolling from a position closer to prone. The therapist can assist him to a position tilted slightly toward prone from side lying and have him roll back by pushing on the mat. As his skill improves, the patient can practice rolling from positions that are progressively closer to prone.

Assuming the Prone-on-Elbows Position

Assuming prone on elbows is another important basic capability. The prone-on-elbows position can be used to move in bed, and it is a key position in some methods of coming to sitting.

There are a variety of methods that a person with a complete spinal cord injury can use to perform this activity. Four methods are presented here: assuming the prone-on-elbows position starting in prone with the shoulders abducted, prone with the shoulders adducted, side lying, or at the end

---

[k] The patient should practice rolling from a position that is *difficult but doable*: tilted from supine just enough to allow him to experience some success in rolling.

[l] The prerequisite skill of extending the elbow using muscle substitution is addressed in Chapter 10.

Problem-Solving Exercise 9–1

Your patient, who has T3 paraplegia (ASIA B) is beginning inpatient rehabilitation. He is 54 years old and mildly obese. He wants to learn to roll in bed independently without using equipment.

- Is this a reasonable goal for this patient to achieve during inpatient rehabilitation, or is he likely to require additional training in this skill after discharge?

- Describe a functional training program appropriate for this patient's goal.
- Describe how you could set this patient up to practice this skill independently while in therapy.

of a roll from supine. The physical and skill prerequisites for these techniques are summarized in Tables 9–5 and 9–6.

From Prone, Shoulders Abducted

When using this method to get onto his elbows, a person starts in the prone position with his arms resting on the mat, as shown in Figure 9–4A. His shoulders are externally rotated and abducted to 90 degrees and his elbows are flexed to approximately 90 degrees.

From the starting position, the person shifts his weight to one side and horizontally adducts and shrugs the opposite shoulder. He then shifts in the other direction and pulls his other arm medially in the same manner. Each time he performs this maneuver, the unweighted elbow is moved a short distance medially. By repeatedly shifting his weight and repositioning his elbows medially, he gradually "walks" his elbows inward until they are positioned vertically under his shoulders.

TABLE 9–5   Assuming Prone on Elbows—Physical Prerequisites

		From Prone, Shoulders Abducted	From Prone, Shoulders Adducted	From Side Lying	At the End of a Roll From Supine
Strength					
Anterior deltoids		☑	☑	√	☑
Middle deltoids				√	√
Posterior deltoids				☑	☑
Biceps, brachialis, and/or brachioradialis				√	
Infraspinatus and teres minor		√	√	√	√
Serratus anterior		•	•	•	•
Pectoralis major		•	•	•	•
Triceps brachii					•
Range of Motion					
Shoulder	Flexion	√	√	√	√
	Abduction	√	√	√	
	External rotation	√		√	☑
	Horizontal adduction	√	√	√	√
Elbow	Flexion	√	√	√	√

√Some strength is needed for this activity, or severe limitations in range will inhibit this activity.
☑A large amount of strength or normal or greater range is needed for this activity.
•Not required, but helpful.

TABLE 9–6 Assuming Prone on Elbows—Skill Prerequisites

	From Prone, Shoulders Abducted	From Prone, Shoulders Adducted	From Side Lying	At the End of a Roll From Supine
Position elbows in extension (p. 158)				√
Maintain elbow extension while flexing shoulders (pp. 158–159)				√
Throw arm(s) across body, elbow(s) extended (p. 164)				√
Roll supine to prone using momentum (p. 165)				√
Weight shift in prone-on-elbows (p. 160)	√	√	√	
Walk elbows in from abducted position (pp. 167–168)	√			
Walk elbows forward from adducted position (p. 168)		√		
Move from side lying to prone-on-elbows (p. 169)			√	√

√ This prerequisite skill is required to perform this activity.

Therapeutic Strategies

To practice using this method to assume the prone-on-elbows position, a patient must be able to weight-shift in this position.

Walking the elbows in from an abducted position is most difficult at the beginning of the task, when the trunk remains on the mat. The task grows easier as the arms become more vertical, approaching the stable prone-on-elbows position. Practice should start in this easier position: starting in prone on elbows with his elbows directly under his shoulders, the patient shifts his weight laterally to unweight one elbow. He moves the unweighted elbow a short distance laterally and shifts his weight back onto it. He should then shift the weight off again and move the elbow back in, returning to the starting position. Moving the elbow back in involves a combined motion of shoulder shrug and horizontal adduction. The therapist can help the patient learn this motion with verbal cueing and by providing resistance at the shoulder and arm.

When the patient has developed the capacity to move an elbow out and back in, he can progress to moving one elbow a short distance laterally, shifting onto it, and moving the other elbow out. He then reverses the steps, walking the elbows back in.

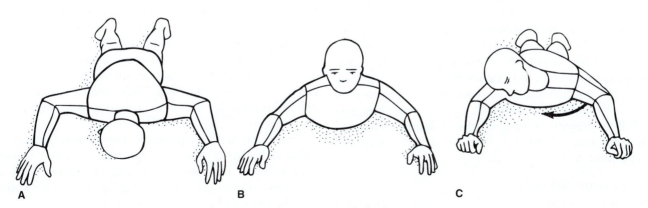

Figure 9–4 Assuming prone-on-elbows position from prone, shoulders abducted. (A) Starting position. (B) Partway up. (C) Weight shifting and moving unweighted arm medially.

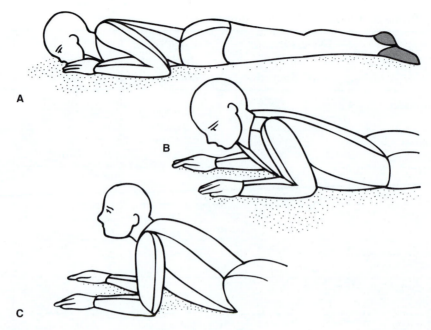

Figure 9–5   Assuming prone-on-elbows position from prone, shoulders adducted. (A) Starting position. (B) Partway up. (C) Prone on elbows.

Walking the elbows out from prone on elbows is relatively easy; bringing them back in is the difficult task. While practicing, it can be tempting for the patient to walk his elbows out too far, reaching a position from which he is unable to return without assistance. The therapist should encourage the patient to walk his elbows out only as far as he can control the motion and return without assistance.

As his skill develops, the patient should walk his elbows out and back over increasing distances. In this manner, he can build up to the point where he can walk his elbows all the way out laterally and back in. At this point, he will be able to assume the prone-on-elbows position from prone.

From Prone, Shoulders Adducted

An alternate method for getting onto the elbows from prone involves shoulder flexion instead of horizontal adduction. The person starts with his elbows flexed and his shoulders adducted (Figure 9–5A).

From the starting position, the trunk is lifted slightly, using forceful flexion of the shoulders. Shifting his weight to one side, the person flexes the unweighted shoulder. This maneuver brings the elbow forward slightly, moving it toward a position under the shoulder. The person then shifts to the other side and pulls the opposite elbow forward. By repeatedly shifting weight to alternate sides and flexing his unweighted shoulders, he "walks" his elbows into position under his shoulders.

Therapeutic Strategies

The skill of walking the elbows forward from an adducted position can be developed in reverse, using an approach comparable to that just described for developing the skill of walking the elbows in from an abducted position. Before practicing, a patient should be able to shift his weight in the prone-on-elbows position.

From a starting position of prone on elbows with the elbows directly under the shoulders, the patient practices walking his elbows back toward his pelvis and then returning to the starting position. As his skill develops, he walks his elbows across increasing distances. In this manner, he gradually builds to the point where he is able to walk his elbows back until he is prone on the mat, and walk them forward from that position to return to prone on elbows.

From Side Lying

When using this method to assume a prone-on-elbows position, the person begins in side lying with the shoulder and elbow of his lower arm (the arm on which he is lying) flexed. If he does not have strong shoulder musculature, he may need to stabilize his hand against his head. Stabilizing his hand in this manner enables him to use this arm more effectively as a lever. Figure 9–6A illustrates the starting position with the hand stabilized against the forehead. The hand can be stabilized in other positions, such as against the chin or the side of the head. Moving to prone on elbows from side lying involves simultaneous use of leverage by the lower arm and momentum from the free arm.

From the starting position, the person pushes the elbow of his lower arm down into the mat using a strong contraction of his posterior deltoids to lift his trunk up and forward over his elbow. Once the lift has been initiated, he can tuck his chin to assist in the motion.

While pushing into the mat with his lower arm, the person forcefully swings his free arm forward, adding

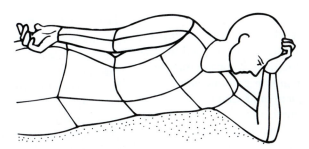

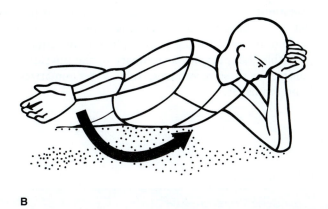

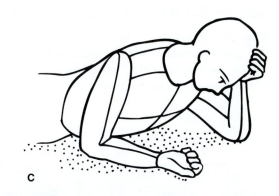

Figure 9–6   Assuming prone on elbows from the side-lying position. (A) Starting position. (B) Partway up, throwing free arm forward. (C) Prone-on-elbows position.

momentum to help move the trunk. On completion of the arm's swing, he can do one of two things with this arm to help pull his trunk up and over his supporting elbow. He can use momentum by reaching or punching the arm at the end of its swing, protracting the scapula. Alternatively, at the end of the free arm's swing, he can stabilize the hand against his supporting elbow. With his hand stabilized in this manner, he can use this arm to pull the trunk, helping to move it to a position over his supporting elbow.

Therapeutic Strategies

Before practicing the skill of moving from side lying to prone on elbows, a patient should be able to shift his weight in the prone-on-elbows position.

Moving from side lying to prone on elbows is most difficult at the beginning, when the patient lifts his trunk from the mat. It becomes easier as the trunk is lifted higher and the supporting arm becomes more vertical. Practice should start where the task is easiest: in the prone-on-elbows position, with one hand stabilized on the chin, forehead, or side of the head. From this position, the patient should lean toward the side of the stabilized (supporting) arm, shifting laterally as far as he can without losing control. He then lifts his body back over the supporting arm. To do this, he uses horizontal abduction of the supporting shoulder. Because the elbow of the supporting arm is stabilized on the mat, horizontal abduction of the shoulder serves to lift the trunk up and over the arm.

The patient can move through larger arcs of motion as his skill increases. When he leans further from vertical, it will become more difficult to return to upright. He may need to use momentum to augment the supporting arm's push. To utilize momentum, he should swing his free arm forward as he pushes his supporting elbow into the mat (Figure 9–6B). As the patient practices leaning and returning to the starting position through increasing arcs of motion, he can gradually progress to the point where he can lean far enough to touch a shoulder to the mat and return to the prone-on-elbows position.

At the End of a Roll From Supine

This method for getting to the prone-on-elbows position is possible for someone with C6 or lower tetraplegia who is both strong in his innervated musculature and skillful in rolling without equipment. Using this technique, the person takes advantage of his body's momentum at the end of a roll, using it to get onto his elbows.

This process is started with a forceful roll. As the person rolls past side lying, he pushes the elbow of his lower arm into the mat. He can use his free arm to assist in the process in either of the two ways described previously: he can reach or punch at the end of the arm's swing, or stabilize the free hand against his supporting elbow and then use this arm to pull. Whichever method is used, these actions must be performed without interrupting the roll from supine. An uninterrupted roll makes it possible for the trunk's momentum to help carry the trunk over the supporting elbow.

Therapeutic Strategies

This method of assuming the prone-on-elbows position can be practiced after the patient has developed at least partial skill in moving from side lying to prone on elbows and has learned to roll from supine without equipment. The therapist can then explain and demonstrate how these two skills can be combined, and encourage the patient to practice. The therapist can provide feedback on the patient's technique and timing, and give assistance as needed. As the patient's skill improves, this cueing and assistance can be reduced.

Coming to Sitting Without Equipment

To dress or transfer out of bed independently, a person must be able to assume a sitting position. If he can do so without equipment, he will be spared the stigma, expense, and restrictions of special equipment.

With Functioning Triceps

An individual with intact upper extremity musculature may be able to come to sitting directly from supine by pushing down on the mat with his hands. If he needs to, he can rock his trunk side to side slightly as he pushes.

Even without fully intact upper extremities, the presence of functioning triceps makes a large difference in the ability to come to sitting. A person with functioning triceps can roll past side lying, plant his hands on the mat, and push himself into a sitting position.

Assuming a sitting posture is a more involved process when functioning triceps are lacking. The three methods described in the following paragraphs do not require triceps. Table 9–7 provides a summary of the physical prerequisites for these techniques. Table 9–8 summarizes the skill prerequisites.

TABLE 9–7 Coming to Sitting Without Equipment—Physical Prerequisites

	Roll and Throw	Straight From Supine, Hands Stabilized	Walking on Elbows
Strength			
Anterior deltoids	☑	☑	√
Middle deltoids	√	√	√
Posterior deltoids	☑	√	√
Biceps, brachialis, and/or brachioradialis		☑	√
Internal rotators			√
Infraspinatus and teres minor	√	√	√
Serratus anterior	•	•	•
Pectoralis major	•	•	•
Triceps brachii	•	•	•
Range of Motion			
Shoulder Extension	☑*	☑*	
Flexion	√		√
Abduction	√	√	√
External rotation	☑*	☑*	
Internal rotation			☑
Horizontal abduction	☑*	☑*	√
Elbow Extension	☑*	☑*	√
Flexion	√	√	√
Forearm Supination	√	√	
Wrist Extension	√	√	
Hamstring flexibility			☑

√ Some strength is needed for this activity, or severe limitations in range will inhibit this activity.
☑ A large amount of strength or normal or greater range is needed for this activity.
• Not required but helpful.
* These motions (shoulder extension, external rotation, horizontal abduction, and elbow extension) must be present in combination.

TABLE 9–8   Coming to Sitting Without Equipment—Skill Prerequisites

	Roll and Throw	Straight From Supine, Hands Stabilized	Walking on Elbows
Weight shift in supine, supported on one elbow and one hand (p. 160)	√	√	
From supine, supported on one elbow and one hand, lift elbow (p. 174)	√	√	
Position elbows in extension (p. 158)	√	√	
Maintain elbow extension while flexing shoulders (pp. 158–159)	√	√	
Dynamic shoulder control in single forearm-supported supine (pp. 160–161)	√	√	
From supine on elbows, lift one elbow (p. 174)	√	√	
From single forearm–supported supine, throw one arm back (pp. 174, 177)	√	√	
Assume prone-on-elbows position (pp. 165–170)			√
Weight shift in prone-on-elbows position (p. 160)	√		√
Move from prone-on-elbows to forearm-supported side lying (pp. 179, 180)	√		√
Dynamic shoulder control in forearm-supported side lying (pp. 160, 161)	√		
From forearm-supported side lying, throw free arm back (pp. 174, 177)	√		
Tolerate upright sitting position*	√	√	√
Dynamic shoulder control in sitting, propped back on one hand (pp. 160, 161)	√	√	
From sitting propped back on one hand, throw free arm back (pp. 174, 177)	√	√	
Weight shift while sitting propped back on two hands (p. 160)	√	√	
From sitting propped back on two hands, walk hands forward (pp. 178, 179)	√	√	
Stabilize hands in pants or under pelvis (p. 182)		√	
With hands stabilized in pants or under pelvis, lift trunk using elbow flexion (p. 182)		√	
Weight shift in supine-on-elbows position (p. 160)		√	
In supine-on-elbows position, walk elbows back (pp. 178, 179)		√	
In prone-on-elbows position, walk elbows to the side (pp. 178, 179)			√
In 90-degree forearm-supported side lying, walk supporting elbow toward legs (p. 181)			√
From forearm-supported side lying, push–pull into sitting position (pp. 181, 182)			√
Extend elbows against resistance†			√
Push with arms to lift trunk from forward lean†			√

√ This prerequisite skill is required to perform this activity.
* Refer to Chapter 11 for a description of this skill and therapeutic strategies.
† Refer to Chapter 10 for a description of this skill and therapeutic strategies.

Rolling and Throwing Arms

This method of assuming a sitting position requires very good flexibility. The shoulders must have greater than normal range in extension. The elbows must extend fully with the shoulders positioned in hyperextension and external rotation.

To come to sitting using this method, the person first assumes the prone-on-elbows position using any of the methods just described (Figure 9–7A). He then shifts his weight onto one elbow. With his unweighted arm, he pushes his trunk up and over the supporting elbow, moving to the forearm-supported side lying position (Figure 9–7B).

From forearm-supported side lying, the person throws his free arm back in an arc, landing on his palm with his elbow fully extended and his forearm supinated (Figure 9–7C). To make the next step possible, the hand must land with the shoulder positioned in external rotation and extreme horizontal abduction and hyperextension (Figure 9–8A). If this shoulder is not in enough extension, it will be higher than the other shoulder (Figure 9–8B). This disparity in shoulder height may make it impossible for the patient to shift his weight onto the higher shoulder.[m]

In the next step, the person shifts his weight onto his extended arm and lifts the other arm (Figure 9–7D). Balancing on his supporting arm, he throws his free arm back. When the palm lands on the mat, the elbow of this arm should be extended, the forearm supinated, and the shoulder horizontally abducted, hyperextended, and externally rotated (Figure 9–7E), Both upper extremities will then be in a position in which the elbows are "locked"; the elbows can remain in extension without muscular effort. An upright sitting posture is then achieved by walking the hands forward. To do this, the person shifts first to one side and then to the other, moving the unweighted hand forward by elevating and protracting the scapula.

Straight From Supine, Hands Stabilized

To assume a sitting position using this method, a person with a spinal cord injury must have very strong elbow flexors. Range-of-motion requirements are the same as those for the method described above.

In the supine position, the hands are stabilized by placing them in the pockets, inside the pants, or under the pelvis. The person then lifts his upper trunk by flexing his elbows forcefully (Figure 9–9B).

Once the person has lifted his upper trunk as high as he can, he moves his elbows posteriorly. Shifting his weight from side to side, he walks his unweighted elbows back until he is in a stable position, supine on elbows (Figure 9–9C).

From the supine-on-elbows position, the individual shifts his weight to one elbow and lifts the unweighted

arm (Figure 9–9D). While lifting, he forcefully contracts the anterior deltoid of his supporting arm, turning his upper trunk so that his shoulders are aligned vertically over the supporting elbow.

From this position, the person comes to sitting in the manner described previously. He throws back first one arm and then the other (Figure 9–9E through G) and walks his hands forward until he reaches an upright sitting posture.

Walking on Elbows

This method of assuming the sitting position does not require the range of motion needed to perform the methods just described. Because neither shoulder hyperextension nor full elbow extension is needed, people who have range limitations can use this method to come to sitting. Moreover, because the person does not position his shoulders in extreme hyperextension while coming to sitting in this manner, he may experience less trauma to his shoulders.

To come to sitting by walking on his elbows, the person first gets into the prone-on-elbows position by using any of the methods described previously. He then walks his elbows to one side. To do so, he shifts his weight first to one side and then to the other, moving the unweighted elbow each time.

The person continues walking his elbows to the side until he reaches a point where his trunk will not laterally flex any further (Figure 9–10B). In the next step, he rotates his pelvis from prone toward side lying. This involves pushing with the elbows (using shoulder flexion with the elbows stabilized on the mat) to roll his pelvis from prone (Figure 9–10C).

With his pelvis tilted from prone, the person can continue walking on his elbows until his shoulders are close enough to his legs. This position will vary, but it is generally such that the trunk is at a 90-degree or smaller angle to the legs (Figure 9–10D).

Shifting his weight onto the elbow that is furthest from his legs, the person lifts his unweighted arm and hooks it behind his legs, placing his forearm behind the knees or thighs (Figure 9–10E). Once his arm is stabilized in this manner, the patient is ready to pull his torso toward his legs.[n] To do so, he repeatedly pulls on his legs while throwing his head toward the legs. The combined pull and head swing should be forceful and abrupt so as to gain maximal momentum. With each pull, the patient drags his supporting elbow further toward his legs. In this manner, he walks his elbow until it is close enough to his legs for him to perform the next step (Figure 9–10F). The target position for the elbow will vary depending on the individual's strength and skill.

Shifting his weight off of his supporting elbow, the person internally rotates this shoulder and plants his palm

<hr>

[m] The amount of shoulder extension required will vary among people; an individual with greater strength and skill will not require as much range.

[n] This step may be omitted if strength and skill allow.

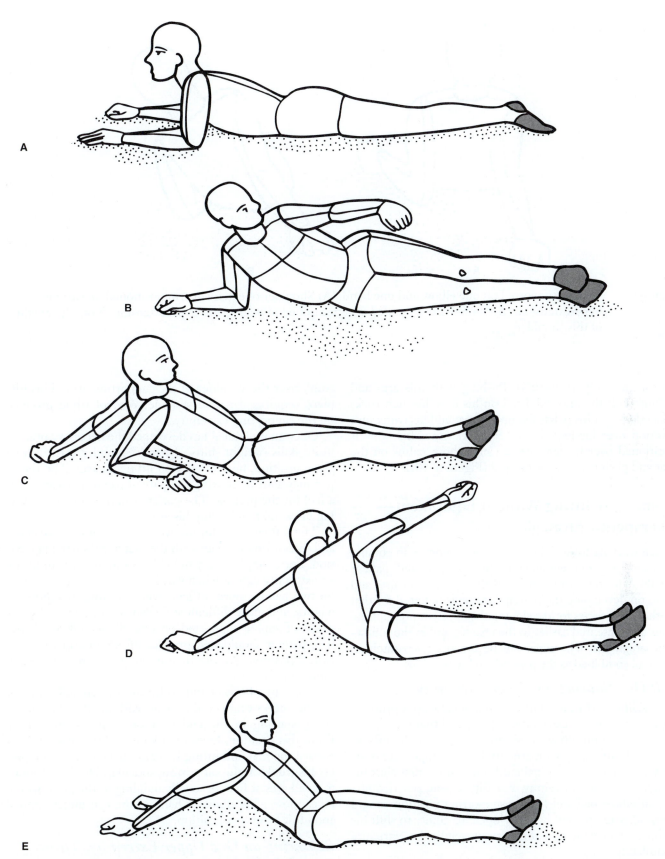

Figure 9–7 Coming to sitting by rolling and throwing the arms. (A) Prone-on-elbows position. (B) Forearm-supported side lying. (C) Supine, supported on one elbow and one hand. (D) Supporting elbow lifted. (E) Sitting, propped back on two hands.

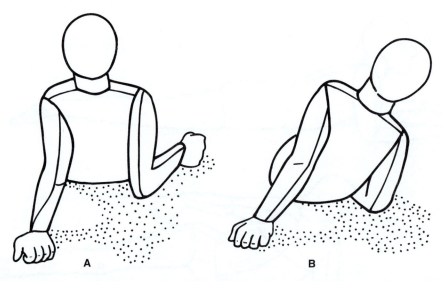

Figure 9–8   Supine, supported on one elbow and one hand. (A) Shoulder of extended arm positioned in extreme hyperextension. (B) Shoulder of extended arm positioned in inadequate hyperextension. Note the height of this shoulder.

on the mat (Figure 9–10G). Pushing with this arm and pulling with the one stabilized on his legs, he then rocks his body to get his pelvis flat on the mat and his trunk into position over his legs (Figure 9–10H). Once his body is positioned over his legs, he can place both palms on the mat and push his torso to upright (Figure 9–10I).

Coming to Sitting Without Equipment— Therapeutic Strategies

When working toward the goal of independence in coming to sitting without equipment, the therapist and patient should determine which method the patient will use, and focus on developing the prerequisite skills required for that method. Strategies for developing the different prerequisite skills are presented earlier in the chapter and in the following paragraphs. The skills can be practiced separately at first and combined as the patient's ability develops.

Lift One Supporting Upper Extremity

This skill is performed when an individual who is propped on two supporting extremities lifts one of them. (Starting in the supine-on-elbows position, for example, he lifts an elbow.) To lift an upper extremity from a supporting position, a person with a spinal cord injury must first shift his weight off of the extremity. For this reason, practice lifting an elbow or hand from a supporting position should occur *after* the patient has developed his ability to shift his weight under control, enough to unweight the extremity completely.

Some functional tasks involve lifting an extremity and pivoting on the supporting shoulder. (see Figure 9–11 for an example). In this maneuver the person shifts his weight and lifts the unweighted extremity, pivoting his

trunk over the shoulder of the supporting arm. This lift-pivot requires dynamic shoulder control while propped on the supporting extremity.

Once an individual has developed the necessary prerequisite skills (weight shifts, dynamic shoulder control) in a given position, he can work on lifting an arm. The therapist may start by moving the patient passively to give him a feel for the motion. The patient can then practice shifting his weight and lifting his arm.

The difficulty of shifting weight off an upper extremity and then lifting it varies with the individual's starting position. For example, many individuals find the task of lifting an extremity easiest when starting in sitting propped back on two hands, more difficult when starting in supine on elbows, and more difficult still when starting from the position of supine supported on one elbow and one hand. The patient should first practice lifting an arm from the easiest position. He can then develop skill in increasingly difficult positions.

A patient who is unable to lift his arm enough to pivot on the supporting shoulder can work on the skill in reverse, starting in the end position with his arm lifted. From this position, he can work on lowering his free arm toward the mat and lifting it again. As he does so, he pivots his trunk on the supporting shoulder. He should move in small arcs at first, gradually building to the point where he can lower his elbow or hand to the mat under control and lift it from that position.

Balancing on One Upper Extremity, Throw Free Arm back

This skill is performed in sitting propped on one hand, supine propped on one elbow, or in forearm-supported side lying. Before practicing this skill in a given position,

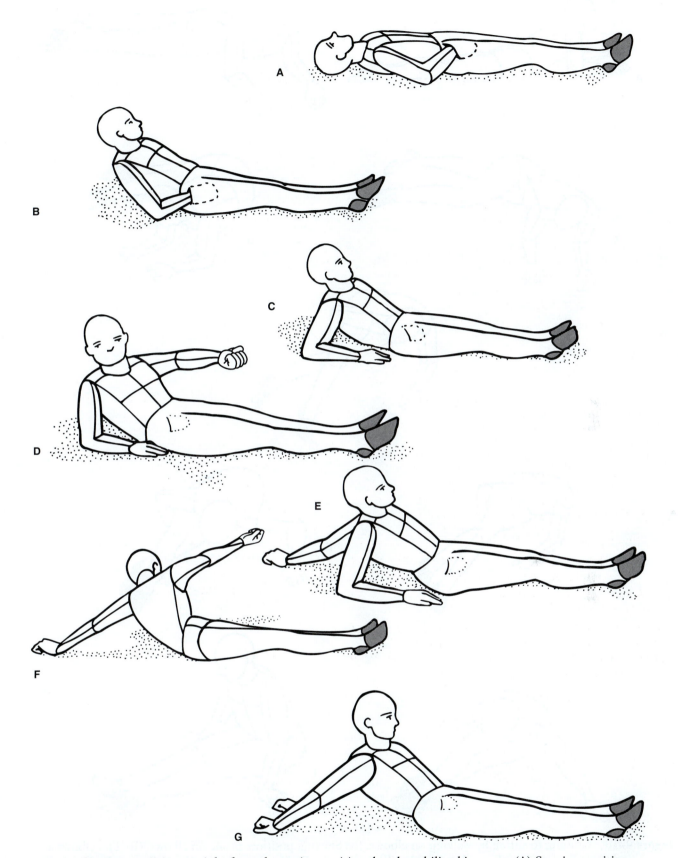

Figure 9–9   Coming to sitting straight from the supine position, hands stabilized in pants. (A) Starting position: supine with hands stabilized in pants. (B) Upper trunk lifted using elbow flexion. (C) Elbows walked back to a stable position. (D) One arm lifted. (E) Free arm thrown back. (F) Second arm lifted. (G) Second arm thrown back.

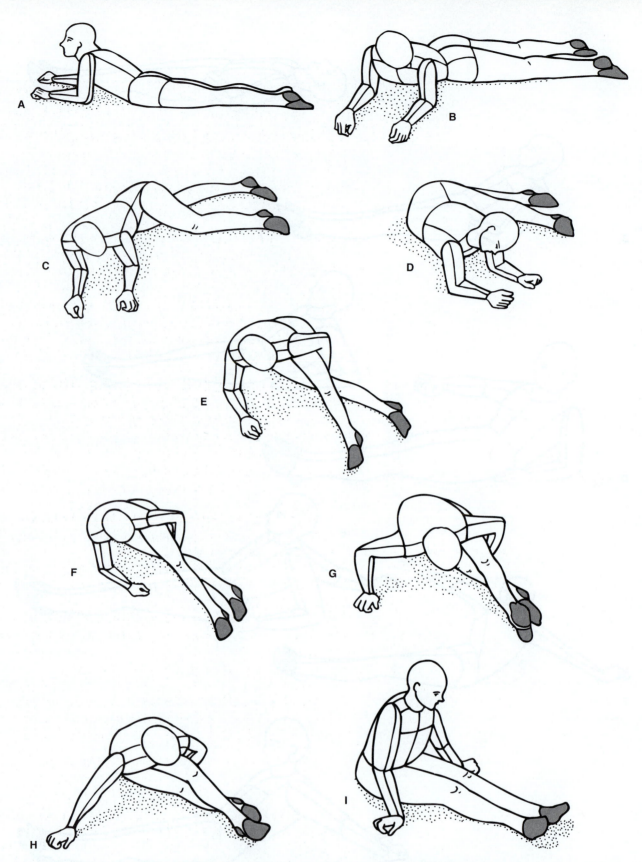

Figure 9–10 Coming to sitting by walking on elbows. (A) Starting position: prone on elbows. (B) The elbows are walked to the side until the trunk will not laterally flex any further. (C) The pelvis is rolled from prone toward side lying. (D) The elbows are walked toward the legs. (E) An arm is hooked around the thighs. (F) The supporting elbow is walked toward the legs. (G) The palm is planted on the mat. (H) The body is rocked into position over the legs. (I) The torso is pushed to upright.

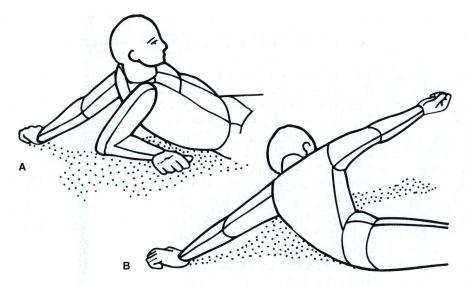

Figure 9–11   Example of lifting an extremity and pivoting on the supporting shoulder: from the position of supine on one elbow and one hand, lift elbow. Trunk pivots on supporting shoulder.

the patient should have developed dynamic shoulder control in that position.

Figure 9–12 illustrates this maneuver performed in forearm-supported side lying. The person with a spinal cord injury balances on one upper extremity and throws his free arm back to a position that allows this extremity to support the trunk. As he throws his arm, his center of gravity moves from over his base of support and he falls in the direction of the swinging arm. For this reason, the palm must land with the arm positioned so that it can accept weight and catch the falling trunk. In the absence of functioning triceps, the final position of the thrown upper extremity is key. The hand should land on the mat slightly medial to the shoulder and the elbow should remain extended. If the hand lands in a position that is too lateral, the arm will not support the trunk. The elbow will flex, causing the person to fall to the mat. If the person is performing this maneuver starting in either forearm-supported side lying or supine propped on one elbow, the hand of the thrown arm should also land in a position that places the shoulder close to the end of its range in extension. This hyperextension is required for a person lacking functional triceps to come to sitting from these positions.

Three factors combine to make it possible for the arm to land with the shoulder positioned appropriately: the starting position of the shoulders, velocity of the swinging arm, and direction of the arm's motion.

When the arm throw is initiated, the shoulder of the thrown arm should be as high as possible. Specifically, the shoulders should be aligned perpendicular to the mat (Figure 9–12B) and the scapula of the supporting arm should be abducted. Then, as the patient's center of gravity shifts and the trunk falls, the shoulder of the thrown arm will fall from as high a position as possible. The further it has to fall, the longer the fall will take. A longer fall

will allow the free arm to swing further, so the hand can land in a stable position medial to the shoulder.

The swinging arm will also be able to move further if it is thrown forcefully. An arm that travels at a high velocity will travel further as the trunk falls, and as a result will land in a better position.

The patient may find it easiest to throw his arm in the direction of shoulder horizontal abduction rather than extension. If the arm is thrown forcefully in the direction of horizontal abduction, momentum will carry it toward the body's midline at the end of the throw.

The motion of the supporting shoulder is also key to the successful performance of this maneuver. As the patient swings his arm into position, he must pivot his trunk on the supporting shoulder (Figure 9–12C). This pivot will make it possible for the shoulders to end in a stable position when the swing is completed (Figure 9–12D).

It can be quite difficult for a patient to learn to throw an arm back while balancing on the other elbow. For this reason, it is advisable to practice first from a position of sitting, propped back on one extended arm. (Figure 9–13). Similar initial positioning and motions are involved, but the more upright posture makes the arm throw easier in sitting. By developing this skill in sitting, a patient can prepare himself for practice in other positions.

During early practice of this skill, the therapist can assist the patient into position, aligned with his free shoulder high. From the starting position, the therapist can move the patient's trunk and free arm passively to demonstrate how the supporting shoulder collapses forward as the trunk falls and the free arm swings back. The patient can then practice the technique with guarding. He is likely to have many failed attempts as he learns the skill. Verbal feedback from the therapist at this point can help him perfect his technique. The guarding and feedback can be reduced as the patient's skill improves.

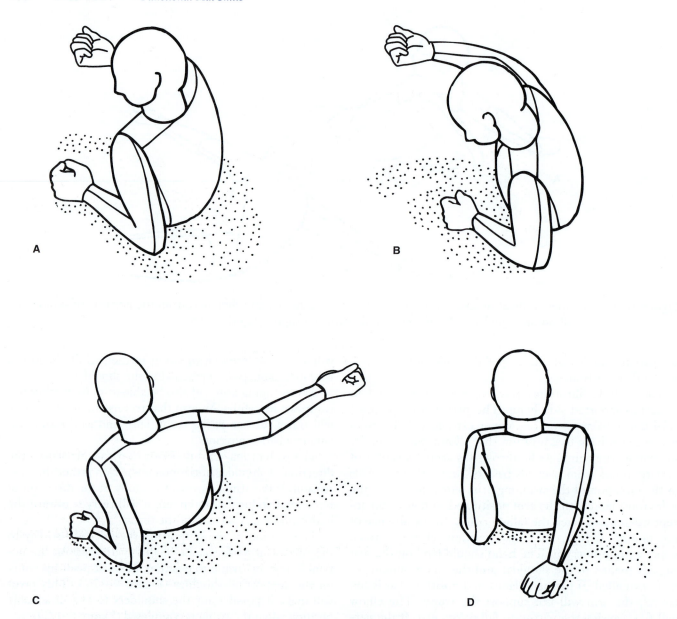

Figure 9–12   From forearm-supported side lying, throw free arm back. (A) Forearm-supported side lying. (B) Ready position to throw: shoulders perpendicular to mat, scapula of supporting arm abducted. (C) Halfway through throw. Trunk pivots on supporting shoulder. (D) End position.

Walk Two Elbows or Hands to New Positions

This skill is performed in the positions of supine on elbows, prone on elbows, or sitting propped on two hands. To walk his elbows or hands to new positions, the individual moves one supporting upper extremity at a time. Practice of this skill in a particular position requires the ability to shift weight in that position. If the patient has difficulty unweighting a hand or elbow enough to move it, he can enhance his weight shift by throwing his head in the direction of the weight shift.

All methods of coming to sitting involve repositioning two supporting elbows or hands by walking them forward, back, or to the side. The positions in which this skill is performed (supine on elbows, prone on elbows, or sitting) and the direction in which the elbows or hands are walked vary with the

method of coming to sitting that the person uses. Practice of this skill should be in positions appropriate to the method of coming to sitting that the individual is working to master.

To practice walking the elbows or hands, the patient starts in supine on elbows, prone on elbows, or sitting propped on two hands with the elbows extended. From the starting position he leans laterally to unweight one arm and moves the unweighted elbow or hand a short distance ° on the supporting surface. The unweighted upper extremity typically is moved using shoulder and scapulothoracic

---

° The elbow or hand should be moved only a short distance each time it is repositioned, to make it possible to maintain stability. As the individual's skill develops, he may find that he can move his supporting upper extremities over larger distances with each "step" without losing his balance.

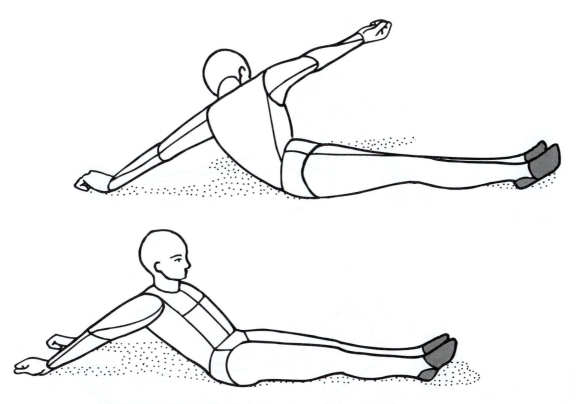

Figure 9–13   Sitting, propped back on one extended arm, throw free arm back.

motions. Once the individual has repositioned one elbow or hand, he shifts his weight onto this upper extremity and repeats the process with the other arm. By repeating these steps, he walks his supporting extremities forward, back, or to the side. The therapist can provide guarding, verbal cueing, manual assistance, or resistance as appropriate.

The difficulty of this skill in a given posture varies with the position of the supporting elbows or hands. The patient should first practice walking his elbows or hands from the easiest position and then develop skill in increasingly difficult positions. For example, when sitting propped back on two hands with the elbows extended, it is easiest to walk the hands forward when they are relatively close to the buttocks, making the trunk almost upright (Figure 9–14A). When the hands are in a more posterior position (Figure 9–14B), the trunk is more reclined and more weight is borne through the hands, making it more difficult to walk them forward. As the individual walks his hands forward toward his buttocks, the task becomes easier. Thus when a patient first practices walking his hands forward while sitting propped on extended arms, he should start with his hands on the mat relatively close to his buttocks. As his skill improves, he can practice walking his hands forward from more posterior starting positions.

Move From Prone on Elbows to Forearm-Supported Side Lying

This maneuver is illustrated in Figure 9–15. To practice, the patient must be able to weight shift in the prone-on-elbows position, and have some dynamic shoulder control in side lying with forearm support. In the absence of functioning triceps, he must also be able to extend one elbow using his anterior deltoid.

Starting in the prone-on-elbows position, the person shifts his weight to one side and plants the hand of his unweighted arm on the mat (Figure 9–15B). He then pushes to rotate his body up and over the supporting arm, ending in the position of side lying with forearm support. The motions of the supporting shoulder are critical to this maneuver. As the patient pushes his torso up and over his arm, the supporting shoulder moves from a position of horizontal adduction to horizontal abduction (Figure 9–15A through C).

The therapist can begin work on this skill by demonstrating and passively moving the patient through the maneuver to give him an idea of the motions involved. The therapist can then assist him into a position of side lying with forearm support, with the "free" hand stabilized against the mat. From this position, the patient can practice rotating his trunk toward prone and back up (Figure 9–16). The power for this motion will come primarily from the "free" arm pushing on the mat. During practice, the patient's motions should be small enough that they remain under his control yet large enough to be a challenge. As his skill increases, he can increase his arcs of motion.

This skill is easiest when the trunk and lower extremities are in a line, with the hips in approximately neutral extension. The hips remain in this position while a person comes to sitting using the technique that involves

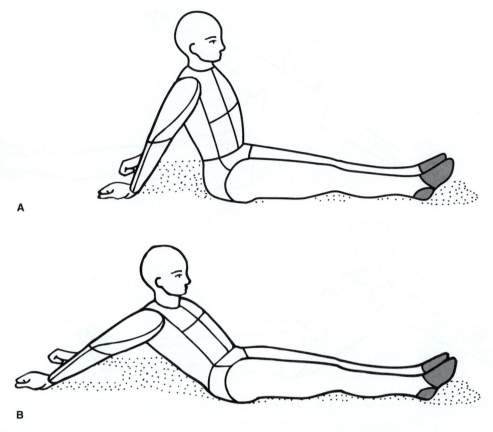

Figure 9–14   Practice walking the hands toward the buttocks is easier with the hands close to the buttocks and the trunk almost upright (A), and more difficult when the hands are further posterior and the trunk is more reclined (B).

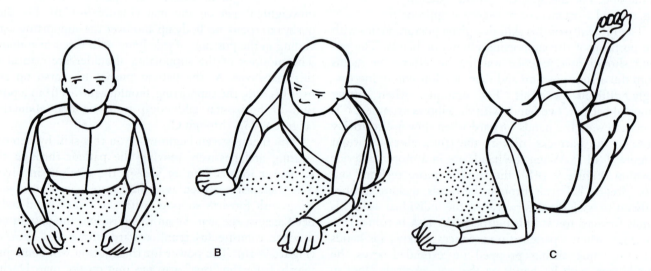

Figure 9–15   Move from prone-on-elbows position to forearm-supported side lying. (A) Prone on elbows. (B) Weight shifted and hand planted. Trunk rotates over shoulder of supporting arm. (C) Supporting shoulder has moved from horizontal adduction to horizontal abduction.

rolling and throwing the arms (Figure 9–7). The maneuver is more difficult when the trunk and lower extremities are angled, as when coming to sitting by walking on the elbows (Figure 9–10). Initial practice should be done in the easier position, with the trunk and lower extremities in a line.

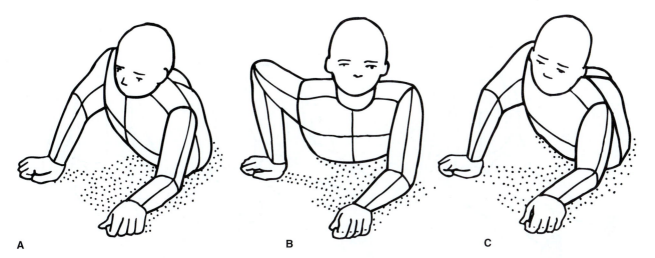

Figure 9–16   In the position of side-lying with forearm support, "free" hand stabilized against the mat. (A) Starting position. (B) Trunk rotates toward prone. (C) Return to starting position.

In 90-Degree Forearm-Supported Side Lying, Walk Supporting Elbow Toward Legs

This skill is one of the steps in coming to sitting by walking on the elbows. Starting in the position shown in Figure 9–17, the individual walks his elbow toward his legs in a series of short moves. To do this, he unweights the elbow and drags it closer to his legs, using his "free" arm to pull on his lower extremities. If he is unable to move the supporting elbow by pulling with his unweighted upper extremity, he can throw his head in the direction of the pull to use momentum to assist in the maneuver. The moves should be timed so that all of the actions (throwing the head, pulling the legs, and moving the supporting elbow) occur simultaneously.

The patient should learn to stabilize and weight-shift in 90-degree forearm-supported side lying before practicing this skill. During initial practice, the therapist can assist the patient with the motion to give him a feel for the maneuver, and provide feedback on his technique. The therapist should emphasize that the motions should be abrupt and forceful. As the patient's skill develops, he can progress to practicing without assistance and feedback.

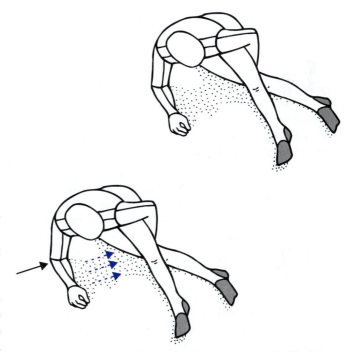

Figure 9–17   In 90-degree forearm-supported side lying, walk supporting elbow toward legs.

From Forearm-Supported Side Lying, Push–Pull Into Sitting Position

Before practicing this skill, a patient must be able to extend one of his elbows against resistance, using either his triceps or muscle substitution. This maneuver begins with the person propped on one elbow in side lying with his hips flexed beyond 90 degrees (Figure 9–10F). The other arm is hooked behind his knees or thighs.

In the absence of functioning triceps, this maneuver may require two steps: the individual repositions the weight-bearing upper extremity to make it easier to extend his elbow using muscle substitution; then he pushes with this arm and pulls with the other to move into sitting. To reposition his weight-bearing upper extremity, he

pulls on his legs to unweight the supporting elbow. At the same time, he internally rotates the shoulder of the supporting arm, placing his palm on the mat. The shoulder should be rotated enough that the elbow points toward the ceiling (Figure 9–10G). Once his hand is planted on the mat, he extends his elbow to push his torso up and over his legs (9–10H). At the same time, he pulls with the other arm. He can use momentum to assist in the motion by throwing his head laterally toward his legs.

Whether the individual uses triceps contraction or muscle substitution to push with his supporting upper extremity, the most difficult part of pushing–pulling into

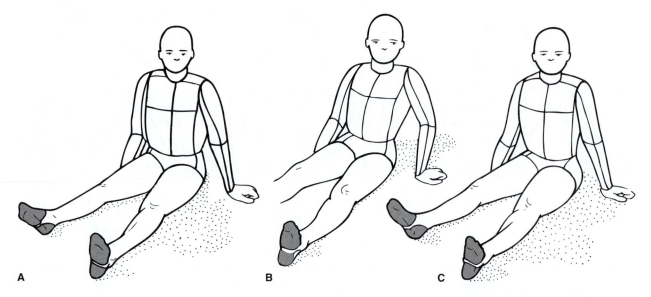

Figure 9–18   In long sitting, practice lowering the trunk to the side. (A) Starting position: long sitting, propped to the side on one arm, other arm hooked around legs. (B) The patient lowers his trunk to the side. (C) Push/pull back to starting position.

sitting is at the beginning. The task becomes easier as his trunk moves up and over his legs. Functional training can begin where the skill is easiest, in the end position: sitting, propped to the side on an arm with its elbow extended. The other arm should be hooked around the legs (Figure 9–18A). From this position, the patient practices lowering his trunk to the side and returning to sitting. He should start with small motions, lowering his trunk slightly and pushing–pulling back up (Figure 9–18B and 9–18C). He can lower his trunk further as his skill increases, gradually building to the point where he can raise his trunk from forearm-supported side lying. During practice, the motions should be small enough that the patient is able to retain control yet large enough to be a challenge.

During initial practice, the therapist can assist the patient with the motions to give him a feel for the maneuvers and provide feedback on his technique. As the patient's skill develops, he can progress to practicing without assistance and feedback.

Stabilize Hands in Pants or Under Pelvis

This prerequisite skill is used in coming to sitting by stabilizing the hands and using elbow flexion to lift the trunk from supine. Learning to stabilize the hands in the pants is a relatively easy task. The patient simply needs to practice working his hands into the front pockets or under the waistband. The pants should be made of a nonstretchy material; sweat pants will not adequately stabilize the hands. The pants must be loose enough for the patient to work his hands in without difficulty. This requirement should not present a problem; if the pants are loose enough to allow independent dressing, they should be suitable for this activity also.

Placing the hands under the pelvis can be a more difficult maneuver. The patient starts with his arms by his

sides with his shoulders internally rotated. Using elbow flexion, he pulls one hand at a time under his pelvis. The therapist can provide assistance during early practice and withdraw this assistance as the patient's skill develops.

In Supine With Hands Stabilized in Pants or Under Pelvis, Lift Upper Trunk Using Elbow Flexion

Initial practice of this skill can be done with the therapist stabilizing the patient's distal forearms instead of with the patient's hands stabilized in his pants or under his pelvis. The therapist can grasp the patient's distal forearms and have him lift his upper trunk (do "sit-ups") using elbow flexion. Practice can start with the shoulders flexed, because this positioning will make the task easier. As the patient grows stronger and more skillful, the therapist can stabilize his arms in progressively lower positions. Once the patient is able to lift his upper trunk with his arms stabilized at his sides, he is ready to practice with his hands stabilized in his pants or under his pelvis.

Coming to Sitting Using Equipment

Weakness, contractures, obesity, spasticity, and inadequate time for full rehabilitation are among the factors that can prevent someone from learning to assume a sitting posture without equipment. In these cases, many can learn to perform this task using equipment.

There are various methods that can be used to come to sitting using a loop ladder attached to the foot of the bed or using loops suspended from a bar over the bed. One method for each is presented in this section. Tables 9–9 and 9–10 summarize the physical and skill prerequisites for these methods. A final alternative method of coming

Problem-Solving Exercise 9–2

Your patient has complete (ASIA A) tetraplegia. She is young, healthy, and highly motivated. She is also dependent in all functional activities. One of her goals is to come to sitting independently in a bed without using equipment.

The patient's muscle test results are as follows.

Muscles	Left	Right
Deltoids (anterior, middle, and posterior)	5/5	4/5
Shoulder internal rotators	5/5	4/5
Elbow flexors	5/5	5/5
Radial wrist extensors	5/5	4/5
Triceps	3/5	2/5
Long finger flexors	0/5	0/5
Abductor digiti minimi	0/5	0/5
Trunk and lower extremity musculature	0/5	0/5

The patient's joint range of motion and muscle flexibility are normal throughout with the following exceptions:

Motions	Left	Right
Shoulder extension	5 degrees	10 degrees
Elbow extension	–5 degrees	–5 degrees
Passive straight-leg raise	80 degrees	70 degrees
Long finger flexors	mild tightness	mild tightness

* Using the ASIA classification system, what is (are) this patient's motor level(s)?
* What method of coming to sitting without equipment is this individual likely to achieve most readily?
* What are the physical prerequisites for this method of coming to sitting?
* What strength and range should the therapeutic exercise program emphasize to facilitate the attainment of this goal?
* What are the skill prerequisites for this method of coming to sitting?
* Describe a functional training program for this patient.

to sitting involves the use of a hospital bed. This alternative should be considered for anyone who either does not have the potential to function on a standard bed or chooses not to pursue this goal.

Loop Ladder

A person with a spinal cord injury who is unable to roll or get into prone on elbows without equipment may be able to come to sitting using a loop ladder.[p] The ladder is attached to the foot of the bed and lies on the mattress (Figure 9–19A).

The starting position is supine, with the loop ladder lying beside the person. The ladder will be used to pull onto the elbow that is closest to the loops. After placing one or both forearms through a loop, the person drives his elbow into the mat while pulling on the loop, lifting his upper trunk over the elbow. The upper trunk should be rotated toward the weight-bearing arm, so that the free (non–weight-bearing) shoulder is higher (Figure 9–19B).

Balancing on one elbow, he removes his arm(s) from the loop and places the forearm of his free arm through the next loop. Pulling on the loop, he unweights his supporting elbow and inches it toward the foot of the bed (Figure 9–19C). When he has moved as far as he can using

that loop, the person moves his free arm to the next loop and repeats the process. In this manner, he walks his supporting elbow around, bending at the hips. This process can be continued until his torso is positioned over his legs.

Someone who routinely uses a loop ladder to come to sitting must plan ahead. When he gets into bed at night, he should place the loops where he will be able to reach them the following morning.

Suspended Loops

Figure 9–20A shows an overhead frame with loops.[q] This equipment is far bulkier, less esthetic, and more difficult to transport than a loop ladder.

Starting in supine, the person places one or both distal forearms through a suspended loop (Figure 9–20B). Pulling on the loop, he raises his shoulders off of the bed (Figure 9–20C). He then places one elbow on the bed, positioned beneath his upper trunk so that he can balance on it (Figure 9–20D).

Balancing on his elbow, the person removes his arm from the first loop and places it through the next one (Figure 9–20E). He then pulls to lift his trunk higher. In doing so, he lifts his supporting elbow off of the bed. While suspended from the loop, he throws his free arm back, ending in the position shown in Figure 9–20F. The thrown upper

---

[p]A loop ladder is a series of loops made of webbing material, sewn end to end. The size and number of loops will vary among individuals.

[q]The ideal number, length, and spacing of the loops will vary depending on the individual's needs.

TABLE 9–9   Coming to Sitting With Equipment—Physical Prerequisites

		Using Loop Ladder	Using Suspended Loops
Strength			
Anterior deltoids		☑	☑
Middle deltoids		√	√
Posterior deltoids		√	√
Biceps, brachialis, and/or brachioradialis		☑	☑
Infraspinatus and teres minor		√	√
Serratus anterior		•	•
Pectoralis major		•	•
Triceps brachii		•	•
Range of Motion			
Shoulder	Extension		√
	Flexion	√	√
	Abduction	√	√
	External rotation		√
	Horizontal abduction		√
Elbow	Extension		☑
	Flexion	√	√
Forearm	Supination		√
Wrist	Extension		√
Combined hip flexion and knee extension		☑	

√ Some strength is needed for this activity, or severe limitations in range will inhibit this activity.
☑ A large amount of strength or normal or greater range is needed for this activity.
• Not required but helpful.

extremity should end in a position that "locks" the elbow: shoulder extended, horizontally abducted, and externally rotated, elbow extended fully, and forearm supinated.

While balancing on his supporting arm, the person moves his other arm to the next loop (Figure 9–20G). Pulling on the loop and throwing his head forward, he unweights his supporting arm and inches the hand forward. When he has moved the supporting hand as far as he can, he balances on this arm and moves his free arm to the next loop. He can then repeat these steps until he reaches an upright sitting posture (Figure 9–20H).

Coming to Sitting Using Equipment— Therapeutic Strategies

When working toward the goal of independence in coming to sitting using a loop ladder or suspended loops, the therapist and patient should determine which method the patient will use and focus on developing the prerequisite skills required for that method. Strategies for developing the different prerequisite skills are presented earlier in the chapter and in the following paragraphs. The skills can be practiced separately at first and combined as the patient's ability develops.

Place Arm Through Loop

This skill is used by people who use loop ladders or hanging loops to come to sitting. Before working on this skill, an individual should be able to position his elbow in extension. To practice with a hanging loop, he must be able to maintain his elbow in extension while he flexes his shoulder.

It can be difficult to place an arm through a loop that is suspended from above. During early training, the task can be made easier by placing the loop on the mat. With the loop in this position, the patient can practice grabbing it and slipping his hand through.

Once a patient has become adept at placing his arm through a loop that is lying on a mat, he can begin working with a hanging loop.[r] To place his hand through a hanging loop, the patient must first bring his hand to the loop, flexing his shoulder while maintaining his elbow in extension. He then slips his hand through the loop. Once the hand is through and the loop is around his forearm, he can internally rotate his shoulder and flex his elbow to "grasp" the loop with his forearm.

[r]Of course, this is necessary only if the patient plans to use hanging loops.

TABLE 9–10 Coming to Sitting With Equipment—Skill Prerequisites

	Using Loop Ladder	Using Suspended Loops
Position elbows in extension (p. 158).	✓	✓
Maintain elbow extension while flexing shoulders (pp. 158, 159).	✓	✓
Place arm through loop (pp. 184, 185).	✓	✓
Pulling on loop ladder, move from supine to single forearm-supported supine (p. 185).	✓	
In single forearm-supported supine, pull on loop ladder and walk supporting elbow toward feet (p. 186).	✓	
Extend elbows against resistance.*	✓	
Push with arms to lift trunk from forward lean.*	✓	
Tolerate upright sitting position†	✓	✓
Lift trunk by pulling on suspended loop (p. 185).		✓
Dynamic shoulder control in single forearm-supported supine (pp. 160, 161).		✓
With one arm through overhead loop, throw free arm back (pp. 185, 186).		✓
Dynamic shoulder control in sitting, propped back on one hand (pp. 160, 161).		✓
In sitting, propped back on one hand, pull on suspended loop and walk supporting hand forward (p. 186).		✓

✓ This prerequisite skill is required to perform this activity.
* Refer to Chapter 10 for a description of this skill and therapeutic strategies.
† Refer to Chapter 11 for a description of this skill and therapeutic strategies.

Practice with a hanging loop should begin with a loop that hangs within easy reach. Once the patient becomes adept at placing his arm through the loop, he can practice with loops hung higher.

Pulling on Loop Ladder, Move From Supine to Single Forearm–Supported Supine

In this maneuver, the person uses a loop ladder lying at his side to lift his trunk and get onto an elbow (Figure 9–19A and 9–19B). With one or both forearms stabilized in a loop, he pulls by flexing his elbow(s) forcefully. At the same time, he extends the shoulder of the arm closest to the loop ladder, driving the elbow into the mat. With these combined motions, the patient lifts his upper trunk up and over the supporting elbow.

Lifting the trunk is most difficult at the beginning of the lift, when the patient is supine on the mat. The task becomes easier as the supporting shoulder approaches a position vertically over the supporting elbow. Practice of the skill should begin in the easier position: starting in forearm-supported supine with one or both forearms placed through a loop, the patient can practice lowering himself slightly toward supine and pulling back up. He should be encouraged to lower himself as far as he can while retaining the ability to control the motion and return to the starting position. As his skill increases, he can move through larger arcs of motion.

From Supine, Lift Trunk by Pulling on Suspended Loop

This skill is illustrated in Figure 9–20C. If a patient has adequate strength, he should be able to master this skill with minimal practice. With his forearm(s) stabilized in a hanging loop, he simply pulls to lift his trunk. If he is unable to position an arm through the loop, the therapist can place the arm for him. If the patient has inadequate strength to lift his trunk from supine, he may be able to practice with pillows or a wedge positioned under his upper trunk. If he is practicing in a hospital bed, he can practice with the head of the bed elevated slightly. As his strength improves, he should practice with his trunk in progressively more horizontal positions.

With One Arm Through Overhead Loop, Throw Free Arm Back

To practice this skill, a patient must be able to tolerate an upright sitting posture.

The endpoint of this maneuver is illustrated in Figure 9–20F. The patient starts in a semireclined position, supporting his trunk with a forearm hooked

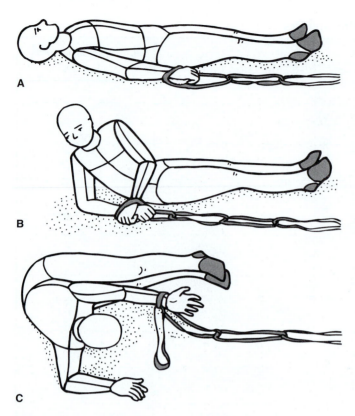

Figure 9–19   Coming to sitting using a loop ladder. (A) Starting position. (B) The upper trunk is lifted by pulling on the loop and driving the supporting elbow into the mat. (C) The supporting elbow is inched toward the foot of the bed. The other arm assists by pulling on the loop ladder.

through a suspended loop. He throws his free arm back, landing with his palm located medial to his shoulder. The thrown arm must land in a position that will enable it to accept weight: elbow extended, shoulder externally rotated and extended, and scapula adducted. To ensure that the arm ends in a proper position, it should be thrown forcefully and in the direction of shoulder horizontal abduction rather than extension.

A patient holding an overhead loop is in a stable position; he does not need to maintain his center of gravity over his base of support. For this reason, throwing an arm while hanging from an overhead loop is not as difficult as doing so while propped on an elbow or hand. Practice should emphasize the force and direction of the throw.

Walk Single Supporting Elbow or Hand to New Position

Both methods of coming to sitting by pulling on loops (loop ladder or suspended loops) involve steps in which the individual is propped on one elbow or hand and repositions it in a series of short moves. To do this, he pulls on a loop to unweight the supporting upper extremity and drags the elbow or hand into a new position (Figures 9–19C and

Figure 9–20F). If the individual is unable to move the supporting hand or elbow by pulling with his unweighted upper extremity, he can use momentum to assist by throwing his head in the direction of the pull.

Practice of this skill should be in positions appropriate to the method of coming to sitting that the individual is working to master. The patient should learn to stabilize and weight-shift in a given position before practicing walking his supporting elbow or hand in that position. During initial practice, the therapist can assist the patient with the motion to give him a feel for the maneuver. The therapist should emphasize that the motions need to be abrupt and forceful. As the patient's skill develops, he can progress to practicing without assistance.

Gross Mobility in Sitting

To get in and out of bed without assistance, a person with a complete spinal cord injury must be able to move his buttocks on the bed while in a sitting posture. This skill can also be used for limited mobility without a wheelchair. This mobility can be useful when the individual is on the floor or the ground, either by choice or after a fall.

Following a complete spinal cord injury, gross mobility in sitting involves pivoting on the arms. The person lifts or unweights his buttocks[s] by leaning forward onto his arms and tucking his head. If he lacks functioning triceps, he must lock his elbows in extension.[t] If his serratus anterior and latissimus dorsi are functioning, he can increase the lift of his buttocks by protracting and depressing his scapulae. While lifting, he uses the head-hips relationship to move his buttocks, swinging his head and upper trunk away from the direction in which he wants his buttocks to move.

The physical and skill prerequisites for gross mobility in sitting are summarized in Tables 9–11 and 9–12.

Gross Mobility in Sitting – Therapeutic Strategies

To practice gross mobility in sitting, a patient must be able to tolerate an upright sitting position, prop on his arms with his elbows extended, and lift or unweight his buttocks in long sitting.[u] Once he has developed these prerequisite skills, he can practice moving his buttocks as described in the following paragraphs.

In Long Sitting, Lift or Unweight Buttocks and Move Laterally

The therapist should explain and demonstrate how the buttocks can be moved laterally by throwing the head and upper torso to the side while lifting. The motion should

---

[s]An actual lift is preferable, but unweighting will suffice if the individual is unable to lift his buttocks off of the mat.
[t]The procedure for locking the elbows is addressed in Chapter 10.
[u]Strategies for developing these abilities are presented in Chapters 10 and 11.

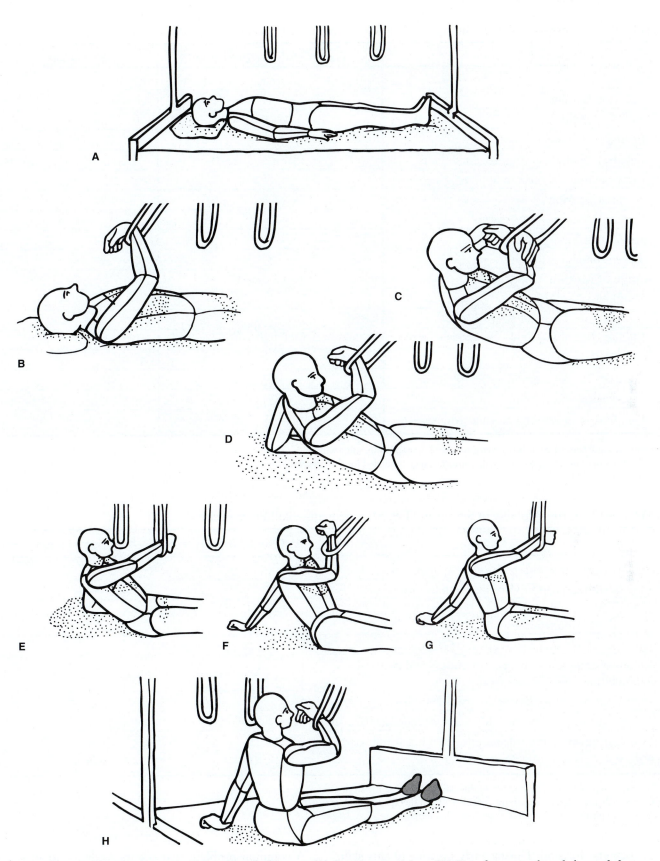

Figure 9–20 Coming to sitting using suspended loops. (A) Starting position. (B) One forearm placed through loop. (C) Upper trunk lifted from bed. (D) Elbow placed on bed. (E) Arm placed through second loop. (F) Trunk lifted and free arm thrown back. (G) Arm placed through third loop. (H) Supporting hand walked forward.

TABLE 9–11   Gross Mobility in Sitting and Leg Management—Physical Prerequisites

	Gross Mobility in Sitting	Leg Management
Strength		
Anterior deltoids	☑	√
Middle deltoids	√	√
Posterior deltoids	√	√
Biceps, brachialis, and/or brachioradialis	√	☑
Infraspinatus and teres minor	√	√
Serratus anterior	√	•
Pectoralis major	•	•
Latissimus dorsi	•	
Triceps brachii	•	•
Range of Motion		
Shoulder Abduction		√
External rotation	☑	
Elbow Extension	☑	√
Flexion		√
Forearm Supination	☑	√
Wrist Extension	☑	√
Combined hip flexion and knee extension	☑	☑

√ Some strength is needed for this activity, or severe limitations in range will inhibit this activity.
☑ A large amount of strength or normal or greater range is needed for this activity.
• Not required but helpful.

TABLE 9–12   Gross Mobility in Sitting and Leg Management—Skill Prerequisites

	Gross Mobility in Sitting	Leg Management
Tolerate upright sitting position.*	√	√
In long sitting, prop forward on extended arms.†	√	
In long-sitting, lift or unweight buttocks by leaning forward on extended arms.†	√	
Control pelvis using head–hips relationship.†	√	
In long sitting, lift or unweight buttocks and move laterally (pp. 186, 188 and 189).	√	
In long sitting, move buttocks forward and back (p. 189).	√	
In long sitting, prop to one side on one extended arm (p. 160).		√
Sitting propped to the side on one extended arm, use free arm to move lower extremity (p. 189).		√

* Refer to Chapter 11 for a description of this skill and therapeutic strategies.
† Refer to Chapter 10 for a description of this skill and therapeutic strategies.
√ This prerequisite skill is required to perform this activity.

be quick and forceful. During early practice of this skill, the patient can lift his buttocks first, then twist to move laterally. He should progress to a single combined lift-and-twist motion. As the patient's skill develops, he should practice moving his buttocks over greater distances.

A common problem that occurs while a patient learns this maneuver is that he raises his head while throwing it to the side, causing the buttocks to drop. The therapist should direct the patient's attention to this problem and encourage him to keep his head low.

Patients also tend to fall forward as they learn the skill. In some cases this is due to the difficulty of keeping the elbows locked in extension during the maneuver. A forward fall also happens when a patient pivots past his balance point. People who fall forward may require additional strengthening, more practice in this activity, or additional practice in the skill of raising the buttocks by pivoting forward on the arms.

During early practice, the therapist can help the patient get a feel for the maneuvers by assisting him with the motions. Once the patient has a feel for the motion, he can practice with guarding, and progress to practicing independently.

In Long Sitting, Move Buttocks Forward and Back

To move his buttocks forward, the person with a spinal cord injury starts in long sitting, propped forward on his arms. He then pushes into the mat to lift or unweight his buttocks and throws his head back forcefully. To move his buttocks back, he starts with his arms behind and slightly lateral to his buttocks. From this position, he pushes into the mat while throwing his head forward forcefully.

During early practice, the therapist can help the patient get a feel for the maneuvers by assisting him with the motions. Once the patient has a feel for the motion, he can practice with guarding, and progress to practicing independently.

Leg Management

An individual who lacks lower extremity function must position his legs passively. Figure 9–21 illustrates the technique for positioning the legs passively. Propping on one

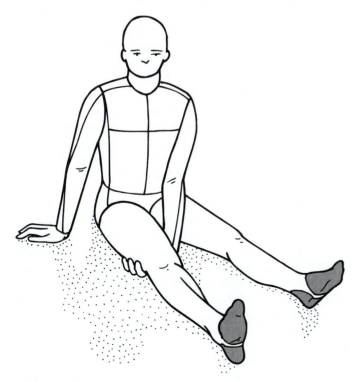

Figure 9–21   Leg management.

arm in the sitting position, the person uses his other arm to move one leg at a time. He does so by pulling his leg toward the supporting arm. If needed, he can add power to his pull by forcefully moving his head and torso in the direction of the pull.

Tables 9–11 and 9–12 summarize the physical and skill prerequisites for leg management on a mat or bed.

Leg Management – Therapeutic Strategies

To practice leg management in sitting, a patient must be able to tolerate an upright sitting position[v] and prop on one arm with the elbow extended. Once he has developed these prerequisite skills, he can practice moving his lower extremities as described in the following paragraphs.

Sitting Propped to the Side on One Extended Arm, Use Free Arm to Move Lower Extremity

To prepare to practice this skill, a patient should develop dynamic stability in long-sitting while propped to the side on one extended arm. In addition to practicing dynamic shoulder control (pivot) as described earlier in the chapter, the patient can practice maintaining his balance while he rotates his trunk, shifts his weight laterally onto the supporting hand, flexes and extends his supporting elbow, and moves his head and free arm in various directions.

During early practice, the therapist can help the patient get a feel for the maneuvers involved in leg positioning by assisting him with the motions. If the patient needs to use head and trunk motions to add force to the pull, therapist should encourage him to perform the motions forcefully, and to synchronize them with the pull. Once the patient has a feel for the motion he can practice with guarding, and progress to practicing independently.

MAT SKILLS FOLLOWING INCOMPLETE SPINAL CORD INJURY: FUNCTIONAL TECHNIQUES AND THERAPEUTIC STRATEGIES

The movement strategies that an individual can use to perform functional tasks after sustaining an incomplete spinal cord injury will depend primarily on his voluntary motor function. A person who retains or regains only sensory function below his injury (ASIA B) will utilize the compensatory techniques that are used by people with complete spinal cord injuries, as just described. A person who has minimal motor sparing or return (ASIA C) is likely to utilize similar movement strategies, but may be able to add trunk or lower extremity motions to make the tasks easier. In contrast, an individual who has significant

---

[v]Strategies for developing upright sitting tolerance are presented in Chapter 11.

motor function below his lesion (ASIA D) will be able to perform mat skills using more normal movement patterns. Someone who is weaker in his upper extremities than in his lower extremities (central cord syndrome) may learn to use his lower extremities and trunk musculature to perform mat skills, without significant contribution from his upper extremities.

Another factor that can have an impact on the performance of mat skills is spasticity. People with incomplete lesions tend to exhibit more spasticity than do people with complete lesions, and spasticity tends to be more severe among those with ASIA B and C lesions.[7-9] Involuntary muscle contractions can interfere with the functional use of voluntary motor function that is preserved below the lesion. When elevated muscle tone interferes with function, the rehabilitation team can work with the patient to reduce the abnormal tone.[w] In addition, the therapist and patient should note the conditions and bodily motions that tend to elicit involuntary muscle contractions. They can then work together in an effort to find ways in which the patient can move without causing these involuntary contractions. In some cases, they may also find ways in which spasticity can be used to enhance the performance of some activities.

Perhaps the most challenging aspect of functional mat training after an incomplete spinal cord injury is determining the methods that the individual can utilize to perform the skills. Each patient has a unique pattern of muscle strength and weakness, spasticity, joint range of motion, muscle flexibility, and body build. It is often difficult to predict what methods of performing mat skills will best suit the individual; some physical maneuvers will be within his potential and others will not. Functional training involves problem solving as the therapist works with the patient to help him discover and develop the movement strategies that will enable him to achieve his functional goals. This may involve compensatory movement strategies, restoration of more normal movement patterns, or a combination of the two.

Rolling

In a person with an intact nervous system, rolling involves coordinated motions of the entire body. The patterns used to roll vary a good deal between adults. In one commonly used rolling pattern, cervical and trunk rotation and reaching with an upper extremity are combined with lower extremity flexion when rolling from supine to prone. Other rolling patterns found in normal adults include pushing with an arm, pushing with one or both legs, and rolling without trunk rotation.[10]

Regardless of the rolling strategy employed, a neurologically intact adult typically utilizes motions of his head, trunk, and both upper and lower extremities. The strategies that a person with an incomplete spinal cord injury

can use to roll will depend largely upon the voluntary motor function that is preserved at and below his neurological level of injury.

Minimal Motor Sparing

When very limited voluntary motor function is present in the trunk and hip musculature, the patient can use head and arm motions to roll using momentum, and can add trunk and hip motions to assist in the maneuver. Preserved function in the abdominal musculature may be used to rotate the trunk partially in the direction of the roll to assist with the motion. Preserved hip musculature can be used to add momentum in the direction of the roll. For example, when rolling toward the right from supine, the individual can flex his left hip as he rocks his body toward the right.

Even musculature that is very weak may be of some benefit. For example, a patient may have hip flexors that are not strong enough to work against gravity but can flex the hip through partial range when he is in the side-lying position. These hip flexors will not be of benefit at the beginning of the roll, when the person remains supine and gravity resists hip flexion. Toward the end of the roll, as he approaches or reaches side lying, however, he will be able to flex his hip and add the momentum of this motion to assist in the roll.

More Extensive Motor Sparing

A person who retains or regains significant innervation of his trunk and hip musculature may be able to roll using normal patterns of motion. Typical rolling in neurologically intact adults involves segmental motions, with either the upper body (head, upper extremities, and upper trunk) or the lower body (lower extremities and lower trunk) leading.[11] There is, however, a good deal of variability in rolling patterns used by normal adults.[10] A patient who has adequate strength to flex his hips, rotate his trunk, and reach his arms across his body while lying supine may be able to roll from supine to prone with normal or near-normal movement patterns. Likewise, an individual who can extend his hips and rotate his trunk from a prone position may be able to learn to roll toward supine with normal or near-normal movement patterns.

Therapeutic Strategies

The patient should practice rolling using compensatory strategies, more normal movement patterns, or a combination of the two, depending on his movement capabilities. Emphasis should be placed on efficient timing and coordination of motions of the head, trunk, and extremities. If needed, the therapist can use demonstration, verbal cueing, tactile cueing, quick stretch, or any combination of these strategies to help the patient learn to perform the motions involved. These inputs should be withdrawn as the patient's rolling ability develops.

Regardless of the rolling strategy used, early practice can begin in the side-lying position, where the task will be

Problem-Solving Exercise 9–3

Your patient has incomplete tetraplegia. He is dependent in all functional activities. He would like to learn to roll from side lying toward prone and supine, so that he can sleep more comfortably.

The patient's pin prick and light touch sensation are intact in the C4 and higher key sensory points, and impaired in C5 and below. His muscle test results are as follows.

Muscles	Left	Right
Trapezius (upper, middle, and lower)	4/5	4/5
Deltoids (anterior, middle, and posterior)	2/5	2/5
Elbow flexors	2/5	2/5
Radial wrist extensors	0/5	0/5
Serratus anterior	1/5	1/5
Pectoralis major (clavicular and sternocostal)	1/5	1/5
Triceps	0/5	0/5
Flexor digitorum profundus	0/5	0/5
Abductor digiti minimi	1/5	1/5
Rectus abdominis (palpable from ribs to pubis)	2/5	2/5
External and internal obliques	2/5	2/5
Hip flexors	2/5	2/5
Hip adductors	2/5	2/5
Quadriceps	2/5	3/5

Muscles	Left	Right
Tibialis anterior	3/5	4/5
Hip abductors	3/5	4/5
Extensor hallucis longus	4/5	4/5
Hamstrings	4/5	4/5
Plantarflexors	4/5	4/5
Gluteus maximus	4/5	4/5

The patient's joint range of motion and muscle flexibility are normal throughout his upper and lower extremities bilaterally. He exhibits elevated muscle tone in all extremities and his trunk: rapid motion (active or passive) of his extremities results in strong involuntary extension of the trunk and all extremities.

- What is this patient's neurological level of injury? What is the lesion's classification, using the ASIA Impairment Scale?
- What movement strategy could this patient use in an attempt to roll from side lying toward prone?
- What movement strategy could this patient use in an attempt to roll from side lying toward supine?
- What strength and range should the therapeutic exercise program emphasize to facilitate the attainment of this goal?
- Describe a functional training program for this patient.

---

easier. As the patient's skill develops, he can practice rolling from progressively supine (when rolling toward prone) or prone (when rolling toward supine) positions.

In addition to functional training, the therapeutic program should include strengthening of the muscles involved in rolling. The strengthening program should emphasize shoulder flexion and extension, scapular protraction and retraction, hip flexion and extension, and trunk rotation. The shoulder girdle and hip strengthening exercises that are appropriate will depend on the strength of the musculature. Exercises may be active, active-assisted, or resisted, and may be performed against gravity or with gravity eliminated. Trunk rotation can be strengthened in side lying or hook lying.[x] In these positions, the patient can rotate his trunk with assistance, independently, or against resistance. As an additional exercise, he may be able to perform sit-ups with rotation. If he does not have adequate strength to perform sit-ups starting with his trunk horizontal, he may be able to do so

starting with his trunk in a less challenging position. For example, his trunk can be elevated by placing wedges behind his back to support him in a semireclined position. If necessary, the patient can be supported with his trunk in a nearly vertical position. As his strength improves, he can perform sit-ups with his trunk starting in progressively horizontal positions.[y]

Coming to Sitting

People with intact nervous systems typically use musculature in the trunk and all extremities to come to sitting. The motions involved vary. One supine-to-sit strategy involves flexing the neck and trunk and pushing with the arms to rise straight from supine. The lower extremities are also involved in the task, serving as an "anchor" as the hip flexors help pull the trunk toward sitting. An alterna-

---

[x]The hook-lying position is supine with the hips and knees flexed and the feet planted on the mat.

[y]As an alternative to working on a mat, the patient may perform sit-ups with rotation on a tilt table. The section on therapeutic strategies for coming to the sitting position (later in this chapter) contains a more detailed description of sit-ups on a tilt table.

tive supine-to-sit strategy involves rolling to the side and pushing to sitting using the arms and trunk musculature. Lower extremity musculature may be used to assist in the roll and to help lift the trunk to sitting. The strategies that a person with an incomplete spinal cord injury can use to assume a sitting position will depend on the voluntary motor function that he has below his lesion.

Minimal Motor Sparing

An individual who retains or regains only minimal voluntary motor function below his lesion will come to sitting using strategies similar to those used by people with complete spinal cord injuries. Spared musculature below the lesion may be used to assist in stabilizing or moving the trunk as the person performs the compensatory motions involved in coming to sitting.

More Extensive Motor Sparing

When adequate voluntary motor function exists below the lesion, a person with an incomplete spinal cord injury may be able to come to sitting using a normal or near-normal movement pattern. The movement strategy that is most effective will depend on the individual's pattern of strength and weakness. If trunk and lower extremity muscles are strong but shoulder girdle musculature is weak, the patient may be able to come to sitting straight from supine by performing a sit-up. If the individual's upper extremity musculature is relatively strong, he may find it easier to roll to his side and then push into a sitting position. A person who has asymmetrical weakness may find it easiest to roll onto his weaker side and use his stronger arm to push to sitting.

Therapeutic Strategies

Because there are so many possible strategies for coming to sitting, the therapist and patient should work together to determine which method will be most effective for the individual involved. Together they can analyze the patient's patterns of strength, weakness, abilities and limitations, and find a method of coming to sitting that best utilizes his capabilities.

Regardless of the method of coming to sitting chosen, the patient can develop his skill by practicing the motions involved. If his goal is to come to sitting using a multistep method similar to one used by people with complete injuries, he may benefit from practicing the various steps and then combining them as his skill develops. If the patient's goal is to come to sitting using a more normal movement strategy (sitting up straight from supine, or rolling to the side and pushing to sitting), he may benefit from practicing the task as a whole without prior practice of the skill's components.

One therapeutic strategy that may be particularly beneficial for developing the ability to come to sitting is practice of the skill in reverse. A patient who is unable to assume a sitting position may find it beneficial to start in sitting and practice lowering his trunk into a more horizontal position. He should lower his trunk backward or to the side, depending on the method of coming to sitting that he plans to achieve. Practice should start with small motions, with the patient lowering his trunk only as far as he is able to control

the motion and return to the starting position. As his skill increases, he can increase the arcs of motion.

In addition to functional training, the therapeutic program should include strengthening of the muscles involved in coming to sitting. The movement strategies used and the patient's pattern of strength and weakness will dictate what muscles should be prioritized in the strengthening program. If he plans to use his upper extremities to help push his trunk to upright, he may benefit from closed-chain exercises in which he bears weight on his palms and uses his arms to lower and raise his trunk from upright. Trunk strengthening exercises are also likely to be beneficial, and can emphasize either flexion or lateral flexion, depending on the method that the patient plans to use to come to sitting. To improve his ability to laterally flex his trunk, the patient can practice lowering his trunk laterally from a sitting position, and returning to sitting. He can start with small arcs of motion at first, and increase the excursion of his motions as his strength improves. The trunk flexors can be strengthened through sit-ups on a mat. The patient can start either with his trunk horizontal or supported in a semireclined position, depending on his ability to flex against gravity.[z] Alternatively, if there are no medical or orthopedic problems preventing upright positioning or weight bearing through his lower extremities, he can perform sit-ups on a tilt table. The patient's legs and pelvis should be secured to the tilt table with straps, and his trunk left free to move.[aa] The table should then be tilted enough toward vertical to enable him to perform sit-ups. As his strength improves, he can work with the tilt table in progressively horizontal positions.

Gross Mobility in Sitting

A person with an intact nervous system has numerous possible movement strategies for moving his buttocks while in a seated position. Using his trunk and leg musculature, he can move his buttocks with or without using his arms to assist. Moreover, he can move in the bed in a variety of other positions, such as scooting in hook lying, or even in side lying.

Following a complete spinal cord injury, gross mobility in sitting involves pivoting on the arms and using scapular and head motions to move the buttocks. A person who has an incomplete cord injury with minimal motor sparing will use essentially the same maneuvers, adding spared trunk or lower extremity musculature to assist in the task. Someone who has an incomplete injury with significant motor sparing may move on a mat or bed using normal or near-normal patterns of motions.

To develop the skill of gross mobility in sitting, the therapist and patient should work together to discover the

---

[z]Strategies for adapting sit-ups on a mat when the abdominal musculature is weak are presented above, in the section on therapeutic strategies for developing rolling following incomplete injury.
[aa]Because of the potential for a drop in blood pressure or postural instability, close monitoring will be required.

movement strategies that will be most effective for this individual. Therapeutic strategies include practice of the skill and its component skills, and exercises to develop the strength and range needed to perform these actions.

Leg Management

People with intact nervous systems move their legs actively during functional activities, and they frequently combine leg repositioning with other elements of functional tasks. For example, when rising from a bed, people with intact nervous systems typically assume a short sitting position at the side of the bed without first assuming a long sitting position. Leg repositioning is performed in concert with trunk motions while rising from supine or side lying to a sitting position at the side of the bed.[12,13]

In contrast, leg management following complete spinal cord injury involves positioning the legs passively using the upper extremities. This repositioning is performed as a separate step rather than as an action performed simultaneously with other motions.

The movement strategies used by a person with an incomplete spinal cord injury will depend on the muscle function below his lesion. He may reposition his legs using his arms only, his legs only, or a combination of leg and arm musculature. Similarly, he may move his legs while performing other components of the functional task, or he may move them as an isolated step in the process.

To develop the skill of moving the legs during functional activities, the therapist and patient should work together to discover the movement strategies that will be most effective for this individual. Therapeutic strategies include practice of the skill and its component skills, and exercises to develop the strength and range needed to perform these actions. Patients who have significant motor return below their lesions may benefit from practicing positioning their legs in concert with other actions involved in the functional task.

Summary

- Mat skills are functional activities that are typically performed on a mat or bed. These skills are required for independent transfers and dressing.
- A person with a complete spinal cord injury who wishes to function independently must learn compensatory strategies for performing mat skills. This chapter presents a variety of techniques that can be used to roll, come to sitting, move the buttocks on a bed, and move the legs during mat activities.
- The movement strategies possible for a person with an incomplete spinal cord injury will depend on the extent of motor sparing or return below his lesion. If he has little or no voluntary motor function below his lesion, he will use movement strategies similar to those used by people with complete injuries. If he has more significant motor function in his trunk and lower extremities,

he may be able to use more normal movement strategies to perform mat skills.
- During rehabilitation, the therapist and patient work together to discover the movement strategies that will enable the patient to perform mat skills most effectively. The therapeutic program then consists of activities directed at developing the strength, range of motion, and skill needed to perform these functional tasks. This chapter presents a variety of strategies for developing the skills involved.
- The therapist and patient should take appropriate precautions during functional mat training to prevent motion of unstable vertebrae, skin abrasions and pressure ulcers, overstretching of the long finger flexors and the low back, and overuse injuries of the upper extremities.

10

Transfer Skills

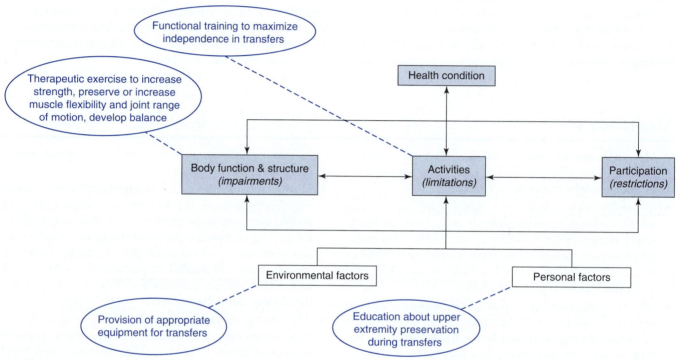

Chapter 10 presents transfer skills and therapeutic strategies for increasing independence in transfers.

Transfers are crucial for independent mobility. A person who can transfer independently can get out of bed in the morning without waiting for assistance and can leave her wheelchair to sit on a couch, get into a car, or get onto the ground. Independent transfer skills also make it possible to get back into a wheelchair after a fall.

This chapter presents a variety of transfer techniques[a] as well as suggestions on how to teach them. The descriptions of techniques and training should be used as a guide, not as a set of hard and fast rules. The exact motions used to perform any activity vary among people because of differences in body build, skill level, range of motion, muscle tone, patterns of strength and weakness, and presence or absence of additional impairments. During transfer training, the therapist and patient should work together to find the exact techniques that best suit that particular individual.

PRECAUTIONS

Following spinal cord injuries, the activities involved in transfer training can cause problems if appropriate precautions are not taken. Transfer activities can result in excessive motion in unstable segments of the spine, skin damage, overstretching of the low back and long finger flexors, and injuries from falls. Over time, transfers may also cause overuse

---

[a] This chapter does not attempt to present all possible transfer techniques. An individual who is unable to master a transfer described in this chapter may fare better with a variation of that transfer or with an altogether different method.

TABLE 10–1   Precautions During Transfers and Transfer Training

Potential Problems	Transfer Activities That Place Patients at Risk	Precautions
Excessive motion at site of vertebral instability, potentially causing additional neurologic and orthopedic damage.	Any activity involving excessive motion or muscular action at or near site of unstable spine. Example: upright activities while the spine remains unstable.	• Strictly adhere to orthopedic precautions. • Check fit of vertebral orthosis with patient in the different postures involved in transfer training. • When the spine is unstable, avoid activities that may cause motion or strong muscular contraction at site of instability.
Skin abrasions and pressure ulcers.	Any activities creating shearing forces on the skin. Example: sliding buttocks on transfer board or mat.	• When possible, instruct patient to lift buttocks instead of sliding. • Vary activities to avoid prolonged periods during which shearing forces are placed on skin. • Choose proper clothing for transfer training (pants rather than hospital gowns).
	Any activities in which the patient's buttocks may forcefully contact the wheelchair. Example: transfers between wheelchair and mat (risk of blunt trauma from contact with wheel).	• Provide careful guarding during practice. • Emphasize the development of control during transfers, with avoidance of contact between the buttocks and wheelchair components that can cause injury.
Impaired tenodesis grasp due to over-stretching of the long finger flexors.	Any activities involving simultaneous wrist and finger extension. Example: weight bearing on palms with fingers extended while practicing short sitting propped forward on two arms.	• With patients who may utilize tenodesis grasp (people with C7 or higher tetraplegia), avoid simultaneous wrist and finger extension. • When bearing weight on palms, maintain interphalangeal joints in flexion.
Overstretched low back, resulting in diminished capacity for functional independence.	Any activities involving simultaneous hip flexion with knee extension in patients with hamstring tightness, placing stress on the low back. Examples: practice lifting legs onto mat or side-approach floor-to-wheelchair transfers when the hamstrings are tight.	• Avoid long itting in patients who lack a minimum of 90 degrees of passive straight-leg raise. • When hamstrings are tight, avoid prolonged practice of activities that involve simultaneous hip flexion and knee extension.
Injury from fall.	Any transfers to or from wheelchair involve some risk of falling.	• Education and training in safe transfer techniques. • Appropriate guarding during functional training.
Overuse injuries of the upper extremities.	Activities involving potentially injurious positions or weight bearing on the upper extremities, performed repetitively over time.	• Education and training in transfer techniques and habits that minimize damaging stresses to the upper extremities.

injuries in the upper extremities. Table 10–1 presents a summary of precautions for transfers and transfer training.

Strategies for Preventing Overuse Injuries

Functional activities that involve weight bearing through the upper extremities are thought to be significant contributors to chronic upper limb pain and injury following spinal cord injury.[1,2] In the presence of lower limb paralysis, weight bearing on the upper extremities cannot be avoided during independent transfers. However, the risk of overuse injury may be reduced by optimizing the techniques used. *To the extent possible*, patients should avoid potentially injurious joint positions during transfers, including end-range wrist extension, end-range shoulder internal rotation combined with abduction or flexion, and end-range shoulder extension combined with internal rotation and abduction. Transfer techniques that involve leaning forward on the upper extremities while depressing and protracting the scapulae may be less injurious than other methods.

Patients should be instructed in strategies they can use after discharge to prevent overuse injuries.[b] These strategies include utilizing transfer techniques that avoid potentially injurious joint positions, minimizing the number of transfers per day, performing transfers to surfaces level with or lower than the sitting surface when possible, varying the direction of transfers, and using a tub bench or roll-in shower for bathing. Transfer boards should be considered for all individuals with spinal cord injury, especially those who are obese, pregnant, or have upper extremity pain or weakness. When one arm is painful, transfers should be performed toward the painful arm when possible.[2–5]

FUNCTIONAL POTENTIALS

After a spinal cord injury, an individual's potential for achieving independence in transfers is determined largely by her voluntary motor function. Table 10–2 presents a summary of the level of independence in transfers that can be achieved by people who have complete spinal cord injuries at different motor levels (motor component of neurological level of injury). When predicting an individual's capacity to develop transfer skills, the clinician should take into consideration the many other factors that affect functional gains.[c] In addition, it is important to recall that these skills take time to develop. The patient is likely to make functional gains during all phases of rehabilitation (inpatient, in home, outpatient), and may continue to do so for months or years after discharge.

[b] Additional strategies for preventing upper extremity overuse injuries are presented in Chapters 8, 9, 11, 12, and 15.

[c] Chapter 8 presents factors that can influence functional outcomes.

TABLE 10–2   Functional Potentials

Motor Level	Significance of Innervated Musculature	Potential for Independence in Transfers
C4 and higher	Inadequate voluntary motor function to contribute to transfers.	Dependent in all transfers.
C5	**Partial innervation of the deltoids** makes it possible to extend the elbows using muscle substitution. Deltoid function plus **partial innervation of the infraspinatus and teres minor** make it possible to "lock" the elbows in extension. **Partial innervation of the biceps brachii, brachialis, and brachioradialis** makes it possible to use elbow flexion to pull. Minimal serratus anterior function is inadequate to stabilize the scapulae against the thorax.	**Typical functional outcomes** Dependent in all transfers. **Exceptional outcomes** **Even:** Independent; those who transfer independently are likely to require transfer boards, and some use boards plus overhead loops.
C6	**Fully innervated deltoids, infraspinatus, teres minor, and clavicular portion of the pectoralis major** allow for stronger elbow extension and "locking" using muscle substitution. **Full innervation of the biceps brachii** allows for stronger pull using elbow flexion. **Partial innervation of the serratus anterior** makes it possible to stabilize the scapulae against the thorax. Scapular protraction allows greater lift of the buttocks. **Partial innervation of the latissimus dorsi** enhances shoulder girdle depression, allowing greater lift of the buttocks. Minimal innervation of the triceps brachii is inadequate to contribute significantly to transfers.	**Typical functional outcomes** **Even:** Some assist to independent in even transfers with or without transfer board. **Uneven:** Some to total assist. **Exceptional outcomes** **Even:** Independent without equipment. **Uneven:** Independent in transfers between the wheelchair and surfaces a few inches above or below the level of the sitting surface; may require transfer board.

TABLE 10–2   (*Continued*)

Motor Level	Significance of Innervated Musculature	Potential for Independence in Transfers
C7	**Partial innervation of the triceps brachii** allows for stronger elbow extension. **Full innervation of the serratus anterior** provides more stable scapulae, stronger protraction and upward rotation. **Partial innervation of the latissimus dorsi and sternocostal portion of pectoralis major** enhance shoulder girdle depression, allowing greater lift of the buttocks.	**Typical functional outcomes** **Even:** Independent in even transfers without equipment. **Uneven:** Independent to some assist in transfers between the wheelchair and surfaces a few inches above or below the level of the sitting surface. **Exceptional outcomes** **Uneven:** Independent in uneven transfers, including transfers between the wheelchair and the floor, using a side-approach transfer.
C8	**Full innervation of the triceps brachii** provides normal strength in elbow extension. **Full innervation of the latissimus dorsi and nearly full innervation of pectoralis major** allow strong shoulder girdle depression. **Nearly full innervation of flexor digitorum superficialis and profundus, and partial innervation of flexor pollicus longus and brevis** provide grasp without muscle substitution, making leg management easier.	**Typical functional outcomes** **Even:** Independent in even transfers without equipment. **Uneven:** Independent in transfers between the wheelchair and surfaces a few inches above or below the level of the sitting surface. **Exceptional outcomes** **Uneven:** Independent in uneven transfers, including transfers between the wheelchair and the floor, using a side-approach transfer.
T1-9	**Fully innervated upper extremities** make all transfers easier to achieve. Trunk musculature inadequate to assist in transfers.	**Typical functional outcomes** **Even:** Independent in even transfers without equipment **Uneven:** Most achieve independence in transfers between the wheelchair and surfaces a few inches above or below the level of the sitting surface; many achieve independence in transfers between the wheelchair and the floor; a side, front, or back approach may be used to transfer from the floor to the wheelchair.
T10 and below	**Partial to full innervation of trunk musculature** (T6–L1) enhances transfer ability.	**Typical functional outcomes** **Even:** Independent in even transfers without equipment. **Uneven:** Independent in all uneven transfers, including between the wheelchair and the floor; a side, front, or back approach may be used to transfer from the floor to the wheelchair.

References for innervation: 6 to 10.

PHYSICAL AND SKILL PREREQUISITES

Every functional activity involves a particular set of skills. Each activity also has requirements for strength, joint range of motion, and muscle flexibility. A deficiency in any of these skill or physical prerequisites will interfere with a person's performance of the activity. Therapeutic programs are designed to develop the strength, range of motion, and skills required to meet patients' goals.

The descriptions of functional techniques presented in this chapter are accompanied by tables that summarize the physical and skill prerequisites. Exact values for the physical prerequisites are not given because the requirements vary among individuals. For example, a person who is thin, coordinated, and has relatively long arms will probably require less anterior deltoid strength to perform a particular transfer than someone who is overweight, uncoordinated, and has short arms.

TRANSFERS FOLLOWING COMPLETE SPINAL CORD INJURY: FUNCTIONAL TECHNIQUES AND THERAPEUTIC STRATEGIES

A person who sustains a complete spinal cord injury has a limited number of muscles with which to function. To transfer from one surface to another, she must utilize the muscles innervated above her lesion to move her entire body. During rehabilitation, she learns how to transfer between her wheelchair and various surfaces by using a variety of compensatory strategies, including muscle substitution, momentum, and the head–hips relationship.[d]

General Therapeutic Strategies

To accomplish a functional goal, the patient must acquire both the physical and skill prerequisites for that activity. For example, when working on a side-approach floor-to-chair transfer, a person with a complete spinal cord injury must develop adequate hamstring flexibility and upper extremity strength as well as the ability to pivot on her arms to lift her buttocks.

When developing skill prerequisites for a functional goal, the patient should start with the most basic prerequisite skills and progress toward more challenging activities. (There is no point in working on lifting the buttocks by pivoting on the arms if the individual cannot maintain an upright sitting position by propping on her arms.) Similarly, patients should practice even transfers before progressing to uneven transfers. As they develop the strength, range of motion, and skills to perform even transfers, they lay the foundation for more advanced transfers.

---

[d] These movement strategies are explained in Chapter 8.

Before asking a patient to attempt a new skill, the therapist should explain and demonstrate the technique. The demonstration should provide a clear idea of the motions involved and the timing of these motions. The patient should also be shown how the new skill will be used functionally.

During transfer training, therapists should remember that every patient has a unique combination of body build, coordination, strength, flexibility, and muscle tone. As a result, patients vary in the manner in which they perform transfers: the exact placement of their hands; the timing of their pushes, pivots, and twists; and the degree to which they must dip their heads to lift their buttocks. What works for one patient may be a total disaster for the next. The challenge of transfer training is finding the timing and maneuvers that best suit each individual.

As a therapist and patient work together on a skill, they can learn from failed attempts by analyzing the problem. Is the patient strong enough to perform the maneuver? Is she flexible enough? Did she pivot too far forward on her arms, or did she fail to pivot far enough? Were her hands too far anterior or not anterior enough?

Trial and error can be another useful strategy for functional training. For example, the best way to determine whether the hands were too far forward in a failed attempt may be to try the maneuver with the hands positioned further back. The relative success of the attempt may provide an answer.

It is important for the therapist and patient to keep in mind that functional training can take a long time; independence in a given transfer may require an extended period of functional training. It is a mistake to give up on a functional goal after only a few trials (assuming that the patient has adequate innervation, of course!). When funding constraints limit the time available for functional training during inpatient rehabilitation, the patient may continue working toward independence in an alternative setting such as at home or in an outpatient clinic.[11]

Basic Skills

Certain skills are required to perform all transfers. The most fundamental of these is the ability to tolerate upright sitting. Individuals who lack functioning triceps must be also able to extend their elbows using muscle substitution, and to lock their elbows in extension. Finally, independent transfers require the capacity to maintain balance in sitting, to push the trunk to upright from a forward lean, control the pelvis using head and shoulder motions, and to manage the lower extremities. The following paragraphs include descriptions of these skills and therapeutic strategies for teaching them.

Tolerate Upright Sitting

When upright activities are first initiated, people with spinal cord injuries may experience orthostatic hypotension. Before an individual can learn to perform any transfers, she must first develop the capacity to tolerate an upright sitting posture. This capacity can be developed through gradual accommodation to progressively upright postures. Strategies for developing upright sitting tolerance are presented in Chapter 11.

Extend Elbows Using Muscle Substitution

When triceps function is absent or inadequate for functional use, the anterior deltoids and clavicular portion of the pectoralis major can be used to extend the elbows.[12,13] This muscle substitution should be taught early in the program; practice can begin before the patient has been cleared for out-of-bed activities. The therapist can manually stabilize one of the patient's hands with the elbow in a slightly flexed position, and ask her to push. When approached in this manner, many patients will utilize muscle substitution without having to think about it. For an individual who is not able to do so, the therapist can cue her to use her anterior deltoid, reminding her verbally ("use this muscle") and touching or tapping over the muscle.

If a patient cannot extend her elbow while the therapist supplies the verbal and tactile cues just described, the following alternative approach can help her learn the motions involved. The therapist positions the patient's elbow in extension and stabilizes her hand. She then asks the patient to hold her elbow straight while she (the therapist) applies resistance over the distal humerus or antecubital fossa in the direction that would cause elbow flexion. To hold her elbow against this force, the patient contracts her anterior deltoid. Once the patient learns to stabilize her elbow using her anterior deltoid, the therapist can use verbal and tactile cues to teach her to extend her elbow with this muscle. Alternatively, the therapist may place the patient's elbow in slight flexion, place her (the therapist's) hand against the patient's antecubital fossa, and ask her to push. ("Push against my hand.") If the patient can tolerate upright sitting, the strategies just described can also be employed while the patient sits on a mat with her hand on the mat lateral to her thigh.

Whichever strategy is employed to teach muscle substitution, the patient's hand needs to be stabilized during the activity. This stabilization (provided by the therapist, the mat, or both) enables the anterior deltoid to work with the arm in a closed-chain position, simulating the muscle's action during a transfer. Once the patient has learned to extend her elbows using muscle substitution, the process can be repeated with the shoulders in a variety of positions.

Lock the Elbows

When pivoting on her arms during a transfer, a person who does not have functioning triceps must "lock" her elbows using positioning and muscle substitution. The position for locking is as follows: shoulders externally rotated, elbows and wrists extended, forearms supinated. Weight is borne on the palms. The elbows are held in extension using the anterior deltoids and shoulder external rotators.

This skill can be practiced in short or (if hamstring flexibility is adequate) long sitting. After demonstrating the technique for elbow locking, the therapist can help the patient position her arms. The patient then holds the locked position while the therapist applies resistance, pushing the elbow toward flexion.

Once the patient has a feel for the position and muscle contraction involved, she can practice locking and unlocking her elbows. If necessary, the therapist can help by supporting the trunk as the patient leans on an arm and practices moving it in and out of position.

Balance in Sitting

During transfers, sitting balance is typically maintained by propping on the upper extremities with the elbows extended. Balance training should begin when a patient can tolerate upright sitting. Practice should occur in short sitting and, if hamstring flexibility is adequate, in long sitting.

Prop Forward on Two Extended Arms in Sitting

Propping forward on extended arms[e] involves leaning forward slightly and supporting the trunk on the arms, with the palms lateral to the thighs and anterior to the hips. Before a patient can practice this skill, she must be able to extend her elbows and hold them in extension against resistance, using either triceps or muscle substitution.

After assisting the patient into position, the therapist asks her to help hold her elbows straight. The patient should also practice positioning her hands and extending her elbows to support her trunk. The therapist can help stabilize the trunk at first, reducing this assistance as the patient's skill improves. The patient will soon be able to support her trunk independently by propping forward on extended arms. To prepare for more advanced activities, she can hold the position as the therapist applies resistance, pushing her shoulders in various directions.

Prop forward on One Extended Arm in Sitting

Before practicing this skill, a patient should be able to prop forward on two extended arms. She can then practice shifting her trunk laterally, with both hands remaining on the mat. At first, the therapist can encourage the weight shift by placing a hand on the lateral surface of one of the patient's shoulders and having her push against it.

The patient should shift under control through increasing arcs of motion until she is able to lean far enough to support her trunk on one arm. She can then lift the unweighted arm and balance in that position. She should practice this with each arm. To increase her skill, she should practice balancing with the supporting arm in various positions and reaching the free arm in different directions.

Unsupported Sitting Balance

An individual with a spinal cord injury will probably never need to sit with both hands in the air to perform a transfer; however, practicing unsupported sitting balance can

---

[e] Throughout this chapter, "extended arms" refers to upper extremities with the elbows positioned in extension.

be a useful therapeutic activity. Developing the ability to use head and arm motions to maintain upright sitting will make other activities easier.

Once a patient can tolerate an upright sitting posture, her first task in working on unsupported sitting balance is finding her position of balance, the position in which her trunk is balanced over its base of support. The therapist should explain and demonstrate how the patient can maintain an upright position with her hands in the air, using hand and head motions: if her trunk starts to fall, the patient moves her hands and head in the opposite direction.

The patient should practice this skill, getting a feel for how her head and arm motions cause her trunk to move. In long or short sitting, the therapist supports the patient at her shoulders and helps her find her balance point. (When the patient's trunk is balanced, the therapist will not feel her pushing forward, backward, or laterally.) The patient will need to experience the loss of balance and learn to regain the balance point using head and arm motions. Her reactions may be slow at first, and she may tend to overcorrect. The therapist can help the process by providing verbal cues. As the patient becomes more adept at maintaining her balance point, the therapist should withdraw the support being provided at her shoulders. To develop the patient's unsupported sitting balance further, the therapist can disturb her balance or have her catch and throw objects. The patient can also practice maintaining her balance while she reaches her arms in different directions.

From a Forward Lean in Sitting, Push Trunk to Upright

To work on this skill, the patient must be able to tolerate upright sitting. She must also be able to extend her elbows against resistance, using either her triceps or muscle substitution.

Probably the best position for working on this activity is short sitting between two mats, with the mats positioned as shown in Figure 10–1. With her hands stabilized on the mat in front of her, the patient lowers her trunk slightly by allowing her elbows to flex a few degrees and then pushes herself back upright. She should lower her trunk only as far as she can maintain full control of the motion and push back to upright. As the patient's ability improves, she should increase the distance of her pushup.

This skill should also be practiced while sitting in a wheelchair. The hands can be placed on or beside the distal thighs.

Control Pelvis Using Head and Shoulders

To perform any transfer independently, a person with a complete spinal cord injury must use the head–hips relationship. By moving her head and upper torso in one direction, she causes her buttocks to move in the opposite direction. Many of the activities described later in this chapter[f] can

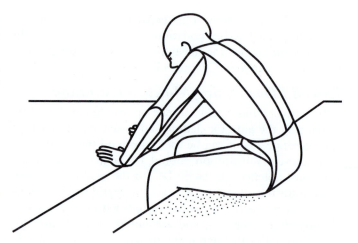

Figure 10–1   Short sitting on mat with second mat placed in front to allow practice pushing trunk to upright from a forward lean.

help develop this ability; however, the therapist and patient may find it helpful to address head–hips control more directly. In doing so, they build a basic skill that is crucial to all transfers.

Quadruped is an excellent position for working on this skill. This is true whether or not upper extremity motor function is intact. In the absence of functioning triceps, the patient's elbows must be locked using muscle substitution.

When first working in quadruped, the therapist assists the patient to her hands and knees, and the patient attempts to maintain the position. The therapist helps her maintain her stability at first, and reduces the assistance as the patient's skill improves. The patient can progress to maintaining the position while the therapist applies resistance in various directions.

Once the patient is able to stabilize herself in quadruped, she can progress to moving her buttocks side to side using head and shoulder motions. She should move only as far as she can control the motion, increasing the arc as her ability improves.

Someone who has innervated triceps can also practice utilizing the head–hips relationship to assume the quadruped position. Starting in prone, the patient places her palms on the mat next to her shoulders. Simultaneously pushing down and forward (cephalad) with her arms, she pushes her head down to lift her buttocks.

If a patient has elbow flexion contractures or inadequate strength to work in quadruped, she may be able to work on head–hips control while positioned on elbows and knees. This activity may be easier if her elbows are supported on a stack of folding mats so that her trunk is in a horizontal position.

Lift the Feet On and Off a Mat

Lifting the legs onto a mat following a transfer involves balancing on one arm and lifting with the other. Propping on one extended arm and leaning away from the wheelchair, the individual places her free hand or forearm

---

[f] The following skills involve the head–hips relationship: move the buttocks in a wheelchair, lift the buttocks by pivoting on extended arms, lift the buttocks and move laterally, unweight the buttocks by leaning forward on extended arms, slide the buttocks laterally while propping on extended arms, and move the buttocks between floor and wheelchair.

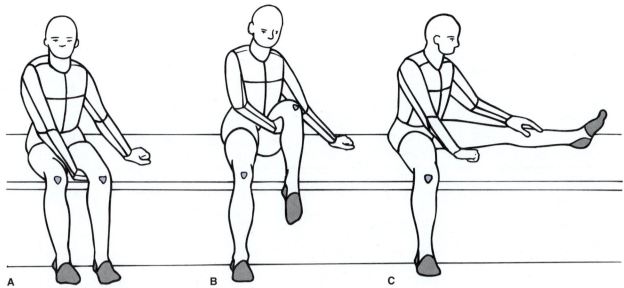

Figure 10–2   Leg management after a transfer. (A) Balancing on one arm, the person places his free arm under the thigh of the leg furthest from the wheelchair. (B) Pulling the leg onto the mat. (C) Straightening the leg on the mat.

under the thigh of the leg furthest from the wheelchair (Figure 10–2A). Balancing on the extended arm, she pulls the thigh onto the mat (Figure 10–2B). She can add power to the lift by leaning away from the leg and throwing her head in the direction of the pull, dropping onto the elbow of the supporting arm, or both. Once her foot is well onto the mat, she straightens her knee by pushing her foot and leg with her hand (Figure 10–2C). She then repeats the process to lift the other leg. Getting the feet back onto the floor involves the same process, done in reverse. If a patient is unable to learn to manage her legs without equipment, she can make the task easier by using either a leg lifter or loops strapped to her distal thighs (Figure 10–3).

The therapist can demonstrate leg management, and provide assistance and verbal cues as the patient practices.

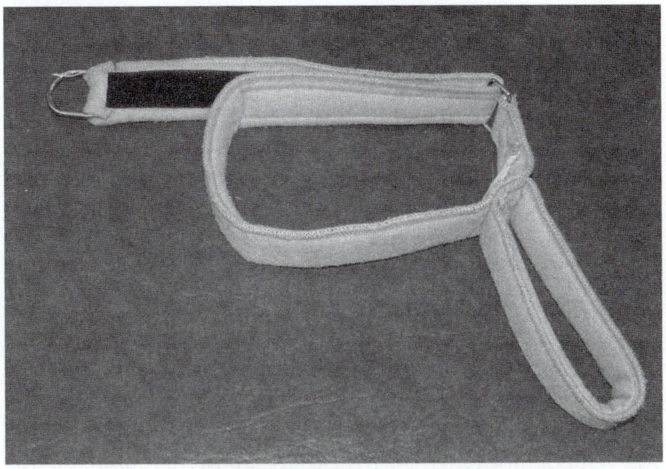

Together they can problem solve regarding optimal placement of the patient's hands, and the timing and force of the movements.

Related Wheelchair Skills

To transfer to and from a wheelchair, an individual must be able to position the chair, engage and disengage the wheel locks, reposition or remove and replace an armrest (if armrests are used), and position the footrests (if they are movable). She must also position her legs, buttocks, and torso in the wheelchair before or after the transfer. The physical and skill prerequisites required to perform these tasks are summarized in Tables 10–3 and 10–4. The following paragraphs describe techniques for performing these prerequisite skills as well as therapeutic strategies for teaching them.

Place an Arm Behind the Wheelchair Push Handle

Many people with spinal cord injuries are able to place an arm behind the wheelchair's push handle using normal motions rather than compensatory movement strategies. An individual who has difficulty with this task may need to use momentum to get her arm into position. Starting with her arm crossed across her torso, she can throw the arm back and up. The motion should be forceful enough to provide adequate momentum to carry the arm to a position behind the push handle.

Therapeutic Strategies
The therapist can help at first by assisting with the throw to give the patient a feel for the motion. An individual who continues to have difficulty can practice with a small wrist weight. The weight will add to the arm's momentum, making it easier to throw the arm back.

Figure 10–3   Loops attached to distal thigh to make leg management easier.

TABLE 10–3   Related Wheelchair Skills – Physical Prerequisites

	Stabilize Trunk In Wheelchair	Move Trunk In Wheelchair	Move Buttocks In Wheelchair	Position Wheelchair	Engage and Disengage Wheel Locks	Position Armrests	Manage Legs	Position Footrests
Strength								
Anterior deltoids	✓	✓	✓	✓	✓	✓	✓	✓
Middle deltoids	✓	✓	✓	✓	✓	✓	✓	✓
Posterior deltoids	✓	✓	✓	✓	✓	✓	✓	✓
Biceps, brachialis, and/or brachioradialis	✓	✓	✓	✓	✓	✓	✓	✓
Range of Motion								
Shoulder Extension	✓	✓	✓			✓		
Shoulder Abduction	✓	✓	✓			✓		
Shoulder Flexion				✓	✓		✓	✓
Elbow Extension	✓	✓	✓	✓	✓			✓
Elbow Flexion	✓	✓	✓			✓	✓	

√ Some strength is needed for this activity, or severe limitations in range will inhibit this activity.

Practice of this skill should start with the patient sitting upright in a wheelchair. Once she has become proficient in this position, she should progress to placing an arm behind a push handle while she leans forward, to the side, or both. As her ability improves, the patient should practice in increasingly tilted positions.

Stabilize the Trunk in a Wheelchair

While sitting in a wheelchair, someone who lacks functional trunk musculature must use her arms for stability when her trunk is in any position other than resting forward on her legs or resting back on the backrest. She must also stabilize her trunk in any situation in which she is likely to be pulled off balance. An example of such a situation is when she lifts one arm to the side. Even such a minor act can shift a person's center of gravity enough to cause her trunk to fall to the side.

To stabilize her trunk in an upright position, a person with a spinal cord injury can simply hook one arm behind a push handle. Alternatively, she can push on her thigh or on an armrest to hold herself upright, using either triceps or muscle substitution to extend her elbow.[g]

Stabilizing the trunk while leaning forward involves similar strategies: the individual can either lean on her

arm(s) or hook one arm behind a push handle. When using the latter strategy, the arm's position is determined by the angle of the trunk's forward lean. Figure 10–4 shows different arm positions that can be used.

Trunk stabilization when leaning to the side can be accomplished by hooking an arm behind a push handle. Alternatively, the individual can hold the armrest away from which she is leaning, using her hand, wrist, or forearm.

Therapeutic Strategies

To practice stabilizing the trunk by holding a wheelchair push handle, a person must be able to tolerate an upright sitting position. It is not necessary for her to be able to place her arm behind the push handle independently.

With her arm hooked behind the wheelchair's push handle, the patient practices holding her body stable. Starting in an upright sitting position, she uses one arm to hold her body upright while she moves the other arm to various positions. This activity can be made more challenging by adding weight to the free arm and by throwing this arm more forcefully.

Once an individual has mastered the skill in upright, she should practice with her trunk leaned in various directions. The degree of lean can increase as she becomes more proficient.

In addition to developing the ability to stabilize her trunk, the patient needs to learn how to adjust her hold on the chair's push handle to allow her trunk to lean (Figure 10–4).

---

[g] The functional techniques and therapeutic strategies for propping on one or two extended arms are described in the preceding section of this chapter.

TABLE 10–4   Related Wheelchair Skills – Physical Prerequisites

	Stabilize Trunk in Wheelchair	Move Trunk in Wheelchair	Move Buttocks in Wheelchair	Position Wheelchair	Engage and Disengage Wheel Locks	Position Armrests	Manage Legs	Position Footrests
Tolerate upright sitting position.*			√		√	√	√	√
Place arm behind push handle (pp. 201, 202).	√	√	√		√	√		
Hold push handle to stabilize trunk (pp. 202, 203).	√	√	√		√	√		
Move trunk in wheelchair (pp. 203–205)		√	√		√		√	√
Manipulate armrests (pp. 207, 208).						√		
Move buttocks on wheelchair seat (pp. 205, 206).			√					
Extend elbows using muscle substitution† (p. 199).	√	√	√		√			
Prop forward on extended arms (p. 199).	√							
Propel wheelchair.*				√				

√ This prerequisite skill is required to perform this activity.
* Refer to Chapter 11 for a description of this skill and therapeutic strategies.
† In the absence of functioning triceps.

When sitting upright, the trunk is stabilized using the upper arm. When moving from upright, the person must relax her arm enough to allow the hold to slide more distally. The therapist can help with initial practice of this skill by lowering the patient's torso while she adjusts her hold on the chair. As her skill improves, the patient can participate in the control of her trunk's descent, leaning progressively further as she relaxes her hold on the push handle. She should work to the point where she can lower her trunk independently and can stop the descent at any point.

Move the Trunk in a Wheelchair

In the absence of functioning trunk musculature, a person with a spinal cord injury uses her arms and head to move her trunk. One way to lean forward while sitting in a wheelchair is to pull on an anterior part of the chair such as the front of the armrest. The person who leans forward in this manner can return to upright by pushing on her thighs, the front of the chair, or the armrests. This push to upright can be accomplished using either the triceps or muscle substitution to extend the elbows.

Momentum can also be used to move the trunk. If the individual throws her head and an arm forward forcefully enough, her body will fall forward. One arm should remain hooked behind the wheelchair's backrest or push handle to provide stability once the trunk has moved forward. This arm should remain relaxed until the trunk has leaned far enough forward; holding too tight will prevent the trunk's forward motion. The arm that remains hooked behind the chair can be used to pull the trunk back into an upright position. The other arm can assist by pushing on a thigh, the front of the chair, or an armrest.

The trunk can also be brought forward by pushing on the wheelchair's tires, behind the seat. The person using this technique should hook one arm behind a push handle for stability and to return to upright.

Any of the methods just described can be combined to bring the trunk forward. For example, an individual may push on a tire with one hand while throwing her head and the other arm forward.

To lean to the side, a person lacking trunk musculature can either pull on an armrest or throw her head and an

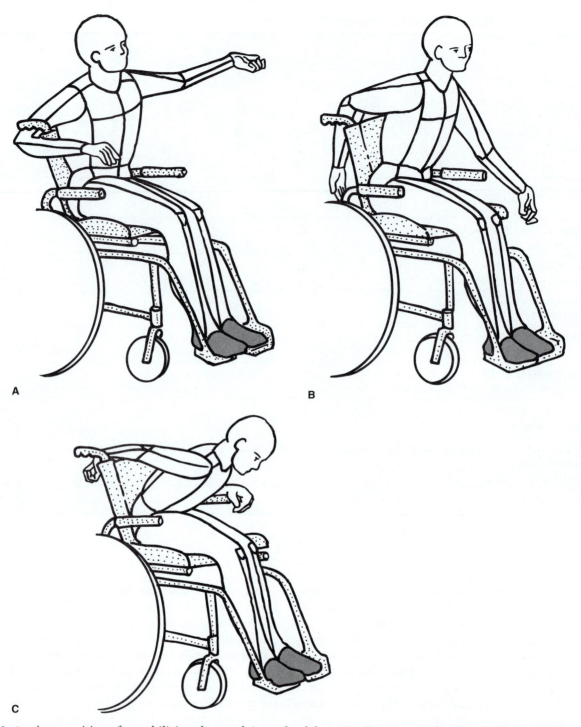

Figure 10–4   Arm positions for stabilizing the trunk in a wheelchair. (A) Sitting upright. (B) Slight forward lean. (C) Pronounced forward lean.

arm to the side and allow their momentum to move her trunk. To return to upright, she can pull on the opposite armrest or push handle.

Therapeutic Strategies
To work on pulling her trunk forward or returning to up-right from a forward lean, a person must be able to toler-ate upright sitting. In contrast, practice leaning the trunk laterally in a wheelchair can begin with the wheelchair

slightly reclined if the patient is not yet able to tolerate fully upright sitting.

When the upper extremities are intact, the patient is likely to require minimal practice to learn to move her trunk using any of the techniques described in the preced-ing paragraphs. Individuals who lack functioning triceps will have greater difficulty, and are likely to find some methods more difficult than others. The therapist and pa-tient should work together to determine which movement strategies are most feasible for that individual. When the patient first begins practice, the therapist can provide assistance with the trunk's motions. As the patient's skill develops, this assistance should be reduced.

A patient learning to use momentum to move her trunk may have difficulty initially because she is reluctant to throw her head and arm forcefully enough to create adequate momentum. The therapist should encourage her to move with abrupt, powerful, and exaggerated motions. The therapist can give the patient a feel for the motion by moving her arm passively. A wrist weight can also be helpful, adding to the arm's momentum and enabling the person to move her trunk. As her skill improves, she should practice without the weight.

When first practicing moving her trunk in a wheelchair, the patient should start with small excursions, moving forward or to the side only as far as she can maintain control and return to upright. As her skill increases, she should move through larger arcs of motion.

Move the Buttocks in a Wheelchair

A person with a complete spinal cord injury uses the head–hips relationship to move her buttocks in a wheelchair: to move her buttocks in one direction, she moves her head and upper torso in the opposite direction. Someone who has intact upper extremity musculature can move on a wheelchair's seat with relative ease. She can simply lift her buttocks by pushing on the armrests or wheelchair seat and throw her head in the direction opposite to where she wants her buttocks to move.

In the absence of functioning triceps, the exact methods used to move the buttocks in a wheelchair are as varied as the people performing them. The descriptions that follow are some examples.

To move her buttocks forward on the seat, a person with a complete spinal cord injury can throw her head back repeatedly and forcefully. She may be able to improve her performance by pushing on the wheelchair's backrest with her elbows while throwing her head.

Another technique that a person can use to move her buttocks out on the wheelchair seat is to lean her head and upper torso back and shimmy, twisting her trunk right and left repeatedly. This shimmying motion is accomplished by throwing the head and arms right and left.

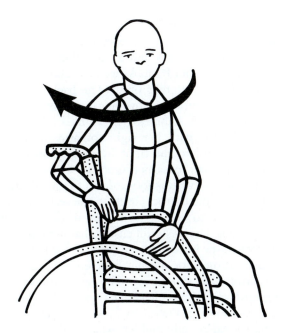

Figure 10–5   Moving the buttocks out in the wheelchair seat. The person twists her head and upper torso to the right and back to move her buttocks forward and to the left.

A third method for moving the buttocks out on the wheelchair seat involves larger twisting motions. Using this approach, a person moves her buttocks forward and to one side by twisting her head and upper torso in the opposite direction. To twist out and to the left, she hooks her right shoulder behind the wheelchair's right push handle and hooks her left hand on the right armrest. Pulling with her arms, she twists her head and upper trunk to the right and back (Figure 10–5). This motion will cause the buttocks to slide to the left and forward. The distance that the buttocks will move depends on the magnitude of the head and upper trunk motion. Someone who is unable to move far enough by twisting to one side can repeat the twist in the opposite direction.

To move her buttocks straight to the side for a short distance, a person with a spinal cord injury can lean in the opposite direction. For example, someone who desires to move to the right can hook her right arm around the chair's right push handle and lean to the left.

Problem-Solving Exercise 10–1

Your patient has C5 tetraplegia, ASIA A. He is practicing the skill of leaning his trunk forward from upright while sitting in a wheelchair. He uses one arm to stabilize himself in the chair while he throws his head and the other arm forward in an attempt to lean forward using momentum. He is unable to lean his trunk forward using this technique.

- What could be causing this problem?
- Describe functional training strategies to develop this patient's ability to lean forward in his wheelchair using momentum.

To move her buttocks laterally over larger distances, an individual can lean her torso forward and to the side, pushing her buttocks back and to the other side. If she is already sitting with her buttocks well back on the seat, the buttocks will move laterally only. (The backrest prevents any rearward motion.) To move her buttocks back and to the left, the person stabilizes her trunk by holding the right push handle with her right forearm or wrist and twists forward and to the right by pulling on the right armrest with her left forearm (Figure 10–6).

This method of twisting forward and to the side can also be used to move the buttocks back on the seat. The person should twist first to one side and then to the other while leaning forward. Doing so will ensure that her buttocks are centered when she has completed the backward motion.

Another method for moving back on the seat involves leaning forward and shimmying. The person leans her body well forward and stabilizes her hands against the front of the armrests, as shown in Figure 10–7. She then shimmies her head and shoulders right and left while pushing her hands forward. The result is a backward motion of the buttocks.

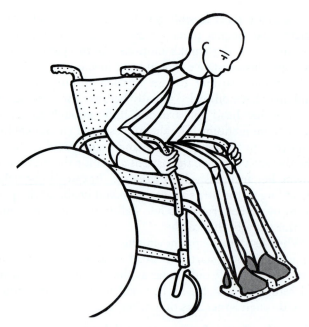

Figure 10–7   Moving the buttocks back in the seat.

Therapeutic Strategies

To practice repositioning her buttocks on a wheelchair seat, a patient must be able to stabilize and move her trunk in the wheelchair. It is difficult at first for people with spinal cord injuries to move their buttocks on their wheelchair seats. The therapist and patient may have to try several of the different methods of performing this task in order to determine which one is most effective for that individual. During early practice using a given method, the therapist can help the patient execute the head and upper torso movements while she tries the maneuvers. This assistance can give the patient a feel for the required force and excursion of the motions. Alternatively, the therapist can aid the process by pulling on the patient's buttocks or legs to enable her to move. This assistance should be timed to coincide with the patient's efforts, and should be just forceful enough to effect some motion. As the patient's skill improves, the therapist can reduce the assistance given.

Position the Wheelchair

During a transfer from a wheelchair to a surface such as a mat, bed, or couch, the wheelchair should be positioned as close to the other surface as possible. The chair should be parked at about a 30-degree angle to the object, with the rear wheel and caster as close as they can get to the other surface. Positioning the wheelchair in this manner will minimize the gap between the surfaces, making the transfer easier and safer.

A patient who has difficulty angling a manual wheelchair as described above should start by positioning the chair parallel to the object, close enough for the rear wheel to touch it. She should then lock the brake closest to the object and push forward on the other wheel to angle the chair.

Floor-to-wheelchair transfers also involve positioning the chair, if it is not already in an upright position. (This is the situation if the person is transferring after having tipped over backwards in the wheelchair.) Moving the wheelchair into an upright position involves engaging the wheel locks and then pulling down on the front of the chair to tip it to upright (Figure 10–8).

Therapeutic Strategies

Before initiating practice positioning a wheelchair next to a mat or other surface in preparation for a transfer, the patient should have begun training in wheelchair

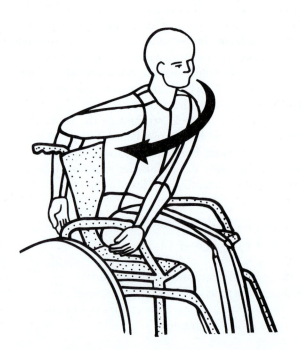

Figure 10–6   Moving the buttocks back and to the left by leaning forward and twisting the head and upper torso to the right.

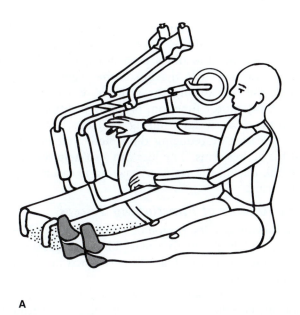 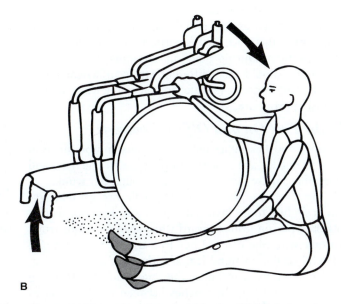

A   B

Figure 10–8   Righting the wheelchair prior to transfer from floor. (A) Engaging the wheel locks. (B) Righting the wheelchair by pulling down on the front of the chair.

propulsion.[h] The therapist can then explain and demonstrate the appropriate wheelchair position and techniques for moving the wheelchair into position, and the patient can practice with assistance and feedback.

Practice righting a wheelchair in preparation for a floor-to-wheelchair transfer requires good balance in longsitting. The therapist can demonstrate the task and assist the patient as needed during practice.

Manage the Wheelchair Parts

Independent transfers involve managing the wheelchair's locks, positioning the armrests, and positioning the footrests.

Engage and Disengage the Wheel Locks

To engage a wheelchair's wheel locks (lock the brakes) while sitting in the chair, the person either pushes or pulls on the locks' levers, depending upon their construction. Disengaging the locks involves the opposite motion. To reach a wheel lock, the person may have to lean forward and to the side. If using a power wheelchair, she turns the motor off and on rather than manipulating wheel locks.

Position the Armrests

Armrest styles vary. Some can be rotated out of the way, either up and back or to the side and back. With these armrest styles, a person can prepare for a transfer by pulling up on the armrest and pushing it out of the way. Other armrests must be removed prior to a transfer. Removing the latter type of armrest involves unlocking it (if locked) and lifting it out of its channels. The lift should be straight upward. Any lateral, forward, or backward pull can jam the armrest in its channels.

If an armrest is removed (as opposed to being rotated out of the way), it can be tempting to place it on the floor after removing it from the wheelchair. The problems with this practice are twofold: the armrest may be damaged and it is likely to be in the wrong place when needed. (It gets kicked under the bed, moved to the other side of the bed, etc.) To preserve her equipment and to save herself the trouble of hunting down misplaced armrests, it is a good idea for someone who uses a wheelchair to get into the habit of storing the armrest on the wheelchair, out of the way but still accessible. An armrest can be hung on one of the wheelchair's push handles, but it may fall off from this position. Alternatively, it can be placed on the wheelchair's seat for storage.

Position the Footrests

If the wheelchair's front rigging is movable, it should be repositioned during transfers so that it does not cause injury or interfere with the transfers. Repositioning the front rigging involves either folding the footplates or swinging the entire footrest mechanism out of the way.

Folding the footplates provides adequate clearance for many transfers. To fold a footplate, a wheelchair user first places her foot on the floor. If she is stabilizing her trunk by holding on to the back of the wheelchair, she needs to shift her hold more distally on the stabilizing arm so that she can lean forward further. She then can reach down with her free hand and fold the footplate by pulling it up. If she cannot grasp the footplate, she can move it by placing her hand or forearm under the plate and pulling upward on it.

During some transfers, such as those between a wheelchair and the floor, one or both footrests are swung out of the way rather than merely folded. To reposition a footrest, the person leans forward and operates the footrest release, using the arm on the same side of the chair as the footrest. The other arm is used to stabilize the trunk.

[h] This skill is addressed in Chapter 11.

Therapeutic Strategies

The therapist can explain and demonstrate techniques for manipulating the wheelchair's parts, and assist the patient as she practices. During functional training, the therapist and patient should trial different styles of wheel locks, armrests, and footrests in order to determine what designs are most appropriate.[i]

Lift the Feet On and Off the Footrests

A person who has intact upper extremity motor function can move one leg at a time by grasping it with one hand and lifting. She can use her other arm to stabilize her trunk.

In the absence of functioning finger flexors, leg management is slightly more involved. To remove her foot from a footrest, a person leans forward while stabilizing her trunk with one arm. She can use her free arm to lift either the ipsilateral or contralateral leg. If lifting the ipsilateral leg, she places her forearm under the thigh and lifts. If lifting the contralateral leg, she reaches between her legs, places her forearm under the contralateral thigh, and lifts. Power can be added to the lift by stabilizing the proximal forearm on top of the other thigh, using this leg as a fulcrum.

Whether the ipsilateral or contralateral leg is lifted, the foot will slide posteriorly off of the footrest as the thigh lifts. If the shoe gets snagged on the heel loop of the footrest, the person can either lift the leg higher or reach down and push her foot off of the heel loop.

Before performing an even transfer, a person with a spinal cord injury should place her feet flat on the floor with the tibias vertical. This can be done by pushing or pulling on the legs to move the feet into position, or by lifting one thigh at a time and letting the unweighted foot swing into position.

To place her foot back on the footrest, the person can use the lifting techniques just described. As her foot gets high enough, she can push it forward with her forearm and place the foot over the footrest.

Therapeutic Strategies

The therapist can explain and demonstrate techniques for moving the feet on and off of the footrests, and assist the patient as she practices.

Even Transfers Without Equipment

Even transfers, also called level transfers, involve moving between two surfaces of equal height. During even transfers, a person with a complete spinal cord injury pivots on her arms, using the head-hips relationship to lift and swing her buttocks. Tables 10–5 and 10–6 summarize the physical and skill prerequisites for even transfers.

An even transfer to a mat or bed can be performed with the legs down (feet on the floor) or up (feet on the mat or bed). In the following descriptions, the legs are down. This is due to the author's preference rather than any particular advantage.

[i] Chapter 11 provides information on wheelchair prescription.

Whenever an even transfer is performed with the legs down, the feet should be positioned with the soles flat on the floor and the tibias perpendicular to the floor. This positioning will maximize the weight accepted through the legs during the transfer. Even in the absence of any motor function, properly positioned lower extremities bear weight during transfers. This makes transfers easier by reducing the weight that the person must lift on her arms. The legs can also help to stabilize the trunk during the transfer, making it easier to pivot on the arms.

In the Absence of Functioning Triceps

The following is a description of a technique for transferring from a wheelchair to a mat. The same technique is used to transfer to a bed, and is performed in reverse to return to the wheelchair.

After moving her buttocks forward in the wheelchair, the person sits upright and positions her hands in preparation for the transfer (Figure 10–9A). Her hands should be anterior to her hips, far enough forward to enable her to lean on them during the transfer. They should not be so far anterior that she cannot pivot on them when leaning forward.

The hand on the wheelchair should be placed next to the person's thigh. The hand on the mat should be positioned far enough away to leave adequate space on the mat for the buttocks at the end of the transfer. This hand should be more anterior than the hand on the wheelchair, to enhance forward stability during the transfer. If possible, the hands should be placed so that the fingers drape over the edge of the supporting surfaces in order to reduce the damaging forces on the wrists.[5] Whether or not the fingers are in this draped position, the interphalangeal joints should be flexed to preserve the tenodesis grasp.

The upper extremities should be positioned for elbow locking: shoulders externally rotated, elbows and wrists extended, and forearms supinated. The person maintains her elbows in extension during the transfer through strong contraction of her anterior deltoids, shoulder external rotators, and clavicular portion of her pectoralis major (if innervated).

To transfer, the person leans forward on her arms, tucks her chin, and rolls her head downward. By pivoting on her arms in this manner, she lifts her buttocks from the wheelchair seat. If any serratus anterior or latissimus dorsi function is present, she should protract and depress her scapulae to increase the height of the lift.

When pivoting on her arms, the person needs to lean forward enough to get adequate clearance of her buttocks. At the same time, she must not pivot so far forward that she moves past her balance point. Doing so will result in a forward fall.

With her buttocks lifted, the person forcefully swings her head and twists her shoulders away from the mat (Figure 10–9B). This twisting motion causes the buttocks to swing toward the mat. It is important for the head to remain down during the transfer to maintain the lift.

Table 10–5   Even Transfers—Physical Prerequisites

	No Equipment	With Board, Upright Method	With Board, Alternate Method	With Board And Loops
Strength				
Anterior deltoids	☑	☑	☑	√
Middle deltoids	√	√	√	√
Posterior deltoids			☑	√
Biceps, brachialis, and/or brachioradialis			☑	√
Infraspinatus and teres minor	√	√	√	√
Serratus anterior	•	•	•	•
Pectoralis major	•	•	•	•
Latissimus dorsi	•	•		
Triceps brachii	•	•	•	•
Range of Motion				
Shoulder Extension				☑
Abduction			√	☑
Flexion	√	√	√	
External rotation	☑	☑		
Internal rotation				☑
Elbow Extension	☑	☑		
Flexion		√		√
Forearm supination	☑	☑		√
Wrist extension	☑	☑		√

√ Some strength is needed for this activity, or severe limitations in range will inhibit this activity.
☑ A large amount of strength or normal or greater range is needed for this activity.
• Not required but helpful.

The sideways motion of the buttocks during the transfer is not accomplished by pushing laterally with the arms; it is achieved by swinging the head and twisting the shoulders. Pushing laterally on the wheelchair will cause the chair to slide. If this problem is to be avoided, the arms must push straight downward throughout the transfer.

In the Presence of Functioning Triceps

Innervated triceps make it easier to support the body's weight on the arms during transfers. If the triceps are strong enough to maintain elbow extension while the individual pivots on her arms, she does not need to lock her elbows with positioning and muscle substitution. The transfer technique just described is used, with the exception that shoulder external rotation and full elbow extension are not necessary.[14]

If adequate strength is present in the wrists and hands, trauma to the wrist may be reduced by avoiding end-range wrist extension when weight is borne on the hands. Alternative hand positions include grasping the wheelchair armrest, placing the hand so that the fingers drape over the edge of the cushion or mat, or weight-bearing on the fist (with the wrist in neutral extension) instead of the palm. The latter position may increase trauma to the metacarpophalangeal joints.[5]

Even Transfers Without Equipment—Therapeutic Strategies

To transfer independently without equipment, a person must be able to tolerate upright sitting, perform the basic skills and wheelchair skills described earlier in this chapter, lift the buttocks by pivoting on extended arms, and move the buttocks laterally while lifting. Functional training involves practice of all of these skill prerequisites, separately

TABLE 10–6   Even Transfers –Skill Prerequisites

	No Equipment	With Board, Upright Method	With Board, Alternate Method	With Board And Loops
Tolerate upright sitting.*	√	√	√	√
Related wheelchair skills (pp. 201–208).	√	√	√	√
Extend elbows using muscle substitution† (p. 199).	√	√		
Lock elbows† (p. 199).	√	√		
Prop forward on two extended arms‡ (p. 199).	√	√		
Prop forward on one extended arm‡ (p. 199).	√	√		
Prop on elbows.§			√	
Unweight buttocks by leaning forward on extended arms‡ (p. 213).	√	√		
Control pelvis using head and shoulders (p. 200).	√	√	√	√
Move buttocks laterally while propping on extended arms‡ (pp. 213, 214).		√		
Lift buttocks by pivoting on extended arms‡ (p. 211).	√			
Lift buttocks and move laterally (p. 211).	√			
Place and remove transfer board (p. 213).		√	√	√
Lift feet on and off of mat (pp. 200, 201).	√	√	√	√
Place arm through loop.§				√

√ This prerequisite skill is required to perform this activity.
* Refer to Chapter 11 for a description of this skill and therapeutic strategies.
† In the absence of functioning triceps.
‡ Arm(s) with elbow(s) positioned in extension.
§ Refer to Chapter 9 for a description of this skill and therapeutic strategies.

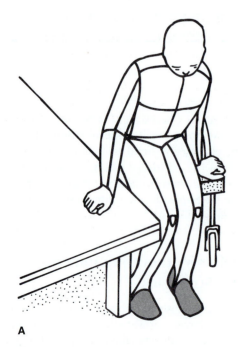

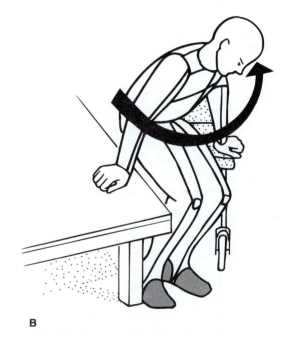

A   B

Figure 10–9   Even transfer without equipment. (A) Starting position. (B) Head thrown down and away from the bed to lift the buttocks up and toward the bed. (The person is shown transferring to a position too close to the end of the mat. The image was drawn in this way to make the legs visible.)

and in combination. Strategies for developing these prerequisite skills are described earlier in the chapter and in the following paragraphs.

Early practice should begin on a mat. When the patient has developed adequate skill in lifting and moving her buttocks, she can practice transfers between the mat and a wheelchair. She should progress to practicing transfers between a bed and a wheelchair, as these transfers are used in daily function.

Lift the Buttocks by Pivoting on Extended Arms

To lift her buttocks, a person must first be able to prop forward on extended arms in sitting and hold this position against resistance.

The patient should be shown how to lean forward over her extended arms while tucking her head and protracting her scapulae. It is often helpful for the therapist to assist her into position, giving the patient a feel for the motion and a sense of just how far she needs to pivot forward to lift her buttocks. The patient should accept full weight on her upper extremities while the therapist helps her lift her buttocks by leaning forward, rolling her head down, and protracting her scapulae. Once in position, the patient can attempt to maintain the lift. As the individual gets a feel for the maneuver, she should progress to practicing with spotting and verbal cueing, and then to practicing independently.

One of the challenges of learning to lift the buttocks is finding the balance point. A person with a complete spinal cord injury must move her body fairly far forward over her arms to lift high enough for a transfer. If she tips too far forward, however, she will fall. When an individual is at her balance point, she has moved as far forward as she can (and thus has lifted as high as she can) without falling. The patient should learn to lift to her balance point and hold there briefly.

Moving past the balance point is not the only cause of falls while performing this maneuver; people lacking triceps can also fall forward due to an inability to stabilize their elbows in extension. To correct this problem, a patient may need further strengthening, practice in locking her elbows, or both.

Often, a patient will develop the ability to pivot and raise her buttocks, but the lift will be inadequate for a transfer without equipment. This problem can occur when the patient does not protract her scapulae enough during the lift, either because of weakness of the serratus anterior or improper technique. If the latter is the case, the therapist can call the person's attention to the problem and provide further instruction. One useful strategy involves placing a hand between the patient's scapulae as she pivots forward on her arms. While pivoting, the patient is asked to push against the therapist's hand by lifting her trunk between her scapulae. If the individual is still unable to perform the motion, the therapist can as-

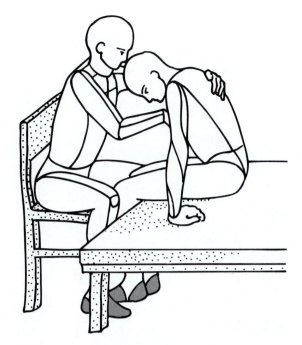

Figure 10–10 Therapist assisting with scapular protraction by lifting the patient's thorax between her scapulae while she pivots forward on her arms.

sist with the scapular protraction during the lift. As the patient pivots forward on her arms, the therapist lifts her thorax between her scapulae (Figure 10–10). The patient should attempt to hold the position. Once she gets a feel for the scapular protraction, she can attempt the motion on her own.

Lift the Buttocks and Move Laterally

Before working on this skill, a person must be able to lift her buttocks by pivoting forward on extended arms.

The therapist should explain and demonstrate how the buttocks can be moved laterally by throwing the head and upper torso to the side while lifting. The motion should be quick and forceful. During early practice of this skill, the patient can lift her buttocks first, then twist to move laterally. She should progress to a single combined lift-and-twist motion. As the patient's skill develops, she should practice moving her buttocks over greater distances.

A common problem that occurs while a patient learns this maneuver is that the she raises her head while throwing it to the side, causing the buttocks to drop. The therapist should direct the patient's attention to this problem and encourage her to keep her head low.

Patients also tend to fall forward as they learn the skill. In some cases this is due to the difficulty of keeping the elbows locked in extension during the maneuver. A forward fall also happens when a patient pivots past her balance point. People who fall forward may require more practice in this activity, strengthening of the anterior deltoids, or additional practice in the skill of raising the buttocks by pivoting on extended arms.

Problem-Solving Exercise 10–2

Your patient has complete (ASIA A) tetraplegia. She is dependent in all functional activities, and is unable to tolerate an upright sitting position. One of her goals is to transfer independently to and from a bed without using equipment.

The patient's muscle test results are as follows.

Muscles	Left	Right
Deltoids (anterior, middle and posterior)	5/5	5/5
Shoulder external rotators	5/5	4+/5
Elbow flexors	5/5	5/5
Radial wrist extensors	5/5	3+/5
Serratus anterior	4/5	4−/5
Triceps brachii	2/5	1/5
Long finger flexors	0/5	0/5
Abductor digiti minimi	0/5	0/5
Trunk and lower extremity musculature	0/5	0/5

Pin prick and light touch on the left are intact in the C2 through C8 key sensory points, impaired in T1, and absent below T1. On the right, pin prick and light touch are intact in C2 through C7, impaired in C8, and absent below. Sensation and voluntary motor function are absent in the anal region.

The patient's joint range of motion and muscle flexibility are normal throughout.

- Identify this patient's motor level(s), sensory level(s), and neurological level of injury using the ASIA classification system.
- What are the physical prerequisites for even transfers without equipment?
- What strength and range should the therapeutic exercise program emphasize to facilitate the attainment of this goal?
- What are the skill prerequisites for even transfers without equipment?
- Describe a functional training program (for the goal of even transfers without equipment) that would be appropriate for this patient at this time.
- How would you progress the patient once she has developed tolerance to upright sitting?

Even Transfers With Board, Upright Method

Weakness, upper extremity pain, contractures, obesity, spasticity, confusion, or low motivation can keep an individual from achieving independence in even transfers without equipment. In these instances, many people can learn to transfer using a transfer board. The board is used to bridge the gap between the wheelchair and the other surface, making it possible to transfer without lifting the buttocks. Tables 10–5 and 10–6 include the physical and skill prerequisites for even transfers using a board.

Like any piece of equipment, a transfer board has disadvantages. Although a board may appear to make a transfer easier, it adds an extra step to the process. Worse, it must be there for the transfer. Someone who depends upon a transfer board will be out of luck if it is ever misplaced or left behind. This is not to say that transfer boards are inherently bad or should never be used. Using a board for transfers may reduce the risk of upper extremity overuse injury.[5] Moreover, many people who are unable to transfer without equipment can gain independence using a board.

The upright method of transferring with a board is similar to an even transfer without equipment. The person first moves her buttocks forward in the chair and positions the transfer board. During the transfer, her hands should

be anterior to her hips, far enough forward to enable her to lean on them. The hand on the wheelchair should be placed next to the thigh, and the hand toward which the individual is transferring should be placed on the board. If the transfer is to be done in one motion, the hand on the board should be far enough away to make room for the buttocks to slide across the board. If the transfer will be performed in several steps, this hand can be placed relatively close to the thigh and repositioned when necessary.

In the absence of functioning triceps, a person locks her elbows using the technique described earlier. The upper extremities are positioned with the shoulders externally rotated, the elbows and wrists extended, and the forearms supinated.[j] If the triceps are strong enough to maintain the elbows in extension during the transfer, this positioning is not necessary.

Although the buttocks do not have to be lifted when using a transfer board, the person does need to shift some weight off of them to make it possible to slide. To unweight her buttocks, a person with a complete spinal cord injury leans forward onto her arms. While doing so, she twists her head and shoulders away from the mat. This

---

[j] If the patient's strength and skill allow, the hands should be positioned to reduce damaging forces to the wrists, as described in the section on transfers without equipment. These hand positions are described in the earlier section on even transfers.

twisting motion causes the buttocks to slide toward the mat. If the individual has sufficient strength and skill, the transfer can be executed in one twist.

Several factors can limit the capacity to slide across the board in one twist. These factors include obesity, arthritic changes in the upper extremities, and inadequate strength or skill. An individual who is unable to transfer in one motion may have to twist repeatedly to move her buttocks across the board. Some find it useful to twist back and forth in rapid succession (shimmying), others perform each twisting motion as a discrete step. Using either of these strategies, each twist of the head and upper torso away from the mat should be forceful, causing the buttocks to slide toward the mat. When moving back into position to prepare for another twist, the motion should not be forceful. A forceful motion toward the mat will cause the buttocks to slide back toward the chair.

Even Transfers With Board, Upright Method—Therapeutic Strategies

To transfer independently with a board using the upright method, a person must be able to tolerate upright sitting, perform the basic skills and wheelchair skills described earlier in this chapter, place and remove a transfer board, unweight the buttocks by leaning forward on extended arms, and slide the buttocks laterally while propping on extended arms. Functional training involves practice of all of these prerequisite skills, separately and in combination. Strategies for developing these skills are described earlier in the chapter and in the following paragraphs.

Place and Remove Transfer Board

To place a transfer board, a person grasps the far end of the board and pulls the near end under her proximal thigh and buttocks. Moving the board back and forth laterally while pulling will help to work the board into position. The board should be angled with the far end higher than the near end, so that it will slide under the thigh instead of being pushed against it. Leaning away from the board will make placement easier.

An individual with impaired grasp can pull on the transfer board using either her forearm or the back of her hand. Nonstandard designs can make board placement and removal easier. For example, a short board or one that has a cutout for the hand may be easier to manipulate. An "offset sliding board" (Figure 10–11) has a small projection that can be useful: with the projection placed against the anteromedial surface of the chair's wheel, the person can slide the board under her thigh using the wheel as a pivot point for the board. If a patient is unable to learn to place and remove a board with any of these features, a loop of webbing can be added to the board to make it easier to manipulate.

A person with good hand function can remove a transfer board by grasping it and pulling it out. In the absence of good hand function, she can use her palm to push

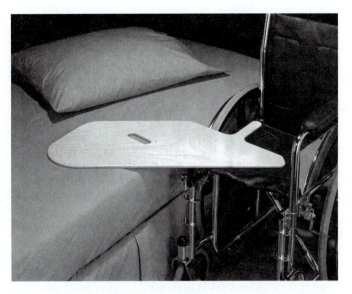

Figure 10–11   Offset sliding board. (Reproduced with permission from Sammons Preston, Bolingbrook, IL.)

outward on the board, pushing either on the top surface or on the sides. Leaning away from the board and working it back and forth will make this task easier.

Functional training in board placement and removal involves instruction and practice. The therapist can provide assistance as needed, reducing this assistance as the patient's skill develops. Training should also include trials with different boards. This will allow the therapist and patient to determine which design is most appropriate for the individual.

Unweight the Buttocks by Leaning Forward on Extended Arms

To develop this skill, a person with a complete spinal cord injury must first be able to prop forward on two extended arms in sitting. Starting in this position, the therapist should instruct the patient to lean forward and tuck her chin. The therapist can facilitate the lean by placing her hands on the anterior surface of the patient's shoulders and having her push against them.

Slide the Buttocks Laterally While Propping on Extended Arms

To perform this activity, the patient must be able to unweight her buttocks by leaning forward on her extended arms. While unweighting her buttocks, she twists her head and upper trunk away from where she wants her buttocks to go. The motion should be forceful and abrupt. Initial attempts are often done without adequate force, and as a result the buttocks do not move. Verbal encouragement to increase the force and excursion of the twist may not work. In these cases, the therapist can help the patient to feel the required motion by assisting her during the attempt, applying force at the patient's shoulders.

Once an individual gets a feel for the head and upper torso motions required, the therapist can help with the lateral slide. Timing the assistance to coincide with the patient's efforts, the therapist applies just enough lateral force to the buttocks to cause motion. As the patient's skill improves, the therapist should reduce the assistance given.

A transfer using a board often requires more than one twist. To make a series of twists possible, the patient moves her head and upper torso back in the other direction between twists. The therapist should instruct her to avoid performing this return motion forcefully, or the buttocks will slide in the wrong direction.

Occasionally, an inexperienced patient twists in both directions with equal force. As a result, the buttocks move back and forth over the same spot. The therapist should give verbal and manual cues to help her correct this problem.

Even Transfers With Board, Alternative Method

Biceps hypertonicity, poor balance, or contractures can make it impossible to prop and twist on the arms with the elbows in extension. Some people who are unable to perform an upright transfer with a board are able to use an alternate method, although finding a method that works for a given individual can be difficult. The therapist and patient will need to be creative in coming up with a solution to the problem.

The following is a description of one alternative method for transferring from a wheelchair to a bed. For clarity, the transfer will be described with the person moving toward the right. Tables 10–5 and 10–6 include the physical and skill prerequisites for even transfers using this method.

After positioning the transfer board, the person turns away from the bed. To do so, she first hooks her left arm behind the wheelchair's left push handle and hooks her right forearm around the wheelchair's armrest. This position is shown in Figure 10–12A. Some people are more successful performing this maneuver with the left hand stabilized against the chair's left wheel.

The person twists her head and shoulders back and to the left by pulling on the push handle and the armrest. This twist causes the buttocks to slide forward and to the right toward the bed (Figure 10–12B). Depending on the individual's strength and ability, positioning the buttocks on the right front corner of the seat may take one or several twists.

From the right front corner of the seat, the person pushes her buttocks across the transfer board toward the bed. To do this, she first places her right palm against the inside of the armrest. Keeping her head low, she pushes on the wheelchair's push handle and armrest and shimmies her head and upper trunk back and forth. This shimmy involves rapid lateral flexion to the right and left alternately.

Once the person has moved her buttocks as far as she can with her arms in the initial position, she can move her arms to a position in which weight is borne on the elbows

on the left side of the wheelchair seat (Figure 10–12C). Keeping her head low, she moves toward the bed by pushing with her arms and shimmying her head and upper trunk. The push and shimmy are continued until the buttocks and thighs are completely on the bed.

To sit up, the person can push on the wheelchair seat, extending her elbows with her anterior deltoids. In the presence of elbow flexion contractures, she may require overhead loops to come to sitting.

Even Transfers With Board, Alternative Method—Therapeutic Strategies

To transfer independently with a board using the alternative method just described, a person must be able to tolerate upright sitting, perform the basic skills and wheelchair skills described earlier in this chapter, and place and remove a transfer board. She must also be able to prop on her elbows,[k] and use head and upper body motions to move her buttocks while in this position. Functional training involves practice of all of these skill prerequisites, separately and in combination. Functional training strategies used to teach upright transfers with a board can be adapted to this transfer.

Problem solving is always an important aspect of functional training. When a patient is unable to perform tasks using standard methods, it becomes even more critical as the therapist and patient work to find alternative strategies to achieve the desired outcome. In working to find alternative methods for transfers, they creatively determine possible ways to accomplish each step of the transfer, and then attempt the novel strategies. If a strategy fails, they analyze the performance to determine whether it is likely to be successful with additional practice, may require minor modifications such as a different placement of the hands, or is unlikely to be successful. In the latter case, they need to think of another solution to the problem.

Even Transfers With Board and Loops

If an individual does not have adequate strength or range of motion to perform a transfer with just a board, she may be able to achieve independence using a board and loops hanging from an overhead frame. Tables 10–5 and 10–6 include the physical and skill prerequisites for even transfers using a board and loops.

Hanging loops should be used only as a last resort. The loops and frame are bulky, unsightly, and not very portable. Moreover, transfers using overhead loops place one shoulder (on the side holding the loop) in a potentially injurious position[5]: abduction combined with internal rotation.

---

[k] Chapter 9 presents strategies for developing dynamic stability in prone-on-elbows. These strategies can be used to develop the ability to prop on the elbows in this transfer.

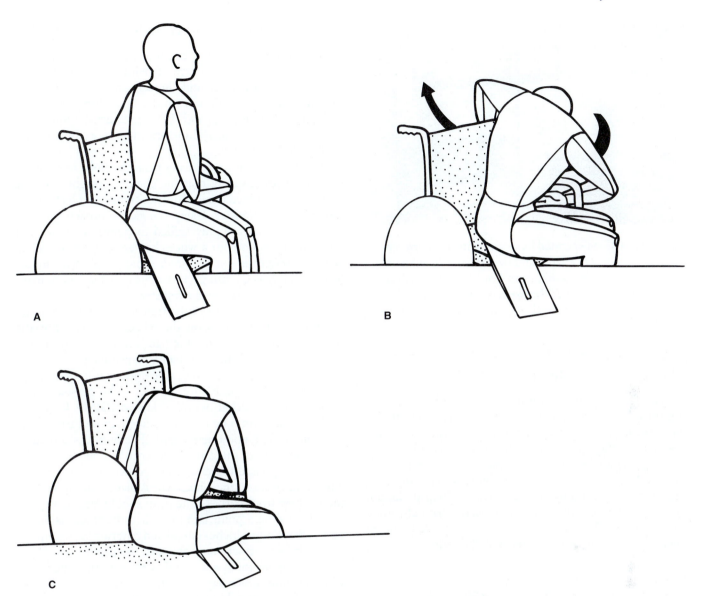

Figure 10–12   Even transfer using sliding board, alternate method. (A) Starting position. (B) Twisting to slide the buttocks out and toward the bed. (C) The transfer is completed with the weight borne on the elbows.

An overhead loop system is shown in Figure 10–13. The exact spacing and length of the different loops will vary between individuals. During transfer training, the therapist and patient should work together to find the optimal configuration of loops for the individual involved.

The following is a description of a wheelchair-to-bed transfer, moving to the left. A transfer in the reverse direction will simply involve reversing the steps.

The person moves her buttocks forward in the chair and places the board. She then positions her hands for the transfer. The left hand should be placed in the nearest loop, palm facing downward. The right hand should be placed on the wheelchair cushion beside the right thigh, well forward on the seat. An alternate position for this arm is over the wheelchair's backrest, with the weight borne above the elbow.

The next step involves positioning the arms and trunk for the transfer. The person leans forward to unweight her buttocks, supporting her weight on both arms. Both elbows should point upward, with the shoulders internally rotated and the elbows flexed (Figure 10–14).

The buttocks are moved toward the bed using the head–hips relationship. While supporting her weight on her hands, the person forcefully throws her head and upper trunk away from the bed. This motion is repeated multiple times. Some are able to perform this transfer using one loop. Others need to reposition their hands to additional loops when they have moved as far as they can from the starting position. An individual repositioning her hands should place her left hand in the next loop and her right hand next to her thigh. She can then resume the twisting motion. The process should continue until the buttocks and thighs are securely on the bed.

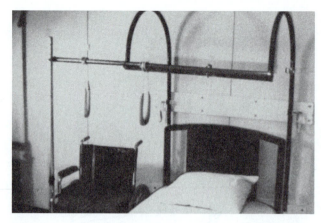

Figure 10–13 Suspended loops for transfers between wheelchair and bed. (Reproduced with permission from Ford J, Duckworth B. *Physical Management for the Quadriplegic Patient*, 2nd ed. Philadelphia: Davis, 1987.)

Even Transfers With Board and Loops—Therapeutic Strategies

To transfer independently using a board and loops, a person must be able to tolerate upright sitting, place and remove the transfer board, and perform the wheelchair skills described earlier in this chapter. She must also be able to place her hands in overhead loops, pull on a loop to lean the trunk forward, and move the buttocks laterally using the head–hips relationship while using a loop to support her trunk. These skills can be practiced separately and in combination. The therapist can assist as needed, and reduce the assistance as the patient's skill develops.

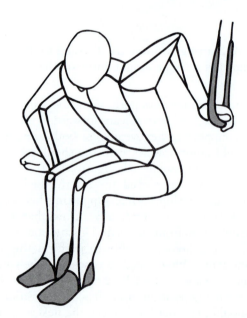

Figure 10–14 Starting position for even transfer from wheelchair to bed using sliding board and overhead loops.

Side-Approach Floor Transfers

This technique for transfers between the floor and a wheelchair has the advantage of being fast. Speed is important when a person finds herself on the street in the middle of an intersection or on the floor during a basketball game. The physical and skill prerequisites required to perform side-approach floor transfers are included in Tables 10–7 and 10–8.

The first step in transferring from the floor to a wheelchair involves ensuring that the chair is upright with the brakes locked. Once the chair is positioned and locked, the individual can transfer. Using the side-approach method, a person utilizes a highly skilled maneuver to move her body from the floor to a wheelchair seat. Because a great deal of strength is not required, some people with motor levels as high as C7 can perform this transfer. Loose hamstrings are necessary for this transfer.

During the actual lift of the transfer, one hand stays on the floor and one stays on the wheelchair seat. For the purpose of this discussion, the hands will be referred to as the floor hand and the chair hand, respectively.

The starting position for a side-approach floor-to-chair transfer is shown in Figure 10–15A. The person sits in front of the wheelchair with her legs at a 30-to 45-degree angle to the chair. The transfer is likely to be easier if her knees are flexed, pointing upward. The buttocks should be slightly in front of the casters, closer to the one behind the person (as opposed to being centered between the casters). The hand closer to the wheelchair is placed on the seat, on the furthest front corner. The palm should face down, and the elbow should point upward. The other hand is placed on the floor, a few inches lateral and anterior to the hip.

To lift her buttocks onto the seat, the person swings her head and upper torso down and away from the wheelchair while pushing downward with her arms. The twist must be forceful and the downward motion of the head must be very pronounced to lift the buttocks high enough. To provide extra lift, the person should protract the scapula of the floor arm at the end of the transfer. She ends in the position shown in Figure 10–15B.

The next task is to assume an upright sitting position. This involves placing the floor hand on the legs and walking it up the legs (Figure 10–15C). Once she has placed her hand on her legs, the person unweights the hand by pushing on the leg and throwing her head back and laterally toward the chair. The other arm can be used to assist in this process, pulling on the armrest or on the push handle of the wheelchair. When the hand on the legs is unweighted, the person quickly moves it and catches her weight on a more proximal handhold. This step is repeated until she achieves an upright sitting position (Figure 10–15D).

The same procedure (with minor changes) is used in reverse when transferring down to the floor. After moving her buttocks to the front of the wheelchair seat, the person positions her legs at a 30-to 45-degree angle to the chair. The hand facing out from the chair becomes the "floor

TABLE 10–7   Uneven Transfers—Physical Prerequisites

	Side-Approach Floor Transfers	Front-Approach Floor Transfers	Back-Approach Floor Transfers	Transfers to and From Low Surfaces	Transfers to and From Higher Surfaces	Bathroom Transfers
Strength						
Anterior deltoids	☑	☑	☑	☑	☑	☑*
Middle deltoids	☑	√	√	√	√	√
Posterior deltoids	√	√	√	√	√	√
Biceps, brachialis, and/or brachioradialis	√					
Infraspinatus and teres minor	√	√	√	√	√	√
Serratus anterior	☑	☑	☑	☑	☑	√
Triceps	√	☑	☑	√	☑	
Pectoralis major		☑	☑		☑	
Latissimus dorsi		☑	☑			
Range of Motion						
Shoulder Extension	☑	√	☑	√	√	
Abduction	☑			√	√	√
Flexion	☑	√		√	√	√
Internal rotation			☑		√	
Elbow Extension	☑	√	√	√	√	☑*
Flexion		√	√	√	√	
Wrist extension	√		√		√	☑*
Combined hip flexion and knee extension	☑					

√ Some strength is needed for this activity or severe limitation in range will inhibit this activity.
☑ A large amount of strength or normal or greater range is needed for this activity.
* In the absence of functioning triceps.

hand." To position this hand, the individual can either walk her hand down her legs or place it directly on the floor while holding onto the wheelchair's push handle, backrest, armrest, or seat with the other hand.

The next step involves moving the buttocks onto the floor. The person slides her buttocks off of the seat by twisting her head and upper torso slightly toward the back of the chair. Once the buttocks have moved from the seat, gravity provides the downward force for the transfer. The person's task at this point is to control the motion so that she lands without trauma to her buttocks. To do so, she slows the downward motion by resisting the upward and chairward twist of her head and upper torso. She should not swing her head and upper trunk up and toward the chair forcefully during the transfer because that would

increase the speed of her descent and result in trauma to her buttocks.

Side-Approach Floor Transfers—Therapeutic Strategies

Before beginning training in side-approach floor-to-wheelchair transfers, a patient should be proficient in even transfers without equipment, and should be skillful in controlling her pelvis using the head–hips relationship. She should also be able to assume the starting position of the transfer.[1] Functional training involves practicing moving

---

[1] The skills needed to assume this position are presented in Chapter 9.

TABLE 10–8   Uneven Transfers—Skill Prerequisites

	Side-Approach Floor Transfers	Front-Approach Floor Transfers	Back-Approach Floor Transfers	Transfers to and From Low Surfaces	Transfers to and From Higher Surfaces	Bathroom Transfers
Tolerate upright sitting position*	✓	✓	✓	✓	✓	✓
Related wheelchair skills (pp. 201–208)	✓	✓	✓	✓	✓	✓
Assume sitting position†	✓	✓	✓			
Assume modified quadruped position (p. 220)		✓				
Assume kneeling position (pp. 220, 222)		✓				
Extend elbows using muscle substitution‡ (p. 199)						✓
Lock elbows‡ (p. 199)						✓
Control pelvis using head and shoulders (p. 200)	✓	✓	✓	✓	✓	✓
Lift buttocks by pivoting on extended arms (p. 211)	✓	✓	✓	✓	✓	✓
Lift buttocks and move laterally (p. 211)	✓			✓	✓	✓
Move buttocks between floor and wheelchair (side approach) (pp. 218–220)	✓					
Lift from floor (front or back approach) (pp. 222, 223)		✓	✓			
Turn body to drop onto wheelchair seat (p. 222)		✓				

✓ This prerequisite skill is required to perform this activity.
* Refer to Chapter 11 for a description of this skill and therapeutic strategies.
† Refer to Chapter 9 for a description of this skill and therapeutic strategies.
‡ In the absence of functioning triceps.

the buttocks between the floor and the wheelchair, and placing the lower extremities in preparation for the transfer.

Move the Buttocks Between Floor and Wheelchair

To lift her buttocks high enough for a floor-to-wheelchair transfer, the person must execute her head and upper torso motions in a forceful and exaggerated manner. As can be seen in Figure 10–15, the head must angle toward the floor for the buttocks to lift high enough. During functional training, the therapist should emphasize the magnitude of the head motion required.

Initially, patients are often reluctant to throw their heads down far enough and with enough force. A therapist can help a patient to get a feel for the maneuver by moving her passively through the motion as she pivots on her arms.

When first working on this skill, it is best to start by transferring between a floor mat and a very low surface such as a short stack of folding mats. The patient should transfer up and down, moving under control in both directions. As her ability improves, she can gradually increase the height of the surface. Transferring between the floor mat and progressively higher stacks of folded mats, she can gradually build up to the full distance from the floor to a wheelchair seat. Mats should be added to increase the height of the transfer only when the individual has mastered the technique at a given height, performing the transfer consistently and with good control.

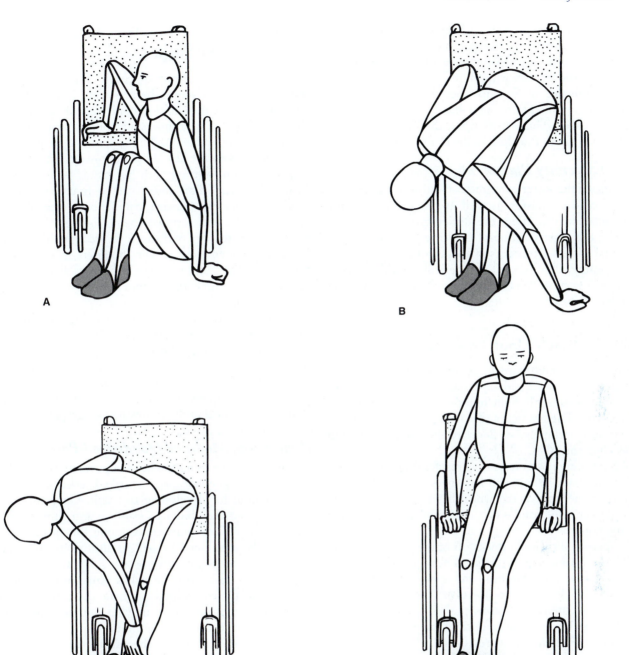

Figure 10–15   Side-approach transfer from the floor to a wheelchair. (A) Starting position. (B) Buttocks onto seat. (C) Walking hand up legs. (D) Sitting upright.

An individual who runs into difficulty with higher transfers may need to throw her head further down to get a better lift. Another possibility is that she needs to protract her scapulae more forcefully as her buttocks approach the level of the higher surface.

The therapist should instruct the patient that when she transfers from a higher to a lower surface, gravity provides the downward force. Instead of forcefully throwing her head up to move her buttocks downward, the patient should resist the downward motion to control her descent.

During functional training, it can be useful to approach the transfer from both directions: in addition to practicing transfers between the floor and higher surfaces, a patient can practice moving between the wheelchair and progressively lower surfaces. During these transfers, her feet should rest on the floor rather than on the piled mats. This position more closely replicates the body's orientation at the end of a floor-to-chair transfer.

Once a patient is consistently able to move between the floor and mats stacked to the height of a wheelchair seat, she is ready for practice with a wheelchair. Because a seat cushion adds height to the transfer, the patient should first practice without it. A cushion can be added when the patient masters the transfer without it.

During practice of floor-to-wheelchair transfers, it is common for a patient to catch her buttocks under the wheelchair's seat. This occurs when the individual transfers from a position too close to the chair.

Lower Extremity Placement

The angle of the lower extremities relative to the chair at the start of the transfer, as well as the position of the knees and feet, can affect the difficulty of the transfer. However, the exact position of the lower extremities that is optimal differs from person to person. During functional training, the therapist and patient should work together to determine the best position for that individual's lower extremities.

Front-Approach Floor Transfers

This transfer technique requires less skill and hamstring flexibility than does a side-approach transfer, but it requires greater strength. Fully innervated upper extremities are necessary. The physical and skill prerequisites required to perform front-approach floor transfers are included in Tables 10–7 and 10–8.

In the starting position for this transfer (Figure 10–16A), the person is side sitting with her knees flexed. The knees are located in front of the wheelchair's casters, centered between them. One hand is on the wheelchair seat, and one is on the floor.

The person lifts her buttocks off of the floor, using the head–hips relationship to do so. Pushing downward on both hands, she twists her head and upper torso down and away from the chair (Figure 10–16B).

In the next step, the person pushes on the chair and raises her trunk to assume an upright kneeling position in front of the wheelchair (Figure 10–16C). While doing so, she must push downward on the chair, as pulling on it will tip it over.

During the next step of the transfer, a forceful downward push on the armrests or (if there are no armrests) seat is used to lift the body (Figure 10–16D). Again, the person must refrain from pulling on the chair. While pushing on the armrests or seat, she tucks her head, protracts her scapulae, and raises her buttocks high above the level of the seat. She then releases one hand and twists, turning and landing on the wheelchair seat.

This transfer is not a particularly good method for returning to the floor. The side approach is faster and easier to perform.[m]

Front-Approach Floor Transfers— Therapeutic Strategies

Before attempting front-approach floor-to-wheelchair transfers, a patient should be proficient in even transfers without equipment, skillful in controlling her pelvis using the head–hips relationship, and able to assume a side-sitting position.[n] She should also be able to push down with her arms to lift her body (depression lift) while in a sitting position, starting with her hands positioned close to her shoulders. This ability can be practiced while sitting in a wheelchair between parallel bars, or while sitting on a floor mat between two chairs (Figure 10–17). If the patient is unable to perform a depression lift with her hands positioned close to her shoulders in this exercise, the parallel bars can be lowered or (if practicing on a mat between two chairs) the patient can sit on a cushion to make the task easier.

Functional training involves practicing the following: moving into modified quadruped with one hand on a wheelchair, assuming a kneeling position, pushing on the wheelchair to lift the body, and turning the body to drop onto the wheelchair seat. These prerequisite skills can be practiced in sequence. Strategies for developing these skills are described in the following paragraphs.

Assume the Modified Quadruped Position

Previous practice using the head–hips relationship to control the pelvis in quadruped, described earlier in this chapter, is helpful for developing this skill. Once the patient has developed the ability to stabilize and shift weight in quadruped, she can practice assuming this position. This skill can be developed by weight shifting in quadruped, moving the pelvis laterally toward side sitting, and then shifting back to return the pelvis into position over the knees. The patient should perform these motions over small arcs of motion at first, moving laterally only as far as she can retain control of the motion and return to midline. As her skill develops, she can increase the distance over which she shifts her weight, gradually building to the point at which she can move into side sitting under control and return to quadruped. Once the patient has learned to move from side sitting to quadruped, she can practice this skill with one hand on the wheelchair (Figure 10–16A and 10–16B).

Assume a Kneeling Position

Starting in modified quadruped (Figure 10–16B), the patient supports her weight on the wheelchair while she walks the hand on the floor toward the chair, and then lifts it onto the chair. Once both hands are on the wheelchair seat, she pushes downward to lift her trunk into an upright

---

[m] In contrast to a side-approach transfer from the floor to a wheelchair, a high level of skill is not required when using a side approach to transfer down from a wheelchair.

[n] The skills needed to assume the side sitting position are presented in Chapter 9.

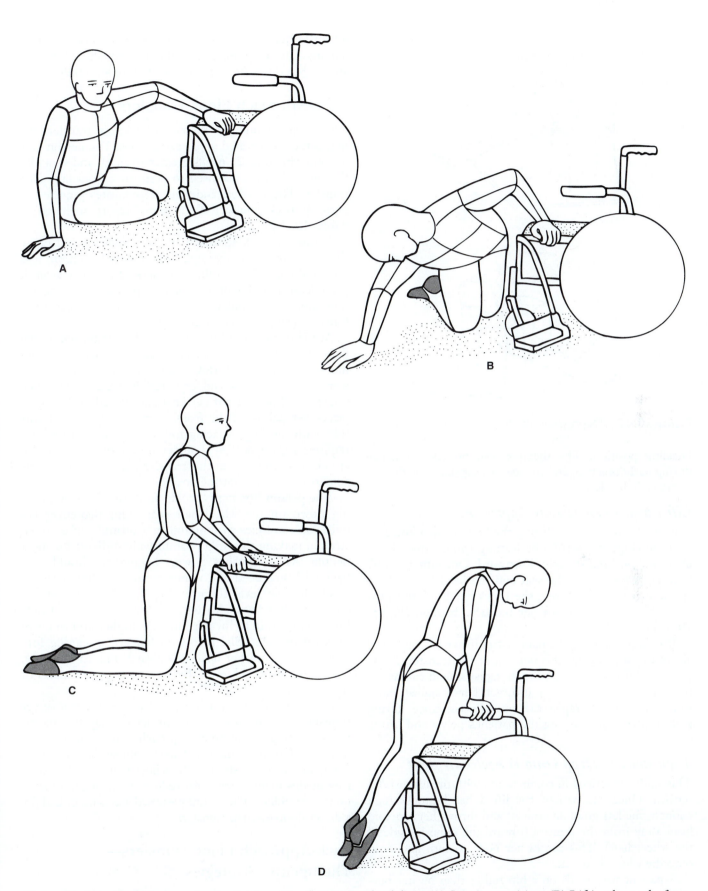

Figure 10–16   Front-approach transfer from the floor to a wheelchair. (A) Starting position. (B) Lifting buttocks from floor. (C) Kneeling in front of wheelchair. (D) Lifting buttocks by pushing down on armrests.

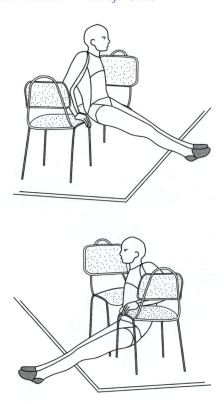

Figure 10–17   Depression lifts between chairs.

kneeling position. The therapist can provide assistance during early practice, and reduce this assistance as the patient's skill develops.

Lift From Floor (Front Approach)

This maneuver involves lifting the body from a kneeling position (Figure 10–16C) by leaning toward the wheelchair and pushing straight downward. Once the person's buttocks have passed the seat and she has lifted as high as she can in this manner, she tucks her head and protracts her scapulae to lift her buttocks further. (Figure 10–16D)

It is important for the patient to lift her buttocks well above the seat during this portion of the transfer. If she does not lift high enough, the therapist should cue her to tuck her head lower and protract her scapulae more forcefully. The therapist can provide assistance during early practice by grasping the patient's pelvis and lifting upward.

Turn Body to Drop Onto Wheelchair Seat

This skill is practiced in combination with the lift just described. Once the patient has lifted her buttocks high enough, she lets go of an armrest and throws her arm and head away from the armrest (toward the opposite side of the wheelchair). This causes her body to turn and drop onto the wheelchair seat.

A patient who lands on a hip rather than on her buttocks may not have lifted high enough. Prior to releasing the armrest, she should lift her buttocks higher by tucking her head lower and protracting her scapulae more. The problem may also occur when the height of the lift is

adequate but the patient does not turn far enough before landing. In these instances, the patient should be instructed to throw her arm and head more forcefully.

Back-Approach Floor Transfers

The third method for floor-to-wheelchair transfers requires fully innervated upper extremities. The person performing this transfer needs greater strength and shoulder flexibility than are required to perform a front-approach transfer. The physical and skill prerequisites required to perform back-approach floor transfers are included in Tables 10–7 and 10–8.

Because a back-approach transfer involves end-range shoulder extension combined with internal rotation, it is potentially injurious to the shoulders.[5] For this reason, it is the least desirable of the transfer approaches and therefore should be avoided if the patient can perform floor transfers using a different method.

At the beginning of this transfer, the person sits on the floor in front of the wheelchair, facing directly away from the chair (Figure 10–18A). Her buttocks should be in front of the casters and centered between them. The transfer will be easier if her knees are flexed. The person places her palms on the front corners of the wheelchair seat, with the fingers facing forward. This hand position requires a great deal of shoulder flexibility. Many people are not able to perform this transfer because they are unable to assume the starting position.

The person lifts her buttocks from the floor by pushing down on the wheelchair seat. This maneuver requires the muscles to function in a position of extreme stretch, making this step prohibitively difficult for most people. As she pushes down, the person should lean back with her head and upper torso until her buttocks reach the seat level (Figure 10–18B). Once the wheelchair seat has been cleared, the person uses the head-hips relationship to lift her buttocks higher and to move back on the seat. She pivots on her arms, leaning forward and curling her head downward (Figure 10–18C). Additional lift is achieved through strong protraction of the scapulae.

People who cannot achieve independence in a direct transfer from the floor to a wheelchair may be able to transfer using an indirect approach: they transfer first from the floor to an intermediate-height surface, such as a stool, and from the stool to the wheelchair seat. Transferring in this manner may also reduce the damaging forces on the shoulders. The techniques used are as described for a direct floor-to-chair transfer.

Back-Approach Floor Transfers—
Therapeutic Strategies

Before undertaking training in back-approach floor transfers, the therapist and patient should weigh the potential benefits of independent floor transfers against the risk of shoulder injury. If back-approach transfers remain

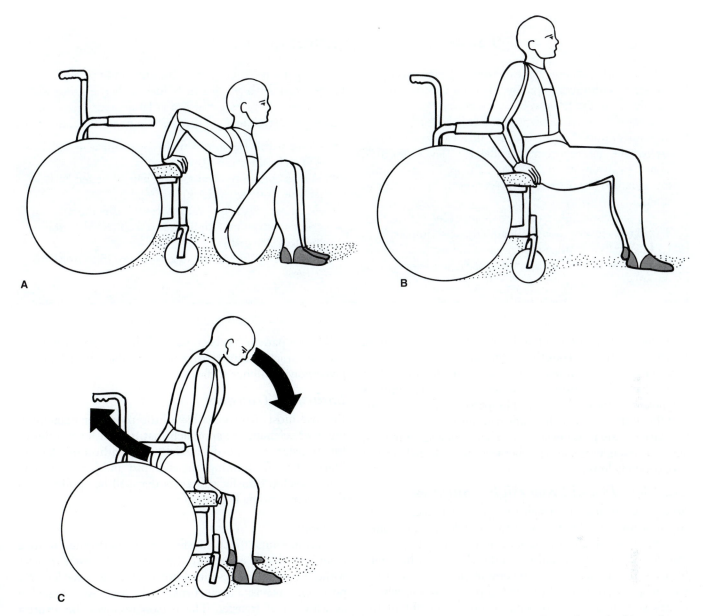

Figure 10–18   Back-approach transfer from the floor to a wheelchair. (A) Starting position. (B) Lifting the buttocks from the floor. (C) Moving the buttocks back on the seat.

a goal, the patient should first become proficient in even transfers without equipment. She should also be able to push down with her arms to lift her body while in a sitting position, starting with her hands positioned close to her shoulders.[o]

Functional training involves practicing the following: assuming the starting position, pushing on the wheelchair to lift the body, and using the head–hips relationship to move the buttocks back on the wheelchair seat.[p] These prerequisite skills can be practiced in sequence.

Lift From Floor (Back Approach)

In this maneuver, the patient sitting in front of a wheelchair lifts her body by leaning back and pushing straight downward. This task requires strength and flexibility rather than a high level of skill. Similar to the side-approach transfer, it can be practiced between the floor and progressively higher stacks of folding mats, or between a pile of floor mats and the wheelchair. As the patient's skill develops, she can practice transferring over progressively larger distances. The therapist can provide guarding and assistance as needed.

Additional Transfers

Transfers To and From Lower Surfaces

To transfer between a wheelchair and a lower surface such as a couch, a person with a complete spinal cord injury uses a method similar to that used for even transfers. The

---

[o] Strategies for developing this capacity are presented in the section on front-approach transfers.
[p] Skills for assuming the starting position (coming to sitting, gross mobility in sitting and leg management) are addressed in Chapter 9, and positioning the buttocks is presented earlier in this chapter.

Problem-Solving Exercise 10–3

Your patient is independent in even and slightly uneven transfers without equipment. He wants to learn to transfer from the floor to his wheelchair.

This individual has 5/5 strength in all of his upper extremity musculature. His hip flexors test 2/5 bilaterally, and all myotomes below this level test 0/5. When he attempts to perform a sit-up, his abdominal musculature has palpable contractions from the ribs to the pubis.

Pin prick and light touch are intact in the C2 through T12 key sensory points bilaterally and impaired in L1 bilaterally. Both sensory modalities are absent below L1 with the exception that sensation is present at the anus.

The patient's joint range of motion and muscle flexibility are normal in all extremities with the following exceptions: shoulder extension is 10 degrees bilaterally and passive straight-leg raise is 70 degrees bilaterally.

- Classify this person's spinal cord injury using the ASIA classification system.
- Which method of floor-to-chair transfer is this patient likely to achieve most readily?
- What strength and range should the therapeutic exercise program emphasize to facilitate the attainment of this goal?
- Describe a functional training program for this patient.

---

difference is that the head and upper torso motions used to lift the buttocks from the lower surface must be more forceful and exaggerated to get an adequate lift. When transferring down from the wheelchair, gravity supplies the power to move the body. The person's task is to control the motion so that she lands without injury.

Once a patient has become proficient in even transfers, she can practice transferring between the wheelchair and progressively lower surfaces.

Transfers To and From Higher Surfaces

To transfer from a wheelchair to a higher surface, the person first locks her brakes with the wheelchair positioned as close as possible to the surface onto which she plans to transfer. If moving toward the right, she places her right hand on the higher surface, several inches in front of the wheelchair seat. The other hand is placed on the wheelchair's seat or armrest, depending on the height of the surface. Placing the hand on the armrest makes a higher transfer possible but increases the risk of the chair sliding to the side during the transfer. Figure 10–19A shows the starting position for the transfer.

While pushing straight down and pivoting on both arms, the person tucks her head and upper torso downward and swings them away from the higher surface. To achieve an adequate lift, the downward motion of the head must be pronounced. To move her buttocks further onto the surface and to gain a more stable position, the person protracts her scapulae strongly.

Once the individual is sitting securely on the higher surface, she leans her torso to a position over this surface. She can then move her hand from the wheelchair to the higher surface and push herself upright.

The maneuvers just described are performed in reverse when transferring from a higher surface to a wheelchair. While the buttocks descend toward the wheelchair, the patient should work to control the motion.

Once a patient has become proficient in even transfers, she can practice transferring between the wheelchair and progressively higher surfaces.

Bathroom Transfers

Because most bathrooms have little room for maneuvering a wheelchair, the approach that is used for a toilet or tub transfer may be dictated by the bathroom's layout. During transfer training, the therapist and patient should work develop transfer strategies that will be applicable in the patient's home bathroom.

Toilet

If space permits, toilet transfers can be performed using a technique that is essentially the same as the even transfer without equipment described previously. The wheelchair is positioned against a front corner of the toilet seat, angled in as with a mat transfer. The person removes the armrest closest to the toilet, positions her legs, moves the footplates out of the way, and gets into position for the transfer. One hand is placed on the far side of the toilet seat and the other is placed on the wheelchair seat next to the thigh. The person then pivots forward on her arms, twisting her head and upper torso down and away from the toilet. The transfer is likely to be slightly uneven, so a higher lift will be required. This can be accomplished by throwing the head and upper torso into a lower position when pivoting the arms. To return to the chair, the same steps are performed in reverse.

In an alternate method, the person straddles the toilet. To use this technique, she approaches the toilet from the front, facing it directly. The footrests are swung out of the way, and the feet are placed on either side of the toilet. The chair is moved into position against the front of the toilet. After the person moves her buttocks forward in the chair, she leans forward and props on her arms (elbows extended) with one hand on either side of the toilet seat. She then pushes down hard with her arms and depresses her

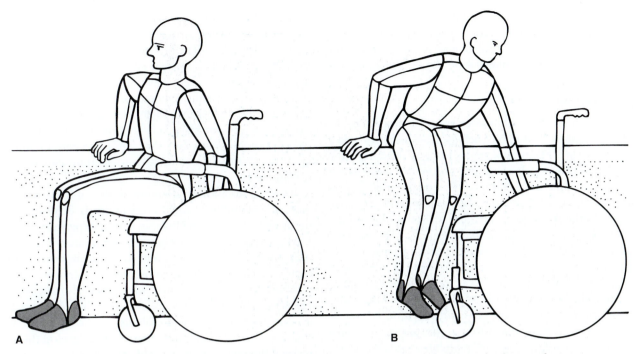

Figure 10–19   Transfer to higher surface. (A) Starting position. (B) Buttocks lifted onto higher surface.

shoulder girdle while leaning forward. This maneuver lifts her buttocks onto the toilet seat. To return to the chair, the person first places her hands on the wheelchair seat, one on each side. She then moves her buttocks back by pushing down with her arms and depressing her scapulae.

Bathtub

Because transfers in and out of bathtubs are potentially injurious to the shoulders, people with spinal cord injuries should utilize tub benches or shower commode chairs and roll-in showers (Figure 10–20).[5]

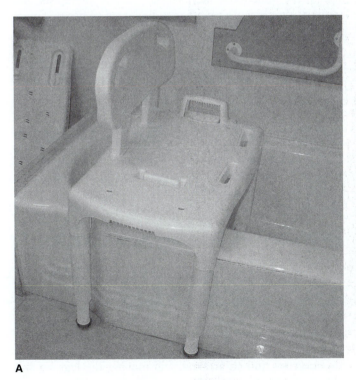

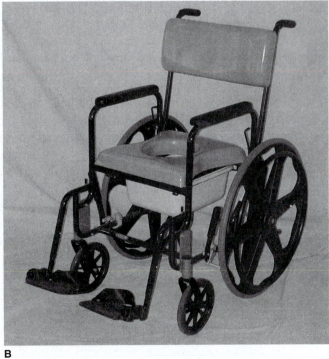

Figure 10–20   Equipment allowing bathing with reduced stress on upper extremities. (A) Tub bench. (B) Shower commode chair. (Reproduced with permission from Activaid.)

Transfers to and from tub benches are performed using techniques similar to those used for even transfers. During functional training, the therapist and patient should try different bench designs to determine which is most appropriate for that individual.

Vehicle Transfers

The skills used for even and uneven transfers described earlier can be applied to transfers between a wheelchair and a car, truck, or van. The person angles her wheelchair as close as possible to the vehicle's seat and moves the armrest and footplates out of the way. With one hand on the vehicle's seat and one on the wheelchair seat, she pivots on her arms and transfers. As the therapist and patient work together on the transfer, they can experiment with different hand positions.

After transferring into a car, the person places her feet in the foot wells and loads the wheelchair. She can load it either behind or next to herself.[q] If the chair has a folding frame, it is likely to be easiest to load the wheelchair behind the front seat (this will be possible with a two-door car). After transferring into the car, the person can turn the chair so that it faces the car (footplates toward the car) and fold the chair. She then lifts the casters through the door and finally pulls the chair into the car. If the chair has a rigid frame, she removes the wheels, folds the backrest, and places the chair and wheels in the car by lifting them across her body.

TRANSFERS FOLLOWING INCOMPLETE SPINAL CORD INJURY: FUNCTIONAL TECHNIQUES AND THERAPEUTIC STRATEGIES

The actions that an individual can use to perform transfers after sustaining an incomplete spinal cord injury will depend primarily on her voluntary motor function. A person who retains or regains only sensory function below her injury (ASIA B) will utilize the techniques that are used by people with complete spinal cord injuries, as just described. A person who has minimal motor sparing or return (ASIA C) is likely to utilize similar movement patterns, but may be able to add trunk or lower extremity actions to make the tasks easier. An individual who has significant motor function below her lesion (ASIA D) may be able to perform transfers using more normal movement patterns.

Another factor that can have an impact on the performance of transfers is muscle tone. People with incomplete lesions tend to exhibit more spasticity than do people with complete lesions, and spasticity tends to be more severe among those with ASIA B and C lesions.[15–17] When elevated muscle tone interferes with function, the rehabilitation team can work with the patient to reduce the abnormal tone.[r] In addition, the therapist and patient should note the conditions and bodily motions that tend to elicit involuntary muscle contractions. They can then work together to find ways in which the patient can transfer without causing these involuntary contractions. For example, the patient may find that she is less likely to experience involuntary contractions if she moves slowly during transfers. On the other hand, the patient and therapist may find that elevated muscle tone can help with certain tasks.

Perhaps the most challenging aspect of transfer training after an incomplete spinal cord injury is determining the methods that the individual can utilize to perform the skills. Each patient has a unique pattern of muscle strength, weakness, tone, and flexibility; joint range of motion; and body build. It is often difficult to predict what transfer methods will best suit the individual; some physical maneuvers will be within her potential and others will not. Functional training involves problem solving as the therapist works with the patient to help her discover and develop the movement strategies that will enable her to achieve her functional goals.

When deciding between transfer techniques, therapists should keep in mind the fact that incomplete spinal cord injuries are associated with a greater potential for motor return than are complete injuries.[18,19] When motor function is preserved below the lesion, use of transfer techniques that utilize this function may help develop more normal movement patterns and enhance the individual's potential for future functional ambulation.[20] Thus therapists and patients should work together to find ways to use this musculature functionally. With each task practiced, a patient should be encouraged to use her trunk and lower extremity musculature to the extent possible. When muscles below the lesion are strong enough that a patient has the potential to learn to perform a task without compensatory strategies, the patient and therapist should work together to develop this ability. When muscles are innervated but too weak to perform a task, their use can be combined with compensatory strategies during functional activities. For example, an individual who has $2+/5$ or weaker strength in her hip flexors will be unable to lift her leg onto a mat or bed using just these muscles. She can, however, utilize this musculature to enhance her performance of the task, flexing her hip actively while lifting the leg with her arm.

Basic Skills and Related Wheelchair Skills

These skills include the various activities performed immediately before or after a person moves to or from a wheelchair: stabilizing and moving the body in a wheelchair, moving the feet on and off of the footrests, repositioning the footrests and an armrest, and moving the legs on and

---

[q] If loading chair with a folding frame in the front, the driver must perform the initial transfer into the passenger side of the car and slide across the seat (bench-style seat) to the driver's side.

[r] Strategies for treating spasticity are presented in Chapter 3.

off of the mat or bed. A person who has only sensory function below her lesion will use compensatory strategies, described earlier in the chapter, to perform these activities. A person who has sparing of voluntary motor function below her lesion will be able to use functioning trunk and lower extremity musculature to perform these skills more easily, with more normal movement patterns, or both.

Therapeutic Strategies

The therapeutic strategies used to develop these skills after incomplete injuries are similar to those used for patients with complete injuries. The patient practices moving her body and manipulating the wheelchair's components, using motions that make maximal use of innervated musculature. The therapist can provide assistance as needed, and engage the patient in problem solving to discover movement strategies that are most effective and efficient.

Even Transfers

People with complete injuries transfer by propping on their arms and using the head–hips relationship to move between surfaces. The transfer techniques that people with incomplete injuries can use depend largely on the motor function present below their lesions. An individual who has minimal sparing in her trunk and lower extremity musculature can utilize techniques similar to those used by people with complete injuries. She is likely to find transfers easier to master, however, because she can use functioning trunk and leg musculature to help lift her weight and maintain her balance.

A person who retains or regains significant innervation of her trunk and lower extremity musculature may be able to transfer using either a stand–pivot or a squat–pivot technique. In these transfer methods, most or all of the weight is supported on the legs.

A stand–pivot transfer involves coming to stand, turning, and sitting on the mat or bed. The arms may or may not be used to assist with these maneuvers. In the sit-to-stand component of the transfer, the individual moves her buttocks forward in the chair, leans her trunk forward, and stands. She can perform each of these actions as a discrete step under control or can combine the forward lean and stand, utilizing momentum to make the task easier.[21] During the stand-to-sit component of the transfer, the individual should control her descent through eccentric contraction of her hip and knee extensors.

In a squat–pivot transfer, the person does not come to a full standing position. Instead, she remains in a "squat" position, leaning her trunk forward and lifting her buttocks enough to clear the wheel. During a squat–pivot transfer, the person can utilize both the head–hips relationship and momentum to enhance her performance as she moves between surfaces. With one hand on the wheelchair and one on the mat or bed, she can use her arms to help maintain her balance while she lifts and turns her buttocks toward the mat or bed.

Therapeutic Strategies

The patient should practice even transfers using techniques that enable her to utilize her innervated musculature and move between surfaces as safely and independently as possible. With the therapist's assistance and guidance, the patient can try various strategies to discover ways in which she can move her body most efficiently between surfaces.

Regardless of the transfer strategy used, the patient may benefit from practicing the different components of the task. If performing a stand–pivot transfer, she can practice coming to stand and returning to sit under control. If she has inadequate strength or control to perform these actions from a wheelchair, she may benefit from practice of sit-to-stand and stand-to-sit from an elevated mat. Practice of these skills will be easiest if the mat is elevated enough that the patient is close to a standing position when her feet are on the floor and her buttocks are on the mat. As her strength and control improve, she can practice with the mat in progressively lower positions until she can stand up and return to sitting under control from a surface the height of her wheelchair seat.

A patient learning a squat–pivot transfer may benefit from practice lifting her buttocks and moving laterally while short sitting on a mat. If she has difficulty with this maneuver, she may benefit from practice lifting her buttocks while sitting on a mat that is elevated slightly. As her strength and control improve, she can practice with the mat in progressively lower positions until she can lift her buttocks and move laterally on a surface the height of her wheelchair seat.

Floor Transfers

Three methods of floor-to-wheelchair transfers are presented earlier in this chapter: side, front, and back approach. Of these transfers, the back approach is most easily adapted to utilize lower extremity musculature. In this transfer, the individual sits facing away from her chair, places her palms on the front of the seat, and pushes down to lift her buttocks. An individual who has some capacity to extend her hips and knees actively can do so while pushing with her arms to lift her buttocks onto the seat.

An alternate floor-to-wheelchair transfer technique utilizes the lower extremities to a greater extent. To perform this transfer, the individual assumes a half-kneeling position in front of the wheelchair, facing sideways to the chair (Figure 10–21). If lower extremity strength is asymmetrical, the stronger limb should be in the forward position (foot planted), as the forward limb will perform most of the work of the transfer. Once she is in a half-kneel position, the person can either place both hands on the wheelchair seat, or place one hand on the seat and one on her knee. Pushing down with her arms and legs, she lifts and turns her buttocks onto the seat. She may find this maneuver to be easier

Problem-Solving Exercise 10–4

Two patients have come to outpatient therapy with the goal of independent even transfers between a wheelchair and a bed. Each has been approved (by their insurance companies) for a limited number of outpatient visits.

Both patients

- Were discharged from inpatient rehabilitation several months ago and have experienced motor return since discharge.
- Are dependent in transfers.
- Can maintain a short-sitting position on a mat without upper extremity support for 2 minutes with supervision.

Their motor and sensory function are as follows:

Patient 1 has 5/5 strength in her biceps bilaterally. Her radial wrist extensors test 2/5 on the right and 1/5 on the left. Her triceps test 1/5 on the right and 0/5 on the left. All other key muscles in the upper extremities test 0/5. All key muscles in both of her lower extremities test 4/5 to 5/5. Voluntary abdominal contraction is palpable from ribs to pubis. Pin prick and light touch are intact (bilaterally) in the C2 through C5 key sensory points, impaired in C6, absent in C7 through T3, and impaired in T4 and below.

Patient 2 has 5/5 strength in his right biceps and 4/5 to 5/5 strength in all other key muscles of his right upper and lower extremities. His left biceps exhibits 5/5 strength. All other key muscles in the left extremities test 3/5. Pin prick and light touch are intact in C5 and higher key sensory points bilaterally. Below C5, pin prick is impaired or absent in all key points on the right, and intact on the left. Light touch is intact on the right, but impaired on the left.

For each of these patients,

- Describe an even transfer technique that would be appropriate for this patient's voluntary motor function.
- Describe a functional training program.

---

if she rocks her head and trunk forward and laterally away from the wheelchair during this lift.

Therapeutic Strategies

The back-approach transfer can be practiced using the strategies presented earlier in the chapter: the patient can practice transferring between the floor and progressively higher stacks of folding mats until she can transfer to and from a surface the height of a wheelchair seat. During this practice, the patient should be encouraged to use her leg musculature as much as possible. She and the therapist can experiment with different placements of her feet (at various distances from the buttocks) to determine the foot position that makes the transfer easiest. They can also try different strategies such as leaning the trunk toward or away from the chair during the lift, or starting the transfer with the elbows (instead of the hands) on the wheelchair seat. Because the legs can be used to support the body's weight, the arms can be repositioned during the transfer.

A patient who plans to learn the half-kneeling transfer approach may benefit from preparatory practice in quadruped, kneeling, and half-kneeling. She can practice assuming each of these positions, as well as stabilizing against resistance applied by the therapist, shifting weight under control, and moving between positions.[22,23] In this manner, she can develop her ability to control her body and move between the various postures involved in the transfer.

The patient can also practice lifting her buttocks from the half-kneel position. This task can be practiced with the patient half-kneeling in front of a stack of folding mats. Initial practice may begin with a stack of mats that is lower than the height of a wheelchair seat. As the patient's ability develops, she can practice lifting her buttocks onto progressively higher stacks. Once she has developed the ability to transfer onto a stack of mats the height of her wheelchair seat, she can practice transferring onto the chair itself.

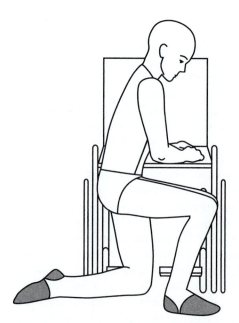

Figure 10–21   Half-kneeling position for floor-to-wheelchair transfer using lower extremities.

Physical Prerequisites

The therapeutic program should include strengthening of the muscles involved in transfers, with emphasis on scapular protraction and depression, elbow extension, and hip and knee extension. Exercise of these muscles in closed-chain positions may be most beneficial because these positions simulate the conditions in which the muscles function during transfers. Innervated muscles in the trunk should also be strengthened[s] to enhance the patient's ability to control her trunk during transfers. Strengthening exercises for limb and trunk musculature should address both concentric and eccentric contractions, since transfers involve both types of contraction.

In addition to strengthening, the exercise program should address range of motion. Range of motion should be preserved or increased as needed for the transfers that the patient is working to achieve.

---

[s] Chapter 9 presents strategies for strengthening trunk musculature.

Summary

- Transfers involve moving the body from one surface to another. The ability to transfer in and out of a wheelchair is a crucial functional skill for anyone who uses a wheelchair for mobility.

- A person with a complete spinal cord injury who wishes to function independently must learn compensatory strategies for performing transfers. This chapter presents a variety of techniques that can be used to perform even and uneven transfers to and from a wheelchair.

- The movement strategies possible for a person with an incomplete spinal cord injury will depend on the extent of motor sparing or return below her lesion. If she has little or no voluntary motor function below her lesion, she will use movement strategies similar to those used by people with complete injuries. If she has more significant motor function in her trunk and lower extremities, she may be able to use more normal movement strategies to perform transfers.

- During rehabilitation, the therapist and patient work together to discover the movement strategies that will enable the patient to perform transfers most effectively. The therapeutic program then consists of activities directed at developing the strength, range of motion, and skill needed to perform these functional tasks. This chapter presents a variety of strategies for developing the skills involved.

- The therapist and patient should take appropriate precautions during transfer training to prevent motion of unstable vertebrae, skin abrasions and pressure ulcers, overstretching of the long finger flexors and the low back, injury from falls, and overuse injuries of the upper extremities.

11

Wheelchairs and Wheelchair Skills

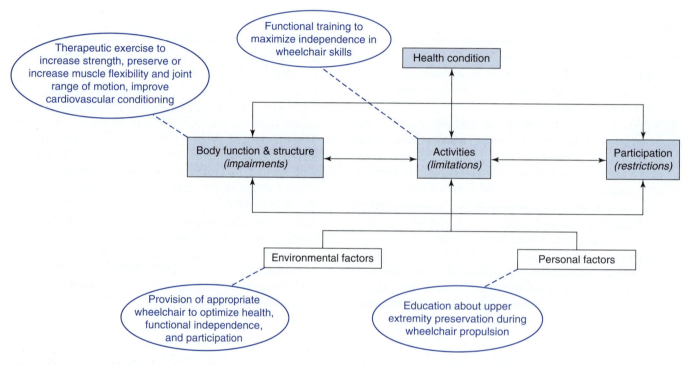

Chapter 11 presents information on wheelchairs, wheelchair skills, and therapeutic strategies for increasing independence in wheelchair skills.

Most people with spinal cord injuries use wheelchairs as their sole means of locomotion. This is true even for those who learn to walk with knee-ankle-foot orthoses (KAFOs) and assistive devices during their rehabilitation.[1] If ambulation is impaired, a wheelchair provides a faster and more energy-efficient means of mobility than does walking. Even people who have such low lesions that they retain active hip flexion and knee extension, and are able to walk with ankle-foot orthoses (AFOs) and assistive devices, find wheelchair mobility to be faster and to require less energy than walking.[2,3]

When ambulation is impaired, an appropriate wheelchair and cushion are essential for preservation of the individual's health and optimization of his functional independence and participation in life situations. After spinal cord injury, the rehabilitation team works with the patient to select a wheelchair and cushion[a] that will best meet his needs. They also work together to develop the patient's ability to function optimally with this equipment. These tasks are inextricably linked; the individual's capabilities influence the selection and adjustment of his wheelchair, and the wheelchair's characteristics, in turn, influence the skills that its user will need to develop.

---

[a] Wheelchair cushions and their selection are addressed in Chapter 5.

This chapter presents information on wheelchair selection and adjustment, wheelchair skills, and training strategies. The descriptions of equipment, techniques, and training presented here should be used as a guide, not as a set of hard and fast rules. The equipment required and motions used to perform any functional task vary among people because of differences in body build, skill level, range of motion, muscle tone, patterns of strength and weakness, and presence or absence of additional impairments. During rehabilitation, the therapist and patient work together to determine the equipment and functional techniques that best suit that particular individual.

PRECAUTIONS

Following spinal cord injury, activities performed in a wheelchair can cause a variety of problems if appropriate precautions are not taken. Table 11–1 presents a summary of precautions for wheelchair use and skill training. These precautions should be taken whenever the individual sits in a wheelchair, starting as soon as out-of-bed activities are initiated. Postdischarge follow-up should include regular maintenance and checks of the wheelchair and cushion, including fit, alignment, and condition, as well as the user's posture, comfort, propulsion techniques, and functional status.[4,5]

TABLE 11–1 Precautions During Wheelchair Use and Skill Training

Potential Problems	Wheelchair Activities That Place Patients at Risk	Precautions
Excessive motion at site of vertebral instability, potentially causing additional neurologic and orthopedic damage	Any activity involving excessive motion or muscular action at or near site of unstable spine. Examples: Upright activities while the spine remains unstable, practice falling backward from wheelie position when spine is not fully healed.	• Strictly adhere to orthopedic precautions. • Check fit of vertebral orthosis with patient sitting in wheelchair. • When the spine is unstable, avoid activities that may cause motion or strong muscular contraction at site of instability.
Skin abrasions and pressure ulcers	Sitting in wheelchair more than 15 to 20 minutes.	• Provide patient with pressure-relieving wheelchair cushion and an appropriately fit and adjusted wheelchair. • Pressure reliefs every 15 to 20 minutes when first sitting, with possible increase in time between reliefs if skin tolerance allows. • Proper sitting posture whenever patient is in wheelchair. • Monitor skin status and adjust sitting time, pressure reliefs, and equipment as indicated.
	Stair negotiation on buttocks.	• Protective padding over buttocks and sacral region during this activity.
Overstretched low back, resulting in diminished capacity for functional independence	Prolonged sitting in wheelchair with lumbar spine in kyphotic posture.	• Proper sitting posture whenever patient is in wheelchair. • Adequate postural support provided by wheelchair and cushion.
Postural deformity	Chronic positioning in wheelchair with improper posture.	• Proper sitting posture whenever patient is in wheelchair. • Adequate postural support provided by wheelchair and cushion. • Access devices (interfaces) of power wheelchairs positioned so that the user can operate them while maintaining good sitting posture.

(Continued)

TABLE 11–1   (*Continued*)

Potential Problems	Wheelchair Activities That Place Patients at Risk	Precautions
Overuse injuries of the upper extremities	Chronic use of manual wheelchair.	• Proper sitting posture whenever the user is propelling the wheelchair. • Lightest possible wheelchair, properly fit and adjusted. • Training in efficient propulsion pattern. • Exercise program to develop strength, endurance, and flexibility in shoulders. • Education regarding all of the above plus avoiding weight gain.[5]
Injury from tip or fall from wheelchair	Reaching outside of base of support; negotiation of environmental obstacles such as inclines, curbs, curb cuts, doorways, or uneven terrain; sports.[6-8]	• Properly fit and adjusted wheelchair, with seat belt and antitipping devices when indicated. • Education and training in safe use of wheelchair and safe falling techniques. • Appropriate guarding during functional training.

Sitting Posture

Because people with spinal cord injuries typically spend a good deal of time sitting in wheelchairs, their posture while using wheelchairs is important. Proper sitting posture (Figure 11–1A and B) will greatly enhance functional status and physical health.

An individual with a spinal cord injury should sit with his buttocks well back on the seat whenever he is in a wheelchair. Habitually sitting with the buttocks forward on the wheelchair seat is likely to stretch the lumbar area (Figure 11–1C). The resulting excessive flexibility in the low back will interfere with the ability to perform functional activities such as independent transfers or rolling in bed.

In addition to stretching the low back, poor sitting posture can lead to the development of pressure ulcers. Pelvic

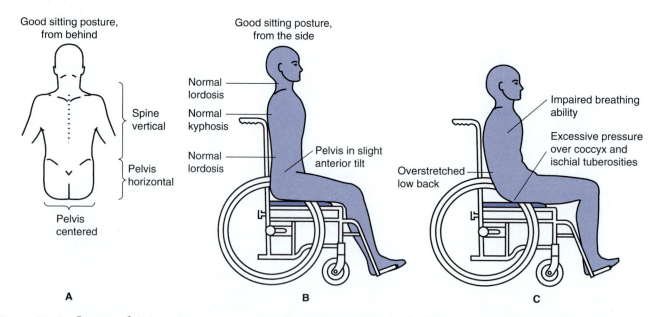

Figure 11–1   Impact of sitting posture on pressure distribution, low-back flexibility, and breathing ability. (A) Good sitting posture, posterior view. (B) Good sitting posture: pressure distributed well, low back protected by proper positioning, and torso positioned to optimize breathing ability. (C) Poor sitting posture: low back overstretched, excessive pressure borne over coccyx and ischial tuberosities, and breathing ability impaired.

obliquity, lateral trunk lean, and posterior pelvic tilt alter the distribution of pressure on the skin,[9,10] resulting in increased risk of skin breakdown over the areas of elevated pressure. Improper positioning can also result in scoliosis, thoracic kyphosis, and forward head. These postural abnormalities can, in turn, lead to reduced functional capacity, upper extremity pain and injury, and impaired respiratory function.

To avoid the development of posture-related problems, the patient should receive instruction on the risks of sitting with his spine and extremities improperly aligned, and should develop the skills needed to maintain appropriate posture. He must also utilize a wheelchair and cushion that provide adequate postural support. The wheelchair and cushion should be configured so that they enable the patient to propel his wheelchair while maintaining proper postural alignment. For example, a power wheelchair with a hand-operated joystick control should be aligned so that the patient can access the joystick without leaning his trunk laterally.

Strategies for Preventing Overuse Injuries

Repetitive stress from manual wheelchair propulsion is a significant contributor to overuse injuries of the upper extremities.[11–21] Because the upper limbs are used to perform virtually all activities when the legs are paralyzed, upper extremity pain is associated with a reduction in functional independence[5,20,22–25] and can interfere with community integration.[26]

Although the link between manual wheelchair use and upper extremity pain has been well established, the solutions to this problem are not as clear. Exercise programs[b] to develop endurance, balanced strength, and normal flexibility in the shoulder girdle musculature may help wheelchair users avoid the development of shoulder pain.[16,18,19] Appropriate sitting posture is also critical for upper extremity preservation. When a person propels a wheelchair while sitting in a position of thoracic kyphosis and forward shoulders, the shoulder joints are subjected to damaging stresses; habitual propulsion in this posture is a likely contributor to shoulder pain.[13] Thus, a properly fitted and adjusted wheelchair may help prevent the development of chronic shoulder pain by providing good postural support. Moreover, training in efficient propulsion techniques, and a wheelchair that is as light as possible and has components and alignment that allow for propulsion with reduced stress on the upper extremities, are likely to be beneficial.[5,12,14,16,21] Finally, follow-up care for people with spinal cord injuries should include monitoring for the development of upper extremity overuse injuries, and appropriate interventions when such injuries occur.[5]

---

[b] Table 8–4 in Chapter 8 includes information on exercises designed to help prevent shoulder overuse injuries.

WHEELCHAIRS

Wheelchair selection involves deciding between numerous options in size, style, and components. Because of the wheelchair's tremendous impact on function and health, its size and features must be chosen carefully. The ideal wheelchair would provide its user with optimal postural support and safety while allowing independent mobility in all environments, with minimal stress to the upper extremities. It would also be affordable, durable, and stylish. Unfortunately, such an ideal wheelchair does not exist, as many of the qualities listed are mutually exclusive. For example, a manual wheelchair with an anterior axle position is easier to propel but will tip over backward more easily. Because each option for wheelchair alignment and components has both benefits and drawbacks, wheelchair selection and adjustment involve compromises. The rehabilitation team should work with the wheelchair user to obtain a chair that best matches that individual's abilities, physical characteristics, home and community environments, lifestyle, preferences, and priorities.[27,28]

When the prospective user has a recent spinal cord injury, wheelchair prescription should be delayed until functional training is well under way. During the weeks and months after injury, an individual's physical status and functional abilities are likely to change dramatically. As a result, his equipment needs will change significantly: a wheelchair that is appropriate for someone just beginning rehabilitation may be unsuitable two months later. If a wheelchair is prescribed prematurely, it is not likely to be optimally matched to the individual's ultimate needs. This is particularly true when there is significant motor return. Unfortunately, the trend toward increasingly shortened inpatient rehabilitation stays necessitates the selection of equipment earlier post injury.

Options

Power Wheelchairs

Power wheelchairs can provide a means of independent mobility for people who are unable to propel manual chairs at home or in the community. Models with power tilt, recline, or tilt and recline are available for people who cannot perform independent pressure reliefs without these features. Different control options are available for power chairs, allowing the user to control the chair using his breath or motions of his upper extremities, head, chin, or mouth. Because of the different control options, power chairs can make independent mobility possible for virtually anyone with a spinal cord injury, no matter how high the lesion.

Power wheelchairs are necessary equipment for many people who cannot function independently using manual wheelchairs. They have drawbacks, however, that make their use problematic for those who are capable of functioning without them. Power chairs are bulky, requiring more space to maneuver than manual wheelchairs. Because they are extremely heavy, power chairs cannot be transported in cars[c] and are restricted to wheelchair-accessible environments. (A manual wheelchair can often be propelled through narrow doorways and taken up and down stairs or curbs independently or with assistance.) Finally, the user does not receive the cardiovascular and muscular conditioning that are gained from propulsion of a manual wheelchair.

Despite the drawbacks of power wheelchairs, a number of factors may make a power chair the most appropriate choice for independent mobility. These factors include inadequate motor function for manual wheelchair propulsion, vocational or educational activities that involve negotiation of long distances or hilly terrain, and medical or orthopedic conditions that preclude the use of a manual wheelchair for functional distances. Moreover, power wheelchairs may be appropriate for people who are at high risk for overuse injuries of the upper extremities due to obesity, advanced age, or a history of upper extremity injury.[29]

People with C4 and higher complete tetraplegia lack the motor function needed to propel a manual chair, and clearly require power chairs. People with C5 tetraplegia are often able to propel manual wheelchairs for limited distances indoors but require power chairs for mobility in the community. Some individuals with C6 tetraplegia function well with manual chairs and choose not to utilize power chairs. Others find that, although they can propel manual chairs over even surfaces, they are unable to function independently in all of the environments that they encounter during the course of a typical day or week. These individuals with marginal propulsion abilities may find manual wheelchair propulsion to be too slow or too tiring and decide that powered mobility is more suitable to their priorities and lifestyles.

Power chairs come in a variety of styles. The major choices in selecting a power wheelchair are its base, seating system, controller, and input device(s). These components are described in the following sections. The commonly prescribed options are summarized in Table 11–2.

[c] For this reason, a manual wheelchair should be prescribed in addition to the power chair, for use when travel in a car is necessary. The exceptions are "transportable" power chairs and power packs that can be added to manual wheelchairs. Both of these can be disassembled and loaded into a car, but they are heavy and difficult to load.

TABLE 11–2   Options Available in Power Wheelchair Components

Components	Options	Characteristics
Power bases	Rear-wheel drive (casters in front)	Largest turning radius.
	Front-wheel drive (casters in rear)	Intermediate turning radius. Tends to "fishtail" (rear of wheelchair swings) at higher speeds.
	Mid-wheel drive (casters in front and rear)	Smallest turning radius.
Seating systems	Stationary (standard)	Simpler mechanics and electronics, less expensive. Does not require long wheel base for stability. Appropriate only for individuals who can perform pressure reliefs independently without tilt or recline feature.
	Tilt	Provides pressure relief while maintaining constant angle between seat and back. Less likely than recline to elicit spasticity, less likely to alter user's sitting posture upon return to upright. Requires long wheel base for posterior stability of chair during tilt.
	Recline	Provides pressure relief by reclining backrest. Knees and hips extend when back reclines, with possible benefits to joint range of motion. Intermittent catheterization easier in reclined position. Creates shear forces on back, although these forces may be minimized with "zero shear" models. Reclining motion may elicit spasticity, causing user's sitting posture to shift. Requires long wheel base for posterior stability of chair during recline.
	Tilt/recline combination	Allows either tilt or recline. Indicated for individuals who need tilt feature for pressure reliefs due to spasticity but need recline feature for intermittent catheterization. Requires long wheel base for posterior stability of chair during tilt or recline.

TABLE 11–2 *(Continued)*

Components	Options	Characteristics
Control options	Proportional	Works like the gas pedal of a car: commands can be graded, with the chair's response proportional to the magnitude of the signal. Example: the rider pushes a joystick over a short arc of motion to make the chair go slowly, pushes the joystick further to go faster.
	Nonproportional (microswitch)	Works like a light switch: commands cannot be graded; the signal can provide an "on" or "off" command to a function. Example: the rider blows (puffs) on a straw to make the chair go forward. The chair's speed is preset, and not proportional to the strength of the puff.
Control options	Momentary	The chair performs a function while the rider delivers the command but stops performing the function when the rider stops. Example: the chair goes forward while the rider holds the joystick forward but stops when the rider releases the joystick.
	Latched	Once signaled, the chair performs a function until it receives a signal to stop. Example: the rider blows on a straw to signal the chair to go forward but does not have to keep blowing to continue going forward.
Access devices (interfaces)	Joystick	Typically proportional control, functioning in momentary mode. Joystick swivels on its base, wheelchair user pushes it forward, backward, right, left, or any angle between these directions to control the direction and speed of the chair's motion. Because of the joystick's simplicity, is the preferred input device for those who are capable of using it. Can be mounted for driving using motions of the hand, chin, mouth, or head. Joystick–user interface can be adapted to maximize comfort and function.
	Proximity head array	Proportional control, typically functions in momentary mode. Sensors embedded in headrest detect wheelchair driver's head position. Driver moves head to control the chair.
	Breath control (sip and puff)	Microswitch control, typically functions in both momentary and latched modes. Wheelchair driver signals chair through a straw, using hard and soft sips and puffs. Can be difficult for some drivers to master because of the relative complexity of the commands.
	Tongue-touch keypad	Microswitch control, functions in latched mode. Sensors embedded in custom-molded device resembling orthodontic retainer worn in roof of mouth. Driver signals chair by contacting sensors with tongue. Can be difficult for some drivers to master because of the relative complexity of the commands.
	Additional input devices	Additional input devices may be used in combination with any of the devices listed above. These devices can be used to signal the chair to stop ("kill switch"), change modes (between driving and reclining, for example), or to perform functions such as legrest control and pressure relief. These switches can be mounted anywhere on the chair, depending on what motions the driver will use to operate the switch. Some of the more commonly used types of auxiliary switches are: *Toggle switch:* switch pivots in one plane, operated by pushing it. *Proximity switch:* sensor detects when body part comes close; operated by moving a body part close to switch. *Button switch:* switch is a button or pad that can be depressed; operated by pressing or hitting it. *Leaf switch:* thin ribbon-like switch, activated when bent; operated by pressing it.

Sources: References 30 to 34.

Integrated Frame and Seat Versus Power Base

Conventional power wheelchairs are made with the seat and frame of the chair constructed as an integrated unit. In more recent designs, the seat and the main chassis of the chair are separate systems. The power base includes the chair's frame, drive wheels, casters, motors, controllers, and battery. A separate seating system is attached to this base.

Seating System

The seating system includes the seat, back, armrests, and legrests of the chair. It is mounted on the wheel base. Seating systems may be stationary or have the capacity to tilt, recline, or both tilt and recline. (Figure 11–2 shows tilt and recline features.) Pressure-relieving and contoured backrests, postural supports, and armrest troughs can be incorporated in the system to promote optimal function, posture, and skin integrity.

Access Device

Access devices, also called input devices or drive controls, are the components that wheelchair riders use to drive their chairs (Figure 11–3). They are also used to direct other functions performed by the chair, such as legrest elevation or seating system tilt or recline, and can be used to interface with environmental control units and computers.

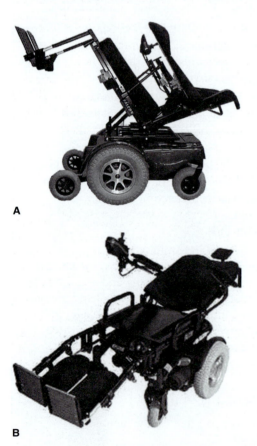

A

B

Figure 11–2   Seating systems showing (A) tilt, and (B) recline functions. (Photos reproduced with permission of Falcon Rehabilitation Products.)

A chair may have one or more access devices, depending on its user's needs and abilities.

Controller

The controller is the electronic "brain" of the wheelchair. It receives the signals sent by the patient through the input device and directs the wheelchair's motors to carry out their various functions. Programmable controllers allow for the adjustment of a variety of parameters, such as maximum speed and rate of acceleration and deceleration.

Manual Wheelchairs

Manual wheelchairs are lighter and smaller than power chairs, so they can be transported in cars and taken into environments that are not accessible to power wheelchairs. Moreover, manual wheelchair propulsion can result in improved physical fitness.[35,36] The muscle strength gained through manual wheelchair propulsion may benefit other areas of function, such as transfers and mat skills. A significant disadvantage of manual wheelchair propulsion is that it can lead to upper extremity pain due to chronic overuse injuries.

Manual wheelchairs are available in standard-weight, lightweight, and ultralight models. Standard weight chairs are heavy, and they have relatively limited options in size, components, and adjustability. Lightweight chairs are somewhat lighter but are still relatively heavy and have limited options. Ultralight wheelchairs are made of durable lightweight materials and are generally available with more options in size, components, and adjustability. Ultralight chairs allow more efficient propulsion, reducing the energy demands on the user[37,38] and making independent propulsion possible for some individuals who are unable to propel standard-weight chairs.[39,40] Recent advances in wheelchair materials include titanium frames, which are lighter than ultralight frames.[29] The lighter weight and superior adjustability of ultralight and titanium wheelchairs may help prevent overuse injuries of the upper extremities.[29] These wheelchairs also tend to look better than other chairs. Their sporty colors and designs can make the user look less impaired, which can facilitate his reintegration into the community.

The components of a manual wheelchair are illustrated in Figure 11–4. Virtually all of these components have several options from which to choose when selecting a wheelchair. The commonly prescribed options for these components are summarized in Table 11–3.

Pushrim–Activated Power-Assist Wheelchairs

Pushrim–activated power-assist wheelchairs (PAPAWs) are a relatively new option for wheeled mobility. A PAPAW is a manual wheelchair with motorized wheels in place of standard drive wheels. When the wheelchair user exerts force on the wheels' pushrims, the motors are activated and add power to the propulsive force. This power assist allows propulsion with less strain on the upper extremities, possibly reducing the risk of overuse injuries.[50–52]

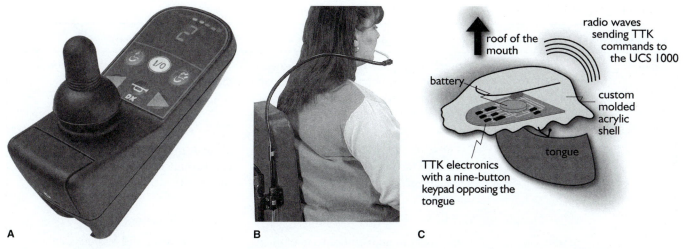

Figure 11–3 Examples of access devices used to drive power wheelchairs. (A) Joystick. (Courtesy of Dynamic Controls.) (B) Breath control. (Courtesy of Therafin.) (C) Tongue-touch keypad. (Courtesy of newAbilities Systems, Inc.)

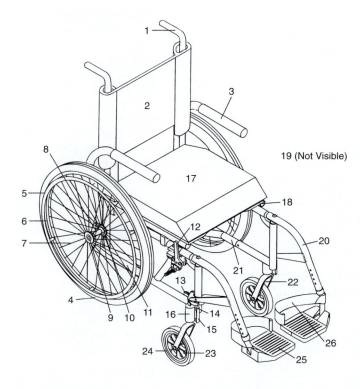

1. Push Handle Backrest Tube	14. Caster Housing Dust Cover
2. Backrest	15. Caster Plate
3. Swing Away Padded Armrest	16. Caster Housing
4. 24" Pneumatic Tire	17. Seat Cushion
5. 21" Aluminum Handrim	18. Seat Sling
6. Aluminum Wheel Rim	19. X-Hinge
7. Spokes	20. Swing Away Footrest/Front End
8. Rear Wheel Hub	21. Crossbrace
9. Quick Release Axle	22. Caster Fork
10. Axle Plate	23. Caster Wheel
11. Rear Frame Component	24. Caster Tire
12. High Wheel Lock	25. Flip-Up Composite Footrest
13. Swing Away Latch Release	26. Heel Loop

Figure 11–4 Manual wheelchair components labeled. (Reproduced with permission from Sunrise Medical, Fresno, CA.)

In addition to allowing propulsion with less strain on the upper extremities, PAPAWs can enhance functional independence. Reported benefits of PAPAWs (versus manual wheelchairs) have included comfort and ease of propulsion, reduced energy cost, and superior performance in laboratory and natural environments, including speed and distance on indoor and outdoor surfaces, and negotiation of carpet, ramps, curb cuts and curbs.[50,53-55] A significant advantage of some PAPAWs is that they can be adjusted to accommodate asymmetrical upper extremity weakness or pain. Disadvantages of PAPAWs include added width, weight, and cost[55] as well as difficulty of propulsion in the event of battery failure.[54]

Selecting Wheelchair Components and Manufacturers

In choosing between the available options for wheelchair components, the prospective owner and the rehabilitation team should weigh the benefits and drawbacks of each option. Trial runs in wheelchairs that have the features under consideration are critical to this choice. Different manufacturers have their own designs for each component, and seemingly minor differences may impact significantly on the wheelchair user's comfort, safety, and ability to function. What seems to be a good option when looking at the manufacturer's literature may turn out to be unsuitable when the chair arrives. Until an individual (particularly one with impaired upper extremity function) tries out a given design, it is often impossible to determine with certainty that he will be capable of using it. Someone who tries a "similar" wheelchair but does not actually sit in, propel, and transfer in and out of the exact model being considered for purchase may find that he cannot function optimally when his own chair arrives.

TABLE 11–3 Options Available in Manual Wheelchair Components

Components	Options	Advantages	Disadvantages
Frame	Folding	Requires less space when folded, does not require good hand function to load into car, provides shock absorption, allows all wheels to contact the ground on uneven terrain.	Heavier, less durable. Propulsion less efficient.
	Rigid	Frame stiffness makes propulsion more efficient. More durable, lighter. Angle between seat and backrest often adjustable.	Wheels must be removed to load into car. Propulsion over uneven terrain more difficult.
Backrest	Fixed height	May be lighter and more durable.	Back height cannot be adjusted.
	Adjustable height	Allows custom adjustment to maximize function and comfort; can change back height as needs change.	May be heavier and less durable.
Backrest	Standard upholstery	Allows convenient folding. Light weight.	Stretches over time, resulting in discomfort and reduced postural support.
	Solid back	Provides superior postural support. Often adjustable in height, depth, and back angle.	Some designs cause wheelchair user to sit in more anterior position on seat, resulting in reduced propulsion efficiency and reduced area for distributing pressure on sitting surface. Must be removed to fold chair.
Seat	Standard upholstery (sling)	Allows folding.	Stretches over time, causing hip adduction and inward rotation, reducing postural stability and comfort, and altering pressure distribution. (Can be stabilized using solid seat insert.)
	Solid	Provides superior postural support. Some models allow folding.	
Wheel attachments	Standard	Less expensive.	Require tools for removal and replacement.
	Quick release	Wheels easily removed and replaced for car transfers or adjusting axle position.	More expensive.
Axle position	Fixed	Lighter.	Axle position cannot be altered.
	Adjustable	Allows custom adjustment for optimal function, posture, and minimizing stress on shoulders.	Anterior and superior axle positions can increase risk of tips/falls.
Wheel camber	Vertical (standard)	Overall chair width narrower.	Less lateral stability than cambered, propulsion over side slope more difficult.
	Cambered	Gives chair superior lateral stability. Reduced rolling resistance and downward turning tendency on side slope make propulsion easier.	Increases overall width of chair.
Wheel locks (Figure 11–5)	High-mount	Easier to reach, can be equipped with extensions to make operation easier.	Can injure thumb, especially during obstacle negotiation.
	Low-mount	Will not injure user's thumb.	More difficult to reach and operate.

TABLE 11–3 (*Continued*)

Components	Options	Advantages	Disadvantages
Wheel design (Figure 11–6)	Wire spokes	Lighter weight.	Require periodic adjustment.
	MAG	More durable, do not lose true, more easily cleaned.	Heavier. Entire wheel or caster must be replaced if damaged.
Antitipping devices	Present on wheelchair	Reduce (but do not eliminate) risk of tipping/falling over backward in wheelchair.	Prevent wheelies, interfere with obstacle negotiation. Anti-tippers cannot be removed or repositioned by person sitting in wheelchair.
	Absent from wheelchair	Allows obstacle negotiation using wheelies.	Greater risk of injury from backward tips/falls.
Handrims	Standard	Durable surface.	Most difficult handrim for propulsion with impaired hand grasp.
	Vinyl coated	Increase friction, making propulsion easier when hand function is impaired.	Surface not durable; gets nicks with sharp edges. Potential for friction burns when descending incline.
	Oval (Figure 11–7)	Ergonomic design makes propulsion easier, reduces hand and wrist pain and risk of friction burns.	Slightly heavier than standard handrims.
	With handrim projections	Handrim projections ("pegs") make propulsion easier when arms are very weak.	Interfere with pushing rhythm, increase overall chair width.
Tires	Pneumatic	Standard pressure: Less rolling resistance. Best shock absorption, providing smoother ride. Treaded pneumatic provide superior traction.	Require more maintenance (puncture, require periodic inflation), make chair's overall width greater.
		High pressure: Least rolling resistance, intermediate width.	Poor traction, very susceptible to puncture.
	Solid	Most durable tires, do not go flat or require inflation, add least width to chair.	Less cushioned ride, "bog down" in sand or soft soil, make obstacle negotiation more difficult.
Caster tires	Pneumatic	Best shock absorption, lower rolling resistance. Do not "bog down" in sand or soft soil. May extend the life of the wheelchair due to shock absorption.	Require more maintenance (puncture, require periodic inflation). Small diameter casters not available.
	Semipneumatic	Intermediate shock absorption, do not puncture or require inflation, do not "bog down" in sand or soft soil.	Heaviest caster tires.
	Solid	Most durable, do not puncture or require inflation, lightest. Some available in softer materials for increased shock absorption.	Less cushioned ride, "bog down" in sand or soft soil, make obstacle negotiation more difficult.
Caster size	Large diameter	Easier to propel over uneven terrain, provide wheelchair with superior forward stability (chair less likely to tip over forward).	Heavier, decreased maneuverability of front end of wheelchair. On chairs with rigid, nonremovable front rigging, may contact feet when swivel.
	Small diameter	Lighter, easier to maneuver on even surfaces. Provide greater clearance between casters and user's heels.	Reduce chair's forward stability, make propulsion over uneven terrain more difficult. Higher rolling resistance.

(Continued)

TABLE 11–3 (*Continued*)

Components	Options	Advantages	Disadvantages
Front rigging	Rigid nonre-movable	Shorter frame length, stronger.	Can interfere with level and floor-to-wheelchair transfers.
	Swing-away detachable footrests	Can be repositioned easily for transfers.	Increase frame length, heavier and less durable than rigid nonremovable.
	Swing-away detachable leg rests (elevating)	Allow propulsion with legs elevated.	Heavy and awkward to reposition, add more to length of chair than all other options, must be removed (not just repositioned) for lateral transfers. Leg elevation in presence of tight hamstrings can cause posterior pelvic tilt.
	Heel loops (on footrests)	Keep feet from sliding off of footplates.	Make removal of feet from footplates more difficult.
Armrests	Present on wheelchair	May reduce risk of developing skin breakdown because of: (1) reduced seating pressure due to partial support of body weight, (2) promotion of upright sitting posture, and (3) enhanced stability promoting the performance of more pressure reliefs. Can be used functionally when reaching for high objects, and when narrowing chair to negotiate narrow doorways.	May restrict mobility. Add to overall weight of chair, can increase overall width. Promote shoulder abduction and internal rotation during propulsion, increasing risk of upper extremity overuse injuries.
	Absent from wheelchair	Preferred by some experienced wheelchair users due to enhanced freedom of trunk and arm motions without armrests.	May increase risk of skin breakdown. Precludes use of armrests for functional tasks.
Armrests	Desk length	Allows closer approach to tables and desks.	
	Full length	Provides support to entire length of forearm.	
Armrests	Fixed		Only stand–pivot or mechanical lift transfers are possible. Add to chair's overall width.
	Removable, swing-away, or pivoting	Can be removed or repositioned for transfers.	Some styles add to chair's overall width. Different styles have varying difficulty of management.
Armrests	Fixed height	Lighter, more durable.	Armrest height cannot be altered.
	Adjustable height	Can be adjusted to the individual to promote optimal posture, can be raised to make standing from wheelchair easier.	Heavier, may be less durable.

Sources: References 6, 7, 30 to 32, 37, 39, and 41 to 49.

240

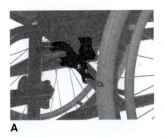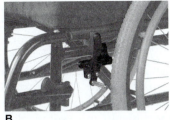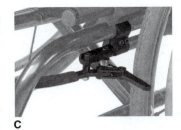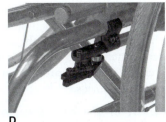

Figure 11–5   Wheel locks. (A) High-mount wheel lock, closed (engaged) position. (B) High-mount wheel lock, open (disengaged) position. (C) Low-mount wheel lock, closed (engaged) position. (D) Low-mount wheel lock, open (disengaged) position. (Reproduced with permission from Sunrise Medical.)

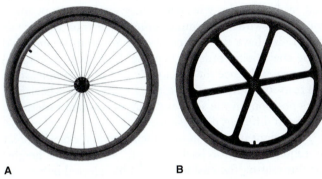

Figure 11–6   Wheel designs. (A) Wire spokes. (B) MAG. (Reproduced with permission from Sunrise Medical.)

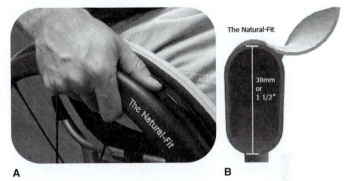

Figure 11–7   Oval handrims. (A) photo shows larger grasping surface and thumb protection built into oval handrims. (B) cross-section of oval handrim. (Reproduced with permission from Three Rivers Holdings, LLC, www.3rivers.com.)

When selecting a wheelchair, the prospective user and the clinicians determine the size, style, and components most suitable to the individual's dimensions, abilities, activities, preferences, and the environments in which he will function. Another important choice is the manufacturer of the wheelchair. The manufacturer of choice will in part be determined by the wheelchair's specifications. Generally, a limited number of manufacturers will produce a chair with the desired characteristics. Other factors to consider when selecting brands include cost, durability, chair weight, the overall dimensions of the chair, availability of replacement parts and service facilities, warranty specifications, and reputation of the manufacturer. When selecting a power wheelchair, the chair's maximum speed, stopping distance, obstacle climbing ability, range, maneuverability, static and dynamic stability, and performance in different climate conditions are also important considerations.[30,31] This information is available from manufacturers.

Although esthetics were not formerly considered to be an important consideration in wheelchair design or selection, the significance of this area is now recognized.[56] Modern wheelchairs come in a variety of colors and styles. Wheelchair selection should include consideration of the chair's esthetics, as it can affect both the user's acceptance of the chair and his integration in the community.

"Wheelchairs have become less institutional-looking. The new chairs are sporty-looking, lighter, faster,

and take up less space, making me look less conspicuous. The first chair I had made me look like a tank."
Dean Ragone[57]
businessman, activist, cervical SCI survivor

Prevention of Overuse Injuries

One critical consideration in selecting a wheelchair is the potential for overuse injuries of the upper extremities. This factor may be particularly important when choosing between a manual, power, or power-assist wheelchair. Especially if the individual has any of the following characteristics, a power or power-assist wheelchair should be considered: marginal potential for manual wheelchair propulsion, preexisting upper extremity pathology, advanced age, obesity, or a home or work environment that will make propulsion difficult.[5]

The wheelchair should be customizable to provide appropriate postural support, allowing adjustment to ensure optimal positioning of the pelvis, spine, and shoulders.[d] The axles of the drive wheels of manual or power-assist

---

[d] This is true for power wheelchairs as well as manual and power-assist wheelchairs.[13]

wheelchairs should allow adjustment to optimize their position relative to the upper extremities. Manual wheelchairs should be as light as possible. These features are recommended to minimize the strain on the upper extremities during propulsion, thus reducing the risk of overuse injuries.[5,21,48]

Additional Considerations Specific to Power Wheelchairs

Wheelchair selection is particularly challenging for the individual with high tetraplegia. Profoundly impaired voluntary motor function will limit his ability to manipulate access devices. It will also limit his ability to correct his sitting posture if it shifts. A shift in sitting posture may result in an inability to reach the chair's access devices, and can cause skin breakdown due to alteration of sitting forces. To complicate the picture further, the individual may have spasticity that is elicited when the chair reclines.

An appropriate wheelchair will enable its user to independently, safely, and comfortably drive the chair, perform pressure reliefs, return to upright after pressure reliefs, and maintain a good sitting posture. The rehabilitation team and wheelchair user work together to determine which combination of components will make this outcome possible. This selection process must involve trial periods and training with the components under consideration to ensure that the individual will be able to function optimally with them.

Probably the most challenging aspect of the selection process is the choice of access device(s). The user must be able to direct his chair to perform all of its necessary tasks. For example, he must be able to signal the chair to tilt or recline enough to achieve adequate pressure relief, and he must be able to return to an upright position. When he is tilted or reclined he will be in a different position relative to gravity and may find it difficult or impossible to operate an access device that he uses without difficulty when sitting upright. For this reason, he may need to drive the wheelchair and perform pressure reliefs with two or more separate access devices.

The various components included in a power wheelchair are often made by different manufacturers. Before prescribing a wheelchair, the rehabilitation team should make sure that the components being recommended are all compatible with each other. They should also take into consideration whether the individual will use the chair's input device to control an environmental control unit or computer. Finally, if the rider will utilize a portable ventilator, the wheelchair prescription must specify the incorporation of a vent tray on the back of the wheel base.

Size Selection

An improperly fit wheelchair can cause deformity, skin breakdown, impaired lower extremity circulation, and physical discomfort. It can also make independent propulsion more difficult, leading to reduced functional status and increased stress on the upper extremities. Table 11–4

presents information on optimal wheelchair dimensions, the benefits of appropriate fit, and the problems that can result from the use of a poorly fitting chair.

Tentative wheelchair dimensions can be determined using a tape measure with the patient sitting or lying on a mat.[e] Figure 11–8 illustrates the measurements to be taken. These measurements are subject to error because of the difficulty inherent in taking linear measures of a three-dimensional person. If the measurements are taken carefully, however, they should make it possible to determine fairly accurately the wheelchair dimensions that will be most appropriate for the individual.

The dimensions of a chair being ordered should be verified by having the wheelchair user sit in and operate a wheelchair with these dimensions. The trial wheelchair should also have the components that are to be included in the chair being ordered because differences in components may influence the fit of the chair. For example, solid backrests or elevating legrests can alter the wheelchair user's position on the seat, and may necessitate ordering a chair with different dimensions.[30]

The height of cushion on which a person sits will affect his requirements for backrest, seat, and armrest height. For this reason, the cushion should be selected before the wheelchair is ordered.

Additional Considerations for People with Incomplete Injuries

Two factors complicate wheelchair selection for individuals with incomplete spinal cord injuries: the potential for motor return and the potential for use of the lower extremities for propulsion.

Potential for Motor Return

Significant motor return is more likely to occur when a spinal cord injury is incomplete. Unfortunately, it is not possible to predict with certainty the amount of motor return or the level of independence in ambulation that a given individual will experience.[f] This uncertainty makes wheelchair selection difficult. For example, a person who has a high lesion with minimal motor sparing may require a power wheelchair with a tilt-and-recline seating system at the time of discharge from inpatient rehabilitation. A year later, he could require the same equipment, a power chair without the tilt–recline feature, a manual chair, or even no wheelchair at all for independent mobility in the community.

Ideally, the patient will be provided with equipment that is appropriate for his current needs, with changes in equipment as his needs change. One option is the use of a

---

[e] Supine is advisable when measuring thigh length ("c" in Figure 11–8), as posterior pelvic tilt in sitting can make it difficult to obtain accurate measurements.
[f] Table 12–15 in Chapter 12 presents factors associated with future ambulatory potential.

TABLE 11–4 Wheelchair Dimensions

Feature	Optimal Dimensions	Benefits of Proper Dimensions	Potential Problems from Improper Dimensions
Seat width	**Less than 1¼ inches** wider than wheelchair user's width at greater trochanters or widest portion of thighs. Hips should not contact wheels, armrests or clothing guards. If the wheelchair user plans to use lower extremity braces or bulky clothing, or if significant weight gain is likely, consider extra width.	Optimal postural support, propulsion efficiency.	**Too wide:** Increased difficulty of wheelchair propulsion, scoliosis, pressure ulcers from improper distribution of pressure over buttocks; overall chair width increased, limiting access through doorways. **Too narrow:** Pressure ulcers from pressure over greater trochanters.
Seat depth	1 to 2 inches less than distance between the posterior aspect of the buttocks and the popliteal fossa.	Optimal postural support, distribution of pressure on buttocks.	**Too deep** (seat too long from front to back): Lumbar kyphosis, impaired circulation below knees. **Too shallow** (seat too short from front to back): Pressure ulcers from excessive pressure on buttocks, due to limited area over which sitting pressure can be distributed.
Seat height	**Measure with cushion in place.** Power chair or manual chair propelled using arms: seat should be high enough to allow proper adjustment of footplates with at least 2 inches of clearance between floor and footplates. Manual chair propelled using legs: feet should rest flat on the floor while the wheelchair user remains in a good sitting posture.	Optimal postural support, safety, functional performance.	**Too low:** Proper leg positioning impossible, causing excessive pressure over ischial tuberosities with resulting pressure ulcers; if low seat height causes inadequate clearance between footrests and floor, footrests more likely to "bottom out" on uneven terrain or at base of inclines, resulting in tips and falls. **Too high:** Elevated center of gravity reduces chair's anteroposterior stability, increasing risk of tips and falls; can limit access to vans by increasing overall height of chair and rider; may make propulsion and transfers more difficult.
Backrest height	**Measure with cushion in place.** Appropriate height will depend on the wheelchair user's ability to stabilize his trunk in a wheelchair. Find optimal fit by experimenting with different back heights.	Optimal postural support, ease and comfort of manual wheelchair propulsion.	**Too high:** Impedes shoulder motion, making manual wheelchair propulsion uncomfortable and more difficult. Impedes posture if combined with inclined seat. **Too low:** Inadequate postural support, with resulting deformity and problems in breathing, skin integrity, and functional status.
Backrest width	Approximately 3/4 inch wider than torso width at level of top of backrest.	Comfort, minimal interference with manual wheelchair propulsion.	**Too wide:** Backrest impedes shoulder motions, increasing difficulty of manual wheelchair propulsion. **Too narrow:** Discomfort, skin damage.

(Continued)

TABLE 11–4 *(Continued)*

Feature	Optimal Dimensions	Benefits of Proper Dimensions	Potential Problems from Improper Dimensions
Footrest-to-seat distance	**Measure with cushion in place and shoes on.** Middle range of adjustable footrest should allow proper adjustment of footrest height with at least 2-inch clearance between floor and footplates.	Optimal pressure distribution, safety.	**Too long:** Inadequate support of feet and legs results in reduced postural support and excessive pressure on posterodistal aspect of thighs. **Too short:** Reduced weight bearing on thighs increases pressure on ischial tuberosities, threatening skin integrity.
Armrest height	**Measure with cushion in place.** In upright sitting posture with arms at sides and elbows flexed 90 degrees, forearms should rest comfortably on armrests. (Measure from wheelchair seat to bottom of elbow.)	Comfort, postural support, pressure reliefs.	**Too high:** Cause scapular elevation, discomfort. **Too low:** Inadequate postural support, inadequate support for glenohumeral joint (relevant for individuals with severe upper extremity weakness), increased risk of skin breakdown due to inadequate postural support.

Sources: References 13, 30, 31, 46, and 47.

rental wheelchair at first, with purchase of a chair once enough time has passed that the individual's ultimate functional potential is more clear. This solution may not be possible because of funding restrictions or a lack of availability of appropriate rental equipment. When it is not possible to delay the purchase of a wheelchair, the patient and rehabilitation team must do their best to select a chair that is most likely to meet both his current and future needs.

Lower Extremity Propulsion

A second consideration in wheelchair selection and adjustment for people with incomplete lesions is the use of the lower extremities for propulsion. An individual who uses

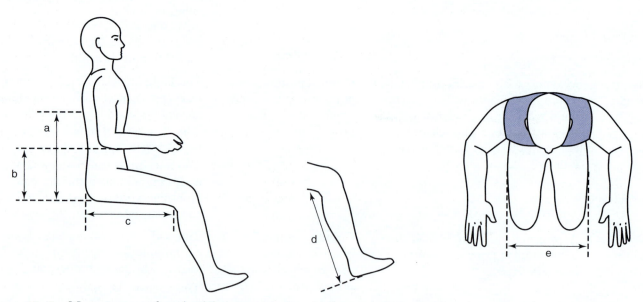

Figure 11–8   Measurements for wheelchair prescription. (a) Seat to inferior border of scapula. (b) Seat to elbow. (c) Posterior aspect of buttocks to popliteal fossa. (d) Posterior thigh to sole. (e) Width at greater trochanters or widest portion of thighs.

his feet for propulsion is likely to require a chair with a lower than standard floor-to-seat height. This feature will enable him to propel without sliding his buttocks forward on the seat; he will be able to maintain a good sitting posture while propelling if his feet can rest flat on the floor while his buttocks remain positioned well back on the seat.

The drawback of a low seat height is that it can make bed transfers more difficult because the person will have to transfer from a low surface to a higher one. A low seat height will also make sit-to-stand transfers more difficult. This problem will be a concern for individuals who both walk and use wheelchairs for their functional mobility. When selecting and adjusting a wheelchair, the patient and rehabilitation team should consider the impact of seat height on propulsion, transfers, and posture.

Examination and Evaluation

When a wheelchair is delivered, the physical therapist should examine and evaluate it, addressing the following questions: Are the chair's dimensions appropriate, and are its features suitable? Does the chair match the prescription? If not, are the substitutions acceptable to both the clinician and the person for whom the chair was ordered? If the wheelchair meets the criteria listed above, the therapist should adjust the wheelchair to ensure that it provides the user with proper postural support and enables him to function optimally.

Adjustment

Proper adjustment of a wheelchair is critical to its user's functional status and health. Improper adjustment can limit the individual's capacity to function independently, and can cause skin breakdown, postural deformity, injury from tips and falls, and increased stress on the upper extremities.

Footrest Height

This adjustment is critical to both posture and pressure distribution. The footrests should be adjusted with the person sitting in the wheelchair on his cushion and wearing shoes. If the cushion is ever changed, the footrest height should be checked and readjusted if needed. The footrests should be positioned at a height that places the thighs parallel to the plane of the seat when the feet are flat on the footplates. This position will help to optimize posture and pressure distribution. Footplates that are positioned too high lift the thighs off the seat, resulting in excessive pressure over the ischial tuberosities. Footplates positioned too low cause excessive pressure on the distal thighs and reduce postural support.

Backrest Height and Angle

If the wheelchair has an adjustable-height backrest, the optimal height should be determined. To find the best backrest height, the wheelchair user can sit in and propel the chair with the backrest adjusted to various heights. He

should also perform functional activities that involve reaching, as backrest height influences a chair's anteroposterior stability. The patient should sit on his cushion during this assessment, as cushion height will influence optimal backrest height. The clinician and wheelchair user should determine which height results in the best posture, comfort, function, and safety. If the angle of the backrest is adjustable, the optimal angle should be determined in a similar fashion.

Armrest Height

The armrests should be positioned so that the rider can rest his arms comfortably on them while maintaining an erect sitting posture. With his back against the backrest and his scapulae in a neutral position (not elevated), he should be able to sit with his forearms on the armrest pads with his shoulders flexed approximately 30 degrees and his elbows flexed approximately 60 degrees.[44] This armrest height promotes proper sitting posture and reduces sitting pressure.

Axle Position

If the manual wheelchair has an axle with adjustable position, the clinician and wheelchair user should work together to find the optimal position. Anteroposterior adjustments can have a profound effect on function, especially in cases where the wheelchair user is only marginal in his propulsion ability.[58] A relatively anterior wheel position makes propulsion easier by increasing the chair's propulsion efficiency, reducing the chair's rolling resistance and tendency to turn downhill,[g] making it easier to turn, and reducing caster flutter (vibration) during propulsion. Anterior placement of the axle also reduces the chair's posterior stability. This reduced stability makes it easier to lift the casters for obstacle negotiation, but also increases the risk of tipping the chair over backward.[6,39,44,48,59,60] Optimal adjustment for an individual may involve finding a balance between propulsion efficiency and stability.[48,58] In general, the axles should be aligned as anteriorly as possible without compromising safety, as this axle position may reduce the risk of upper extremity overuse injuries.[5,12,48]

Vertical axle adjustments can affect the tilt of the seat and backrest: a more superior axle position effectively tilts the seat and backrest backward.[h] A slight backward tilt of the seat (referred to as seat angle, positive seat slope, or posterior inclination) can be helpful to the wheelchair user who has difficulty maintaining trunk stability. If the wheelchair has an adjustable-angle backrest, the seat and backrest angles can be adjusted separately.

---

[g] Sidewalks usually have a cross slope, with the sidewalk surface tilting slightly toward the street. A wheelchair being propelled over this slope tends to turn in the downhill direction, making propulsion more difficult.
[h] Moving the axle superiorly is the same as moving it UP relative to the back of the seat. This adjustment can also be conceptualized as moving the back of the seat DOWN relative to the position of the axle.

There is disagreement in the literature about the optimal angles of the seat and backrest in terms of postural support and function[61,62] as well as whether tilting the seat from horizontal increases the risk of skin breakdown.[59,63]

Vertical axle adjustments can be combined with change in the height of the caster fork to alter the seat height without changing the tilt of the seat. (In other words, the seat can be raised or lowered without altering its angle.) A lower seat will result in better anteroposterior stability.[6] A relatively low seat height may also help prevent overuse injuries of the upper extremities. When the patient is sitting in a good posture with his hands resting on the highest point of the pushrims, his elbows should be flexed between 100 and 120 degrees.[5,21]

Unfortunately, axle position adjustments that benefit propulsion and posture can interfere with transfers to and from the wheelchair. Moving the wheels to an anterior or superior position reduces the distance that the seat extends anterior to the wheels. This reduces the space available for lateral transfers to and from the wheelchair.[58] For the individual who is marginal in both transfer and propulsion skills, optimal wheelchair adjustment will involve finding a balance between transfer and propulsion abilities.

Alterations in axle position change the position of the wheel locks relative to the wheels, interfering with the locks' function. Thus the locks must be adjusted after the axles have been positioned. Axle position also affects the orientation of the casters, which impacts on wheelchair propulsion. When adjustments are made in a wheelchair's axle position, the caster angle should be adjusted to achieve a vertical orientation of the caster stems.[39,48,58]

Wheel Alignment

A manual chair's rear wheels should be aligned so that the distance between their front and rear aspects is equal. If the two wheels are angled so that they are closer to each other in the front than in the back (toe-in) or are closer in the back than in the front (toe-out), propulsion will be more difficult. To check this alignment, the therapist should measure the distance between the right and left wheels' rims at the height of the axle. This measurement should be taken at the front and rear aspects of the wheels.[39]

Tire Pressure

If the casters or rear wheels have pneumatic tires, they should be inflated to their recommended pressures. Underinflated tires can increase rolling resistance, making propulsion more difficult.[39,49]

Adjustments Specific to Power Wheelchairs

In addition to many of the adjustments just described, the adjustment of a power wheelchair includes the chair's access devices. The access devices should be positioned where they enable the rider to utilize them most effectively. If either a joystick or toggle switch is used, it may require modification to enhance the rider's ability to manipulate it. During the period of training in wheelchair skills, a fair number of adjustments may be required. The patient and rehabilitation team must work together to find the spatial orientation and physical configuration of the access devices that enable the patient to utilize them efficiently and comfortably to perform all of the chair's actions.[64]

The control parameters also require adjustment to suit the needs of the individual involved. A number of adjustments can be made, including the chair's maximum speed, turning speed, rate of acceleration and deceleration, and rate of tilt or recline. These parameters can be set to accommodate the individual's skill level, preferences, and physical response to motion. Optimal settings are likely to change as training progresses.

FUNCTIONAL POTENTIALS

The motor function that an individual has following spinal cord injury will influence to a large degree the manner in which he will be able to utilize a wheelchair. Table 11–5 presents a summary of the level of independence in wheelchair skills that can be achieved by people who have

Problem-Solving Exercise 11–1

Your patient has C7 tetraplegia, ASIA B. She propels her wheelchair independently over even surfaces for long distances, and is interested in learning how to negotiate small (1-to 2-inch) curbs. She has difficulty "popping" her casters from the floor.

- Assuming that the wheelchair has adjustable rear wheel axles, what adjustment could you make to the axle position to make it easier to lift the chair's casters from the floor?

- What effect will this change in axle position have on the chair's stability?
- What could be added to the chair to make it safer (assuming that they are not already present)? What impact will this addition have on curb negotiation?
- What effect will the change in axle position have on the patient's ability to propel the chair?
- What effect could the change in axle position have on transfers?
- So should you move the wheels or not?

TABLE 11–5 Functional Potentials

Motor Level	Significance of Innervated Musculature	Potential for Independence in Wheelchair Skills
C3 and higher	Inadequate voluntary motor function to utilize upper extremities to propel manual wheelchair or control power chair using hand-held joystick.	**Typical functional outcomes** **Propelling manual wheelchair:** Unable to propel chair. **Driving power wheelchair:** Independent driving power chair using motions of the head or chin, tongue, or breath to access the input device. **Pressure reliefs:** Independent in pressure reliefs using power tilt and/or recline. **Positioning in wheelchair:** dependent.
C4	Inadequate voluntary motor function to utilize upper extremities to propel manual wheelchair. **Full innervation of trapezius and partial innervation of rhomboids and levator scapulae** enhances capacity for (limited) postural control. When some voluntary motor function is present in the C5 myotome, this musculature plus that listed above makes it possible to utilize a hand-held joystick to control power wheelchair in exceptional cases. (Using the ASIA classification system, people with a C4 motor level can have limited function in the C5 myotome.)	**Typical functional outcomes** **Propelling manual wheelchair:** Unable to propel chair or perform pressure reliefs. **Driving power wheelchair:** Independent driving power chair using motions of the head or chin, tongue, or breath to access the input device. **Pressure reliefs:** Independent in pressure reliefs using power tilt and/or recline. **Positioning in wheelchair:** Dependent. **Exceptional functional outcomes** **Power wheelchair:** Independent in driving power chair and controlling specialty seating system using hand-held joystick. **Positioning in wheelchair:** Able to shift trunk laterally from upright and return to upright from *slight* lateral lean.
C5	**Partial innervation of the deltoids** makes it possible to extend the elbows using muscle substitution. **Partial innervation of the biceps brachii, brachialis, and brachioradialis** plus partial innervation of the deltoids makes it possible to use elbow and shoulder flexion to pull. Minimal serratus anterior function is inadequate to stabilize the scapulae against the thorax.	**Typical functional outcomes** **Propelling manual wheelchair:** Independent to some assist indoors on uncarpeted level floors; may use either high-friction or pegged handrims; manual wheelchair propulsion ability inadequate for mobility in the community. **Obstacle negotiation:** Unable to propel over uneven surfaces or obstacles. **Driving power wheelchair:** Independent using hand-held joystick. **Pressure reliefs:** Independent in power wheelchair using power tilt and/or recline; some assist to independent in pressure relief in manual wheelchair using lateral lean method. **Positioning in wheelchair:** Some assist to dependent in positioning buttocks and trunk in wheelchair. **Exceptional functional outcomes** **Pressure reliefs:** Independent in pressure reliefs without specialty seating system. **Positioning in wheelchair:** Independent in positioning buttocks and trunk in wheelchair.

(Continued)

TABLE 11–5   (*Continued*)

Motor Level	Significance of Innervated Musculature	Potential for Independence in Wheelchair Skills
C6	**Fully innervated deltoids, infraspinatus, teres minor, and clavicular portion of the pectoralis major** allow for stronger elbow extension using muscle substitution. **Fully innervated deltoids, biceps brachii, brachialis and brachioradialis** allow strong shoulder and elbow flexion for pulling. **Partial innervation of the serratus anterior** makes it possible to stabilize the scapulae against the thorax. Scapular protraction and stability enhance propulsion capability and capacity to position self in wheelchair. **Partial innervation of the latissimus dorsi** enhances shoulder girdle depression, allowing greater lift of the buttocks during pressure reliefs. Minimal innervation of the triceps brachii is inadequate to contribute significantly to wheelchair skills.	**Typical functional outcomes** **Propelling manual wheelchair:** Independent indoors on uncarpeted level floors; may use high-friction handrims; manual wheelchair propulsion ability likely to be inadequate for mobility in the community. **Obstacle negotiation:** Some to total assist negotiating mild obstacles such as carpeted floors, sidewalks, 1:12 grade ramps. **Driving power wheelchair:** Independent using hand-held joystick. **Pressure reliefs:** Independent in power wheelchair either without specialty seating system or using power tilt and/or recline. Some assist to independent in pressure relief in manual wheelchair using depression, forward lean, or lateral lean method. **Positioning in wheelchair:** Some assist to independent in positioning buttocks and trunk in wheelchair. **Exceptional functional outcomes** **Propelling manual wheelchair:** Independent on even and slightly uneven surfaces for long distances, allowing independent mobility in the community using a manual wheelchair. **Obstacle negotiation:** Independent in negotiation of mild obstacles such as 1:12 grade ramps, slightly uneven (outdoor) terrain, 2- to 4-inch curbs. **Pressure reliefs:** Independent in pressure relief in manual wheelchair using depression, forward lean, or lateral lean method. **Positioning in wheelchair:** Independent in positioning buttocks and trunk in wheelchair.
C7	**Partial innervation of the triceps brachii** allows for stronger elbow extension. **Full innervation of the serratus anterior** provides more stable scapulae, stronger protraction and upward rotation. **Partial innervation of the latissimus dorsi and sternocostal portion of pectoralis major** enhance shoulder girdle depression, enhancing propulsion, pressure reliefs, and positioning in wheelchair.	**Typical functional outcomes** **Propelling manual wheelchair:** Independent indoors and outdoors on level terrain for long distances, allowing independent mobility in the community using manual wheelchair. **Obstacle negotiation:** Independent to some assist negotiating 1:12 ramps. Some to total assist negotiating unlevel terrain and curbs. **Pressure reliefs:** Independent. **Positioning in wheelchair:** Independent in positioning buttocks and trunk in wheelchair. **Exceptional functional outcomes** **Obstacle negotiation:** Independent in negotiation of mild obstacles such as ramps with slightly steeper than 1:12 grade, slightly uneven (outdoor) terrain, 4-inch curbs.

TABLE 11–5   (*Continued*)

Motor Level	Significance of Innervated Musculature	Potential for Independence in Wheelchair Skills
C8	**Full innervation of the triceps brachii** provides normal strength in elbow extension. **Full innervation of the latissimus dorsi and nearly full innervation of pectoralis major** allow strong shoulder girdle depression, enhancing propulsion, pressure reliefs, and positioning in wheelchair. **Partial innervation of the long finger flexors allows grasp of wheelchair handrims,** resulting in greater ease in wheelchair propulsion and obstacle negotiation.	**Typical functional outcomes** **Propelling manual wheelchair:** Independent indoors and outdoors on level terrain for long distances, allowing independent mobility in the community using manual wheelchair. **Obstacle negotiation:** Independent negotiating 1:12 ramps. Some assist negotiating unlevel terrain and curbs. **Pressure reliefs:** Independent. **Positioning in wheelchair:** Independent in positioning buttocks and trunk in wheelchair. **Exceptional functional outcomes** **Obstacle negotiation:** Independent in negotiation of mild obstacles such as ramps with grade slightly steeper than 1:12, slightly uneven (outdoor) terrain, 4-inch curbs, narrow doorways. Can fall safely.
T1 and lower	**Fully innervated upper extremities** make all wheelchair skills easier to achieve. (Innervation of trunk musculature associated with lower levels of injury enhances performance.)	**Typical functional outcomes** **Propelling manual wheelchair:** Independent indoors and outdoors on level terrain for long distances, allowing independent mobility in the community using manual wheelchair. **Obstacle negotiation:** Independent negotiating 4- to 6-inch curbs, uneven terrain, ramps with grade steeper than 1:12, narrow doorways; can descend stairs backward holding handrail, ascend on buttocks and bring chair; can fall safely and return wheelchair to upright while remaining in chair. **Pressure reliefs:** Independent. **Positioning in wheelchair:** Independent in positioning buttocks and trunk in wheelchair. **Exceptional functional outcomes** **Obstacle negotiation:** Independent in negotiating curbs higher than 6 inches, ascending stairs while remaining in wheelchair, descending stairs in wheelie.

Sources: References for innervation: 65 to 69.

complete spinal cord injuries at different motor levels (motor component of neurological level of injury). When prognosticating about an individual's capacity to develop wheelchair skills, the clinician should take into consideration the many other factors that also impact on functional gains.[i]

PHYSICAL AND SKILL PREREQUISITES

Each method of performing a functional activity involves a particular set of skills. Each activity also has strength, joint range of motion, and muscle flexibility requirements. A deficiency in any of these skills or physical requirements will impair a person's performance of the activity.

The descriptions of functional techniques that follow are accompanied by tables that summarize the physical and skill prerequisites. Exact values for the physical prerequisites are not given because the requirements vary among individuals. For example, someone who is very skillful in curb negotiation will require less strength for this activity than another person who is less skillful and must use sheer strength rather than momentum.

PRACTICE IN DEPARTMENT AND "REAL WORLD"

The physical therapy department in a rehabilitation center should be equipped with curbs of varying heights, stairs, and a ramp. This equipment is useful for initial practice of obstacle negotiation; however, practice should not end with mastery of these artificial obstacles. Many obstacles that a wheelchair user will encounter outside of the department will be more difficult to negotiate. For example, ascending a cement curb from a street is likely to be more difficult than ascending a wooden curb from a linoleum floor. The "real world" is full of uneven sidewalks, long and steep staircases, heavy doors, and uneven surfaces such as grass and sand. Functional training should include practicing wheelchair skills outside of the department so that the individual will be better prepared to function in the "real world" after rehabilitation.

WHEELCHAIR SKILLS FOLLOWING COMPLETE SPINAL CORD INJURY: FUNCTIONAL TECHNIQUES AND THERAPEUTIC STRATEGIES

Someone who uses a wheelchair for independent mobility must possess a variety of skills. These skills include propulsion of the wheelchair over even surfaces and negotiation of obstacles, as well as the more basic skills of pressure reliefs, positioning the trunk and buttocks within the wheelchair, and handling the chair's parts. Chapter 10 addresses the skills required for positioning, and the management of wheelchair parts.

General Therapeutic Strategies

To accomplish a functional goal, a patient must acquire both the physical and skill prerequisites for that activity. For example, when working on driving a power wheelchair with a hand-held joystick, a person with a spinal cord injury must develop adequate strength in his shoulder girdle, as well as developing the ability to push the chair's joystick in various directions.

When developing skill prerequisites for a functional goal, the patient should start with the most basic prerequisite skills and progress toward more challenging activities. (A person had best develop skill in maintaining a wheelie before attempting to negotiate stairs in this position!) Before asking a patient to attempt a new skill, the therapist should explain and demonstrate the technique.[j] The demonstration should provide a clear idea of the motions involved and the timing of these motions.

The characteristics of the wheelchair will have a strong impact on the individual's ability to function. For this reason, wheelchair selection, adjustment, and skill training are intertwined processes. Therapists should remember that every patient has a unique combination of body build, coordination, strength, flexibility, and muscle tone. As a result, patients vary in the wheelchair features and adjustment that they will find most functional and comfortable. Moreover, each person is unique in the exact motions that he uses and the timing of these motions as he ascends a curb or rights his wheelchair after a fall. The challenge for the patient and therapist is finding the equipment components and adjustments that best suit each individual, and the movement strategies that will allow him the greatest independence.

As a therapist and patient work together on a skill, they can learn from failed attempts by analyzing the problem. Is the patient strong enough to perform the maneuver? Did he drop his casters too early or too late as he attempted to ascend the curb? Did he approach the curb with adequate speed?

It is important for the therapist and patient to keep in mind that functional training can take a long time. It is a mistake to give up on a functional goal after only a few trials. (Assuming that the patient has adequate innervation, of course!) When funding constraints limit the time available for functional training during inpatient rehabilitation, the

---

[i] Chapter 7 presents factors that can influence functional outcomes.

[j] This demonstration can also be provided by another person with a spinal cord injury if someone is available who has similar impairments but a higher level of functional ability. Alternatively, the patient may watch a videotaped demonstration of the skill.

patient may focus on pressure reliefs and basic propulsion during inpatient rehabilitation, and continue working toward independence in more advanced skills in an alternative setting such as an outpatient clinic or in the home.[70]

Tolerate Upright Sitting

When upright activities are first initiated, people with spinal cord injuries may experience orthostatic hypotension. This is a transient problem that is most prevalent among people with lesions above T6.[71–73] Especially after prolonged bed rest, moving directly to an upright sitting position can cause a drop in blood pressure, with resulting dizziness, vomiting, and loss of consciousness. Before an individual becomes independent in any wheelchair skills, he must first develop the capacity to sit upright in a wheelchair without experiencing these problems. Although upright sitting tolerance involves physiological accommodation rather than skill development, it is included in this chapter because all wheelchair skills depend upon it.

Tolerate Upright Sitting–Therapeutic Strategies

The development of upright sitting tolerance involves gradual accommodation to elevation of the head and torso above horizontal. A reclining wheelchair is useful for this process. When a recently injured person is first placed in this type of wheelchair, the chair's back can be almost fully reclined and the legrests elevated. As the patient adapts to sitting, the wheelchair's back can be raised in small increments to increasingly vertical positions,[k] and the legrests can be lowered.

Thigh-high antiembolic stockings and an abdominal binder[l] can be worn initially to reduce orthostatic hypotension by facilitating venous return. Unless it is required to enhance the individual's breathing ability,[m] the binder can be discontinued once the patient has accommodated to sitting. The patient can be weaned gradually from its use through loosening over a period of days.

During the period of adjustment to upright sitting, mild dizziness is common and will need to be tolerated. If the patient becomes very nauseated, or begins to lose consciousness, vision, or hearing, these symptoms can be eliminated by elevating the legs, tipping the wheelchair

back into a more reclined position, or both. It is important to remember that the above-described symptoms are not dangerous and to treat them accordingly.[n] A calm attitude on the therapist's part can result in an easier and more rapid adjustment to sitting.

While the patient adjusts to sitting, he can perform strengthening exercises and begin working on wheelchair propulsion. He can also practice stabilizing his trunk and leaning from side to side in the wheelchair, controlling the motion by pulling on the armrests.

Positioning in the Chair

The ability to position one's self and to maintain that position within a wheelchair is one of the most basic requirements for the independent use of a wheelchair. To use a wheelchair independently, a person needs to be able to maintain an upright sitting posture.[o] He should also be able to reposition his trunk and buttocks in the chair so that he can adjust his posture in the event that his position shifts during the day.

With Functioning Biceps and Deltoids

Chapter 10 presents techniques for stabilizing the trunk in a wheelchair and for moving the trunk and buttocks. These techniques require functional strength in the biceps and deltoids.

In the Absence of Functioning Biceps and Deltoids

Without functioning biceps and deltoids, the potential for stabilizing and moving the trunk is limited; however, a person with high tetraplegia can gain some skills in this area. To maintain an upright sitting posture, a person with a high lesion can hold his head upright and his scapulae adducted. A person with functioning trapezius, sternocleidomastoid, and cervical paraspinal musculature (present with C4 tetraplegia) can make limited adjustments in his trunk's position, tilting his trunk laterally by throwing the head and shoulders. For example, he can tilt his trunk to the left by repeatedly throwing his head to the left while simultaneously elevating his right scapula. These neck and scapular motions are performed forcefully to maximize momentum. This technique can be used to tilt to the side from an upright position or to return to upright from a slight lateral lean.

---

[k] Rehabilitation professionals should be mindful of the potential for damaging pressure on the skin overlying the sacrum when the wheelchair is in a reclined position. Strategies to protect the skin in this position include frequent pressure reliefs, and cushioning on the backrest that minimizes or eliminates sacral pressure.

[l] An abdominal binder is an elasticized band that encompasses the entire abdomen.

[m] See Chapter 6 for respiratory issues.

[n] Orthostatic hypotension should not be confused with autonomic dysreflexia, which is a dangerous condition. Autonomic dysreflexia is characterized by a rise in blood pressure rather than a fall and is brought on by noxious stimulation below the lesion. Its management is addressed in Chapter 3.

[o] An individual who is unable to do so without equipment may use a strap or lateral supports, but this equipment may interfere with independent pressure reliefs.

TABLE 11–6   High-Lesion Skills: Positioning in Wheelchair and Control of Power Wheelchair–Physical Prerequisites

	Positioning in Wheelchair	Hand-held Joystick	Chin-Control and Head-Control Joystick	Mouth-Control Joystick or Tongue-Touch Keypad	Breath Control	Proximity Head Array
Strength						
Cervical paraspinals	✓	✓	✓			✓
Sternocleidomastoid	✓		✓			✓
Trapezius	✓	✓−	✓			✓
Anterior deltoids	•	•				
Middle deltoids	•	•				
Posterior deltoids	•	•				
Serratus anterior	•	•				
Oral musculature				✓	✓	
Biceps, brachialis, and/or brachioradialis		✓−				
Range of Motion						
Cervical — Lateral flexion	✓−					✓−
Cervical — Rotation			✓−			✓−
Cervical — Flexion			✓−			✓−
Cervical — Extension	✓−		✓−			✓−
Scapular — Elevation	✓−					
Scapular — Abduction		✓−				
Scapular — Adduction		✓−				

✓− At least 2−/5 to 2/5 strength is needed for this activity, or severe limitations in range will inhibit this activity.
• Not required but helpful.
✓ At least 3/5 strength is needed for this activity.

The physical and skill prerequisites required for positioning in the chair in the absence of functioning biceps and deltoids are presented in Tables 11–6 and 11–7.

Positioning in the Chair–Therapeutic Strategies

Chapter 10 presents therapeutic strategies for individuals who have adequate strength in their deltoids and biceps to use their upper extremities to position themselves in their wheelchairs. Training strategies for patients who lack this strength are presented in the following section.

Sitting in a Wheelchair, Move Trunk Using Head and Scapular Motions

To practice this skill, the patient should be able to tolerate upright or nearly upright sitting. During initial practice, the patient can work on moving laterally from a midline sitting position. The therapist can demonstrate the technique and then manually guide him through the motions. The patient then practices throwing his head and shoulder vigorously and repeatedly in one direction at a time. In this manner, he can practice moving laterally past his balance point in one direction and then the other.

TABLE 11–7   High-Lesion Skills: Positioning in Wheelchair and Control of Power Wheelchair–Skill Prerequisites

	Positioning in Wheelchair	Hand-held Joystick	Chin-Control and Head-Control Joystick	Mouth-Control Joystick or Tongue-Touch Keypad	Breath Control	Proximity Head Array
Sitting in wheelchair, move trunk using head and scapular motions (pp. 252, 253)	✓					
Place hand on joystick (p. 255)		✓				
Move joystick in all directions using arm and scapular motions (p. 256)		✓				
Signal wheel chair using chin, head, or tongue motions (pp. 256, 257)			✓	✓		
Signal wheelchair by sipping and puffing in appropriate pattern (p. 257)					✓	
Signal wheelchair by moving head toward/away from sensors in headrest (pp. 256, 257)						✓
Drive power wheelchair (p. 257)		✓	✓	✓	✓	✓

✓ This prerequisite skill is required to perform this activity.

Early training should also include practice in returning upright from a lateral lean. This practice should start with the patient sitting with a *slight* lean, in a position barely lateral to midline sitting. The therapist should encourage him to return his trunk to upright using vigorous head and scapular motions.

Once the patient is able to move both toward and away from an upright position, he can combine practice of the two skills, shifting a short distance to the side and returning to upright. As his ability improves, he can gradually increase the arc of motion. He should practice moving laterally toward and away from upright over increasing arcs until he achieves his maximal capability.

Pressure Reliefs

The ability to perform pressure reliefs is probably the most important functional skill that a person with a spinal cord injury can acquire. When someone with a complete injury sits for more than a few minutes, he requires periodic relief of pressure over his buttocks to prevent skin breakdown. This is true regardless of the quality of cushion on which he sits.[10] An individual who cannot perform pressure reliefs independently must depend upon assistance from others throughout the period of sitting.

The purpose of a pressure relief is to reduce the pressure on tissues that have been bearing weight, allowing circulation in areas that have been ischemic during weight bearing. When sitting with good posture, the bulk of weight bearing occurs on the ischial tuberosities. It is the skin over these bony prominences that must be relieved during a pressure relief.

People vary in their requirements for pressure relief. During rehabilitation, each must discover his skin's requirements for the duration of each pressure relief and the length of time that can pass between reliefs.

Sitting Push-up

Perhaps the quickest and most effective method of pressure relief is the sitting push-up. Someone with adequate strength in his triceps can eliminate pressure over his ischial tuberosities by lifting his buttocks completely off of the supporting surface. To do so, he places his hands lateral to his buttocks on the wheelchair's seat, armrests, or wheels. He then lifts his body by pushing down, extending his elbows and depressing his shoulders. A disadvantage of this method is that it may subject the upper extremities to damaging forces.[74]

Weight Shift

Pressure reliefs do not require complete elimination of pressure on the ischial tuberosities. A person with a spinal cord injury can perform an effective pressure relief by leaning forward enough to unweight his ischial tuberosities[9,75] or by leaning to one side and then the other, unweighting one side at a time.[9] Pressure reliefs performed by shifting weight forward or laterally instead of lifting the buttocks in a push-up may be less damaging to the upper extremities.[74,76]

Power Tilt or Recline

A person with a power tilt or recline feature on his wheelchair can perform pressure reliefs independently by using an access device to signal his chair to tilt or recline. He can use the same device that he uses to drive the chair, or he may use one or more alternate inputs. Regardless of the number of switches used, he must be able to direct the chair to tilt or recline fully and return to upright after the pressure relief.

Pressure Reliefs—Therapeutic Strategies

Training in the performance of pressure reliefs should begin as soon as possible after out-of-bed activities are initiated. Early emphasis on this skill may promote the development of good pressure relief habits.[P]

Patients who have wheelchairs without power tilt or recline features must learn to relieve the pressure on their buttocks either by performing sitting push-ups or by shifting their weight laterally or forward. Strategies for developing these skills are presented in Chapter 10.

[P] Chapter 5 presents additional information on skin care, including patient education and training.

A patient who performs pressure reliefs by tilting or reclining his power wheelchair must first learn to utilize the wheelchair's access device. (He must learn to place his hand on the joystick and move it, for example.) These prerequisite skills and therapeutic strategies for developing them are presented in the section that follows on driving power wheelchairs. Once a patient has begun learning to use the wheelchair's access device, he can practice tilting or reclining the wheelchair and returning it to upright.

Tilt or Recline Power Wheelchair and Return to Upright

If the patient utilizes a power wheelchair with a tilt or recline feature, the manner in which he signals the chair to perform this function will depend on the type of access device used. This will, in turn, be influenced by the patient's ability to utilize the various devices available. Functional training goes hand in hand with equipment selection and adjustment as the therapist and patient analyze the available options, select the input device that appears to best match the patient's abilities, and try the device.

An access device that does not require the patient to move against gravity will be as easy to utilize whether the patient is sitting upright or is tilted or reclined. Tongue-touch keypads and sip-and-puff devices are examples. With these devices, functional training involves instruction in the manner in which the individual will give commands to the chair, and practice of the skills involved.

Problem-Solving Exercise 11–2

Your patient has normal joint range of motion and muscle flexibility throughout his upper and lower extremities bilaterally. His upper extremity muscle test results are as follows:

Muscles	Left	Right
Trapezius (upper, middle, and lower)	4/5	4/5
Deltoids (anterior, middle, and posterior)	2+/5	2+/5
Elbow flexors	2+/5	2+/5
Radial wrist extensors	0/5	0/5
Serratus anterior	1/5	1/5
Pectoralis major (clavicular)	1/5	1/5
Triceps	0/5	0/5
Flexor digitorum profundus	0/5	0/5

The patient is learning to perform pressure reliefs by tilting the seating system of a power wheelchair, controlling the chair using a hand-held joystick. He can independently place his hand on the joystick and can move the joystick through its full excursion in all directions when the seating system is in its upright position. When he attempts to perform a pressure relief, however, his hand falls off of the joystick after he has tilted approximately 45 degrees from upright. He is then unable to lift his hand to place it back on the joystick to tilt further or to return to upright.

- Why is the patient unable to maintain his hand on the joystick while he tilts the chair through its full excursion?
- What equipment changes could enhance this patient's ability to perform a pressure relief and return to upright independently?
- What muscle strength could the therapeutic exercise program emphasize to facilitate the attainment of this goal?
- Describe a functional training activity for this patient.

An input device that is accessed through upper extremity motions may be more difficult to utilize when the patient sits in a tilted or reclined position. As the seating system tilts or reclines from upright, the user's body moves relative to the line of gravity, and the input device may also move relative to gravity. For example, a hand-held joystick is likely to be manipulated using arm motions performed in a horizontal plane when the seat is upright. The plane of motion of the joystick moves as the seat tilts back, and the patient must move his hand and arm against gravity to push the joystick forward. As a result, a person with severely limited upper extremity strength may be unable to signal the chair to perform a tilt through its full excursion, or return to upright from a tilted position. When this is the case, the patient can practice tilting and returning to upright over a small arc of motion, increasing the excursion as his ability increases. He may also improve his performance by strengthening his shoulder and elbow musculature. An alternative solution is the use of a different input device to control the chair's tilt function.

Driving a Power Wheelchair

A variety of options are available to enable people with limited physical capabilities to control power wheelchairs. Access devices commonly used to drive are joysticks, proximity head arrays, breath control, and tongue-touch keypads. These inputs, and the manner in which the wheelchair driver uses them, are described in Table 11–2. The physical and skill prerequisites required to drive a power wheelchair using these input devices are summarized in Tables 11–6 and 11–7.

Driving a Power Wheelchair–Therapeutic Strategies

Functional training involves practice of the prerequisite skills appropriate to the input device used: place a hand on the joystick and move it in all directions using arm and scapular motions; move the joystick in all directions using head, chin, or tongue motions; or signal the wheelchair by moving the head relative to sensors in the headrest, sipping and puffing in the appropriate pattern, or pressing the tongue against a tongue-touch keypad. Regardless of the type of input device, the person must also practice driving the wheelchair.

Place Hand on Joystick

A person who has enough strength in his deltoids and biceps to move well against gravity should be able to learn to place his hand on his wheelchair's joystick without difficulty. He may require only a demonstration and brief practice.

Someone with limited ability to move against gravity in elbow flexion and shoulder flexion and abduction may be able to learn this skill, but will require more practice. An individual with such pronounced upper extremity

weakness places his arm on the joystick using a combination of scapular, shoulder, and elbow motions. The maneuvers used are determined by the arm's starting position. If the arm is initially positioned hanging down outside of the armrest, the person elevates his scapula to lift his arm. By partially abducting and internally rotating his shoulder, he places his elbow in a gravity-reduced position for elbow flexion. He can then place his hand on the joystick by flexing his elbow.

If the person's arm is positioned in his lap, he uses a combination of scapular elevation and retraction, shoulder abduction and external rotation, and elbow flexion to place his hand on the joystick. Alternatively, he can use these motions to position his hand outside of the armrest, then lift it onto the joystick using the maneuver described above.

When an individual has limited ability to move his shoulder and elbow against gravity, practice of the required motions may begin with the arm suspended in a sling or supported by a skateboard placed on a board (Figure 11–9). Using this equipment, the patient can practice moving repeatedly through gravity-eliminated arcs. As his strength and skill improve, he can progress to moving up a slight slope and increase the slope as appropriate. With different positions of the sling or board, he can work on moving his shoulder and elbow through the various motions required to place his hand on a joystick. In this manner, he can build the strength required for this skill.

Skill training can begin with the patient working on moving his hand onto the joystick from a position just lateral to the stick. As his ability improves, he can move his hand from positions progressively lateral and inferior to the joystick. In this manner, he can gradually develop the ability to lift his hand onto the joystick, starting with his arm hanging at his side lateral to the armrest. The ability to perform this skill with the arm initially positioned in the lap can be developed using the same strategy: the patient begins by repeatedly placing his hand from a position just medial to the joystick. As his skill builds, he works from progressively medial and inferior starting positions.

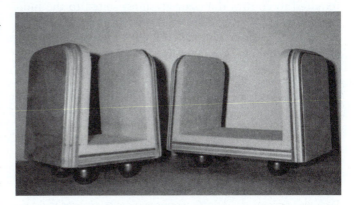

Figure 11–9 Skateboards.

Move Joystick in All Directions Using Arm and Scapular Motions

When a joystick is mounted for hand control, it is mounted in a vertical or nearly vertical position. To control his wheelchair, the person must be able to move his hand in all directions in a horizontal or nearly horizontal plane. Independent placement of the hand on the joystick is not necessary for practicing this skill. Practice in moving a joystick should be done with the wheelchair's motor off or disconnected from the wheels (clutch disengaged).

People with good scapular and shoulder control are not likely to need much training to master this skill. They may require only a demonstration and brief period of practice. Individuals with weaker proximal musculature require more extensive training. Before learning to push a joystick, they must develop the ability to perform the necessary motions. Practice may begin with the arm suspended in an overhead sling or supported by a skateboard placed on a board. Using this equipment, the patient can practice moving his hand in all directions in the horizontal plane. Backward and forward motion can be accomplished using scapular adduction and abduction.[q] Glenohumeral rotation and horizontal adduction and abduction are used for lateral motions. Diagonal motions are performed by combining these glenohumeral and scapular motions.

The patient can practice using a joystick once he is able to move his hand well with his arm supported by a sling or skateboard. If he remains unable to move the joystick, the therapist can facilitate practice by making the task easier. This can be done by suspending the arm in an overhead sling or mobile arm support, splinting the elbow and wrist, and strapping the hand to the joystick.[r] These "crutches" can be removed[s] as the patient's skill improves with practice.[64, 77]

Particularly if the patient has very limited upper extremity strength, the training period with the wheelchair is likely to involve a fair amount of equipment adjustment. The joystick can be moved in any plane: it can be placed in a more medial, lateral, anterior, posterior, superior or inferior position; rotated in the horizontal plane; or tilted from vertical in any direction. By altering the joystick's position, the therapist can place it so that the motions required to control the chair are most suited to the individual's patterns of strength and weakness. In addition to placing the joystick optimally in space, the therapist can alter the joystick/user interface. The stick can be made taller or thicker, or a grip shaped like a ball, a "T" or a

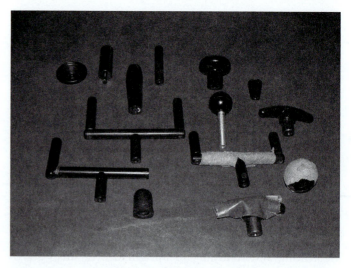

Figure 11–10   Examples of joystick attachments (also called extensions) that can accommodate different manipulation abilities. Attachments in lower right corner have been wrapped in high-friction material.

goal post can be added to enhance the individual's capacity to manipulate it (Figure 11–10). The therapist and patient should work together to determine the joystick position and configuration of the joystick/user interface that will be most comfortable and functional.

Move Joystick in All Directions Using Head, Chin, or Tongue Motions

When a joystick is mounted for head control, the headrest is the interface between the patient and the joystick. The patient controls the wheelchair by pushing the headrest backward or to the side. When a joystick is mounted for chin or mouth control, it is placed in a position close to horizontal; the end of the joystick moves in a nearly vertical plane. To control his wheelchair, the person moves the end of the joystick in all directions within this plane. With chin control, neck and jaw motions are used to move the stick up, down, laterally, and diagonally. With mouth control, the patient uses his tongue to push the joystick.

The therapist should explain and demonstrate the motions and allow the patient to practice pushing the stick in all directions. Practice moving the joystick should be done with the wheelchair's motor off or disconnected.

Mastery of this ability is likely to be more a matter of equipment adjustment than skill development. The therapist and patient should work together to determine the joystick position, and configuration of the joystick/user interface, that will be most comfortable and functional.

Signal Wheelchair by Moving Head Toward and Away From Sensors in Headrest

If the patient is learning to use a proximity head array, the therapist should explain and demonstrate how head motions can be used to signal the chair by activating sensors

---

[q] In the absence of active scapular abduction, the patient can adduct actively using the middle trapezius and allow passive abduction upon relaxation of the trapezius.

[r] These strategies can also be employed while the patient is practicing driving the wheelchair.

[s] These "crutches" should be removed one at a time as skill increases. With each removal, the patient's performance can be expected to deteriorate temporarily until his skill improves.

in the headrest. The patient can practice initially with the wheelchair's motor off or disconnected.

Signal Wheelchair by Sipping and Puffing in Appropriate Pattern

If the patient is learning to use breath control, the therapist should explain and demonstrate the sipping and puffing pattern and allow the patient to practice. The patient will need to develop both the technique of delivering hard and soft sips to the straw with the appropriate force, and will need to learn the "code" of sips and puffs that are used to signal the chair. Initial practice should be done with the wheelchair's motor off or disconnected. The equipment typically includes a visual display that can be used to provide feedback to the patient about the signal that he has provided.

Signal Wheelchair by Pressing Tongue Against Sensors in Tongue-Touch Keypad

The therapist should show the patient the sensors embedded in the tongue-touch keypad, and explain how it works. The patient will need to develop his skill in contacting the desired sensors with his tongue, and will need to learn how the sensors are used to signal the chair. Initial practice should be done with the wheelchair's motor off or disconnected. The equipment typically includes a visual display that can be used to provide feedback to the patient about the signal that he has provided.

Drive Power Wheelchair

Before practicing driving a power wheelchair, a person should have developed some initial skill in signaling the wheelchair using the access device. Driving practice should begin in a large area that is free of obstacles and potential victims. A therapist should be present to override the controls when necessary. Ideally, the wheelchair will have a "kill switch" that can be used to stop the chair if a collision is imminent.

When training first begins, the controller should be adjusted so that the chair's maximum velocity, turning speed, and rates of acceleration and deceleration are all slow. These parameters can be adjusted as the patient's skill improves.

During early work on driving, emphasis should be placed on gaining control of the chair. The patient should practice starting, stopping, and maneuvering in all directions. Once he has mastered these tasks, he can progress to driving over greater distances, maneuvering around obstacles, and driving over inclines, uneven terrain, and doorsills.

Once an individual has gained some ability to control his chair, he can practice without constant supervision. He may first practice within the department, where assistance is available when needed. As his skill and confidence improve, he can practice in other areas, further removed from assistance. When driving a chair independently, the wheelchair user should have a means of effecting an "emergency stop." If he is driving with a hand-held joystick, and if he is

consistently able to remove his hand from the joystick while driving, he can stop the chair by lifting his hand from the joystick. Otherwise, he will need a separate "kill switch," typically a leaf switch or button switch that can be activated using head or scapular motions.

Propulsion of Manual Wheelchair With Standard Handrims

A person with functioning finger flexors can propel his wheelchair by grasping the handrims and pulling forward or backward. The following descriptions of techniques for propelling forward, backward, and turning are appropriate for people who lack functional finger flexors. In these techniques, friction is used to move the handrims. The physical and skill prerequisites required to propel a manual wheelchair with standard handrims are summarized in Tables 11–8 and 11–9.

Forward

To propel forward, a person who cannot grasp starts by placing his palms against the lateral surface of the handrims. His elbows are flexed and his shoulders are internally rotated slightly. Using elbow extension and combined shoulder adduction, external rotation, and flexion, he stabilizes his palms against the handrims and pushes forward.[t] In the absence of functioning triceps, the anterior deltoids are used to extend the elbows.

Regardless of whether the upper extremities are fully innervated, the wheelchair user should propel in a manner that is least injurious to his upper extremities. He should propel with long and smooth strokes, starting with his hands well back on the handrims and pushing until they are well forward (Figure 11–11). The direction of the push should be forward rather than down toward the wheels' axles.[12] As the person reaches back between strokes, he should allow his hands to drift down and back in a semicircular pattern while the wheelchair glides forward. By using this propulsion pattern and minimizing the frequency of his pushes, the wheelchair user may subject his upper extremities to lower levels of damaging forces.[5,21,78,79]

Backward

Backward propulsion without innervated finger flexors can be accomplished by reversing the technique for forward propulsion. The person places his palms on the outer surface of the handrims, squeezes in, and pulls back (Figure 11–12A).

In an alternate method of backward propulsion, the person places his palms on top of the tires with his hands facing backward, just posterior to his buttocks. He pushes

---

[t] People who cannot grasp the handrims must use a medially directed force to stabilize their palms against the handrims. This requirement makes wheelchair propulsion less efficient than propulsion with intact upper extremities.[88,89]

TABLE 11–8   Propulsion of Manual Wheelchair With Standard Handrims–Physical Prerequisites

		Forward	Backward, Pulling Handrims	Backward, Pushing Tires	Turning
Strength					
Trapezius		√	√	√	√
Anterior deltoids		☑	√	√	√
Middle deltoids		√	√	√	√
Posterior deltoids		√	√	√	√
Infraspinatus, teres minor		√		√	√
Pectoralis major, teres major		•	•		•
Biceps, brachialis, and/or brachioradialis		√	√	√	√
Serratus anterior		•			•
Triceps		•		•	•
Hand musculature (active grasp)		•	•	•	•
Range of Motion					
Scapular	Elevation			√	
	Depression			√	
	Abduction	√			
	Adduction	√	√	√	√
Shoulder	Flexion	√	√		√
	Extension	√	√	√	√
	Internal rotation	√	√		√
	External rotation	√		☑	√
	Abduction			√	
Elbow	Flexion	√	√		√
	Extension	√	√	√	√

√ Some strength is needed for this activity, or severe limitations in range will inhibit this activity.
☑ A large amount of strength or normal or greater range is needed for this activity.
• Not required, but helpful.

backward on the tires by extending his elbows, using either triceps or anterior deltoids. (Figure 11–12B)

Someone who is unable to extend his elbows against the resistance supplied by his chair's wheels may be able to propel backward using a third method, illustrated in Figure 11–12C. When using this method, the person starts by placing his palms against the medial-superior surfaces of his tires, posterior to his buttocks. His shoulders should be externally rotated and elevated and his elbows locked[u] in

extension. By depressing his scapulae, he then pushes the wheels backward.

Turning

The technique used to turn will depend upon the turning radius desired. Turning in a long arc simply involves pushing harder with one hand than the other, or pushing one wheel while applying resistance to the other. To turn sharply, the wheelchair user can pull one wheel backward while he pushes the other one forward. The techniques for pushing the wheels forward and backward are the same as those described in the preceding paragraphs.

---

[u] Elbow locking is addressed in Chapter 10.

TABLE 11–9   Propulsion of Manual Wheelchair With Standard Handrims–Skill Prerequisites

	Forward	Backward, Pulling Handrims	Backward, Pushing Tires	Turning
Maintain upright sitting position*	√	√	√	√
Place palms against standard handrims (pp. 259, 260)	√	√		√
Push standard handrim(s) forward (pp. 260, 261)	√			√
Pull standard handrim(s) backward (p. 261)		√		
Place palms on tires, behind seat (p. 261)			√	
With palms on tires behind seat, propel wheelchair backward using elbow extension and scapular depression or using only scapular depression (p. 262)			√	
Propel manual wheelchair over even surfaces (p. 261)	√			

* Refer to Chapter 10 for a description of this skill and therapeutic strategies.
√ This prerequisite skill is required to perform this activity.

Propulsion of Manual Wheelchair With Standard Handrims–Therapeutic Strategies

Practice of manual wheelchair propulsion can begin as soon as the individual is able to tolerate an upright or near-upright position. Individuals with intact upper extremities can typically begin practice propelling after receiving a brief explanation of propulsion strategies. Patients with impaired hand function are likely to benefit from practice of the prerequisite skills separately and in combination, and progress

to propelling the wheelchair. Strategies for developing the prerequisite skills are described in the following paragraphs.

Place Palms Against Standard Wheelchair Handrims

Most people who have the physical potential to propel a manual wheelchair are able to place their palms against their chairs' handrims without practice. A few, however, have difficulty recognizing when their palms are in contact with the handrims. These patients require training in this prerequisite skill.

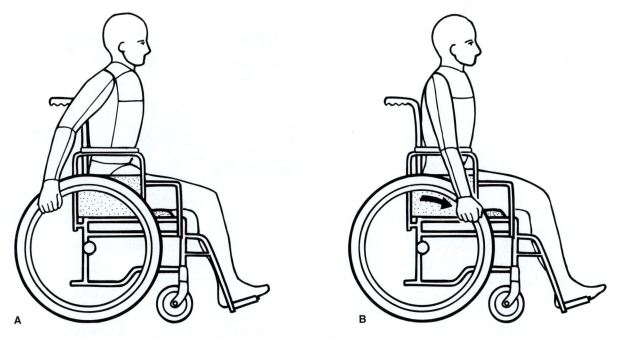

A   B

Figure 11–11   Efficient wheelchair propulsion using long strokes.

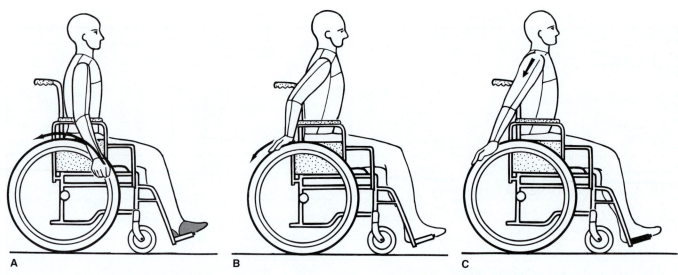

Figure 11–12   Backward propulsion without innervated finger flexors, using standard handrims. (A) Squeezing in and pulling back on handrims. (B) Pushing back on tires using elbow extension. (C) Pushing back on tires using scapular depression.

When training is required, the patient should be encouraged to focus on alternative sensory cues to recognize when his hands are placed appropriately. He can concentrate on proprioceptive and tactile sensations from his hands and arms while the therapist places his hands passively on the chair's handrims. He can progress to placing his hands with assistance and finally, practice placing his hands without help.

Push Standard Handrim(s) Forward

To practice this skill, a patient should be able to place his palms against the wheelchair's handrims. Most people with intact upper extremity musculature are able to push their wheelchair handrims forward without extensive training. At most, they may require brief instruction and practice. People who lack functioning finger flexors require more training to acquire this skill. They must learn to compensate for their lack of active grasp, moving the handrims by pressing their palms inward against the rims and pushing forward. Handrims with a high-friction surface will make this task easier. During early practice, therapists can move their patients' hands passively to give them a feel for the motions involved. The patient can then assist with the motions and progress to pushing without assistance.

Because moving a wheelchair's handrims involves moving the wheelchair, this skill is difficult for many who have impaired upper extremity function. The therapist can make the task easier by placing the chair's casters in a trailing position (Figure 11–13). If an individual remains unable to move his handrims despite this positioning, the therapist can assist with the chair's motion. While the patient attempts to push the handrims forward, the therapist pushes the chair, providing just enough force to enable him to move the wheelchair. As his ability and strength improve, the assistance should be decreased.

The functional training strategy just described is appropriate if the individual is on the verge of being able to propel

without assistance. This approach has the advantage of enabling the patient to develop propulsion skills using the type of handrims that he will ultimately use. Unfortunately, this training strategy does not allow for independent practice.

When a patient lacks the strength to propel his wheelchair without assistance, the therapist can make the task easier by wrapping the chair's handrims with rubber tubing (Figure 11–14). The tubing provides small handholds for the patient, making it easier to push the handrims. Because the handholds are small, he must use the same motions to propel the chair as he would without the tubing: he squeezes in and pushes forward. Thus, while he practices pushing his chair with the handrims wrapped, he develops the musculature and skills required for propulsion without tubing.[v]

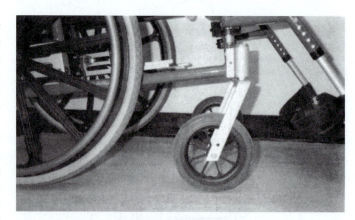

Figure 11–13   Caster in trailing position.

---

[v] One nice thing about rubber tubing is that it deteriorates. Thus as the patient's strength and skill are improving, the tubing is gradually disintegrating. Often, the individual's readiness to progress to propulsion without tubing coincides with the tubing's deterioration. This can make the transition to propulsion without tubing easier.

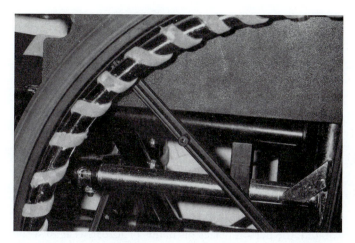

Figure 11–14   Wheelchair handrim wrapped in rubber tubing.

Some people initially lack the strength to push a chair, even with the handrims wrapped in tubing. When this is the case, the therapist may resort to placing pegged handrims on the patient's chair. Handrim projections (pegs) can enable a weak individual to propel his chair, making practice possible. The patient should grow stronger with practice and may eventually build his strength enough to enable him to propel with standard handrims. The disadvantage of practicing with pegged handrims is that the motions used are different from those used to propel with standard handrims. Instead of squeezing in and pushing forward, the wheelchair user simply pulls forward on the handrim projections.[w] Because the musculature and skills involved are different, the transition from pegged to standard handrims will be more difficult than a transition from wrapped to unwrapped standard handrims.

Regardless of the type of handrim used, wheelchair propulsion practice should begin on hard and smooth floor surfaces such as linoleum tile. Propelling over this type of surface is easier than propelling over carpet.[80, 81]

Propel Manual Wheelchair Over Even Surfaces

Once an individual is able to push his handrims forward, with or without assistance, he is ready to begin work on forward wheelchair propulsion. The therapist should explain and demonstrate propulsion techniques described earlier that minimize injurious forces on the upper extremities. During early practice, the therapist should give the patient feedback on his propulsion technique.

The therapist and patient should remember that wheelchair propulsion is difficult initially if upper extremity musculature is impaired. Pushing is likely to be too slow to be functional at first, but the patient should keep at it. The only way to become more proficient is to practice.

Once an individual is able to propel his chair forward and turn without assistance, he can practice independently. He should be encouraged to push to therapies and meals during the day, and can propel during his free time in the evenings. In addition to practicing propulsion, the patient can exercise on an arm cycle ergometer to improve his wheelchair propulsion endurance.[82]

Pull Standard Handrim(s) Backward

Before working on this skill, a patient should be able to place his palms against the wheelchair's handrims.

Most people with intact upper extremity musculature are able to pull their wheelchair handrims backward without extensive training. At most, they may require brief instruction and practice.

People who lack functioning finger flexors require more training to acquire this skill. They must learn to compensate for their lack of active grasp, moving the handrims by pressing their palms inward against the rims and pulling backward. During early practice, therapists may move their patients' hands passively to give them a feel for the motions involved. The patients can then assist with the motions and progress to pulling their handrims backward without assistance.

This skill is difficult for many people who have impaired upper extremity function. The therapist can make the task easier by positioning the chair's casters anteriorly (Figure 11–15). If an individual remains unable to move his handrims despite this positioning, the therapist can provide assistance. As the patient's ability and strength improve, the assistance should be decreased.

Place Palms on Tires, Behind Seat

A patient must be able to place his arms behind his chair's push handles before he begins work on this skill.[x] Once he has acquired that prerequisite skill, learning to place his palms on the tires should require only demonstration and a brief period of practice.

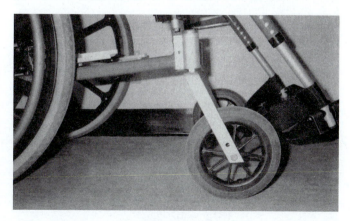

Figure 11–15   Caster positioned anteriorly.

---

[w] Functional techniques and therapeutic strategies for propulsion using pegged handrims are presented later in the chapter.

[x] Strategies for developing the ability to place the arms behind the push handles are described in Chapter 10.

With Palms on Tires Behind Seat, Propel Backward Using Elbow Extension and Scapular Depression

To practice this skill, a patient should be able to place his palms on his wheelchair's tires, behind the seat. An individual who lacks functional strength in his triceps must be able to extend his elbows using muscle substitution.[y]

During initial practice, the therapist may move the patient's arms passively to give him a feel for the motions. With the casters positioned anteriorly (Figure 11–15), the patient can then assist with the motions and progress to pushing the wheels backward without assistance.

With Palms on Tires Behind Seat, Propel Backward Using Scapular Depression

People who are unable to propel their wheelchairs backward using combined elbow extension and scapular depression may learn to do so using scapular depression alone. To practice this skill, a patient should be able to place his palms on the wheelchair's tires, behind the seat. Training can be done using the strategy just described for backward propulsion using elbow extension and scapular depression.

Propulsion of Manual Wheelchair With Handrim Projections

Inadequate strength or range of motion can make propulsion with standard handrims impossible or prohibitively difficult. Handrim projections, also called pegs, may make propulsion easier in these instances. The physical and skill prerequisites

---

[y] Strategies for developing the skill of elbow extension using muscle substitution are described in Chapter 10.

required to propel a manual wheelchair with pegged handrims are summarized in Tables 11–10 and 11–11.

Forward

To propel forward using pegged handrims, each palm or forearm is placed behind a peg. Using shoulder and elbow flexion, the wheelchair user pulls forward on the pegs. Propulsion will be more efficient if he uses long strokes, starting with his hands on pegs that are posterior to his buttocks (Figure 11–16).

Backward

Backward propulsion can be accomplished by pulling back on the handrim projections. With his shoulders internally rotated, the person places his hands or forearms against the front aspects of anteriorly located pegs. He then pulls back using glenohumeral extension and scapular adduction.

An individual who is strong enough may be able to propel backward by pushing against the backs of his tires, as described earlier.

Turning

Turning is accomplished in the same manner as turning a wheelchair with standard handrims. Using the techniques described above, the person pushes one wheel harder than the other or pushes one wheel forward while pulling the other backward.

Propulsion of Manual Wheelchair with Handrim Projections–Therapeutic Strategies

Practice of propulsion with pegged handrims can begin as soon as the individual is able to tolerate an upright or near-upright position. The patient can practice the prerequisite

---

TABLE 11–10   Propulsion of Manual Wheelchair With Pegged Handrims–Physical Prerequisites

		Forward	Backward	Turning
Strength				
Trapezius		√	√	√
Anterior deltoids		√	√	√
Middle deltoids		√	√	√
Posterior deltoids		√	√	√
Biceps, brachialis, and/or brachioradialis		√	√	√
Pectoralis major, teres major			√	
Range of Motion				
Scapular	Adduction		√	
Shoulder	Flexion	√	√	√
	Extension	√	√	√
	Internal rotation		√	
Elbow	Extension	√	√	√

√ Some strength is needed for this activity or severe limitations in range will inhibit this activity.

TABLE 11–11   Propulsion of Manual Wheelchair with Pegged Handrims–Skill Prerequisites

	Forward	Backward	Turning
Maintain upright sitting position[*]	√	√	√
Place palms or forearms against handrim projections (p. 263)	√	√	√
Pull handrim projections forward (p. 263)	√		√
Pull backward on handrim projections (pp. 263, 264)		√	√
Propel manual wheelchair over even surfaces (pp. 261, 263)	√		

[*] Refer to Chapter 10 for a description of this skill and therapeutic strategies.
√ This prerequisite skill is required to perform this activity.

skills separately and in combination, and progress to propelling the wheelchair. Strategies for developing the prerequisite skills are described in the following paragraphs.

Place Palms or Forearms Against Handrim Projections

Most people who have the physical potential to propel a manual wheelchair are able to place their palms or forearms against their chairs' handrim projections without practice. A few, however, have difficulty recognizing when they have made contact with the pegs. When this is the case, the patient should be encouraged to focus on alternative sensory cues. The wheelchair user can concentrate on proprioceptive and tactile sensations from his hands and arms while the therapist places his palms or forearms passively against the handrim projections. He can progress to placing his hands with assistance and finally practice placing his hands without help.

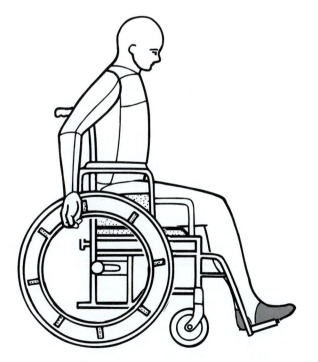

Figure 11–16   Forward propulsion using pegged handrims.

Pull Handrim Projections Forward

Once a patient has developed the ability to place his palms or forearms against his chair's handrim projections, he can work on pulling them forward. During early practice, therapists can move their patients' arms passively to give them a feel for the motions involved. Patients can then assist with the motions and progress to pushing without assistance.

Because moving a wheelchair's handrims involves moving the wheelchair, this skill is difficult for many people who have impaired upper extremity function. As is true with standard handrims, initial practice with pegged handrims should begin on a smooth floor surface such as linoleum. The therapist can make the task easier by placing the chair's casters in a trailing position (Figure 11–13). Propulsion will also be easier if the handrim projections are positioned symmetrically on the two sides of the chair. If an individual remains unable to move his handrims despite this positioning of the casters and pegs, the therapist can assist with the chair's motion. While the patient attempts to push the handrims forward, the therapist pushes the chair, providing just enough force to enable him to move the wheelchair. As the patient's ability and strength improve, this assistance should be decreased.

If a patient is able to propel his wheelchair forward easily, he is probably ready to work with standard handrims.

Propel Manual Wheelchair Over Even Surfaces

Once an individual is able to push his handrims forward, with or without assistance, he is ready to begin work on forward wheelchair propulsion. The training strategy is the same as described for propulsion with standard handrims.

Pull Backward on Handrim Projections

Before practicing this skill, a person should be able to place his palms or forearms against the anterior aspects of his chair's handrim projections.

Training in this skill should begin with a demonstration of how a wheelchair can be propelled backward by placing the hands or forearms in front of anteriorly located handrim projections and pulling backward. During early practice, therapists may move their patients' arms passively to give them a feel for the motions involved. Patients can then assist with the motions and progress to pulling without assistance. The strategies just described for pulling forward can be utilized: casters positioned (anteriorly) to make the task easier, handrim projections symmetrical, and assistance provided as needed.

Wheelies–Functional Techniques and Therapeutic Strategies

A wheelie is a maneuver in which the wheelchair's casters are lifted off of the ground and the wheelchair rests on its rear wheels. It is not a functional goal in and of itself. Rather, it is a prerequisite skill, used to negotiate uneven terrain and curbs, and in some circumstances to descend steep ramps and stairs. Some individuals also use wheelies for pressure relief.

During much of functional training in wheelie skills, hands-off (noncontact) guarding is best. If the therapist's hands remain on the push handles while the patient works to maintain his balance or move in a wheelie position, the therapist is likely to make corrections for him. This will deprive the patient of practice and can make it difficult for him to discern when he has moved off of his balance point. Hands-off guarding can be performed as shown in Figure 11–17 or using a strap attached to the wheelchair's frame.[z] The therapist should allow the chair to fall a short distance when it moves too far from the balance point, so the patient can feel that he has lost his balance and needs to make corrections.

Maintain Balance Point in Wheelie Position

The balance point in a wheelie is the position in which a wheelchair is on its rear wheels and is in equilibrium, falling neither forward nor backward. A patient need not be able to assume his balance point independently before beginning practice in maintaining this position.

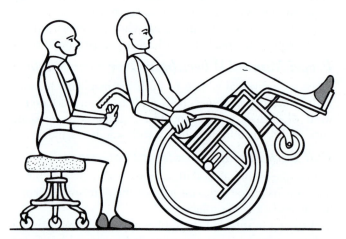

Figure 11–17 Noncontact guarding for wheelie practice.

The first step in teaching a person how to maintain his balance point in a wheelie is showing him where that point is located. If the individual has an inaccurate understanding of where his balance point is located, he will be unable to maintain the correct position. (If his notion of the balance point is tilted forward from the correct position, he will resist tipping his chair back far enough. As a result, he will constantly fall forward.) To teach a person where his balance point is located, the therapist can demonstrate in his own chair and then tip the patient back[aa] and allow him to feel the position.

After showing the patient his balance point, the therapist should teach him how to control his chair in a wheelie. With the therapist guarding closely, the patient can pull his handrims forward and back while in a wheelie position, paying attention to the effects that these maneuvers have on the chair's position (Figure 11–18). Gross motions are acceptable at this point; the purpose of this exercise is to familiarize the patient with the control motions.

Once the patient has learned how to tip his chair forward and back in a wheelie, he is ready to begin working on maintaining his balance point. The therapist can assist the patient to the balance point and encourage him to keep the chair balanced. The patient is likely to overcorrect at first. He should be encouraged to maintain his balance with smaller corrections. The therapist should spot closely but quickly progress to noncontact guarding.

Fear is often the largest barrier to learning this skill. Someone who is afraid of falling over backward is unlikely to allow himself to remain tipped far enough back to balance. He will attempt to maintain the chair's wheelie in a position tilted too far forward and, as a result, will not be able to balance. This tendency is compounded by the fact that wheelchairs balance at a point that is tilted further back than most would expect. A patient may feel as though he is about to fall backward when he is at his balance point. Therapists can help by attending to their patients' feelings during functional training. The therapist should remain reassuring and calm, and should encourage the patient to relax. When assisting a fearful patient to his balance point, the therapist should avoid quick, jerky motions that may increase the patient's fear. In addition, the therapist can assure the patient that he will catch him if he starts to fall.

If a patient is able to get into a balanced wheelie position without assistance, he can practice maintaining that position independently, using safety rigging to prevent falls. Figure 11–19 illustrates a setup in which the wheelchair's push handles are secured to suspended straps. The straps are attached with enough slack to allow the patient to move slightly past his balance point but without enough slack to allow him to fall to the floor.

[z] If using a strap, the therapist should hold it so that there is enough slack to allow the patient to move past his balance point, but if the chair tips too far back the therapist will be able to prevent a fall by pulling on the strap.

[aa] The therapist should take care to show the patient his true balance point. The balance point is easily found if the therapist pays attention to the force that he must exert on the chair to keep it tipped back on the rear wheels. At the balance point, the chair will remain in position (briefly) without any assistance from the therapist. If the chair is tipped too far back or forward, the therapist will have to apply force to keep the chair from tipping further back or forward, respectively.

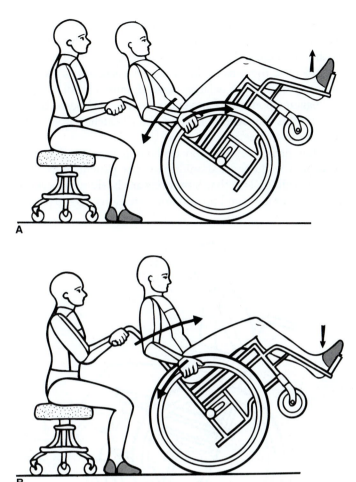

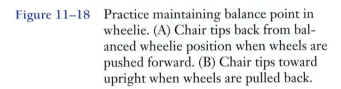

Figure 11–18   Practice maintaining balance point in wheelie. (A) Chair tips back from balanced wheelie position when wheels are pushed forward. (B) Chair tips toward upright when wheels are pulled back.

Assume Wheelie Position

To assume a wheelie position, the wheelchair user essentially tips his chair over backward. This skill may be easier to acquire if the patient has initiated (not necessarily completed) training in maintaining his balance in a wheelie. This prior exposure to wheelies can give him an understanding of how far back he must tip his chair, and it can make him less fearful about falling over backward.

A wheelchair's construction and alignment influence the difficulty of this task. An ultralight wheelchair with its axles positioned relatively anteriorly is easy to tip backward. A heavier wheelchair or more posteriorly located axles makes the task more difficult.

With intact upper extremities and an ultralight wheelchair, the wheelie position can be attained easily from a stationary position. The wheelchair user grasps[bb] the handrims posteriorly and pulls them forward abruptly and

---

[bb] An individual who lacks functioning finger flexors moves his handrims using friction, pressing in on the rims instead of grasping them.

Figure 11–19   Safety rigging for independent practice of achieving and maintaining wheelie position.

forcefully. If an individual is unable to lift his casters in this manner, he may be able to do so by throwing his head back when he pulls the handrims.

Impaired upper extremity function, a heavy wheelchair, or posteriorly located axles make it more difficult to tilt a chair back. People who are unable to "pop a wheelie" from a stationary position may be able to accomplish the task using the following technique: grasp the handrims anteriorly, pull backward, then abruptly and forcefully reverse the direction of pull. The person may find the task easier if he throws his head back when he pulls the handrims forward.

During early practice, the therapist should encourage the patient to use abrupt, forceful motions. The aim is to disturb the wheelchair's balance, tipping it over backward. The patient will not accomplish this if he "eases into" his motions. To gain enough momentum to tilt his chair, he may need to exaggerate his motions at first. He can refine his motions as he develops a feel for the maneuver.

An individual who is unable to lift his casters may be pulling the handrims in the wrong direction, throwing his head in the wrong direction, or timing his maneuvers incorrectly. The therapist should observe him as he makes his attempts, and give him feedback on his technique.

For some, this skill takes a good deal of practice to achieve. Independent work will make this extensive practice feasible. Safety rigging, described earlier and illustrated in

Figure 11–19, is required to keep the patient from falling backward. With this safety rigging, an individual who has been instructed and has received some initial practice and feedback can independently practice attaining his balance point.

Glide Forward in Wheelie Position

Before beginning training in this skill, a person should be able to assume and maintain his balance point in a wheelie.

To initiate a forward glide in a wheelie, the wheelchair user positions his chair at its balance point (Figure 11–20A) and tips the chair forward slightly. The forward tilt will make the chair start to fall forward (dip; Figure 11–20B). The person counteracts this fall and propels the chair by pushing forward on the handrims (Figure 11–20C). He should allow the rims to slide through his hands as his chair glides forward in its balance point (Figure 11–20D). From the balance point, he can repeat the dip and push. By repeating this sequence of actions, the wheelchair user glides forward in a wheelie.

After demonstrating and explaining how to glide in a wheelie, the therapist should allow the patient to practice with guarding. The chair's motions are likely to be jerky at first, with exaggerated up and down motions. As the patient

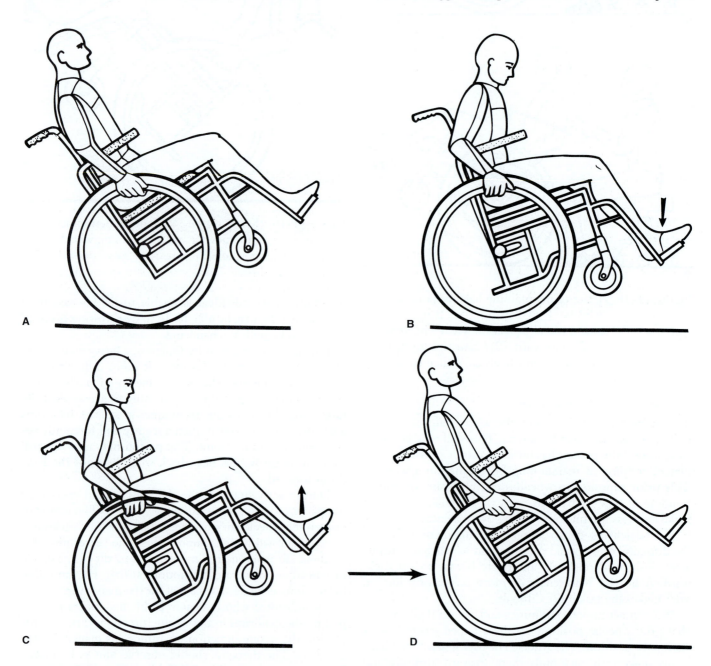

Figure 11–20   Forward glide in a wheelie. (A) Starting position: balanced wheelie position. (B) Wheelchair falls forward slightly. (C) Forward push on handrims propels chair forward and lifts casters. (D) Glide in balance point.

gains skill and confidence, the therapist should encourage him to smooth out the motion. The patient should also work to gain *control* of his glide; to use a glide functionally, he will need to be able to glide at various speeds, turn, and stop his chair at will. With practice, he should gain the capacity to glide faster and with greater control and less vertical motion of the casters.

Turn in Wheelie Position

Before initiating practice of this skill, the patient should be able to assume and maintain his balance point in a wheelie.

Turning in place while balanced on two wheels can be accomplished by pushing one handrim forward while pulling the other back. To turn while propelling forward or backward in a wheelie, the wheelchair user can push or pull one handrim more forcefully than the other. As he turns, he must make adjustments as necessary to keep his chair in a balanced position.

After demonstrating and explaining how to turn in a wheelie, the therapist should allow the patient to practice with guarding. At first, the chair's motions are likely to be jerky, with excessive vertical motions of the casters. As the patient gains skill and confidence, the therapist should encourage him to smooth out the motion.

Propel Backward in Wheelie Position

To practice this skill, a patient should be able to assume and maintain his balance point in a wheelie.

Propelling backward in a wheelie is like gliding forward, with the actions performed in reverse. From a balanced wheelie position, the wheelchair user tips his chair back slightly. The backward tilt will make the chair start to fall backward. The person counteracts this fall and propels the chair backward by pulling back on the handrims.

After demonstrating and explaining how to propel backward in a wheelie, the therapist should allow the patient to practice with guarding. At first, the chair's motions are likely to be jerky. As the patient gains skill and confidence, the therapist can encourage him to smooth out the motion.

Negotiating Inclines in a Manual Wheelchair

Ramps, curb cuts, and hills present similar challenges to wheelchair users: propelling up a slope involves a risk of tipping/falling over backward, and requires greater force than does propelling on a horizontal surface. Descending a slope in a wheelchair involves controlling the chair as gravity causes it to roll downhill. To be safe when descending a ramp or hill in a wheelchair, the wheelchair user should maintain control of the chair for the entire length of the slope; he should be able to steer to the right or left and stop at will. If he does not have this level of control, he may eventually collide with someone or something that gets in the way. There is no guarantee that a clear path will stay clear as a wheelchair descends a slope.

The physical and skill prerequisites required to negotiate inclines in a manual wheelchair are included in Tables 11–12 and 11–13.

Ascending

Fully innervated upper extremities make ramp ascension easier but are not required for this activity. Someone with C6 tetraplegia may be able to negotiate mild slopes. More and stronger innervated musculature will make it possible to negotiate steeper and longer inclines.[83]

Propulsion up an incline is accomplished on four wheels, using variations of the techniques described previously for forward propulsion. The techniques are altered to enable the wheelchair user to propel up the ramp without tipping over backward or rolling backward between pushes. To ascend a ramp without tipping over backward, the wheelchair user pushes forward forcefully but avoids jerking the wheels abruptly. A forward lean of the head and (when possible) trunk will also help prevent backward tipping. To avoid rolling backward between pushes, he uses shorter strokes and repositions his hands rapidly between pushes.

Descending on Four Wheels

When descending a slope, the wheelchair user keeps the chair under control by resisting its motion. He can slow or turn the chair by applying resistance to the handrims.

A person with functioning hand musculature can control the chair by gripping the handrims loosely and allowing them to slide through his hands. His grip should provide enough resistance to the handrims to slow and control the chair's descent. An individual who lacks functioning finger flexors can control the chair's descent by pressing his palms against the handrims, slightly in front of his hips.

Descending in a Wheelie Position

Many ramps and curb cuts are steep, with an abrupt angle at the bottom where they meet the street or sidewalk. When a person descends such a ramp or curb cut on four wheels, the footplates may "bottom out," striking the street or sidewalk. The chair comes to an abrupt stop, and the rider may be thrown out of the chair. This problem can be avoided by descending the slope in a wheelie.

Descending an incline in a wheelie is an easy skill to master for anyone who can glide on two wheels. The wheelchair user approaches the slope in a wheelie, then grips the chair's handrims loosely and allows them to slide through his hands as he descends the slope. His grip should provide just enough resistance to slow and control the chair's descent. Good hand function is required for this skill.

Negotiating Inclines in a Manual Wheelchair—Therapeutic Strategies

Practice in negotiation of inclines should begin on a gentle slope, as this will make the task easier. However, training should not be limited to the gentle 1:12 grade of

TABLE 11–12   Negotiation of Inclines and Uneven Terrain–Physical Prerequisites

	Ascend Incline	Descend Incline on Four Wheels	Descend Incline in Wheelie Position	Negotiate Uneven Terrain on Four Wheels	Negotiate Uneven Terrain in Wheelie
Strength					
Trapezius	✓	✓	✓	✓	✓
Anterior deltoids	☑	✓	✓	☑	☑
Middle deltoids	✓	✓	✓	✓	✓
Posterior deltoids	✓	✓	✓	✓	✓
Infraspinatus, teres minor	✓			✓	
Pectoralis major, teres major	•	•	✓	•	✓
Biceps, brachialis, and/or brachioradialis	✓	✓	✓	✓	✓
Serratus anterior	•			•	✓
Triceps	•		✓	•	✓
Hand musculature (active grasp)	•	•	✓	•	✓
Range of Motion					
Scapular — Abduction	✓		✓	✓	✓
Scapular — Adduction	✓		✓	✓	✓
Shoulder — Flexion	✓		✓	✓	✓
Shoulder — Extension	✓	✓	✓	✓	✓
Shoulder — Internal rotation	✓	✓	✓	✓	✓
Shoulder — External rotation	✓			✓	
Elbow — Flexion	✓	✓	✓	✓	✓
Elbow — Extension	✓		✓	✓	✓
Finger — Flexion			✓		✓

√ Some strength is needed for this activity, or severe limitations in range will inhibit this activity.
☑ A large amount of strength or normal or greater range is needed for this activity.
• Not required, but helpful.

a standard public incline. Many if not most ramps found in the community are far steeper than this. People undergoing rehabilitation should develop the skills needed to ascend and descend slopes as steep as possible within their potentials.

Propel a Manual Wheelchair up a Slope

To practice this skill, a person should be fairly proficient in wheelchair propulsion. Before attempting to ascend a ramp, the patient should be shown proper technique: forceful pushes with rapid repositioning of the hands between pushes, and a forward lean to reduce the risk of tipping backward. The patient should be encouraged to move his hands simultaneously and symmetrically, and to use shorter strokes than he uses for propulsion over even surfaces.

Practice in ramp negotiation should begin on an incline with a very gentle slope. Initially, the patient may not be able to push the chair forcefully enough to ascend. When this is the case, the therapist can assist, applying just enough force to the chair's push handles to enable the patient to push up the ramp with maximal effort. The assistance should be reduced as the patient's ability improves with practice.

People learning to push their wheelchairs up ramps often reposition their hands too slowly between pushes, allowing their chairs to roll backward excessively. Guarding is required to ensure safety at this point. While guarding, the therapist should allow a slight backward roll between pushes. The chair's motion, combined with verbal cueing, can provide feedback to the patient regarding his technique.

TABLE 11–13   Negotiation of Inclines and Uneven Terrain–Skill Prerequisites

	Ascend Incline	Descend Incline on Four Wheels	Descend Incline in Wheelie Position	Negotiate Uneven Terrain on Four Wheels	Negotiate Uneven Terrain in Wheelie
Propel wheelchair over even surfaces (p. 261)	√			√	
Propel wheelchair up a slope (pp. 268, 269)	√				
Descending slope on four wheels, control wheelchair by applying friction to handrims (p. 269)		√			
Assume wheelie position (pp. 265, 266)			√		√
Maintain balance point in wheelie position (p. 264)			√		√
Descending slope in wheelie, control wheelchair by applying friction to handrims (p. 269)			√		
Negotiate uneven terrain on four wheels (p. 270)				√	
Propel wheelchair forward (glide) in wheelie position (pp. 266, 267)			√		√
Turn in wheelie position (p. 267)					√
Propel backward in wheelie position (p. 267)					√
Negotiate uneven terrain in wheelie position (p. 270)					√

√ This prerequisite skill is required to perform this activity.

As a patient's skill in ascending slopes increases, the assistance given should be reduced. Once the individual masters a slope of a particular grade, he should progress to steeper slopes. Training in ramp negotiation can continue in this manner until the patient has reached his maximal potential.

Descending a Slope on Four Wheels, Control Wheelchair by Applying Friction to the Handrims

This skill should be practiced after a patient has become proficient in propulsion over even surfaces. During functional training, emphasis should be placed on controlling the chair's descent. To negotiate a ramp safely, a person must be able to stop the chair or turn while descending. This is possible only if he maintains control throughout the descent rather than releasing the handrims and trying to regain control when the need arises.

Practice in descending ramps should begin on gentle slopes at low speeds. Once an individual has developed the ability to slow, stop, and turn a manual wheelchair while slowly descending a gentle slope, he can progress to practicing at higher speeds and on steeper inclines.

Even on a mild incline and at a slow speed, a patient may be unable to control his chair's descent at first. When this is the case, the therapist can help to slow the chair. The therapist should resist the chair's downhill motion just enough to enable the patient to control the chair with maximal effort. This assistance can be reduced as his ability improves.

Descending a Slope on Two Wheels, Control Wheelchair by Applying Friction to the Handrims

This skill can be taught using the functional training strategies used to teach ramp descent on four wheels. Before beginning training, the patient should be skillful in gliding forward and turning in a wheelie.

Problem-Solving Exercise 11–3

Your outpatient has complete T8 paraplegia. His range of motion is normal in all extremities, and his strength is normal in all musculature innervated above the lesion. He reports that he has fallen twice while descending steep curb cuts. On both occasions, his footplates hit the pavement at the bottom of the curb cut and his chair tipped over forward.

- What technique can this person learn for safe descent of curb cuts?
- What are the physical prerequisites for this skill?
- What strength and range of motion should the therapeutic exercise program emphasize to facilitate the attainment of this goal?
- Describe a functional training program for this patient.

Negotiating Uneven Terrain in a Manual Wheelchair

Slightly uneven terrain, such as bumpy asphalt or a well-groomed lawn, may be negotiated using the same techniques as are used for propulsion over even surfaces. Propulsion will be more difficult on uneven surfaces, requiring more strength. Someone who is only marginally functional pushing on even surfaces will not be able to propel on uneven terrain.

Very uneven terrain is more challenging. A wheelchair's casters tend to get caught in ruts or bog down in gravel or sand. Because the greatest difficulty in propelling over uneven terrain involves catching or sinking of the casters, uneven surfaces are often easier to negotiate with the casters off the ground. The wheelchair user assumes a wheelie position and maintains it as he propels over the rough surface.

The physical and skill prerequisites required to negotiate uneven terrain in a manual wheelchair are included in Tables 11–12 and 11–13.

Negotiating Uneven Terrain in a Manual Wheelchair–Therapeutic Strategies

Once a patient has mastered propulsion over even surfaces, he should practice on slightly uneven terrain, such as a level sidewalk that is in good condition. As the patient's strength and skill improve, he can progress to more challenging surfaces such as grass, sand, gravel, and sidewalks in disrepair. The patient should practice negotiating the various surfaces that he is likely to encounter after his rehabilitation.

Negotiating Uneven Terrain on Four Wheels

To practice this skill, the patient should be proficient in propulsion over even surfaces. Propelling over slightly uneven terrain is primarily a matter of pushing hard. If the wheelchair's progress is impeded by a tough spot, such as a clump of grass, the person may be able to get past it by backing up and ramming the obstacle.[cc] The therapist can provide feedback and assistance as needed as the patient practices.

Negotiating Uneven Terrain in a Wheelie

The challenge of negotiating uneven terrain in a wheelie is maintaining one's balance. While pushing hard to propel his chair over irregularities in the supporting surface, the wheelchair user must compensate for the effects that these irregularities have on the chair's equilibrium. Before beginning work on this skill, a patient should be proficient in propulsion forward, backward, and turning in a wheelie on even surfaces. During practice on uneven terrain, the therapist can provide guarding, feedback, and assistance as needed.

Negotiating Curbs in a Manual Wheelchair

Although ramps and curb cuts have become fairly common, many public places remain inaccessible to wheelchairs. Certainly most private residences are inaccessible. It is likely that many places where an individual wants to go will not have ramps or will have ramps that are obstructed or placed in inconvenient locations.

Curb negotiation skills can be used to get over a variety of obstacles that block a wheelchair's path with a vertical obstruction. Examples of such obstacles include curbs at the junctures between streets and sidewalks, irregularities in sidewalks, elevated thresholds or weather stripping in doorways, and entranceways in which the floor on one side of the doorway is higher than on the other side.

Ideally, someone who uses a wheelchair for mobility in the community will be able to negotiate tall curbs – the taller the better. Any skill in curb negotiation will be helpful, however, no matter how limited. Even the ability to negotiate a 1-inch curb will be useful, making it possible to get over weather stripping or an irregularity in the sidewalk.

The height of curb that an individual will be able to master will be influenced by his lesion level as well as his strength and skill. It is possible for people with tetraplegia as high as C6 to ascend 2-inch and even 4-inch curbs using either of the following methods. Curb negotiation is challenging, however, with such a high lesion. It is more readily accomplished by people with fully innervated upper extremities. For many people with paraplegia, independent

---

[cc] Alternatively, he can pop his casters from the ground to lift them over the obstacle. Strategies for developing this skill are described above.

negotiation of 6-inch or higher curbs is a reasonable goal. The physical and skill prerequisites required to negotiate curbs in a manual wheelchair are included in Tables 11–14 and 11–15.

Ascending From Stationary Position

This curb ascension technique utilizes strength more than momentum. It requires less space than ascending using momentum because it does not involve a running start. It also requires less skill; the timing of motions is not as critical. However, this technique is more limited: higher curbs can be negotiated using momentum.

To ascend a curb from a stationary position, the wheelchair user approaches it front-on and stops a few inches shy of the curb (Figure 11–21A). From this position, he pops his casters onto the curb: starting with his hands well back on the handrims, he pulls forward forcefully and abruptly (Figure 11–21B). To lift his casters, he may need to throw his head back simultaneously with the pull.

Once the casters are on the curb, the person backs his chair until the casters are at the edge (Figure 11–21C). Positioning the chair in this manner makes it possible to gain some momentum in the next step.

When the casters are positioned appropriately, the wheelchair user places his hands well back on the handrims (Figure 11–21D). He then pulls forward forcefully and throws his head and trunk forward. If the wheels hit the curb with enough force, the chair will ascend (Figure 11–21E). During this step, the trunk may fall forward. This should not pose a problem; the person can return to an upright sitting position once the chair is past the curb.

TABLE 11–14 Negotiating Curbs–Physical Prerequisites

		Ascend From Stationary Position	Ascend Using Momentum	Descend Backward	Descend in Wheelie
Strength					
Trapezius		√	√	√	√
Anterior deltoids		☑	☑	√	√
Middle deltoids		√	√	√	√
Posterior deltoids		√	√	√	√
Infraspinatus, teres minor		√	√		
Pectoralis major, teres major		•	•	•	√
Biceps, brachialis, and/or brachioradialis		√	√	√	√
Serratus anterior		•	•	•	•
Triceps		•	•	•	√
Hand musculature (active grasp)		•	•	•	√
Range of Motion					
Scapular	Abduction	√	√	√	√
	Adduction	√	√	√	√
	Downward rotation	√	√		
Shoulder	Flexion	√	√		
	Extension	√	√	√	√
	Internal rotation	√	√	√	√
	External rotation	√	√		
Elbow	Flexion	√	√	√	√
	Extension	√	√	√	√
Finger	Flexion				√

√ Some strength is needed for this activity, or severe limitations in range will inhibit this activity.
☑ A large amount of strength or normal or greater range is needed for this activity.
• Not required, but helpful.

TABLE 11–15   Negotiating Curbs–Skill Prerequisites

	Ascend From Stationary Position	Ascend Using Momentum	Descend Backward	Descend in Wheelie
Position trunk in wheelchair*	√	√	√	
Propel manual wheelchair over even surfaces (p. 261)	√	√	√	
From stationary position, lift casters from floor (p. 275)	√			
Pop casters onto curb from stationary position (p. 275)	√			
Position casters at edge of curb (p. 275)	√			
Ascend curb from stationary position (p. 275)	√			
Lift casters off floor while chair moves forward (p. 275)		√		
Pop casters onto curb while chair moves forward (pp. 275, 276)		√		
Ascend curb using momentum (pp. 276, 277)		√		
Backing down curb, control rear wheels' descent (p. 277)			√	
Lower casters from curb by turning wheelchair (p. 277)			√	
Assume wheelie position (pp. 265, 266)				√
Glide forward in wheelie (pp. 266, 267)				√
Descend curb in wheelie position (p. 277)			√	

* Refer to Chapter 10 for a description of this skill and therapeutic strategies.
√ This prerequisite skill is required to perform this activity.

Ascending Using Momentum

Ascending a curb using momentum involves finesse rather than sheer muscle power. It is faster than ascending from a stationary position because the wheelchair user does not stop in front of the curb before ascending. Taking advantage of momentum also makes it possible to get up higher curbs than can be ascended from a stationary position.

Using this method, some people with C6 tetraplegia can ascend low curbs. An exceptionally skillful person with fully innervated upper extremities can ascend 10-inch or higher curbs.

To ascend a curb using momentum, the wheelchair user approaches it head-on, with speed. At the last moment, he pops his casters up onto the curb: without slowing the chair, he reaches back and pulls forward on the handrims abruptly and forcefully. He may need to throw his head back at the same time to lift the casters. The caster pop

should be timed so that the casters lift over the curb and land just before the rear wheels hit the curb. Momentum will carry the chair up the curb if the maneuver is timed correctly and the curb is approached with adequate speed.

Descending Backward

This method of descending curbs does not involve a wheelie. Thus, it is the method of choice for people who cannot glide in a wheelie. It is, however, most appropriate for lower curbs. On higher curbs, the chair may tip over backward.

To descend a curb backward, the wheelchair user first backs his chair to the edge of the curb (Figure 11–22A). After the wheels pass the curb's edge, he controls the chair's descent by resisting the handrims' motion. Leaning the trunk and head forward will reduce the likelihood of the chair tipping over backward when the wheels hit the ground (Figure 11–22B).

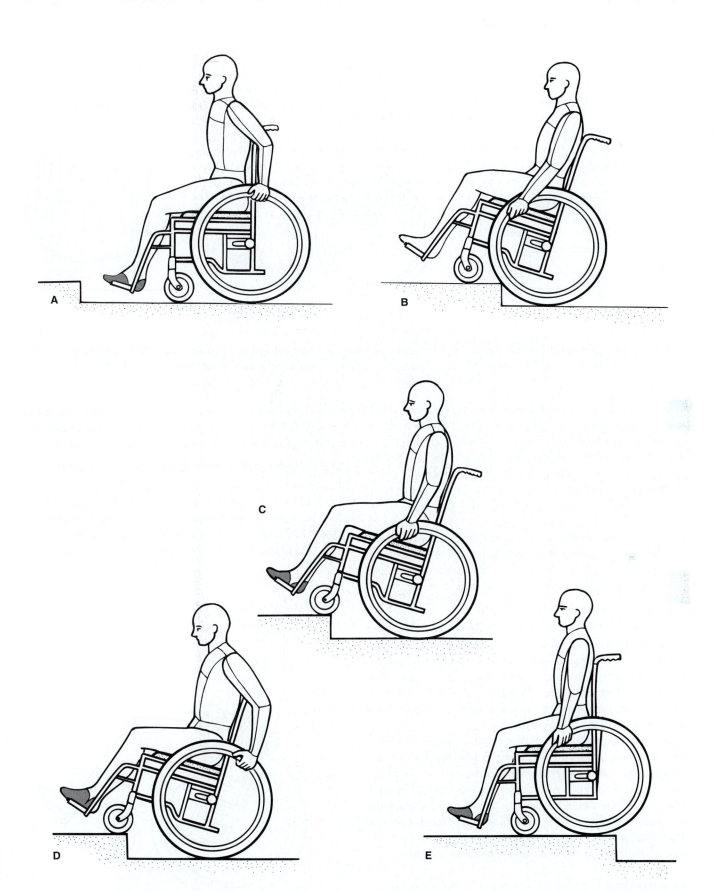

Figure 11–21   Ascending curb from stationary position. (A) Starting position: facing the curb, a few inches from curb. (B) Casters popped onto curb. (C) Casters backed to edge of curb. (D) Hands placed well back on handrims. (E) Curb ascended.

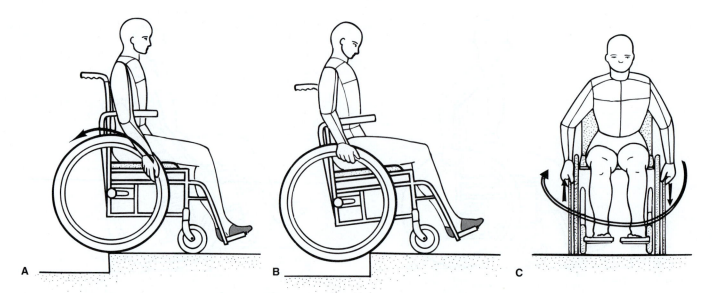

Figure 11–22 Descending curb backward. (A) Starting position: chair backed to edge of curb. (B) Controlling chair's descent. (C) Turning the wheelchair in a tight arc to lower casters from curb.

After lowering the chair's rear wheels, the wheelchair user removes the casters from the curb. He can roll the casters straight back off of the curb *only* if the curb is a very low one. If he rolls his chair straight back from too high a curb, the footplates will catch on the curb.

Most curbs are high enough that backing the casters off is not possible. To avoid catching his footplates on the curb, the wheelchair user lowers the casters by turning the chair rather than backing up (Figure 11–22C). He should turn his chair in a tight arc, pushing one wheel forward while pulling the other back. Once the casters move past the curb, they will drop safely to the lower surface.

Descending in a Wheelie Position

Descending curbs in a wheelie is faster than descending backward. To descend backward, the individual must interrupt his chair's forward motion to turn around and approach the curb backward, and must turn again after descending the curb. Descending in a wheelie does not involve this interruption of forward motion. Good hand function is required for this method.

To descend a curb using this method, the wheelchair user pops his chair into a wheelie position as he approaches the curb. He glides toward the curb in a wheelie and maintains that position as the chair descends the curb (Figure 11–23). The wheelie may be maintained after the curb has been descended, but that is not necessary for safe curb negotiation. The casters should, however, remain elevated until after the rear wheels have landed.

Negotiating Curbs in Manual Wheelchair– Therapeutic Strategies

During functional training, the therapist and patient should work together to determine which methods of ascending and descending curbs are most feasible for that individual.

A patient who has the potential to master more than one method may benefit from doing so, as this will enable him to utilize different strategies in different environments.

Ascending Curb From Stationary Position

To ascend a curb from a stationary position, a person needs to lift the casters from the floor, place them on the curb, back the wheelchair up to position the casters at the edge of the curb, and then ascend the curb from that position. These prerequisite skills can be practiced separately

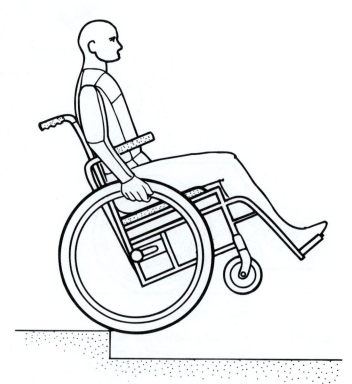

Figure 11–23 Descending curb in a wheelie.

or in combination. Strategies are described in the following paragraphs.

From Stationary Position, Lift Casters From Floor

Before learning to lift his casters from the floor, the patient should be proficient in forward propulsion over even surfaces. He need not be able to assume or to maintain a balanced wheelie position.

Lifting a wheelchair's casters from the floor is a lesser version of assuming the wheelie position; the same maneuvers are used, but they are performed less forcefully. To teach a patient to lift his casters, the therapist can use the training strategies presented earlier for teaching a patient to assume a balanced wheelie position.

Pop Casters Onto Curb From Stationary Position

Training in this skill should begin after the patient has acquired the ability to lift his wheelchair's casters from the floor from a stationary position. Once an individual can lift his casters consistently, he can practice popping his casters onto small (1-inch) curbs. As his skill develops, he can progress to taller curbs.

Position Casters at Edge of Curb

A person with the physical potential to ascend curbs should be able to master this prerequisite skill with minimal practice. During training, the therapist should emphasize placing the casters right at the edge of the curb (Figure 11–24A). This position maximizes the distance between the curb and the chair's rear wheels (Figure 11–24B), making it possible to gain more momentum for ascending the curb.

Ascend Curb From Stationary Position

Once a wheelchair user has lifted his casters onto a curb and positioned them at the edge, he grasps[dd] the chair's handrims posteriorly and pulls forward forcefully. To add to the chair's forward momentum, he throws his head and (if possible) trunk forward as his chair approaches the curb. This added momentum is especially important with higher curbs or when the individual's upper extremity musculature is impaired.

Training should start on a small (1-inch) curb. As the person's skill improves, he can progress to taller curbs. The curb height should be increased in small increments, with the patient progressing only when he is able to ascend a curb of a given height consistently.

Ascending Curb Using Momentum

Training in ascending a curb using momentum should begin with practice lifting the casters from the floor while the chair moves forward. Once a patient has learned this skill, he can practice popping the casters onto the curb while the chair moves forward, and ascending the curb. Strategies for developing these skills are described in the following paragraphs.

Impaired upper extremity function, a heavy wheelchair, or posteriorly located axles will make it difficult to accomplish this task. These factors, however, will not necessarily prevent acquisition of this skill.

Lift Casters off Floor While Chair Moves Forward

Lifting a wheelchair's casters while propelling forward is more difficult than doing so from a stationary position. Patients should learn to lift the casters from a stationary position first, to gain understanding of and skill in the actions used. They can then progress to "popping" the casters while propelling forward.

The therapist should explain and demonstrate how to propel forward and, without stopping, lift the casters by grasping[ee] the handrims posteriorly and pulling them forward abruptly and forcefully. The therapist can then guard the patient as he practices. An individual who is unable to lift his casters may be pulling his handrims with inadequate force or in the wrong direction, throwing his head in the wrong direction, or timing his maneuvers inappropriately. The therapist should observe as he makes his attempts, and give him feedback on his technique.

During early practice, the patient can work at low speeds. As his skill develops, he can increase his speed.

Pop Casters Onto Curb While Chair Moves Forward

To pop a wheelchair's casters onto a curb while propelling forward, the wheelchair user must lift the casters high enough to clear the curb and time the maneuver appropriately: the casters must lift before the footplates hit the curb

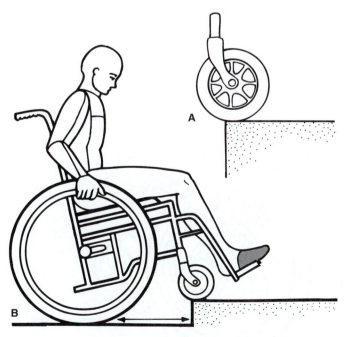

Figure 11–24   Positioning casters at edge of curb. (A) Correct caster position. (B) Caster position maximizes distance between curb and rear wheels.

[dd] A person who lacks functioning finger flexors moves his handrims using friction, pressing in on the rims instead of grasping them.
[ee] A person who lacks functioning finger flexors moves his handrims using friction, pressing in on the rims instead of grasping them.

and must lower just after crossing the curb. After a patient has developed the ability to lift his casters while propelling forward, he should work on his timing. He can practice popping his casters over a mark on the floor by propelling toward the mark, and popping his casters just before his footplates reach it. When he is consistently able to time his caster lift in relation to a floor mark, he will be ready to work on curbs.

Curb training should begin on a small (1-inch) curb, with the patient progressing to higher curbs as his skill develops. Once he has developed some skill in popping his casters onto a curb of a given height, he can practice this maneuver concurrently with ascending the curb using momentum.

Ascend Curb Using Momentum

Before initiating practice in ascending curbs using momentum, a patient must have developed some skill in popping his casters onto a curb while his chair moves forward, but he need not have perfected this maneuver.

To ascend a curb using momentum, a wheelchair user approaches it front-on and pops his casters onto the curb at the last moment. Timing is crucial; the casters should lift over the curb and land just before the rear wheels hit. If the maneuver is timed correctly and the wheelchair has approached the curb with enough speed, momentum will carry the chair up the curb. During functional training, the therapist should carefully observe the patient's timing so that he can provide feedback. He should also encourage the patient to be aware of the timing.

For most people, a good deal of practice is required to learn this skill. Training should start on a small (1-inch) curb. As the patient's skill improves, he can progress to taller curbs. The curb height should be increased in small increments, with the patient progressing only when he is able to ascend a curb of a given height consistently.

Close guarding is required as the patient works on ascending curbs using momentum.[ff] If the chair is not tipped back enough or if it drops too early as it approaches the curb, the casters will hit the curb's vertical surface (Figure 11–25A). The chair will stop abruptly, and the rider may be thrown forward out of the chair. If the casters drop too late, the rear wheels will hit first while the chair is still tipped back (Figure 11–25B). Again, the chair is likely to stop abruptly. On a tall curb, an abrupt stop can cause the chair to tip over backward.

Use of a seat belt during curb negotiation practice will enhance safety, preventing forward falls out of the wheelchair. Until the patient has mastered curb negotiation, the therapist should also provide close guarding. Because a patient can fall forward or backward during this activity, the therapist must be prepared to catch in either direction. The therapist can guard from behind, following closely as the patient propels toward the curb. Alternatively, the therapist can guard

---

[ff] This is not meant to imply that guarding is not required during practice of other curb negotiation skills. Guarding will be required during practice of any obstacle negotiation until the patient has developed adequate skill to function independently and safely.

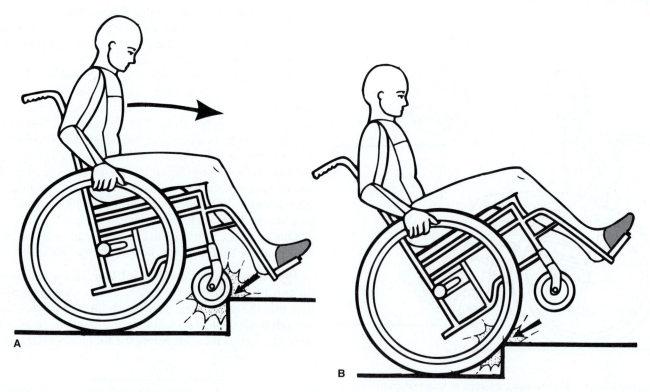

Figure 11–25   Problems resulting from improper technique when ascending curb using momentum. (A) Caster strikes curb's vertical surface. (B) Rear wheel strikes curb while chair is still tipped back.

from the front. This involves standing beside the curb prepared to catch when the patient reaches it.

Descending Curb Backward

After an individual succeeds in popping his casters onto the curb or ascending the curb, he can practice getting back down. These skills can then be practiced concurrently.

Backing Down Curb, Control Rear Wheels' Descent
Backing a wheelchair down a curb under control requires the ability to apply a strong forward force on the wheels. A patient should be skillful in manual wheelchair propulsion before beginning practice backing down a curb.

Functional training in this skill should emphasize developing control. The patient should practice backing just past the curb's edge and then resisting the chair's motion as gravity pulls it downward. Training should begin on small (1-inch) curbs, progressing to higher curbs as skill develops.

Lower Casters From Curb by Turning Wheelchair
To perform this maneuver, a person need only be able to turn his wheelchair in a tight arc. Anyone who is able to propel a manual wheelchair independently should be able to learn, with minimal practice, to lower his casters from a curb by turning his chair.

Descending Curb in a Wheelie Position

Before practicing this skill, a patient must be able to glide forward in a wheelie with good control. Training should begin with small (1-inch) curbs, progressing to higher curbs as the patient's skill develops. The therapist should guard closely to ensure the patient's safety, and provide feedback as needed to improve his technique.

Negotiating Stairs in a Manual Wheelchair

Why should a person who uses a wheelchair learn to negotiate stairs in this day and age? Although most public buildings have elevators, most private buildings do not. Someone who wants to visit friends and relatives, or the second floor of his own home, is likely to have to negotiate stairs. And even public buildings with elevators *do not* have functioning elevators when there is a power outage or a fire.

Independent stair negotiation is more convenient than assisted stair negotiation; someone capable of helping may not always be available. Independent stair negotiation can also be safer. An attendant, family member, or helpful stranger can slip or lose his grip. A wheelchair user who can ascend and descend stairs without help will be in control, rather than dependent on the skill, strength, and sobriety of another.

The physical and skill prerequisites required to negotiate stairs in a manual wheelchair are included in Tables 11–16 and 11–17.

Ascending on Buttocks

This method of ascending stairs is slow but requires less strength than ascending in a wheelchair. In rare cases it is possible for an individual with C8 tetraplegia to perform this skill, but it is more feasible for people with fully innervated upper extremities. Ascending stairs on the buttocks requires the ability to transfer independently between a wheelchair and the floor.[gg]

The first task in ascending stairs on the buttocks is a transfer from the wheelchair to a low step (Figure 11–26A). The transfer can be to the lowest step or to the one above it, depending on the individual's ability. Once on the step, the person positions his buttocks securely on the step, with his legs facing down the steps and the knees bent. The step-to-step transfers that follow will be easiest to perform if the legs are aligned with the body's midline, instead of leaning to the side. To maintain this alignment, the person can position his feet laterally and lean his knees against each other.

After aligning his buttocks and legs on the step, the person props on one arm and grasps the chair with the other hand. He then turns the chair so that it faces away from the stairs, with the rear wheels against the lowest step. Tilting the chair back, he places the push handles on the highest step that they will reach (Figure 11–26B).

From this point, the individual ascends the stairs by transferring up one step at a time and pulling the chair along. To transfer up a step, he places both hands on the next higher step and leans back while pushing down (Figure 11–26C). As his buttocks clear the edge of the higher step, he lifts them onto the step by depressing his shoulders and tipping his head forward.

Once the person has transferred up a step, he moves his legs. He should place them with the knees flexed and the feet flat on a lower step (Figure 11–26D). Positioning the legs in this manner will make it easier to transfer to the next step.

It may be possible to transfer up a step before moving the chair. As the individual moves further up the stairs, he must bring the chair along. To pull the wheelchair up a step, he first places his buttocks well back on the step and positions his legs as just described. He then places his free hand (the one farthest from the chair) slightly lateral to his trunk on the step above the one on which he sits. Propping on this arm, he leans back and pulls the chair up a step, placing the push handles on the step above the one on which he sits (Figure 11–26E and F).

Once a person has brought his wheelchair up onto the steps so that the wheels rest on a step, he must hold the chair to keep it from falling down the stairs. If he lets go even briefly, it will fall. Maintaining a hold on the chair while transferring from step to step can be accomplished by bearing weight through the push handle when transferring. The force on the push handle must be directed straight downward.

Ascending stairs involves repeating the process of pulling the wheelchair up a step, transferring up, and repositioning the legs. Once the person has reached the landing at the top of the stairs, he pulls the wheelchair onto the landing. He then rights the chair (away from the edge, please!) and transfers into it.

[gg] Transfers between the wheelchair and floor are presented in Chapter 10.

TABLE 11–16   Negotiating Stairs–Physical Prerequisites

	Ascend on Buttocks	Ascend in Wheelchair	Descend on Buttocks	Descend in Wheelchair Holding Rail	Descend in Wheelie
Strength					
Fully innervated upper extremities	●	☑	●	●	√
Anterior deltoids	☑	☑	☑	☑	√
Middle deltoids	√	√	√	√	√
Posterior deltoids	√	√	√	√	☑
Biceps, brachialis, and/or brachioradialis	☑	√	☑	☑	☑
Serratus anterior	☑	☑	☑		√
Latissimus dorsi	☑	☑	☑		
Triceps	☑	☑	☑	●	√
Hand musculature (active grasp)	√	●	√	●	√
Range of Motion					
Scapular Abduction	√	√	√	√	√
Adduction	√	√	√		√
Downward rotation	√	√	√		
Upward rotation	√	√	√	√	
Shoulder Flexion	√	√	√	√	
Extension				√	√
Internal rotation	√	√	√	√	√
External rotation				√	
Elbow Flexion	√	√	√	√	√
Extension	√	√	√	√	√
Finger Flexion	√		√		√

√ Some strength is needed for this activity, or severe limitations in range will inhibit this activity.
☑ A large amount of strength or normal or greater range is needed for this activity.
● Not required, but helpful.

Ascending in a Wheelchair

Ascending stairs in a chair is faster than ascending on the buttocks. Moreover, the person does not risk traumatizing his skin on the stairs and will not get his clothes wet or dirty. *Strong*, fully innervated upper extremities are required.

Ascending stairs in this manner requires the use of either a seat belt (preferably) or a belt that encircles the proximal thighs and the wheelchair seat. The wheelchair user backs up to the stairs, grasps the rail(s), and pulls on the rail(s) to tip the chair back. He lowers himself until the chair's push handles rest on a step (Figure 11–27A).

To ascend a step, the person first places his hands on the step above the one on which the push handles rest (Figure 11–27B). He then lifts his buttocks and the wheelchair by pushing down forcefully (Figure 11–27C). He will feel the chair's resistance reduce substantially as the wheels get up over the edge of the step.

Once an individual has lifted his wheelchair up a step, he moves his hands to the next step. To keep the chair from falling back down the stairs, he must move his hands one at a time. This involves balancing first on one arm and then the other and moving the free hand up a step.

The stairs are ascended one step at a time by repeatedly pulling the wheelchair up a step and repositioning the hands to the next step. Once an individual has reached the landing at the top of the stairs, he pulls the wheelchair well onto the landing. After pulling his chair a safe distance from the top of the stairs, he can right the chair

TABLE 11–17 Negotiating Stairs–Skill Prerequisites

	Ascend on Buttocks	Ascend in Wheelchair	Descend on Buttocks	Descend in Wheelchair Holding Rail	Descend in Wheelie
Transfers between wheelchair and floor*	✓		✓		
Position buttocks and legs on step*	✓		✓		
Sitting on step or floor, tilt wheelchair back to position to ascend or descend stairs (p. 283)	✓		✓		
Sitting on step, stabilize wheelchair by pushing down through push handles (p. 283)	✓		✓		
Transfer up a step while stabilizing wheelchair (p. 283)	✓				
Sitting on step, position buttocks and legs while stabilizing wheelchair (p. 283)	✓		✓		
Sitting on step or landing, pull wheelchair up (p. 283)	✓				
Sitting on floor, pull wheelchair to upright position (p. 283)	✓		✓		
Lower chair into position to ascend stairs in wheelchair (p. 284)		✓			
Sitting in wheelchair tilted back onto steps, reposition hands (p. 284)		✓			
Sitting in wheelchair, push on step to lift wheelchair up a step (p. 284)		✓			
Return wheelchair to upright (p. 293)		✓			
Sitting on a step, lower wheelchair down a step (p. 283)			✓		
Sitting on a step, transfer down a step while stabilizing wheelchair (p. 283)			✓		
Sitting in wheelchair holding stair handrail(s), lower chair down stairs (p. 284)				✓	
Assume wheelie position (pp. 265, 266)					
Glide forward, back, and turn in wheelie (pp. 266, 267)					✓
In wheelie, position wheels at top of step (p. 284)					✓
In wheelie, stabilize wheelchair against step (p. 284)					✓
Descend step, remaining in wheelie position (p. 285)					✓

* Refer to Chapter 10 for a description of this skill and therapeutic strategies.
✓ This prerequisite skill is required to perform this activity.

while remaining in it. Alternatively, he can get out of the wheelchair, return it to an upright position, and perform a floor-to-chair transfer.

Descending on Buttocks

To descend stairs on his buttocks, the wheelchair user performs in reverse the sequence of maneuvers used to ascend stairs on his buttocks.

Descending in a Wheelchair, Holding Rail

Using this technique to descend stairs, a wheelchair user holds the rail and lowers the chair backward. Because he stays in his wheelchair, he does not risk traumatizing his skin on the stairs or getting his clothes wet or dirty. This skill would be very helpful in the event of an emergency because it enables a person to descend stairs safely and quickly without assistance.

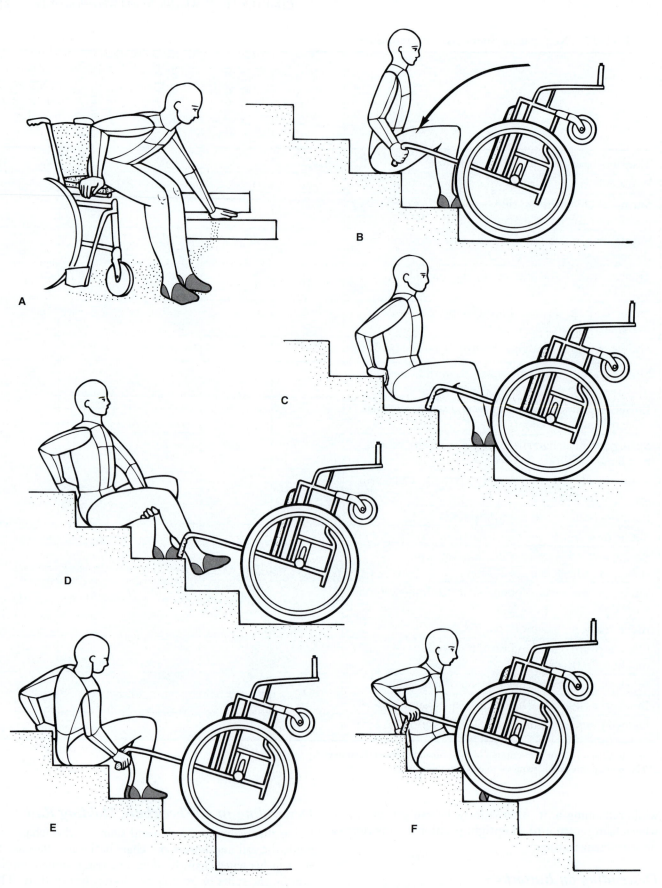

Figure 11–26 Ascending stairs on buttocks. (A) Transferring to step. (B) Tilting wheelchair back onto step. (C) Transferring up a step. (D) Repositioning legs. (E) Pulling wheelchair up a step. (F) Transferring up a step while stabilizing wheelchair.

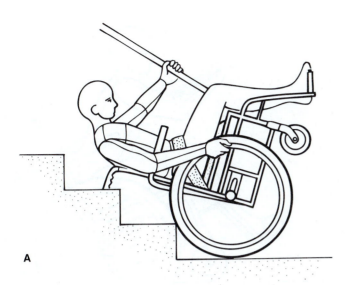

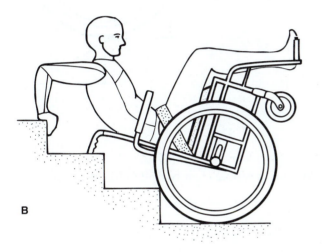

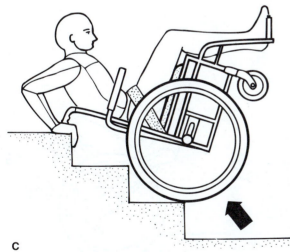

Figure 11–27   Ascending stairs in wheelchair. (A) Chair lowered onto step. (B) Hands positioned for ascending step. (C) Ascending step.

Virtually anyone with fully innervated upper extremities should be able to master this technique. Full use of the upper extremities, however, is not required for the exceptional individual.

To descend stairs using this method, the wheelchair user positions his chair close to one rail at the top of the stairs, facing away from the stairs (Figure 11–28A). He grasps the rail firmly with both hands.[hh] The hand of the arm closest to the rail should be positioned lower on the rail than the other hand.

Pulling on the rail, the person moves his chair to the edge of the top step. As the wheels move past the edge, he leans his trunk forward. Maintaining his grasp on the rail, he controls the chair's descent (Figure 11–28B). As the chair progresses down the stairs, he moves his hands down the rail, sliding one hand at a time.

Descending in a Wheelie

This stair negotiation technique involves maintaining the chair in a wheelie position during the descent. The wheelchair user faces down the stairs and holds the wheelchair's handrims rather than the stair rails. This technique is safest when each step has a large horizontal surface (depth, or run) and a small vertical rise.[ii] It is also safer on a small series of stairs rather than a long flight.

Like descending holding a rail, descending stairs in a wheelie is fast and does not require the person to leave the chair. Its greatest advantage is that it makes it possible to descend stairs quickly when rails are absent. Descending in a wheelie is more difficult, however, and involves a greater risk of falling. This maneuver can be performed only by people with fully innervated upper extremities who are *exceptionally* proficient in wheelchair skills.

When using this method, the person maintains a wheelie as he lowers the chair down one step at a time. He first approaches the stairs in a wheelie and positions the wheels at the edge of the top step (Figure 11–29A). From this position, he propels forward until the tires move over the edge and he feels the chair begin to descend. At this point, he stops pushing forward and works to control the chair's descent as gravity pulls it down the step (Figure 11–29B). He maintains control by gripping the handrims loosely and allowing them to slide through his grasp. When the wheels reach the next step, he can stabilize the chair by pulling back on the handrims until the wheels press against the vertical surface of the higher step (Figure 11–29C). He is then ready to repeat the process on the next step. In this manner, the wheelchair user descends the stairs one step at a time.

[hh] On a narrow stairway, it may be possible to reach both rails. A person may then choose to position his chair in the center of the stairs and hold both rails as he lowers himself.

[ii] The dimensions of each step should be such that there will be room for the wheels to rest on it. As a rule of thumb, the run of each step should be *at least* half the diameter of the wheel. Steps with a higher rise may require a larger run, as they will cause the wheels to rest further forward on the run.

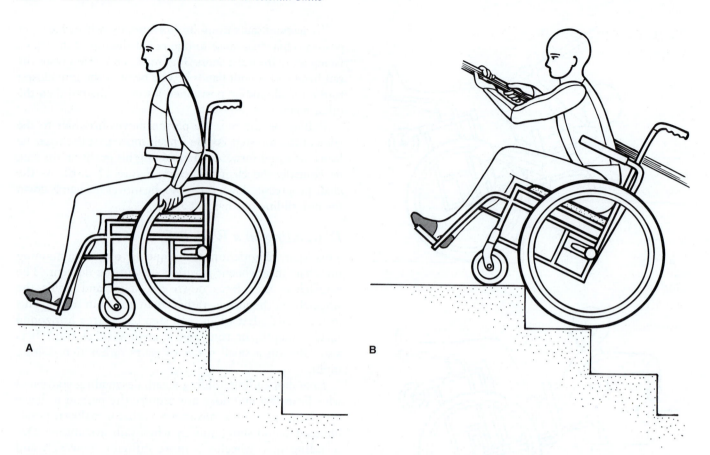

Figure 11–28   Descending stairs in wheelchair, holding rail. (A) Starting position: chair backed to top step. (B) Lowering wheelchair down stairs.

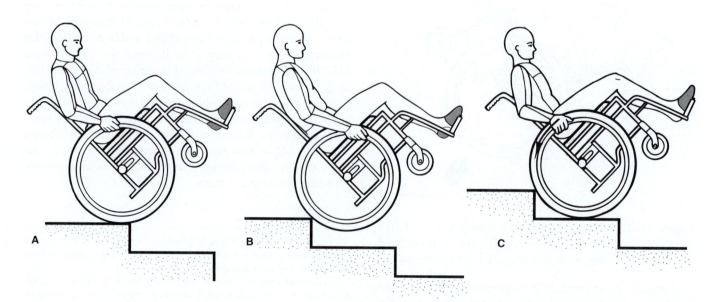

Figure 11–29   Descending stairs in a wheelie. (A) Starting position: in wheelie, wheels positioned at edge of top step. (B) Controlling chair's descent. (C) Stabilizing wheelchair by pulling wheel against stair.

Negotiating Stairs in a Manual Wheelchair–Therapeutic Strategies

The therapist and patient should work together to determine which methods of ascending and descending stairs are most feasible for the individual. A patient who has the potential to master more than one method may benefit from doing so, as this will enable him to utilize different strategies in different circumstances.

During the practice of any stair negotiation technique, the therapist should guard the patient. When the patient is practicing ascending or descending on his buttocks, the therapist should also ensure that the wheelchair does not fall down the stairs. Skin integrity is another concern when negotiating stairs on the buttocks. A strap-on specialty cushion that pads the person's buttocks and sacral area (Figure 11–30) can help protect the skin during this activity.

Ascending and Descending on Buttocks

The prerequisite skills for negotiating stairs on the buttocks, presented in the following paragraphs, can be practiced in combination. These prerequisite skills all require good dynamic balance in sitting propped on one or two arms (addressed in Chapter 10).

Transfer Between Wheelchair and Step or Floor
Chapter 10 presents techniques and therapeutic strategies for transfers to and from a wheelchair.

Sitting on Step or Floor, Tilt Wheelchair Back to Position to Ascend or Descend Stairs
A person with intact upper extremity musculature and good balance in sitting propped on one arm should find it easy to position his wheelchair in preparation to ascend or to descend stairs on his buttocks. He simply grasps a push handle and pulls it to turn and tip the chair. A brief period of practice should be sufficient to master this maneuver.

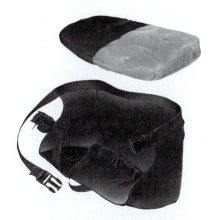

Figure 11–30   Strap-on specialty cushion protects skin overlying buttocks and sacral area during practice of stair negotiation on buttocks. (Reproduced with permission of Sunrise Medical.)

Sitting on Step, Stabilize Wheelchair by Pushing Down Through Push Handles
During functional training, the patient should be encouraged to push straight downward through the chair's push handle. An obliquely directed push may cause the chair to slide on the step. Practice should start with the patient sitting on a step that is close to the base of the stairway. A wheelchair is easier to stabilize in this location because it is supported by the floor. After brief practice at the base of the stairs, the patient can progress to practicing on higher steps.

Transfer Up or Down a Step While Stabilizing Wheelchair
Training in this skill should begin after the patient can stabilize his wheelchair while sitting on stairs. He must also be proficient in using the head–hips relationship and performing step-high back-approach uneven transfers to and from the floor.[jj]

Before an individual becomes skillful in this maneuver, he may have difficulty stabilizing his chair while transferring. While concentrating on the transfer between stairs, the inexperienced patient may apply an obliquely directed force to the chair's push handle, causing it to slide. The therapist should encourage him to push straight downward through the push handle as he transfers.

Practice should begin on a low step, where the chair is supported by the floor. As the patient's skill develops, he should progress to transferring from higher steps. After he has developed some skill in transferring up or down a step while stabilizing his chair, he can practice this skill concurrently with the skill of moving the chair up or down a step.

Sitting on Step, Position Buttocks and Legs While Stabilizing Wheelchair
Training in this skill should begin after the patient can stabilize his wheelchair while sitting on stairs. He should also be independent in gross mat mobility and leg management.[kk] Practice should begin on a low step, where the chair is supported by the floor. As the patient's skill develops, he should practice on higher steps.

Sitting on Step or Landing, Pull Wheelchair Up or Lower It Down a Step
A patient with good dynamic balance in one-hand-supported short-sitting should learn to move his wheelchair between steps with minimal practice. The patient is likely to find the task easier if he leans away from the chair as he pulls it up or lowers it.

Sitting on Floor, Pull Wheelchair to Upright Position
To right a wheelchair while sitting on the floor, a person with a complete spinal cord injury first gets into a long-sitting position. Propping on one arm, he pulls upward on

---

[jj] Training strategies for the head–hips relationship and transfer skills are presented in Chapter 10.
[kk] Training strategies for gross mat mobility and leg management are presented in Chapter 9.

one of the wheelchair's push handles to right the chair. Alternatively, he can engage the wheel locks and pull downward on the front of the chair. A patient with good dynamic balance in one-hand-supported long sitting should learn to right his wheelchair with minimal practice.

Ascending in a Wheelchair

The prerequisite skills for ascending stairs in a wheelchair, presented in the following paragraphs, can be practiced separately or in combination.

Lower Chair Into Position to Ascend Stairs in Wheelchair

Someone who has the physical potential to ascend stairs in a wheelchair should learn with minimal practice to lower his chair into position. If a patient has difficulty at first, he can practice lowering and raising himself through a small arc of motion, gradually increasing the arc as his skill and confidence develop (Figure 11–31).

Sitting in Wheelchair Tilted Back Onto Steps, Reposition Hands

In this maneuver, a person who is sitting in a wheelchair that is tilted back onto a step moves his hands from one step to another. This task is made challenging by the fact that he must support himself and the chair while he does so. To do this, he supports himself on one hand at a time, repositioning his free hand to the step above.

Practice should start at the base of the stairway, where a wheelchair is easier to stabilize. After brief practice at the base of the stairs, the patient can progress to practicing on higher steps.

Sitting in Wheelchair, Push on Step to Lift Wheelchair Up a Step

Lifting a wheelchair up a step while sitting in the chair is more a matter of strength than skill. This maneuver will be easier to learn if the patient is skillful in back-approach uneven transfers[II] and can reposition his hands between steps.

Training should start at the base of a stairway, with the patient belted into a wheelchair that is tilted back onto the stairs. He may find the maneuver easier if he lifts one wheel at a time up the step. A patient who has difficulty pulling his chair up the steps may first practice raising and lowering his chair over a single step at the base of the stairs.

Descending in Wheelchair, Holding Rail

This maneuver is easy to learn, requiring neither great amounts of strength nor skill. The greatest obstacle to overcome during functional training is fear: understandably, many people are afraid at first that they will lose control of the chair and fall down the stairs.

To reduce a patient's fear during functional training, the therapist should stress the maneuver's safety and make a point of modeling comfort while demonstrating the technique. The therapist should also make it clear to the patient that he is guarding carefully during practice. The patient may feel more secure during initial practice if it takes place on a short (two- or three-step) stairway. He can progress to working on longer stairways as his comfort level increases.

Descending in Wheelie Position

The prerequisite skills for descending stairs in a wheelie position, presented in the following paragraphs, can be practiced separately and then in combination.

In Wheelie, Position Wheels at Top of Step

Before working on this skill, a patient must be proficient in gliding forward, backward, and turning in a wheelie. Functional training then simply involves demonstration and practice. A patient who has difficulty positioning his chair at the top edge of a step may start with practice positioning the chair relative to a mark on the floor. He can progress to positioning his chair at the top edge of a low (1-inch) curb, then practice on higher curbs, and finally, work on positioning his chair at the top of a series of steps.

In Wheelie, Stabilize Wheelchair Against Step

To practice this skill, a patient should be proficient in maintaining a balanced wheelie position. The patient should work on stabilizing his chair against a curb before practicing against a step, as this will make guarding easier.

After demonstrating the technique, the therapist can position the patient in a wheelie with the back of the chair's wheels resting against a curb. Once positioned, the patient can practice stabilizing the chair by pulling back on the wheels' handrims. He can work on maintaining the chair's position, and lowering and raising (tilting) the chair through small arcs of motion (Figure 11–32).

Once an individual is able to stabilize his chair well, he should learn to get his chair into position. Starting in a

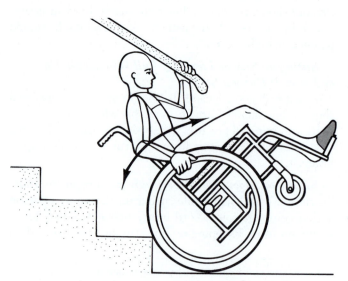

Figure 11–31   Practice lowering wheelchair into position to ascend stairs in wheelchair.

[II] These transfers are presented in Chapter 10.

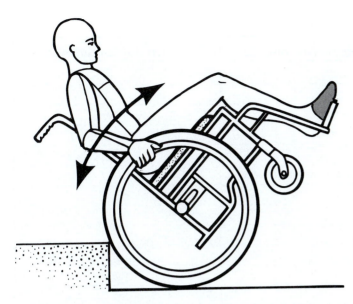

Figure 11–32   Practice stabilizing wheelchair against a curb.

wheelie with the chair a few inches from the curb, he should practice backing until the wheels make contact with the curb, then practice stabilizing the wheels. Once he can perform these maneuvers well at a curb, he can practice on the bottom step of a stairway.

When a patient has developed skill in stabilizing his chair against a curb and descending a curb while remaining in a wheelie, he can practice the two skills concurrently.

Descend Step, Remaining in Wheelie Position

A patient should be able to stabilize his wheelchair against a step in a wheelie position before beginning practice in this skill. He should also be skillful in balancing, gliding, and descending curbs in a wheelie.

When descending a curb in a wheelie, one does not have to remain in the wheelie position; once the chair's rear wheels have reached the base of the curb, the casters can drop without threat to the rider's safety. In contrast, one must remain in a wheelie when descending steps forward. If the chair tips forward before it has reached the bottom of the steps, it and the rider will fall down the stairs. It is this risk of falling that makes descending stairs in a wheelie hazardous to all but the most skillful riders.

During functional training, the patient should develop the ability to descend a step under control, remaining in a wheelie during and after the descent. He should develop his skill on curbs first because practice there will be safer than on stairs. The patient may start on low curbs, progressing to higher curbs as his skill develops. Once he is consistently able to remain in a wheelie while and after descending a step-high curb, and can stabilize his wheelchair against the step, he can practice on a small series of steps. He can start on stairs with a small vertical rise per step, progressing to higher steps and longer stairways as his skill improves.

Negotiating Narrow Doorways

Many doorways in private homes are too narrow for wheelchairs to pass through. This is especially true of bathroom doors and of doors in mobile homes. Even if an individual has the financial resources to adapt his own home, he is likely to encounter narrow doorways when he leaves his home.

Fully innervated upper extremities and a wheelchair with a folding frame are needed to negotiate narrow doorways using the techniques described in this section. The physical and skill prerequisites are presented in Tables 11–18 and 11–19.

Sitting on an Armrest

In preparation for getting his wheelchair through a narrow doorway, the person positions his chair. If possible, his footplates should extend into the doorway and the doorjamb should be within reach (Figure 11–33A). After positioning the chair, he removes a foot from one footplate and folds the footplate up (Figure 11–33B). (Otherwise the footplates will collide as the chair narrows, limiting the amount that the chair can be narrowed.)

Once the chair is positioned, the person places his hands on the armrests so that he can transfer onto an armrest. The hand toward which he plans to transfer should be well forward, to leave room for his buttocks. The transfer is achieved by pushing down forcefully and throwing the head down and away from the armrest (Figure 11–33C).

After transferring to the armrest, the wheelchair user props with one hand on the opposite armrest. With his free hand, he grasps the seat and pulls upward forcefully and abruptly (Figure 11–33D). As he does so, he shifts his weight off of his supporting hand. When he pulls on the chair in this manner, it narrows slightly. Repeated pulls will narrow the wheelchair to the desired width.

Once he has narrowed his chair sufficiently, the wheelchair user is ready to move through the doorway. Still balancing on one arm, he pulls on the doorjamb (Figure 11–33E) or propels through the door by pushing the handrims with his free hand.

After passing through the door, the person transfers back into the wheelchair's seat. With one hand on each armrest he pushes down and tucks his head to lift his buttocks, and swings his head laterally toward the armrest on which he has been sitting.

Remaining on the Seat

This technique provides a means of narrowing a chair for the many users who choose not to use armrests on their folding-frame chairs. A chair's width cannot be reduced a great deal using this method, so it is not useful with very narrow doorways.

Reducing a wheelchair's width while remaining seated involves rocking the chair side to side while pulling up on the sides of the seat. The wheelchair user initiates the process by throwing his head to one side, simultaneously

TABLE 11–18   Negotiating Narrow Doorways–Physical Prerequisites

		Sitting on Armrest	Remaining on the Seat
Strength			
Fully innervated upper extremities		✓	✓
Range of Motion			
Scapular	Abduction	✓	
	Adduction	✓	
	Downward rotation	✓	
	Upward rotation	✓	
Shoulder	Flexion	✓	
	Extension	✓	
	Internal rotation	✓	✓
Elbow	Flexion	✓	✓
	Extension	✓	
Finger	Flexion	✓	✓

✓ Some strength is needed for this activity, or severe limitations in range will inhibit this activity.

pulling up on the opposite side of the seat. (If rocking to the left, he throws his head to the left and pulls up on the right side of the seat.) The head motions and pulls on the seat must be performed forcefully and abruptly. As this maneuver is repeated, the chair rocks to one side and then the other. With each rock and pull, the chair narrows slightly. Once the chair's width has been reduced sufficiently, it can be propelled through the doorway.

Negotiating Narrow Doorways–Therapeutic Strategies

Sitting on an Armrest

The prerequisite skills for negotiating narrow doorways while sitting on an armrest, presented in the following paragraphs, can be practiced separately and in combination. All

of these skills require good dynamic balance in short sitting propped on one or two arms (addressed in Chapter 10).

Transfer to Armrest

To practice transferring to an armrest, a patient should be adept in even and slightly uneven transfers without a sliding board and in using the head–hips relationship to move his buttocks.[mm]

The therapist should demonstrate and then have the patient practice transferring from his wheelchair seat to the armrest. The patient should be encouraged to push down hard and throw his head and upper trunk down and to the side to lift his buttocks. Emphasis should be placed on exaggerated motions of the head and upper trunk.

[mm] These skills are addressed in Chapter 10.

TABLE 11–19   Negotiating Narrow Doorways–Skill Prerequisites

	Sitting on Armrest	Remaining on the Seat
Transfer to armrest (pp. 286, 288).	✓	
Maintain balance while sitting on armrest (p. 288).	✓	
Narrow wheelchair while sitting on armrest (p. 288)	✓	
Sitting on armrest, pull doorjamb to move narrowed wheelchair through door (p. 288). *or* Sitting on armrest, propel narrowed wheelchair (pp. 288, 289).	✓	
Transfer from armrest to wheelchair seat (p. 289).	✓	
Narrow wheelchair by rocking side to side (p. 289)		✓
Propel wheelchair over even surfaces (p. 261)		✓

✓ This prerequisite skill is required to perform this activity.

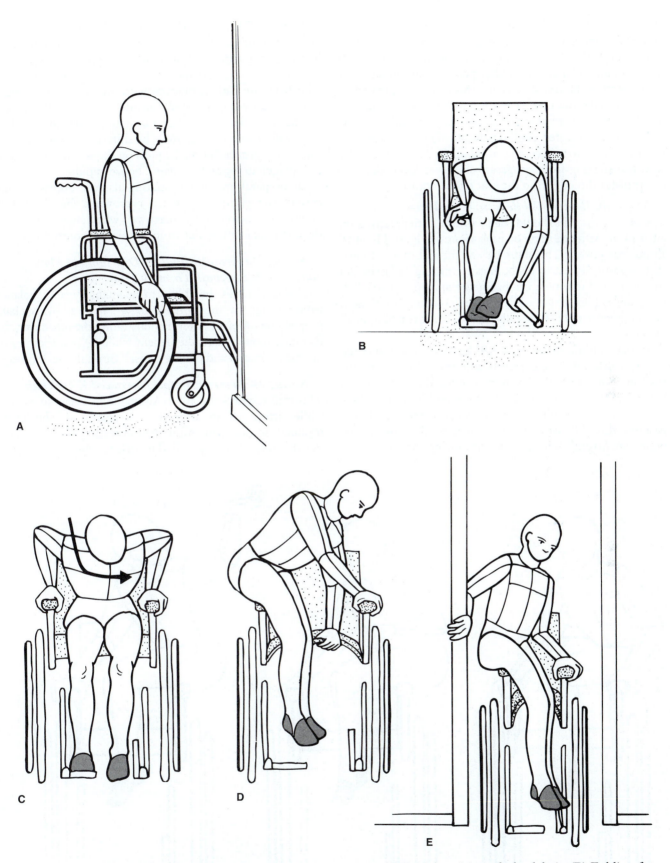

Figure 11–33 Negotiating narrow doorway, sitting on an armrest. (A) Initial position of wheelchair. (B) Folding foot plate after removing foot. (C) Transferring onto armrest. (D) Narrowing wheelchair by pulling upward on the seat. (E) Pulling on doorjamb to pull wheelchair through doorway.

During initial practice, many patients will be able to get onto their armrests with only guarding. These individuals can develop their skill by practicing with spotting until they become independent. Other patients have more difficulty learning the transfer. When this is the case, the therapist can make the task easier by placing cushions on the wheelchair's seat, reducing the distance that must be traversed in the transfer. As the patient's skill increases with practice, he can reduce the number of cushions on the seat, transferring from progressively lower levels until he can transfer directly from the seat to the armrest.

Maintain Balance While Sitting on Armrest
Practice of this skill should start with the patient sitting on an armrest, with one hand on each armrest (Figure 11–34A). From that position, he shifts his weight and lifts the hand that is propped next to his buttocks. Once he can maintain this position, the patient can begin working on dynamic balance, shifting his weight while propping on one arm. Finally, he can practice maintaining his balance while reaching in all directions.

Initial training in this skill will be most practical if the patient works on it concurrently with transfers to the armrest: he can alternate transferring onto the armrest and balancing there. Once he has become skillful in maintaining his balance while sitting on an armrest, he should practice this skill with the chair narrowed. This can be done concurrently with practice narrowing the chair.

Narrow Wheelchair While Sitting on Armrest
To practice this skill, a patient must be able to maintain his balance while sitting on an armrest, propped on one arm. The therapist should demonstrate narrowing the wheelchair, then have the patient practice with guarding. The patient should be encouraged to pull forcefully and abruptly upward on the wheelchair seat while maintaining his balance. The chair will be easier to narrow if he shifts his weight off of his supporting arm each time he pulls on the seat. He should be encouraged to regain his balance between pulls.

In preparation for negotiating narrow doorways, the patient can combine practice narrowing the chair with practice balancing on the narrowed wheelchair. To reopen the chair, he can transfer from the armrest onto the seat.

Sitting On Armrest, Pull on Doorjamb to Move Narrowed Wheelchair Through Door
This skill requires the ability to maintain dynamic balance while sitting on the armrest of a narrowed wheelchair, propped on one arm. After demonstrating the maneuver, the therapist should guard the patient while he practices grasping the doorjamb and pulling himself through the doorway.

Sitting on Armrest, Propel Narrowed Wheelchair
This skill requires the ability to maintain dynamic balance while sitting on an armrest of a narrowed wheelchair, propped on one arm. After demonstrating the maneuver, the therapist should guard the patient while he practices

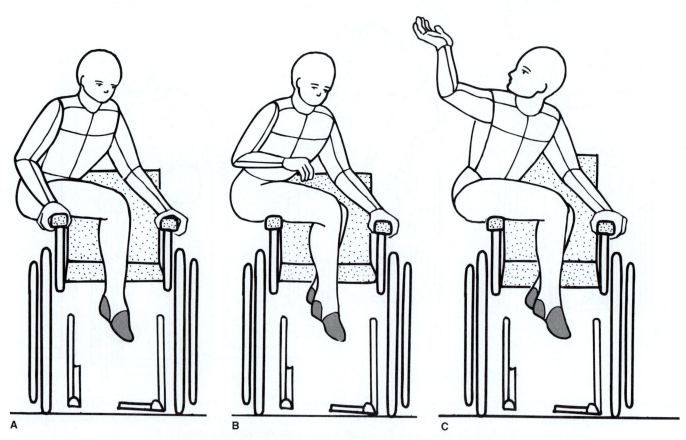

Figure 11–34 Practice maintaining balance while sitting on armrest.

propelling the chair by pushing on one handrim at a time with his free hand.

Transfer From Armrest to Wheelchair Seat

Before practicing this skill, a patient should be adept in even and slightly uneven transfers without a sliding board and in using the head-hips relationship to move his buttocks.[nn] A patient who has these prerequisite skills should be able to transfer from an armrest to the wheelchair seat without difficulty, after a brief period of practice with guarding. During initial practice, the wheelchair should remain open. As his skill develops, the patient can progress to transferring onto the seat of a narrowed wheelchair.

Remaining on the Seat

Training in this skill begins with practice narrowing the seat by rocking side to side. Once a patient can narrow his wheelchair adequately in this manner, he can propel through the doorway.

Narrow Wheelchair by Rocking Side to Side

The therapist should demonstrate this technique and have the patient practice with guarding. The patient should be

---

[nn] These skills are addressed in Chapter 10.

encouraged to use forceful and abrupt motions, synchronizing his head throws with upward pulls on the seat.

Falling Safely in a Manual Wheelchair

Many obstacle negotiation skills involve propelling the chair with the casters lifted off the ground. These activities involve a risk of falling; a person who negotiates curbs independently or propels his chair in a wheelie is likely to fall eventually. To minimize the risk of injury, anyone who learns to lift his casters off the ground should learn to respond appropriately when falling. Tables 11–20 and 11–21 present the physical and skill prerequisites for falling safely in a wheelchair.

Falling backward involves some risk, but appropriate action during the fall may reduce the risk of injury. When falling backward, a wheelchair rider should tuck his head and hold the wheels. When a person falls in this manner, he is not likely to injure himself or even experience discomfort. The chair's push handles, not the person's back or head, take the brunt of the force when the chair lands.[oo]

[oo] A wheelchair that lacks push handles, has a low backrest, or has a backrest with badly stretched upholstery will not provide this protection during a fall.

TABLE 11–20 Falling Safely and Returning to Upright–Physical Prerequisites

	Falling Safely	Block Lower Extremities While Falling Safely	Return to Upright While Remaining in Wheelchair
Strength			
Fully innervated upper extremities	•	✓	✓
Sternocleidomastoid	✓		
Biceps, brachialis, and/or brachioradialis	✓		
Hand musculature (active grasp)	•		
Range of Motion			
Scapular Abduction		✓	✓
Adduction			✓
Upward rotation			✓
Shoulder Flexion			✓
Extension			✓
Internal rotation		✓	✓
External rotation			✓
Abduction			✓
Elbow Flexion	✓	✓	✓
Extension	✓	✓	✓

✓ Some strength is needed for this activity; severe limitations in range will inhibit this activity.
• Not required but helpful.

TABLE 11–21   Falling Safely and Returning to Upright–Skill Prerequisites

	Falling Safely	Return to Upright While Remaining in Wheelchair
While falling backward in wheelchair, tuck head and hold wheels (p. 290) or Tuck head and block legs (p. 290)	√	
After falling backward in wheelchair, position self in chair (p. 291)		√
Sitting in overturned wheelchair, lift upper trunk from floor and engage wheel locks (p. 291)		√
Sitting in overturned wheelchair, balance on one hand (pp. 291, 293)		√
Sitting in overturned wheelchair, rock chair to upright (p. 293)		√

√ This prerequisite skill is required to perform this activity.

When the wheelchair lands, the legs' momentum may cause the person's knees to hit his face. An alternate method of falling can prevent this. Using this method, the wheelchair user tucks his head and maintains his hold on one wheel. He quickly reaches his free arm across his legs and grasps the opposite armrest or seat. This arm blocks his thighs as they fall, keeping his knees from hitting his face (Figure 11–35).

Falling Safely in a Manual Wheelchair– Therapeutic Strategies

Falling safely is a simple ability, without any true skill prerequisites. Functional training in this instance is more a matter of developing a new habit than of acquiring a new skill. For most people, the automatic reaction when tipping over backward in a wheelchair is to turn and reach out a hand, with the elbow extended. A person who reaches in this manner when he falls will land on his palm, taking the force of the fall through his upper extremity. In the process, he may injure himself. During functional training, this automatic reaction must be replaced by a safer falling technique.

Fear can be a barrier to developing the habit of falling safely. To reduce a patient's fear, the therapist should model comfort with falling and demonstrate that it does not hurt. The therapist can also help the patient overcome his fear by introducing the fall gradually. The patient can first practice the appropriate actions to take when falling, using either of the techniques just described. He can then perform these maneuvers while the therapist simulates a fall, lowering the chair backward from a balanced wheelie position (Figure 11–36A). At first, these simulated falls can be slow, with warning, and over a small arc. As the

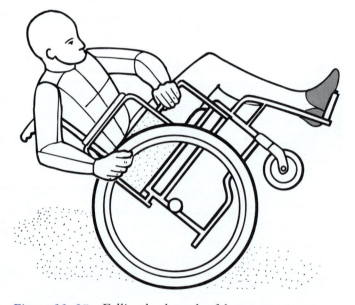

Figure 11–35   Falling backward safely.

patient's tolerance to this activity increases, the therapist can increase the speed and distance of the chair's "fall" and finally, omit the warning.

In the activity just described, the therapist should remain in control of the wheelchair, preventing a true fall. Once the patient develops some tolerance to falling and demonstrates the ability to respond appropriately, he can practice true falls. A fearful patient can develop his tolerance to falling by building up the distance over which he falls. Starting with a short fall onto a pile of floor mats, he can fall over progressively larger distances as his tolerance and habit develop (Figure 11–36B).

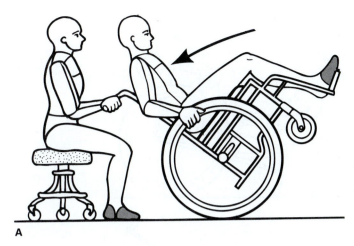

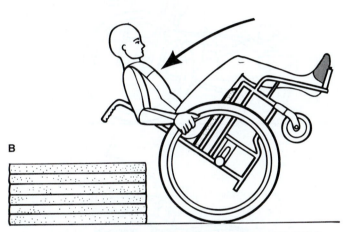

Figure 11–36   Practice safe falling technique. (A) With therapist assisting. (B) Onto floor mats.

Fall Recovery

After someone has fallen safely in his wheelchair, he faces the task of getting back up. One option is to get out of the chair, place it in an upright position, and transfer back into it. A faster alternative involves staying in the chair while pushing it back to upright. Fully innervated upper extremities are required to perform this maneuver. Tables 11–20 and 11–21 present the physical and skill prerequisites for returning the wheelchair to upright after a fall.

Righting a wheelchair while remaining in it requires proper positioning: buttocks on the seat and legs looped over the front edge of the seat (Figure 11–37A). If the wheelchair user is wearing a seat belt or has held on during his fall, he should be fairly well positioned already. If he has slid out slightly or if his legs have fallen off of the seat, he will need to position himself in the chair before righting it. To move his buttocks back onto the seat, he pulls on the wheels. He can then grasp his legs and position them, looping them over the seat.

Once positioned appropriately, the person locks the chair's brakes. He will probably need to lift his trunk to

reach the wheel locks. He can do this by pulling on an armrest or the frame of his wheelchair (Figure 11–37B). With his trunk lifted and the wheel locks engaged, the person should place one hand on the floor (Figure 11–37C). For simplicity, this hand is called "the supporting hand" in the rest of this description. The other hand is called "the free hand."

The supporting hand should be positioned directly beneath the trunk, so that weight can be shifted onto it. Balancing on this hand, the person releases the chair. He then reaches his free hand across his body and grasps the opposite wheel (Figure 11–37D).

Righting the chair from this position involves rocking it forward repeatedly and walking the supporting hand around to the side and toward the front of the wheelchair. Rocking the chair is accomplished by bending the elbow of the supporting arm and then extending it (Figure 11–37E and F). The push against the floor should be forceful and abrupt enough to thrust the chair toward an upright position. Each time the chair rocks forward, the supporting hand is inched forward around the side of the chair.[pp] When the chair falls back from its forward rock, the person balances on his supporting arm and repeats the process.

As the wheelchair user rocks the chair and inches his supporting hand forward, his chair gradually assumes a more upright position (Figure 11–37G). Eventually, he will reach a position from which he can thrust hard enough to rock the chair forward past its balance point, returning it to an upright position (Figure 11–37H).

Fall Recovery–Therapeutic Strategies

The prerequisite skills for returning a wheelchair to upright after falling backward, presented in the following paragraphs, can be practiced separately and in combination.

After falling backward in wheelchair, position self in chair; sitting in overturned wheelchair, lift upper trunk from floor and engage wheel locks

The therapist should explain and demonstrate these skills, then assist and provide verbal cueing as needed during practice. These maneuvers may be awkward when the person is sitting in an overturned chair, but a patient who has the physical potential to right his chair after a fall should be able to master these skills without a great deal of practice.

Sitting in Overturned Wheelchair, Balance on One Hand

Before beginning training in this skill, a patient must have good dynamic balance when sitting propped back on one arm.[qq]

---

pp This maneuver will be easier if the armrest has been removed, particularly if the wheelchair user is short.
qq This skill is addressed in Chapter 9.

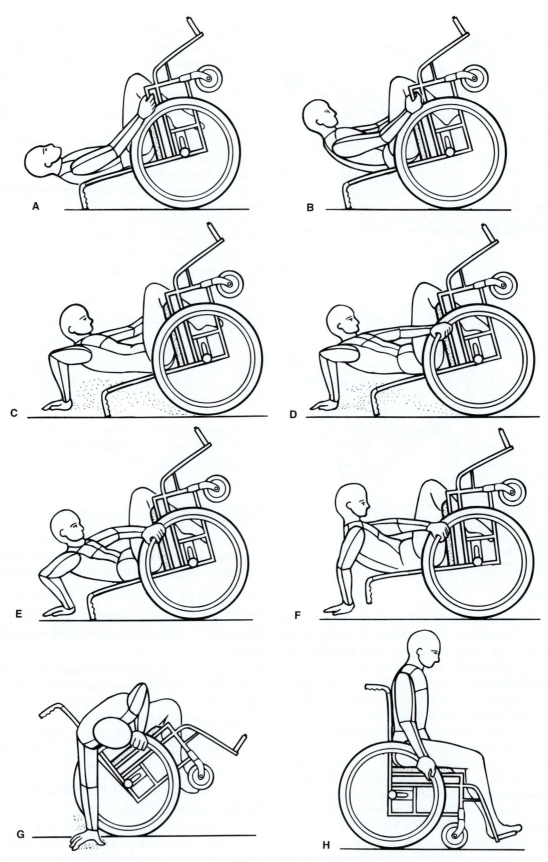

Figure 11–37 Returning to upright after fall. (A) Starting position: buttocks on seat, legs looped over front edge of seat. (B) Trunk lifted by pulling on front of wheelchair. (C) Hand placed on floor. (D) Opposite wheel grasped. (E and F) Rocking wheelchair toward upright by pushing with supporting arm. (G) Hand inched forward. (H) Upright.

Appropriate hand placement is the key to balancing on one hand while sitting in an overturned wheelchair. The hand should be positioned directly behind the trunk, so that the person can support his weight on it. The patient should practice placing his hand, shifting his weight onto it, and releasing the other hand's grasp on the chair. When he has developed the ability to release the chair and balance on one hand, he should practice reaching his free hand toward the opposite wheel.

Sitting in Overturned Wheelchair, Rock Chair to Upright

Before beginning training in this skill, a patient must have good dynamic balance when sitting in an overturned wheelchair propped back on one arm.

Starting in the position shown in Figure 11–37D, the patient should practice rocking the chair toward upright. The therapist should encourage him to use forceful and abrupt motions to thrust the chair upward from the floor. When the patient has rocked the chair forward enough to unweight his supporting hand, he should inch this hand forward around the side of the chair. He should reposition the hand rapidly and over short distances, so that he can support himself and maintain his balance when the chair rocks back. The therapist can facilitate practice at first by assisting with the chair's forward rock, pulling up on the chair's push handles while the patient pushes. The therapist can also help support the chair if the patient does not regain his one-hand support quickly enough when the chair rocks back. As the patient's skill develops, this assistance should be withdrawn.

Pushrim–Activated Power-Assist Wheelchairs–Functional Techniques and Therapeutic Strategies

Pushrim–activated power-assist wheelchairs (PAPAWs) are propelled using the same movement strategies as are used to propel manual wheelchairs with standard handrims. During functional training, the patient should practice propelling forward, backward, and turning on even surfaces. Practice should begin in an open area away from other patients, to avoid collisions. The therapist should be present to ensure the patient's safety. As the patient develops the ability to consistently and safely control the chair, he can progress to propelling in more confined spaces and in the presence of other people. He can practice negotiating inclines, uneven terrain, and small curbs as well. Functional training should also include manipulation of the controls (switching between indoor and outdoor power modes, for example). Finally, the patient should practice removing and replacing the wheels and batteries, so that he can perform these tasks during car transfers or change to standard drive wheels.

If the PAPAW allows adjustment of settings such as pushrim sensitivity and amount of power delivered to aid propulsion, the settings should be adjusted to optimize the patient's performance. As the patient's skill and strength develop and he begins negotiating outdoor surfaces and obstacles, the settings can be changed accordingly.

The various brands of pushrim–activated systems differ in the adjustments that they allow, amount of power that they deliver, communication/coordination between wheels, and pushrim sensitivity.[54] A PAPAW can compensate for asymmetrical weakness if it has wheels that communicate with one another,[84] or pushrim sensitivity that can be adjusted on each side.[55] PAPAWs also differ in features such as overall weight and maximal weight of a single component (relevant during car transfers, for example).[54] The therapist and patient should trial the equipment and determine which is most suitable for that individual, taking into account the patient's performance in all areas as well as his unique functional needs and preferences.

WHEELCHAIR SKILLS FOLLOWING INCOMPLETE SPINAL CORD INJURY: FUNCTIONAL TECHNIQUES AND THERAPEUTIC STRATEGIES

The actions that an individual can use to perform functional tasks after sustaining an incomplete spinal cord injury will depend primarily on his voluntary motor function. A person who retains or regains only sensory function below his injury (ASIA B) will utilize the techniques that are used by people with complete spinal cord injuries, as just described. A person who has minimal motor sparing or return (ASIA C) is likely to utilize similar movement patterns but may be able to add trunk or lower extremity motions to make the tasks easier. An individual who has significant motor function below his lesion (ASIA D) may be able to function independently without a wheelchair. If he does use a wheelchair, he is likely to be able to use his lower extremities to perform many wheelchair skills.

Another factor that can have an impact on the performance of wheelchair skills is spasticity. People with incomplete lesions tend to exhibit more spasticity than do people with complete lesions, and spasticity tends to be more severe among those with ASIA B and C lesions.[85–87] Involuntary muscle contractions can interfere with the functional use of muscles that remain innervated. When elevated muscle tone interferes with function, the rehabilitation team can work with the patient to reduce the abnormal tone.[TT] In addition, the therapist and patient should note the conditions and bodily motions that tend to elicit involuntary muscle contractions. They can then work together in an effort to find ways in which the patient can utilize a wheelchair without causing these involuntary contractions. In some cases, they may also find ways in which abnormal muscle tone can be used to enhance the performance of

---

[TT] Strategies for treating spasticity are presented in Chapter 3.

Problem-Solving Exercise 11–4

Your outpatient, who has C6 tetraplegia (ASIA A), lives in an urban environment. Prior to her injury, she used public transportation to travel to and from work and other activities in her community. While she was in inpatient rehabilitation, she developed the ability to propel her ultralight manual wheelchair independently over even surfaces for up to 500 feet but remains unable to negotiate longer distances, uneven surfaces, inclines, or other obstacles without assistance. She is also unable to utilize public buses independently because she cannot push her wheelchair onto their lifts. Her stated goals for therapy are to become independent in community mobility and return to work. She has expressed interest in trying power-assist wheels.

- What are the advantages and disadvantages of power-assist wheels for this individual?
- How might you obtain power-assist wheels for this patient to try?
- Assuming that you are able to obtain power-assist wheels, describe a functional training program for their use.
- What other equipment option might be appropriate to discuss with this patient?

some activities. For example, this author had a patient (with C4 tetraplegia, ASIA C) who exhibited spasms in his trunk muscles that were brought on by tactile stimulation of his thighs: when the anterior aspect of either thigh was touched, the patient's trunk flexed laterally toward the side that had been touched. The patient learned to elicit these spasms to shift his trunk laterally from midline and to return to midline from a lateral lean.

Use of a Power Wheelchair

A person who has motor return below his lesion may have the capacity for more actions that he can use to access input devices. The therapist and patient should work together to determine what body motions can be utilized and which input devices will enable him to function most independently and comfortably.

Manual Wheelchair Propulsion Over Even Surfaces

When motor sparing or return occurs in one or both of an individual's lower extremities, he may be able to use them to propel a manual wheelchair. He may propel his wheelchair using only his legs, or any combination of one or both arms and one or both legs.

The patient should be encouraged to maintain good sitting posture while propelling his wheelchair, with his buttocks well back on the seat. To use a single leg to propel forward, he should reach his foot forward and plant his heel on the floor. He can then pull the chair forward using knee flexion. Backward propulsion involves performing the reverse of these actions, and turning can be accomplished by exerting a laterally or diagonally directed force while propelling. If using two legs to propel, the patient should move his legs reciprocally: one leg pulls while the other reaches out.

Strategies for functional training are similar to those presented above for people with complete lesions. The

therapist can demonstrate and provide assistance as needed. If propulsion is very difficult for the individual, the therapist can make the task easier at first by prepositioning the casters, altering the handrims if necessary, and having the patient practice on a smooth floor surface such as linoleum. The patient should be encouraged to propel himself to his various activities in the course of the day. With practice, he should become faster and more proficient.

Negotiating Obstacles in Manual Wheelchairs

An individual who has significant motor sparing or return in one or both legs is likely to find negotiation of inclines, curbs, and uneven terrain easier if he approaches these obstacles backward.

Inclines

Inclines can be negotiated using one or both legs, with or without one or both arms. Descending and ascending steep inclines is likely to be easiest and safest if performed with the chair facing down the slope. This position eliminates the risk of falling over backward down the ramp. It also enables the wheelchair rider to push with his foot or feet to provide power for ascending the incline or controlling the descent.

Strategies for functional training are similar to those presented earlier for people with complete lesions. The therapist can demonstrate and provide assistance as needed. Practice should start on mild and short inclines, and progress to progressively steeper and longer ramps as the patient's skill develops.

Curbs

A wheelchair rider can ascend curbs backward using one or both legs and one or both arms, using all of his extremities that are strong enough to contribute to the effort. To ascend a curb backward, the individual backs his

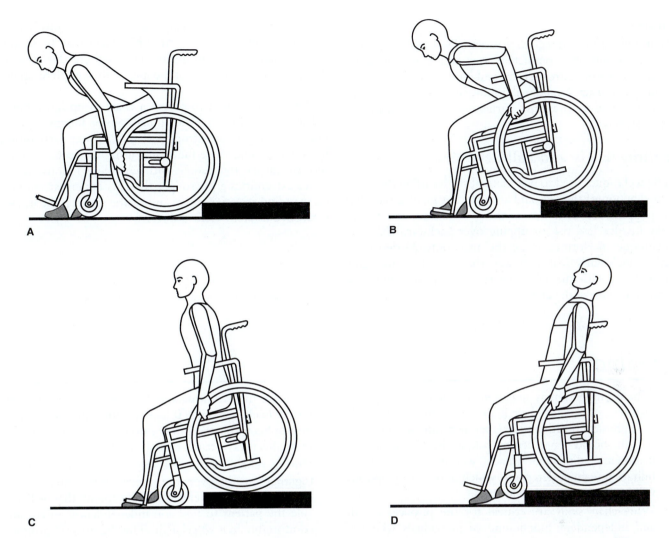

Figure 11–38   Ascending curb using upper and lower extremities. (A) Starting foot, trunk, and hand position. (B) Push/pull rear wheels onto curb. (C) Casters positioned at edge of curb. Foot, trunk, and hand position in preparation for lifting casters onto curb. (D) Push/pull casters onto curb.

chair to the curb so that the rear wheels contact the curb. He then plants his foot or feet on the floor in a position posterior to his knees, leans his trunk forward, and grasps the chair's handrim(s) (Figure 11–38A). The forward lean unweights the chair's rear wheels, making it easier to lift them onto the curb. The forward lean also makes it possible to reach further forward/inferiorly on the handrims.

While maintaining a forward lean, the individual pushes with his foot or feet and pulls on the handrim(s) to roll the rear wheels up onto the curb (Figure 11–38B). After positioning the rear wheels on top of the curb, he continues rolling the chair to position the casters at the edge of the curb (Figure 11–38C).

Once the casters are positioned at the edge of the curb, the patient plants his foot or feet at the base of the curb, leans back to unweight the casters, and positions his hand(s) anteriorly on the push rims. To lift the casters onto the curb, he simultaneously pulls on the handrim(s) and pushes with his foot or feet (Figure 11–38D). The curb can be descended by performing the same motions in reverse.

Strategies for functional training are similar to those presented earlier for people with complete lesions. The therapist can demonstrate and provide assistance as needed. Curb negotiation training should start on short (1-inch) curbs, and progress to progressively higher curbs as the patient's skill develops.

Uneven Terrain

To negotiate slightly uneven terrain, an individual may simply propel his chair using the technique that he utilizes over even surfaces, pushing/pulling harder to move the wheels over irregularities in the surface. Alternatively, he may find it easier to propel his chair backward over uneven terrain. If the casters sink into soft soil or get caught on an irregularity in the surface, he can try leaning backward to shift his weight off of the casters.

Stairs

Stair negotiation strategies are essentially the same as those used by people with complete lesions, although functioning trunk or lower extremity musculature may make some maneuvers easier. Functional training involves the same approaches as were presented earlier for patients with complete lesions.

Falling Safely and Fall Recovery

The techniques used to negotiate obstacles using the combined action of the legs and arms do not involve wheelies or popping the casters from the ground and, as a result, may involve less risk of tipping over backward than the techniques performed using the arms only. Moreover, if the wheelchair's seat is lower than standard to allow propulsion with the legs, the resulting lower center of gravity will make the chair more stable.

If a patient is likely to perform any activities involving a risk of tipping over backward in his wheelchair, he should learn to fall safely. The techniques used are the same as those described above for people with complete spinal cord injuries.

The method used to return a chair to upright after a fall will depend on the individual's motor function. If his upper extremities are stronger than his lower extremities, he is likely to be more functional using the technique described earlier for people with complete lesions. If his lower extremities are stronger than his upper extremities, he may find it easier to get out of the chair, right it, and perform a floor-to-chair transfer.[ss]

[ss] Floor-to-wheelchair transfers are presented in Chapter 10.

Summary

- When ambulation is impaired, the selection and adjustment of a wheelchair is necessary for the individual's physical health and independent functioning. The patient should play a central role in the wheelchair selection and adjustment process, working with the rehabilitation team to determine which of the many options will be most appropriate for him.

- Wheelchair skills are critical for the physical health and independent functioning of individuals who use wheelchairs for mobility. This chapter presents techniques for positioning the trunk in a chair, pressure reliefs, propulsion over even surfaces, negotiation of obstacles, falling safely, and returning the chair to upright after a fall.

- The manner in which a person with a spinal cord injury utilizes a wheelchair will depend on the extent of motor sparing or return below his lesion. If he has little or no voluntary motor function below his lesion, he

must use muscles innervated above the lesion to perform wheelchair skills. If he has significant motor function in his trunk and lower extremities, he may be able to use his legs or trunk to assist in these activities.

- During rehabilitation, the therapist and patient work together to discover the movement strategies and equipment components and adjustment that will enable the patient to function independently, safely, and comfortably in a wheelchair. The therapeutic program then consists of activities directed at developing the strength, range of motion, and skill needed to perform these functional tasks. This chapter presents a variety of strategies for developing the skills involved.

- The therapist and patient should take appropriate precautions to prevent motion of unstable vertebrae, pressure ulcers, overstretching of the low back, postural deformity, upper extremity overuse injuries, and injury due to tips or falls.

Suggested Resources

ORGANIZATIONS

Rehabilitation Engineering and Assistive Technology
   Society of North America (RESNA): *www.resna.org*
Rehabilitation Engineering Research Center (RERC) on
   Transportation Safety: *www.rercwts.pitt.edu*
Rehabilitation Engineering Research Center on Wheeled
   Mobility: *www.mobilityrerc.catea.org*

WEB SITES

ABLEDATA: *www.abledata.com*
Spinal Cord Injury Peer Information Library on
   Technology (SCI PILOT): *www.scipilot.com*
The Wheelchair Site: *www.thewheelchairsite.com*
USA Tech Guide, United Spinal Association:
   www.usatechguide.org
WheelchairNet: *www.wheelchairnet.org*

12

Ambulation

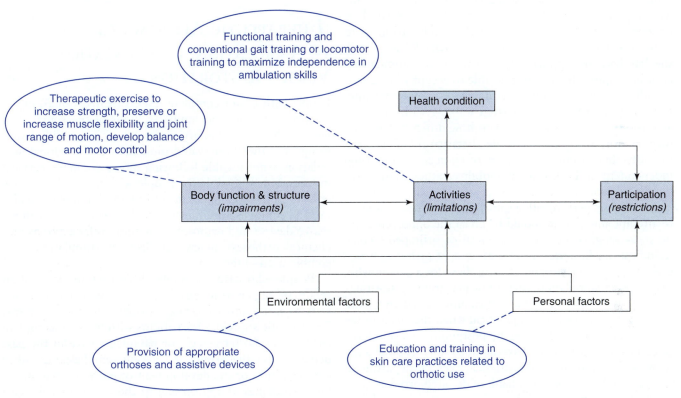

Functional training and conventional gait training or locomotor training to maximize independence in ambulation skills

Therapeutic exercise to increase strength, preserve or increase muscle flexibility and joint range of motion, develop balance and motor control

Health condition

Body function & structure *(impairments)*

Activities *(limitations)*

Participation *(restrictions)*

Environmental factors

Personal factors

Provision of appropriate orthoses and assistive devices

Education and training in skin care practices related to orthotic use

Chapter 12 presents information on ambulation skills, orthoses, and therapeutic strategies for increasing independence in walking and related activities.

Ambulation is a priority concern for many people following spinal cord injury. Especially during the early weeks and months after injury, much of a patient's questioning often centers on her future capacity to walk.[1] Walking can be an emotionally charged issue, with significance far beyond the pragmatic consideration of independent mobility. For many, it symbolizes power, competence, and potency. The inability to walk may be experienced as inadequacy, failure, and incompetence.

AMBULATION AFTER COMPLETE INJURY: TO WALK OR NOT TO WALK?

Walking is clearly a priority for patients. However, it is an area of controversy for many health professionals.[1] Ambulation with assistive devices and knee–ankle–foot orthoses or hip–knee–ankle–foot orthoses is a good deal slower than normal ambulation and is profoundly more energy-consuming.[1–9] In contrast, the speed and energy costs of wheelchair propulsion[a] are similar to those of normal walking.[9] As a result, people with complete spinal cord injuries are likely to abandon their ambulation skills after rehabilitation.[5,10–13] This is true even for people who can walk with two ankle–foot orthoses and assistive devices.[14]

A reasonable question arises: If research and experience have shown that a person with a complete spinal cord injury is likely to abandon ambulation, why should the rehabilitation team spend time, money, and energy on gait training? The answer is twofold.

First, although most patients with complete injuries give up ambulation following rehabilitation, some *do not*.[9,15–17] Is it ethical to deny people the opportunity to walk because they *probably* will give it up? If we do, some would-be walkers will never get the chance. Second, a patient may receive psychological benefit from gait training even if she ultimately uses a wheelchair. Until she has had the opportunity to experience ambulation after her injury, she may not be able to accept wheelchair mobility. ("They wouldn't let me try. I know if I could just try. . . .") Once she has tried walking with orthoses and assistive devices and has seen how difficult it is, she may be more ready to accept the alternative. Wheelchair mobility then becomes a matter of choice, representing independent and convenient mobility rather than symbolizing disability.

Ideally, any person with a spinal cord injury who wishes to attempt ambulation should be given the opportunity to do so as long as there is no medical or orthopedic contraindication. Because of the high cost of orthoses, however, it is hard to justify purchasing them for a person who may give up ambulation after a few gait training sessions. Offering the opportunity for gait training to patients with spinal cord injuries is more practical when the cost can be minimized. This can be done by postponing the purchase of orthoses until patients have demonstrated the capacity to walk functionally. If the physical therapy department has adjustable orthoses or a bank of donated orthoses, patients can begin gait training without purchasing them. The individual's equipment can then be purchased toward the end of gait training, after she has shown the ability and drive required to walk independently.

Although patients should be given the opportunity to try walking, they should not be pressured into it if they are not interested. Unlike transfers, mat activities, and wheelchair skills, walking with orthoses is not a "survival" skill required for independent living.[b] Similarly, gait training should not supersede functional training in survival skills. If a patient has limited funding for functional training, more practical skills should take precedence.[c]

When a patient with a complete spinal cord injury expresses interest in attempting ambulation, she should be given a clear understanding of the potential usefulness of this skill. The therapist should provide the patient with a realistic assessment of her potential for functional ambulation, and explain both the difficulty of ambulation with orthoses and assistive devices and the low rate of continued ambulation after completion of rehabilitation. The patient should also receive an explanation of the potential for injury from falls or excessive stress on the upper extremities, and the negative impact that these injuries could have on her activities and participation.

THERAPEUTIC APPROACHES TO AMBULATION: COMPENSATION VERSUS RESTORATION

People with motor complete lesions (ASIA A or B) in the cervical, thoracic, and lumbar regions of the spinal cord have inadequate voluntary motor function for ambulation using only their innervated musculature. Functional ambulation is not feasible following motor complete cervical injuries, but is possible for people with lesions below this level if they use compensatory strategies. These strategies include compensatory movement skills combined with assistive devices and orthoses (sometimes referred to as mechanical orthoses), functional electrical stimulation, or a combination of the two.

People who have incomplete lesions at any level often retain or regain voluntary motor function adequate for walking using normal or near-normal movement patterns. Therapeutic strategies for patients with motor incomplete (ASIA C or D) tetraplegia or paraplegia have in the past depended on the extent of paralysis, emphasizing either compensation or the development of more normal movement strategies as appropriate to the extent of voluntary motor function present.

In recent years, new rehabilitation strategies have been developed that are intended to promote restoration of walking by tapping into the plasticity of the central nervous system. These new approaches, often called "locomotor training,"[d,18–20] are designed to provide central pattern generators in the spinal cord with sensory input that mimics normal ambulation. Strategies include therapist- or

---

[a] For people with paraplegia, the speed and energy requirements of wheelchair propulsion are comparable to those of normal ambulation. People with tetraplegia are likely to propel more slowly and with greater difficulty.
[b] This is not meant to imply that patients should be forced to pursue survival skills if they are not motivated to do so. However, therapists should make every effort to convince them of the need to learn these skills.

---

[c] When a patient is determined to walk, the therapeutic program may reflect a compromise between the patient's desire for ambulation and the need to develop other functional skills.
[d] The term *locomotor training* is also commonly used with a broader meaning, referring to training in ambulation using any of a variety of strategies, including conventional gait training, over-ground training using body weight support, and body weight–supported treadmill training (BWSTT).[138] In this chapter, the term will refer to programs that include BWSTT.

robotic-assisted ambulation on treadmills or over ground, typically with body weight reduction during much of the training.[e] Research has demonstrated that these strategies lead to improvements in over-ground ambulatory ability in subjects with motor incomplete injuries, and that conventional gait training of equal intensity yields equivalent results.[21–23] Thus both locomotor training and conventional gait training remain legitimate approaches to the restoration of ambulation following motor incomplete spinal cord injury. In contrast, locomotor training has to date been ineffective in restoring functional ambulation in patients with motor complete injuries.[21–25] Until alternative therapies are developed that can enhance restoration of locomotion in patients with motor complete spinal cord injuries, compensation will remain the therapeutic approach most appropriate for this population.

This chapter presents information on therapeutic strategies for developing functional ambulation in patients with complete and incomplete spinal cord injuries. The descriptions of equipment, ambulation techniques, and gait training

---

[e] These therapeutic approaches are discussed in greater detail at the end of this chapter, in the section on strategies for patients with incomplete injuries.

should be used as a guide, not as a set of hard and fast rules. The equipment required and motions used to walk and perform other ambulation-related skills vary between people because of differences in body build, skill level, range of motion, muscle tone, patterns of strength and weakness, and presence or absence of additional impairments. During functional training, the therapist and patient should work together to find the exact equipment and movement strategies that best suit that particular individual.

PRECAUTIONS

Following spinal cord injury, ambulation can cause problems if appropriate precautions are not taken. Table 12–1 presents a summary of precautions for gait training with orthoses.

LOWER EXTREMITY ORTHOSES

When motor function is inadequate for ambulation, mechanical orthoses can be used to provide stability and, in some cases, motion to the joints of the lower extremities. An orthosis can prevent, limit, cause, or resist movement of the joints that it crosses.[26] Table 12–2 presents the

TABLE 12–1   Precautions During Ambulation and Ambulation Training

Potential Problems	Ambulation Activities That Place Patients at Risk	Precautions
Excessive motion at site of vertebral instability, potentially causing additional neurologic and orthopedic damage	Any activity involving excessive motion or muscular action at or near site of unstable spine. Example: Upright activities while the spine remains unstable.	• Strictly adhere to orthopedic precautions. • Check fit of vertebral orthosis with patient in upright postures.
Pressure ulcers	Use of orthoses.	• Assess fit of orthoses and shoes to ensure that skin is not subjected to excessive pressure. • Ensure that any orthotic joints allowing motion are aligned with anatomic joints, to prevent shear forces and friction on skin from orthoses moving relative to limb. • Assess fabrication of orthoses and shoes to ensure that skin does not come in contact with sharp or rough surfaces. • When orthoses are first worn, gradually increase wearing time. • Monitor skin status for signs of damage from orthoses. Teach patient to inspect skin before donning and after doffing orthoses.
Injury from fall	Ambulation with orthoses and assistive devices involves some risk of falling.	• Education and training in safe ambulation and falling techniques. • Appropriate guarding during gait training. • Provide patient with properly functioning orthoses and assistive devices.

TABLE 12–2   Orthotic Control Terminology

Control	Impact on Movement
Stop	Prevents motion beyond a certain degree in a given direction.
Hold	Prevents motion in either direction in a given plane.
Assist	Causes the joint to move in a given direction.
Lock	Prevents motion of a joint when locked, allows motion when unlocked.
Adjustable or variable	Allows the control provided at the joint to be adjusted.

terminology used to describe the different types of control that an orthosis can provide. Lower extremity orthoses can be made of metal, plastic, or a combination of the two. Orthoses in each of these classes (metal, plastic, and metal–plastic) can provide each type of control: they can limit (stop), prevent (hold), or cause (assist) motion in the joints that they span.

Orthotic Prescription

A large variety of lower extremity orthoses are available for restoring ambulation after spinal cord injury. When prescribing an orthosis, the rehabilitation team selects the anatomic joints that the orthosis will span, the control that it will provide at each joint, and the orthotic components and materials that will be most appropriate for the individual.

Considerations for Orthotic Prescription

When an orthosis is used to aid in ambulation, its purpose is to provide stability during stance, enhance swing, or both. When choosing between various orthotic designs, the control that a given orthosis can provide is of primary importance; an orthosis should be selected that best meets the individual's biomechanical needs. These needs can be determined by assessing the patient's capacity for lower extremity and trunk control during ambulation. If the individual is able to walk without orthoses, the therapist should perform a careful gait analysis[f] to identify the gait deviations that may require orthotic intervention. When determining biomechanical needs, the therapist should take into consideration the patient's voluntary motor function, muscle tone, and range of motion.

A second consideration in choosing between orthotic designs is adjustability. Especially when a patient receives her

first orthosis, adjustability can be useful because it allows the rehabilitation team to "fine tune" the appliance for the individual, optimizing the patient's gait pattern, standing balance, and ability to stand from a sitting position. Adjustability also makes it possible to alter the control that the orthosis provides as the patient's needs change. Metal orthoses typically allow greater adjustability of joint control than do plastic orthoses. A disadvantage of an adjustable joint is that it is likely to add weight and bulk to the orthosis.

A third consideration when selecting orthoses is weight. The weight of an orthosis influences the energy cost of walking; heavier orthoses increase the oxygen consumed per meter of ambulation.[27] If all other things are equal, a lighter orthosis may result in the ability to walk greater distances before tiring. Plastic orthoses are lighter than metal orthoses.

A fourth consideration in orthotic prescription is the potential for damage to the patient's skin. A plastic or combined metal–plastic orthosis, because of its intimate fit, can exert excessive pressure on the skin if the patient's limb swells. These types of orthoses can also cause skin maceration if the patient perspires excessively. Thus metal orthoses are indicated for patients who have fluctuating edema or excessive perspiration in their lower extremities.

Additional considerations in orthotic prescription include durability, ease of donning and doffing, cosmesis, cost, and impact on other functional activities such as transfers. Unfortunately, the funding source should also be considered in orthotic selection; third-party payers frequently provide limited funding for orthoses.[g]

Choosing Between Orthotic Options

For any biomechanical deficit, there are a variety of possible orthotic solutions. For example, a patient who is unable to dorsiflex her ankles during swing due to muscle weakness could utilize metal, plastic, or metal–plastic ankle–foot orthoses (AFOs) to assist dorsiflexion or stop plantarflexion. Moreover, each of these types of orthosis has a number of different designs that could provide the needed control. The various orthotic options differ in their adjustability, weight, risk of causing skin breakdown, durability, ease of donning and doffing, cosmesis, cost, and impact on overall functional independence. Clinicians involved in prescribing orthoses should investigate the benefits and drawbacks of the various orthotic options. Orthotic prescription should then be based on an analysis of the advantages and disadvantages of each option, taking into consideration the needs and priorities of the patient.

When possible, it can be helpful to try orthoses before ordering them. Since most lower extremity orthoses that are appropriate for people with spinal cord injuries are

---

[f] Chapter 7 includes information on the examination of ambulation after spinal cord injury. A thorough presentation of gait analysis is beyond the scope of this text. The following references provide comprehensive information on gait analysis: 139 to 142.

[g] Limited funding may necessitate selection of less expensive orthotic options. In addition, consideration should be given to orthoses that allow adjustment to accommodate future changes in status, as funding may not be available for replacement orthoses.

custom-made, it is generally not possible to obtain trial orthoses that are *identical* to the ones being ordered. It may be possible, however, to utilize a *similar* orthosis for a trial period. Many physical therapy departments have a collection of adjustable or donated orthoses that can be used for these trials.[1] During the trial period, the clinicians and wearer should note the influence of the orthosis on the individual's gait pattern, endurance in ambulation, standing balance, and performance of other tasks, such as sit-to-stand or car transfers. Although a trial orthosis cannot perfectly replicate a custom-made one, its use can provide some information on the impact that an orthosis will have on the individual's capacity to function.

Orthotic selection is a team process. Physical therapists, orthotists, and prospective wearers play key roles, each bringing a different perspective and knowledge base. Physical therapists contribute an understanding of the pathomechanics of gait as well as knowledge about the patient's physical status, functional capacity, and vulnerabilities relevant to orthotic use. Orthotists bring information on the characteristics of the currently available orthotic components, materials, and designs. Prospective orthotic wearers bring their preferences, values, and priorities. The physical therapist, orthotist, and prospective wearer should work together to determine the orthotic design that will be most appropriate for the wearer.

Ankle–Foot Orthoses

Ankle–foot orthoses (AFOs) are primarily used for people who have the ability to stabilize their knees in stance using their quadriceps but need orthotic control at their ankles. The control needed at the ankle will depend on the motor function present.

When the dorsiflexors are weak, a dorsiflexion assist at the ankle will prevent excessive plantarflexion during swing. By moving the ankle into neutral dorsiflexion during swing, an AFO can prevent toe drag and position the ankle for heel-first contact at the beginning of stance. A dorsiflexion assist will also allow plantarflexion after heel strike, resulting in a more normal gait pattern.

In the presence of elevated tone in the gastrocnemius and soleus, a plantarflexion stop should be used instead of a dorsiflexion assist. The reason for this is twofold. First, a dorsiflexion assist can elicit spasticity by providing a quick stretch to the plantarflexors. A plantarflexion stop will not cause this problem. Second, plantarflexors with elevated tone are likely to overpower a dorsiflexion assist and place the ankle in a plantarflexed position. A plantarflexion stop will prevent this motion, enhancing foot clearance during swing and reducing the occurrence of knee hyperextension during stance. The disadvantage of a plantarflexion stop is that it increases the flexion moment at the knee during early stance,[28] increasing the demand on the quadriceps. Modification of the shoe's heel may be required to avoid excessive knee flexion during loading response.[14]

Weakness in the plantarflexors may necessitate a dorsiflexion stop to prevent excessive dorsiflexion (and resulting knee flexion) as the person's center of gravity passes anterior to her ankle. A stop limiting dorsiflexion to 10 degrees will provide adequate stability, increase walking speed,[29] and allow a relatively normal gait pattern.[30]

In addition to controlling ankle motions, an AFO can be used to provide control at the knee. When the quadriceps are weak, an AFO that stops dorsiflexion can help to prevent knee flexion during stance. This type of orthosis is often called a floor reaction AFO[h] because it utilizes floor reaction forces to control the knee.[31] An AFO that prevents plantarflexion can have the opposite effect on the knee: an ankle held in a neutral or slightly dorsiflexed position can prevent genu recurvatum.[32]

Metal Orthosis With Double-Action Ankle Joint

One type of orthotic ankle joint that is frequently used because of its adjustability is a double-action ankle joint, also called a dual-channel ankle joint, double-adjustable ankle joint, or bichannel adjustable ankle. This metal ankle has channels located anterior and posterior to the joint's axis (Figure 12–1).

A double-action ankle joint can be used to limit, prevent, or assist motion in the sagittal plane.[33,34] The control it provides will depend on the contents of the channels; pins (small metal rods) in the channels stop motion and springs in the channels assist motion. The pins and springs are held in place by set screws. The control provided by the orthotic joint can be adjusted

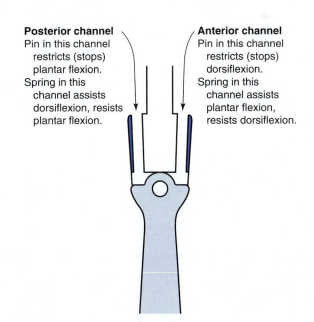

Posterior channel
Pin in this channel restricts (stops) plantar flexion.
Spring in this channel assists dorsiflexion, resists plantar flexion.

Anterior channel
Pin in this channel restricts (stops) dorsiflexion.
Spring in this channel assists plantar flexion, resists dorsiflexion.

Figure 12–1   Double action ankle joint, interior view.

---

[h] Also called a ground reaction AFO.

TABLE 12–3 Double-Action Ankle Joints: Control Options and Adjustment

Control	Pin or Spring Location	Adjustment
Dorsiflexion stop	Pins in anterior channels	**To allow more dorsiflexion:** Turn set screws in anterior channels counterclockwise.
		To allow less dorsiflexion: Turn set screws in anterior channels clockwise.
Plantarflexion stop	Pins in posterior channels	**To allow more plantarflexion:** Turn set screws in posterior channels counterclockwise.
		To allow less plantarflexion: Turn set screws in posterior channels clockwise.
Hold	Pins in posterior and anterior channels, adjusted to prevent any motion in sagittal plane	**To hold the ankle in a more dorsiflexed position:** Turn set screws in anterior channels counterclockwise, reposition ankle to the more dorsiflexed position, then turn set screws in posterior channels in clockwise direction.
		To hold the ankle in a more plantarflexed position: Turn set screws in posterior channels counterclockwise, reposition ankle to the more plantarflexed position, then turn set screws in anterior channels in clockwise direction.
Dorsiflexion assist	Springs in posterior channels	**To increase force of dorsiflexion assist:** Turn set screws in posterior channels in clockwise direction.
		To reduce force of dorsiflexion assist: Turn set screws in posterior channels in counterclockwise direction.
Free motion in sagittal plane	Anterior and posterior channels left empty	

by tightening or loosening the set screws, turning them clockwise or counterclockwise, respectively.[i] The type of control that the orthosis provides can be altered by changing the contents of the channels. For example, a plantarflexion stop can be converted to a dorsiflexion assist by removing the pins from the posterior channels and replacing them with springs. Table 12–3 summarizes the control options and adjustment for a double-action ankle joint.

Plastic

Custom-molded plastic AFOs are commonly prescribed because they are lighter than metal AFOs. They can also be worn with a variety of shoes, making them more cosmetically acceptable to many wearers.[34] A plastic AFO can provide the same types of control that metal orthoses can provide.

A plastic AFO can be made with or without an articulating ankle. When an articulating ankle is incorporated in the orthosis, the ankle's design and materials determine the control that it provides and the degree to which it can be adjusted. When an AFO does not contain an articulating

ankle, the control that the orthosis provides is determined by its trim lines[j] and materials.

Knee–Ankle–Foot Orthoses

Knee–ankle–foot orthoses (KAFOs) are used when orthotic stabilization is required at the knees and ankles. This stabilization may be required due to muscle weakness or deficits in proprioception.[34] KAFOs are often used by people who lack muscular stabilization not only of the knees and ankles but of the hips and trunk as well. These individuals use compensatory motions of their upper bodies to control their hips and the portions of their trunks that are not innervated.

Conventional Metal KAFOs

A conventional metal KAFO has double uprights that are connected posteriorly by two thigh bands and a calf band. Anterior thigh and leg cuffs and a knee cap stabilize the leg in the orthosis. Typically, drop-ring locks are used at the knees. The ankles typically stop plantarflexion. Dorsiflexion may be stopped or left unrestricted.

[i] The medial and lateral set screws should be adjusted the same amount. Otherwise the orthotic ankle will be subjected to excessive stress.

[j] This term refers to the edges of the orthosis. An AFO with more anterior trim lines extends more anteriorly around the ankle, so that the orthosis encases more of the circumference of the lower leg and ankle. An AFO with more posterior trim lines does not extend as far anteriorly around the lower leg and ankle.

Scott–Craig KAFOs

A Scott–Craig KAFO (Figure 12–2) is designed to provide maximal stability at the ankle and foot, making it possible to balance in standing without upper extremity support.[1] A T-shaped foot plate is embedded in the sole of the shoe, extending from the heel to the level of the metatarsal heads. This plate provides excellent anteroposterior and mediolateral stability, making the shoe a stable base for the rest of the orthosis. An adjustable double-stop ankle[k] holds the ankle immobile in 5 to 10 degrees of dorsiflexion, placing the hips in a stable position during stance.[l] The optimal angle for a given individual's ankle is determined during initial gait training.

The knee locking mechanism of a Scott–Craig orthosis is a pawl lock with a bail control.[m] The bail control is a U-shaped lever that circles around the back of the leg, attached medially and laterally at the mechanical knee joints. Upward pressure on the bail control unlocks the orthotic knee, allowing flexion. The wearer who is in a sitting position can unlock the orthotic knee by pulling upward on the

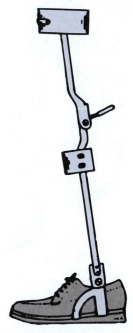

Figure 12–2   Scott-Craig orthosis. (Reproduced with permission from Lower-Limb Orthotics [1986], Sidney Fishman, PhD, and Norman Berger, eds, Prosthetic-Orthotic Publications, New York.)

bail. Alternatively, she can unlock the knees while she sits down from a standing position. To do so, she stands with the bails positioned on top of the sitting surface and then sits down. When the sitting surface pushes upward on the bails, the knees will unlock.

In addition to the knee locking mechanism and the specialized shoe and ankle, a Scott–Craig KAFO has two metal uprights, a single posterior thigh band, a hinged pretibial band, and a cushioned heel. The sole of the shoe is shaped to allow both stability and a smooth roll-over in stance. After the orthotic user has developed her ambulatory skills and the optimal ankle position has been determined, a sturdy plastic AFO can be substituted for the components below the knee.[32,35,36]

Advances in orthotic materials allow fabrication of KAFOs that are lighter than was previously possible. These orthoses should be designed to provide the same joint positioning as is provided by classic Scott–Craig orthoses.[37] An orthosis with a long sole plate and an ankle that is positioned rigidly in dorsiflexion makes walking easier for people with complete paraplegia who require KAFOs. The stability provided by these features makes it possible to maintain a balanced standing posture without upper extremity effort. (Once in a balanced standing posture, the individual may be able to balance with both hands lifted.) Additionally, the magnitude of the vertical oscillations of the individual's center of gravity during gait are less than occur with KAFOs that allow free dorsiflexion. The end result is that less energy is consumed during ambulation.[32,35]

Stance-Control KAFOs

In recent years, a new type of orthotic knee has been developed that stabilizes the knee during stance but allows knee flexion during swing. Several designs of KAFOs made with this type of knee (stance-control KAFOs, or SCKAFOs) are on the market, although they are not yet in common use. They may allow more normal-appearing and energy-efficient ambulation, but to date research has been sparse.[37–40] Elevated muscle tone may interfere with their functioning. Minimal hip and knee strength requirements for safe and functional use of these orthoses are as yet unclear and may vary between orthotic designs.

Hip–Knee–Ankle–Foot Orthoses

Hip-knee-ankle-foot orthoses (HKAFOs) provide orthotic control to the hips and joints caudal to this point. The various types of HKAFO differ most in the type of hip control that they provide. During gait, they can lock the hips in extension, allow a limited range of flexion and extension, or cause reciprocal motion at the hips. They all require the use of assistive devices for ambulation. HKAFOs are less functional than KAFOs in terms of capacity for stair and curb negotiation, transfers in and out of cars, and toileting.[41]

---

[k] A double-stop ankle is a double-action ankle joint with anterior and posterior stops.
[l] When the feet are flat on the floor and the ankles are held in dorsiflexion, the hips are placed in an anterior position. The effect of hip position on stability is discussed later in this chapter.
[m] Alternatively, drop-ring locks can be used.[143] Drop-ring locks are engaged and disengaged manually.

Conventional HKAFOs

A conventional HKAFO is made of the components used in KAFOs plus locking hip joints and a pelvic band to provide hip and pelvic stability. A spinal orthosis can be added to provide trunk stability. Because of the orthotic stabilization at the hips, ambulation with conventional HKAFOs is limited to a swing-to or swing-through gait.[33] Because of their weight and the high energy requirements of ambulation with these orthoses, conventional HKAFOs are rarely prescribed for adults with spinal cord injuries.[42]

Hip Guidance Orthoses

A Hip Guidance Orthosis (HGO), also called a ParaWalker, allows free flexion and extension of the hips within a limited range. This metal orthosis includes metal foot plates, locking knees, hip joints with flexion and extension stops, a pelvic band, and a chest strap. The wearer walks with a reciprocal gait by unweighting one leg at a time and allowing gravity to pull the unweighted leg forward like a pendulum suspended at the hip.[41,43] The wearer relies heavily on her arms during ambulation.[44,45] This type of orthosis has limited usefulness in terms of functional ambulation.[41]

Reciprocating Gait Orthoses

A Reciprocating Gait Orthosis (RGO) is a type of HKAFO that immobilizes the knees, ankles and feet and causes reciprocal motions of the hips during ambulation.[n] The orthosis consists of plastic KAFOs with locking knees and reinforced ankles, attached proximally to a molded pelvic band with thoracic extensions (Figure 12–3). Hip motions are controlled by cables that transfer forces between the hips. Motion at one hip causes motion in the opposite direction to occur in the contralateral hip: to take a step forward, the wearer shifts her weight off of the leg and extends the contralateral hip.[35,36,46] This hip extension is accomplished using scapular retraction and back extension.[47]

Alternative HKAFO designs that reciprocally link sagittal plane hip motions include the Advanced Reciprocating Gait Orthosis (ARGO), which couples the hips through one cable, and the Isocentric Reciprocating Gait Orthosis (IRGO), which utilizes a bar and tie rod mechanism to couple the hips.[48–50] The various designs of reciprocating gait orthoses (RGO, ARGO, and IRGO) enhance stance stability by preventing simultaneous bilateral hip flexion.[45,51] However, they have several disadvantages when compared to KAFOs. They are more expensive,[15,42,52] and require more frequent maintenance. They are bulkier and more cumbersome, making donning, doffing and transfers more difficult. These disadvantages are not counterbalanced by functional advantages; as is true with KAFOs and other types of HKAFO, ambulation with reciprocating gait orthoses is slow and requires a high energy expenditure.[8,42,46,47,49] Reciprocating gait

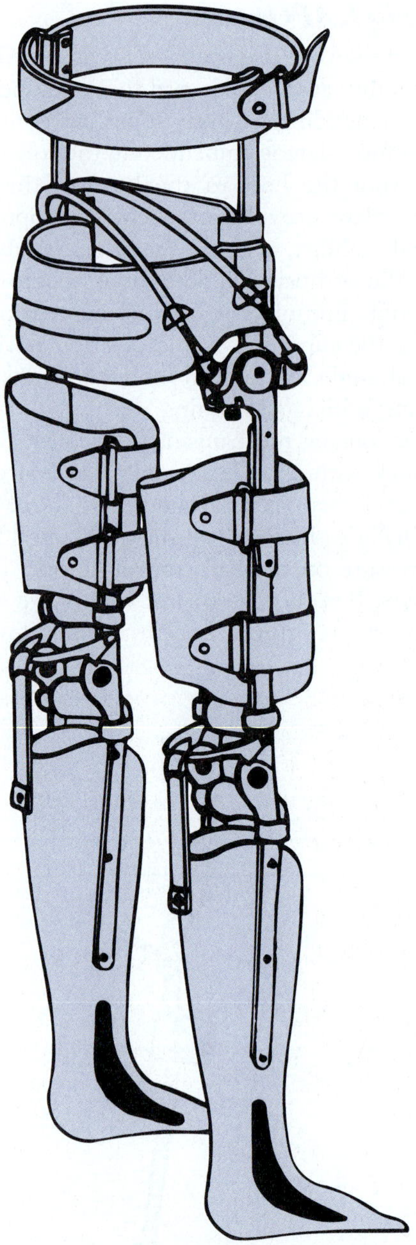

Figure 12–3   Reciprocating gait orthosis. (Reproduced with permission from Nick Rightor, CO, and the LSU Medical Center. [1983]. In *LSU Reciprocating Gait Orthosis: A Pictorial Description and Application Manual.* Chattanooga, TN: Fillauer, Inc.)

orthoses are more likely to be used for exercise than for functional mobility.[11]

FUNCTIONAL POTENTIALS

After a spinal cord injury, an individual's potential for achieving independence in ambulation and the orthotic support that she will require are determined largely by her

---

[n] One study reports incorporating stance-control KAFOs into reciprocating gait orthoses,[144] but this orthotic design is not in common use.

voluntary motor function. People with more intact voluntary motor function in their lower extremities are able to bear less weight on their arms while walking. This decreased dependence on the arms for support reduces the energy costs of ambulation.[6,7,53,54]

With complete injuries, the voluntary motor function present in the lower extremities is determined by the level of the lesion; thus lesion level has a strong impact on ambulatory potential. Table 12–4 presents a summary of the level of independence in ambulation that can be

TABLE 12–4   Potential for Functional Ambulation Following Complete Spinal Cord Injury

Motor Level	Significance of Innervated Musculature	Potential for Independence in Ambulation
C8 and higher	Inadequate voluntary motor function for functional ambulation.	Functional ambulation not feasible.
T1-T9	**Fully innervated upper extremities** make it possible to lift the body's weight using elbow extension and scapular depression. Trunk musculature inadequate to provide trunk control.	**Ambulation potential:** Unlikely to walk functionally; may walk for exercise, independently or with assistance. **Assistive devices:** Forearm crutches or walker. **Orthoses and movement strategies:** KAFOs with locked knees and ankles held in slight dorsiflexion are required for ambulation; swing limb advancement and hip and trunk stability during stance are achieved using compensatory movements of the head and upper extremities. Alternative orthoses: HKAFOs, various designs.
T10-T12	**Partial innervation of trunk musculature** (T6-L1 innervation) enhances ambulation ability. Lack of lower extremity motor function limits ambulation potential.	**Ambulation potential:** Independent functional ambulation within the home and for limited distances in the community is possible, although *most choose wheelchairs for mobility* due to the high energy requirements of ambulation. **Assistive devices:** Forearm crutches or walker. **Orthoses and movement strategies:** KAFOs with locked knees and ankles held in slight dorsiflexion are required for ambulation; swing limb advancement and hip stability during stance are achieved using compensatory movements of the head and upper extremities; trunk stability during stance is achieved using trunk musculature and/or compensatory movements, depending on the motor function present in the trunk. Alternative orthoses: HKAFOs, various designs.
L1	**Full innervation of trunk musculature** enhances ambulation ability. **Minimal innervation of psoas major** may provide active hip flexion (<3/5 strength*) during swing.	**Ambulation potential:** Independent functional ambulation is possible within the home and for limited distances in the community; *most choose wheelchairs for mobility* due to the high energy requirements of ambulation. **Assistive devices:** Forearm crutches or walker. **Orthoses and movement strategies:** KAFOs with locked knees and ankles held in slight dorsiflexion are typically required for ambulation; swing limb advancement is accomplished using either compensatory movements (for swing-through or swing-to gait) or active hip flexion (for four-point gait); hip stability during stance is achieved using compensatory movements of the head and upper extremities; trunk stability during stance is achieved using trunk musculature. Alternative orthoses: HKAFOs, various designs.

(Continued)

TABLE 12–4 (*Continued*)

Motor Level	Significance of Innervated Musculature	Potential for Independence in Ambulation
L2	**Partial innervation of psoas major, iliacus, sartorius, and pectineus** provide active hip flexion (≥3/5 strength*) for swing limb advancement. **Partial innervation of sartorius and gracilis** provide limited capacity for knee flexion for swing limb advancement (relevant only if AFOs are used instead of KAFOs.) **Minimal innervation of the quadriceps** (<3/5 strength*) inadequate to contribute significantly to ambulation.	**Ambulation potential:** Independent functional ambulation is possible within the home and for limited distances in the community; *most choose wheelchairs for mobility* due to the high energy requirements of ambulation. **Assistive devices:** Forearm crutches or walker. **Orthoses and movement strategies:** KAFOs with locked knees and ankles held in slight dorsiflexion are typically recommended for ambulation; swing limb advancement is accomplished using either compensatory movements (for swing-through or swing-to gait) or active hip flexion (for four-point gait); hip stability during stance is achieved using compensatory movements of the head and upper extremities; trunk stability during stance is achieved using trunk musculature. Potential for ambulation with ground-reaction AFOs.
L3	**Fully innervated iliacus and pectineus, and nearly full innervation of psoas major and sartorius** provide strong hip flexion for swing limb advancement. **Partial innervation of sartorius and gracilis** provide limited capacity for knee flexion for swing limb advancement (relevant only if AFOs are used instead of KAFOs.) **Partial innervation of the quadriceps** (≥3/5 strength*) provides potential for active knee control during stance.	**Ambulation potential:** Potential for independent community ambulation; many choose wheelchairs for long distances due to the high energy requirements of ambulation. **Assistive devices:** Forearm crutches or walker. **Orthoses and movement strategies:** If quadriceps strength is adequate for knee control (typically ≥4/5), the knee may be left unbraced; AFOs with plantarflexion stops or dorsiflexion assists are required to allow toe clearance during swing; dorsiflexion stops are needed to prevent excessive ankle dorsiflexion during late stance. If quadriceps strength is not adequate for knee control (typically <4/5), KAFOs with locked knees and ankles held in slight dorsiflexion are usually recommended for ambulation; swing limb advancement is accomplished using either compensatory movements (for swing-through or swing-to gait) or active hip flexion (for four-point gait); hip stability during stance is achieved using compensatory movements of the head and upper extremities; trunk stability during stance is achieved using trunk musculature. Alternative orthoses if quadriceps strength is inadequate for knee stability: ground-reaction AFOs.
L4	**Fully innervated sartorius and gracilis** provide limited capacity for knee flexion for swing limb advancement. **Fully innervated quadriceps** provides knee control during stance. **Partial innervation of the tibialis anterior and peroneus tertius** allows active dorsiflexion (≥3/5 strength*) during swing limb advancement and potential for eccentric control of ankle plantarflexion during early stance. **Partial innervation of tensor fascia latae, gluteus medius, and gluteus minimus** provide limited capacity for hip abduction, likely to be inadequate to stabilize the pelvis in the frontal plane during stance.	**Ambulation potential:** May ambulate independently within the community; if significant weight is borne on the upper extremities (because of hip extensor and abductor weakness), likely to choose wheelchairs for long distances due to the high energy requirements of ambulation. **Assistive devices:** Forearm crutches or canes. **Orthoses:** AFOs with dorsiflexion stops are required to prevent excessive ankle dorsiflexion during late stance; if dorsiflexor strength is inadequate to provide eccentric control of plantarflexion after initial contact, or if dorsiflexors fatigue during ambulation and toe drag results, a dorsiflexion assist may be required.

TABLE 12–4   *(Continued)*

Motor Level	Significance of Innervated Musculature	Potential for Independence in Ambulation
L5	**Nearly full innervation of the tibialis anterior** provides ankle dorsiflexion during swing and eccentric control of plantarflexion during early stance. **Nearly full innervation of the tensor fascia latae and partial innervation of the gluteus medius and gluteus minimus** provide stronger hip abduction for stabilization of the pelvis in the frontal plane during stance. **Partial innervation of the hamstrings** enhances the capacity for active knee flexion for swing limb advancement. **Nearly full innervation of peroneus tertius and extensor digitorum longus, and partial innervation of the tibialis posterior, peroneus longus and brevis, extensor hallucis longus, flexor digitorum longus, and flexor hallucis longus** provide limited capacity for stabilization of the subtalar joint and foot during stance.	**Ambulation potential:** Independent community ambulation. **Assistive devices:** Standard canes. **Orthoses:** AFOs with dorsiflexion stops are indicated to prevent excessive ankle dorsiflexion during late stance.
S1	**Full innervation of the tensor fascia latae, gluteus medius, and gluteus minimus** provides strong hip abduction for stabilization of the pelvis in the frontal plane during stance. **Nearly full innervation of the hamstrings** provides strong knee flexion for swing limb advancement. **Nearly full innervation of the hamstrings and partial innervation of the gluteus maximus** provide sagittal plane stability for the hip in early stance. **Partial innervation of the gastrocnemius and soleus** provide active plantarflexion ($\geq$3/5 strength*), with potential for eccentric control of dorsiflexion during midstance and terminal stance. **Full innervation of peroneus tertius and extensor digitorum longus, tibialis posterior, peroneus longus and brevis, and extensor hallucis longus; partial innervation of the flexor hallucis longus; and nearly full innervation of the flexor digitorum longus** provide strong inversion and eversion for stabilization of the subtalar joint and foot during stance.	**Ambulation potential:** Community ambulation. **Assistive devices:** No assistive devices, or standard cane(s). **Orthoses:** If plantarflexor strength is inadequate to control the forward progression of the tibias during late stance, AFOs with dorsiflexion stops are indicated.

(Continued)

TABLE 12–4   *(Continued)*

Motor Level	Significance of Innervated Musculature	Potential for Independence in Ambulation
S2	**Full innervation of the hamstrings and gluteus maximus** provides strong hip extension for stabilization of the hip in the sagittal plane during early stance. **Full innervation of the gastrocnemius and soleus** provides strong plantarflexion for eccentric control of dorsiflexion during midstance and terminal stance.	**Ambulation potential:** Community ambulation. **Assistive devices:** None. **Orthoses:** None.

KAFOs, knee–ankle–foot orthoses; HKAFOs, hip–knee–ankle–foot orthoses; AFOs, ankle–foot orthoses
* Strength grades indicate strength in key muscles according to American Spinal Injury Association classification system.
Sources: References 6, 7, 41, 52, 53, and 55 to 62.

achieved by people who have complete spinal cord injuries at different motor levels (motor component of the neurological level of injury).

With incomplete lesions, ambulatory potential is related more to the degree of completeness than the neurological level of injury. Greater preservation or return of voluntary motor function below the lesion leads to a better potential for functional ambulation.

In predicting an individual's capacity to walk, the clinician should take into consideration the many other factors that also affect functional gains. These include muscle tone, range of motion, pain, motivation, age, physical condition, medical complications, obesity, access to services and equipment, and physical coordination.[7,41,52,53,63–67]

PHYSICAL AND SKILL PREREQUISITES

Every functional activity involves a particular set of skills. Each activity also has strength, joint range of motion, and muscle flexibility requirements. A deficiency in any of these skill or physical requirements will impair a person's performance of the activity. Therapeutic programs are designed to develop the strength, range of motion, and skills required to meet patients' goals.

The descriptions of ambulation skills that follow are accompanied by tables that summarize the physical and skill prerequisites. Exact values for the physical prerequisites are not given because the requirements vary among individuals. For example, a person who is very skillful in coming to

Problem-Solving Exercise 12–1

Your patient has L5 paraplegia, ASIA A. He uses forearm crutches to walk without orthoses, bearing excessive weight on his upper extremities. When he attempts to walk without the crutches, he is unstable because of excessive knee flexion during late stance.

The patient's joint range of motion and muscle flexibility are normal throughout. His light touch and pin prick sensation are normal in the C2 through L5 dermatomes, impaired in S1, and absent below. Proprioception is normal in his upper extremities, hips, knees, and ankles. The muscle test results are as follows:

Muscles	Left	Right
Abdominals and upper extremities	5/5	5/5
Hip flexors	5/5	5/5

Muscles	Left	Right
Hip abductors	4/5	4/5
Quadriceps	5/5	5/5
Hamstrings	4/5	4/5
Ankle dorsiflexors	5/5	5/5
Long toe extensors	4/5	4/5
Ankle plantarflexors	2/5	2/5

- What is the most likely cause of this patient's knee instability during late stance? Explain your answer.
- Would AFOs or KAFOs be most beneficial for this patient? Why?
- What control should these orthoses provide? Explain.

stand from the floor may require less hamstring flexibility for this activity than does someone who is less skillful.

PRACTICE IN DEPARTMENT AND "REAL WORLD"

Independence in ambulation over even surfaces will enable a person to walk indoors in a single-level home or work environment. To walk in the community, obstacle negotiation skills are necessary. The physical therapy department in a rehabilitation center should be equipped with curbs of varying heights, stairs, and a ramp. This equipment is useful for the initial practice of obstacle negotiation; however, practice should not end with mastery of these artificial obstacles. Many obstacles that a patient will encounter outside of the department will be more difficult to negotiate. For example, ascending a cement curb from a street is likely to be more difficult than ascending a wooden curb from a linoleum floor. The world is full of carpeted floors, uneven sidewalks, long and steep staircases, and uneven surfaces such as grass and sand. Functional training should include practicing ambulation skills outside of the department so that the patient will be better prepared to function in the "real world" following rehabilitation.

AMBULATION WITH KNEE-ANKLE-FOOT ORTHOSES FOLLOWING COMPLETE SPINAL CORD INJURY: FUNCTIONAL TECHNIQUES AND THERAPEUTIC STRATEGIES

Complete spinal cord injury at and above the L3 or L4 neurological level of injury results in a loss of adequate voluntary motor function to control the knees and ankles during ambulation. KAFOs can provide a stable base during stance by immobilizing the ankles and knees. During gait training with KAFOs and assistive devices, the patient learns to use compensatory movement strategies to walk and perform other gait-related tasks.

Functional ambulation involves more than walking over even surfaces. To use KAFOs functionally at home, an individual must be able to balance in standing, walk over even surfaces, rise from a wheelchair and sit back down, fall safely and get up from the floor, and don and doff the orthoses. To walk in the community, she must also be able to walk over obstacles. This chapter presents descriptions of these ambulation skills using two KAFOs and forearm (Lofstrand) crutches,[o] as well as suggestions on how to teach these skills.

General Therapeutic Strategies

To accomplish a functional goal, the patient must acquire both the physical and skill prerequisites for that activity. For example, when working on ambulation with a swing-through gait, she must develop adequate strength and range in the extremities, as well as the ability to balance in standing, advance the lower extremities by pushing down on forearm crutches, and regain and maintain a balanced standing posture.

When developing skill prerequisites for a functional goal, the patient should start with the most basic prerequisite skills and progress toward more challenging activities. (A person had best develop the ability to maintain an upright standing posture before attempting to take a step.)

Before asking a patient to attempt a new skill, the therapist should explain and demonstrate the technique.[p] The demonstration should provide a clear idea of the motions involved and the timing of these motions. The therapist should also explain how the new skill will be used functionally.

During functional training, the therapist should remember that every person with a spinal cord injury will perform a particular activity differently. Each has a unique combination of body build, coordination, strength, and flexibility, and these characteristics influence the manner in which she performs functional tasks. For example, each person is unique in the exact motions that she uses and the timing of these motions as she stands up from the floor. What has worked for the last patient may be a total disaster for the next. The challenge of functional training is finding the timing and maneuvers that best suit the individual involved.

As a therapist and patient work together on a skill, they can learn from failed attempts by analyzing the problem. Is the patient strong enough to perform the maneuver? Is she flexible enough? Is she shifting her weight too far or not far enough? Are her crutches placed appropriately?

Equipment

The parallel bars or crutches should be adjusted to the appropriate height. The standard height for assistive devices is used: as the patient stands in a balanced posture with her shoulders relaxed and her hands on the parallel bars or on the crutches, her elbows should be in 20 to 30 degrees of flexion.

The therapist must evaluate the orthoses carefully to make sure that they fit and function well and are aligned appropriately. The ankles should be held in slight dorsiflexion, and the knees should lock securely in full extension. The orthoses must not exert excessive pressure on any area of the skin. Before the patient dons the orthoses the first time, the therapist should check for potential sources of trauma to the skin, such as rough seams in

---

[o] This chapter does not attempt to present all possible ambulation skills. An individual who is unable to master a skill described in this chapter may fare better with a variation of that technique or with an altogether different method.

[p] This demonstration can also be provided by another person with a spinal cord injury if someone is available who has similar impairments but a higher level of functional ability. Alternatively, the patient may watch a videotaped demonstration of the skill.

leather components or nail points protruding from the soles of the shoes. During gait training, the therapist and patient should check the patient's skin frequently for problems caused by abrasion or excessive pressure. The skin is at risk wherever it comes in contact with the orthosis.

Parallel Bars

Anyone with a complete spinal cord injury who lacks functioning hip extensors will be very unstable when she first gets onto her feet using KAFOs. For this reason, the most sensible place to initiate gait training is in the parallel bars. This equipment provides stable support for early practice; however, the very stability that makes parallel bars a secure place to begin standing and walking can cause problems. They will support a person's weight regardless of whether she pulls, pushes, or leans on them. No other assistive device can provide this degree of support. A patient who develops the habit of leaning laterally or pulling on parallel bars is likely to have difficulty making the transition to ambulation with other assistive devices.

To prepare a patient for the eventual transition to ambulation outside of the parallel bars, the therapist should encourage her to avoid leaning laterally or pulling on the bars. This should be stressed from the beginning of gait training, to avoid the development of bad habits. When pressing on the bars, the patient should direct the force vertically downward. By maintaining her hands in an open position while standing and walking, she can avoid inadvertently pulling on the bars.

No matter how careful a patient and therapist have been to avoid developing bad habits in the parallel bars, the transition from bars to crutches is a challenging one because crutches provide much less stable support than do parallel bars. Even someone who walks independently and skillfully in the parallel bars is likely to require close guarding, even significant assistance, when she first ventures out of the bars. The therapist should keep the difficulty of this transition in mind. Deterioration in the patient's performance when she first practices with crutches is not necessarily an indication that she should utilize a walker or return to the parallel bars for further preparatory practice.[q]

Guarding

Guarding is required during much of gait training to ensure the patient's safety. The challenge of guarding well is to keep the patient safe without interfering with her gait or motor learning.

Contact guarding while walking with a person with a complete injury is best done from behind. A therapist who stands behind the patient is less likely to get in the way of her head and trunk motions and feet as she steps. When

practicing stairs or curbs, the therapist is likely to find it easier to guard the patient when standing below her.

When a patient loses her balance while walking, the natural reaction for many therapists is to pull her pelvis (via a gait belt) up and toward the therapist. This guarding technique is not effective for people with complete spinal cord injuries because a backward tug on a patient's pelvis will throw her hips into an unstable position. Uncontrolled forward flexion of the trunk on the hips (jackknifing) is likely to result.

A therapist should guard in such a way that the patient's balance is restored, not hindered, when assistance is given. When a person lacking innervated hip extensors loses her balance while walking with KAFOs, the therapist should push her pelvis forward and pull her upper trunk back. These forces will return her to a balanced standing posture (Figure 12–4).

When a therapist makes a postural correction for a patient or catches her when she starts to lose her balance, the patient should be made aware of this assistance. Especially if the therapist has a hand on an area with impaired sensation, the patient may not realize that the therapist has assisted her. As a result, she will not realize that she has made an error that needs to be corrected.

There are two ways in which a therapist can make a patient aware of her mistakes and of the assistance being given. First, the therapist can provide verbal feedback. ("I had to catch you just now. You were falling to the left.") Verbal feedback is especially important when a patient first attempts a skill. In the second strategy, the therapist guards

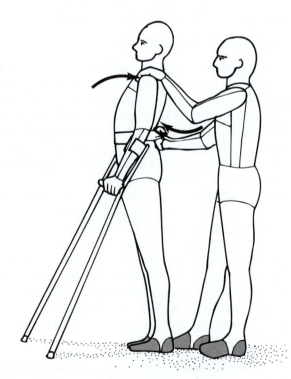

Figure 12–4   Forces applied when helping a patient maintain or return to a balanced standing posture.

in a way that enables the patient to feel her mistakes: when the patient starts to jackknife or lose her balance to the side, the therapist does not catch her or correct her posture until she has fallen far enough that she can sense what has happened.[r] In addition to detecting when she has begun to fall, the patient can practice responding to the instability and regaining her balance. This strategy for guarding is not appropriate when the patient first attempts a skill. Standing for the first time, or walking outside of the parallel bars for the first time, can be frightening enough as it is. The therapist should begin allowing partial falls only after the patient has overcome her initial fear of the activity.

Close guarding is required during most of gait training. At some point, however, a person who plans to walk independently must practice walking without spotting. The transition from walking with guarding to walking alone can be a test of nerves for both the patient and the therapist. To ease this transition, and to maximize the patient's safety throughout the process, the shift should be gradual. As (and *only* as) an individual demonstrates that she can safely perform a skill unassisted, the therapist's guarding should be withdrawn. The patient and therapist first progress from walking with contact guarding to walking with the

therapist's hands hovering inches away. They then progress to walking with the therapist standing nearby, ready to provide assistance if needed. When both parties are ready, the patient walks alone.[s] In this manner, the patient and (perhaps more so) the therapist can be weaned from guarding.

Balanced Standing

Balanced standing is the most basic ambulation skill; before a person can walk, she must be able to remain upright in a standing position. In the absence of innervated lower extremities, posture is the key to balanced standing. The position of stability is illustrated in Figure 12–5A. The person wearing KAFOs stands with her pelvis forward so that her weight line falls posterior to her hip joints. This position results in an extension moment at the hips. Since hip extension is restricted by the Y ligaments, the hips are stable in this posture.

In contrast to extension, hip flexion is not limited by ligaments. In the absence of muscular control, the hips will flex without restriction if a flexion moment exists at the hips. Thus if a person who lacks hip extensors changes her posture so that her weight line falls anterior to her hips, she will lose her stability at the hips; she will "jackknife" as a result of this unrestricted hip flexion (Figure 12–5B).

[r] This is not to say that the patient should be allowed to plummet halfway to the floor each time she starts to lose her balance. A few inches of free fall is generally enough to catch a person's attention.

[s] Before walking alone, the patient must be proficient in falling safely.

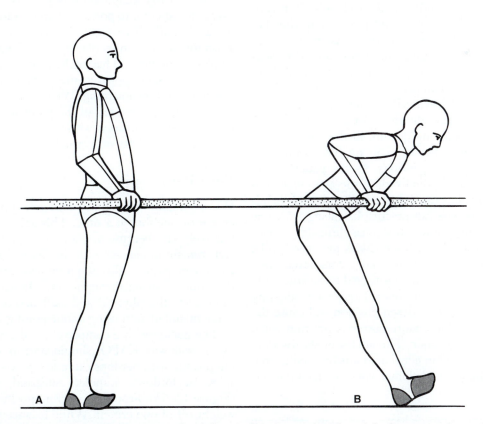

Figure 12–5   Balanced standing. (A) Position of stability: pelvis forward with weight line posterior to hip joints. (B) "Jackknifing": stability lost if weight line passes anterior to hips.

Attaining and maintaining a balanced standing posture is accomplished using the head-hips relationship. With her hands stabilized on parallel bars or forearm crutches, the person can push her pelvis forward by retracting her scapulae and throwing her head back. Tucking the head forward and protracting the scapulae will move the pelvis posteriorly.

Functional ambulation requires the ability to stand, at least briefly, with one or both hands lifted. This ability is required to move the crutches, open doors, and to reach for objects.

Balanced Standing—Therapeutic Strategies

Training in balanced standing should include practice maintaining a balanced standing posture as well as weight-shifting while standing upright. Before a patient begins practice in balanced standing, she should have had prior practice using the head-hips relationship to control her pelvis.[t]

Maintaining Balanced Standing

The therapist should demonstrate and explain the balanced standing posture, showing how head and shoulder motions can be used to move the pelvis and stabilize the hips. The patient should stand with her head erect, chest forward (scapulae retracted), and pelvis forward. Her feet should be a few inches apart.

During early training, the patient gains an awareness of her pelvic motions in standing and develops skill in controlling these motions. She should practice moving her pelvis using head and scapular motions. As she moves in and out of a balanced posture, she should attend to sensory cues that tell her of the position of her pelvis. Practice should include experiencing how her hips jackknife when her weight line falls anterior to her hips.

During initial training, the therapist can assist the patient to a balanced standing posture in the parallel bars. The therapist can help her to maintain the posture and give her feedback and suggestions. As the patient's skill develops, the therapist should reduce the assistance provided. Once the patient can balance well with both hands on the parallel bars, she can practice balancing with one hand, then both hands, lifted. If she has difficulty balancing, the alignment of the orthotic ankles may need to be adjusted. Aligning the ankles in a more dorsiflexed position will cause the pelvis to be positioned more anteriorly when the feet are flat on the floor. Conversely, aligning the ankles in a more plantarflexed position will cause the pelvis to be positioned in a more posterior position when the feet are flat on the floor. The ankles of the two orthoses should be aligned in equal amounts of dorsiflexion; asymmetrically aligned ankle joints will cause lateral instability in standing.

---

[t] Strategies for developing skill in controlling the pelvis using head and shoulder motions are presented in Chapter 10.

When a person with a spinal cord injury walks, her feet do not always land where she wants them to. A patient will be better prepared for ambulation if she learns to balance, at least briefly, with her feet in less than optimal positions. Training in standing balance, then, should be done with the feet in various positions. The patient should start with her feet in the easiest position (close to parallel and a few inches apart) and progress to balancing with her feet in more challenging positions.

Initial practice of standing balance should take place in the parallel bars. Once the patient has progressed to walking in the bars and is ready to start working with forearm crutches, she should practice standing with crutches. Because crutches provide less stable support than do parallel bars, balancing with them is more challenging.

Weight Shift in Standing

Before practicing weight shifts while standing with a given assistive device (parallel bars or forearm crutches), the patient should be adept in maintaining a balanced standing posture using that assistive device.

The patient can begin weight shifting with lateral shifts, with her feet side by side a few inches apart. As her skill improves, she can progress to shifting her weight with her feet in other positions. If she is to walk with a four-point gait, the patient must develop the ability to stand with one foot diagonally in front of the other and shift her weight onto the forward foot.

During early weight-shifting practice, the therapist can assist the patient into position in the parallel bars and guard her as she shifts her weight. The therapist can help her get a feel for the motion by placing a hand against the patient's trunk or shoulder and having her push against the hand. As the patient's skill improves, the therapist can withdraw the resistance and the guarding. When gait training in the parallel bars has progressed to the point where the patient is ready to start ambulation with forearm crutches, she should practice weight shifts with crutches.

Four-Point Gait

When walking with a four-point gait, a person moves one crutch or one foot at a time. This gait pattern is slow but relatively safe because at least three points (crutches and feet) remain in contact with the floor at all times. A four-point gait pattern also requires less energy expenditure than does a swing-through gait.[7] Tables 12–5 and 12–6 summarize the physical and skill prerequisites for independent ambulation using a four-point gait pattern.

The person with a complete spinal cord injury preparing to walk with KAFOs should start in a balanced standing posture with her hips extended, pelvis forward, lumbar spine in lordosis, scapulae retracted, and head erect (Figure 12–6A). From this starting position, she shifts her weight off of one crutch. While balanced on her feet and one crutch, she lifts the unweighted crutch and moves it forward (Figure 12–6B).

Problem-Solving Exercise 12–2

Your patient has T12 paraplegia, ASIA A. She has just started gait training with Scott-Craig KAFOs. When she stands in the parallel bars, she frequently loses control: her trunk falls forward rapidly, flexing at the hips.

- What is this type of loss of control called? Why does it occur?
- Describe the movement strategy that the patient could utilize in an attempt to avoid this uncontrolled motion.

- What range of motion limitation could be contributing to the difficulty that this patient has when standing?
- What orthotic adjustment could make balanced standing easier for this patient? Describe how you would make this adjustment.
- Describe how you should guard this patient.

TABLE 12–5   Ambulation Over Even Surfaces–Physical Prerequisites

	Four-Point Gait	Swing-Through Gait	Swing-to Gait	Drag-to Gait	Stepping Back or to the Side
Strength					
Trapezius	√	√	√	√	√
Deltoids	√	☑	√	√	√
Biceps, brachialis, and/or brachioradialis	√	√	√	√	√
Serratus anterior	☑	☑	☑	☑	☑
Pectoralis major	☑	☑	☑	•	☑
Latissimus dorsi	☑	☑	☑	√	☑
Triceps	☑	☑	☑	√	☑
Wrist and hand musculature	•	√	√	•	•
Abdominals	•	•	•	•	•
Quadratus lumborum	•				•
Iliopsoas	•				
Range of Motion					
Scapular — Elevation	√	√	√		
Scapular — Depression	√	√	√	√	√
Scapular — Abduction	√	√	√	√	√
Scapular — Adduction	√	√	√	√	
Scapular — Downward rotation	√	√			
Shoulder — Flexion	√	√	√	√	√
Shoulder — Extension	√	√			
Elbow — Extension	☑	☑	☑	√	√
Hip — Extension	☑	☑	☑	☑	
Knee — Extension	☑	☑	☑	☑	☑
Ankle — Dorsiflexion	√	√	√	√	√

√ Some strength is needed for this activity, or severe limitations in range will inhibit this activity.
☑ A large amount of strength or normal range is needed for this activity.
• Not required but helpful.

TABLE 12–6 Ambulation Over Even Surfaces–Skill Prerequisites

	Four-Point Gait	Swing-Through Gait	Swing-to Gait	Drag-to Gait	Stepping Back or to the Side
Control pelvis using head–hips relationship.*	✓	✓	✓	✓	✓
Balanced standing (p. 312).	✓	✓	✓	✓	✓
Weight shift in standing (p. 312).	✓	✓	✓	✓	✓
Lift and move one crutch (p. 314).	✓			✓	✓
Step forward with one leg (pp. 314–316).	✓				
Step to side or back with one or two legs (p. 319).					✓
Lift and move two crutches (p. 316).		✓	✓	(✓)	
Swing-through step (p. 316).		✓			
Swing-to step (pp. 317–319).			✓		
Drag-to step (pp. 318, 319).				✓	
Distance/efficient ambulation (p. 319).	✓	✓	✓	✓	

* Refer to Chapter 10 for a description of this skill and therapeutic strategies.
✓ This prerequisite skill is required to perform this activity.

After moving a crutch, the person steps with her contralateral foot. (For simplicity, the leg that is moving or about to be moved will be called the swing leg.) To step, she shifts her weight off of the swing leg, presses down on the crutches, and elevates the swing side of her pelvis (Figure 12–6C).

Elevation of the swing side of the pelvis can be accomplished by hip-hiking actively using the latissimus dorsi, quadratus lumborum, or abdominal musculature if these muscles are innervated. The person can supplement this muscular action with the head–hips relationship: while shifting her weight and pushing on her crutches, she tucks her head down and laterally away from the swing leg. As the torso pivots on the shoulders, the swing side of the pelvis lifts.

With one side of the pelvis lifted, gravity causes the leg to swing forward as a pendulum (Figure 12–6D). If the individual's hip flexors are innervated, she can use them to step actively.

After stepping, the person regains a balanced standing posture, pushing her pelvis forward by lifting her head and retracting her scapulae (Figure 12–6E). From the balanced standing posture, she repeats the process just described and steps with her other leg.

Four-Point Gait—Therapeutic Strategies

Before practicing walking, a patient should have gained some skill in balanced standing. Training in walking with a four-point gait pattern should include practice lifting and moving one crutch, and stepping forward with one leg. These skills can be practiced in combination, with the patient repositioning her crutches and stepping in the appropriate sequence.

Lift and Move One Crutch

To lift a crutch while standing, a person must be able to maintain a balanced standing posture and weight shift while using crutches. She will be better prepared to practice moving a crutch if she has practiced lifting a hand while standing in the parallel bars.

The patient should practice lifting and placing one crutch at a time while the therapist guards and provides assistance as necessary. As her skill improves, the assistance can be withdrawn.

Step Forward With One Leg

Balanced standing and weight shifting are prerequisites for stepping forward with one leg. To practice stepping using a given assistive device (parallel bars or forearm crutches), the patient should be adept in standing and shifting weight using that assistive device. She should also be skillful in the use of the head–hips relationship before attempting to step with one leg.

Practice should start with the patient standing in the parallel bars with one hand in front of the other. (The hand opposite the stepping leg should be more anterior.) From this position, she practices shifting her weight off of the leg and lifting her pelvis on the unweighted side. When her pelvis tilts (lifts on the unweighted side)

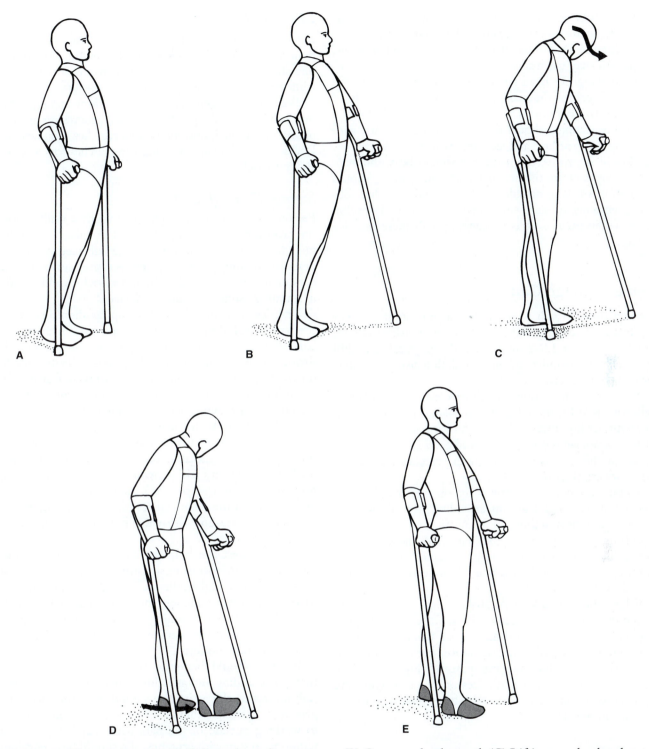

Figure 12–6   Four-point gait. (A) Balanced standing posture. (B) One crutch advanced. (C) Lifting one leg by elevating pelvis on that side. Head tucked down and laterally away from swing leg. (D) Once lifted, leg swings forward as a pendulum. (E) Balanced standing posture with one leg advanced.

enough to lift the foot off the ground, the leg swings forward as a pendulum or by muscle action, depending on whether or not the iliopsoas is innervated.

The patient elevates her pelvis by hip-hiking actively, or using the head–hips relationship, or a combination thereof. Whichever method she uses, the therapist can help her to learn the motion by demonstrating, assisting with the motion, and providing verbal and tactile feedback during practice.

A patient with innervated quadratus lumborum, latissimus dorsi, or abdominals can lay the groundwork for stepping by practicing elevating her pelvis in the side-lying position. Utilizing quick stretch and resistance, the therapist can facilitate motor learning and strengthening.

If using the head–hips relationship to elevate her pelvis, the patient may use exaggerated motions when first practicing, tucking her head far down and to the side. As she develops a feel for the maneuver, she can reduce her head and upper trunk motions.

Practice stepping should begin in the parallel bars, with the therapist guarding and assisting as needed. As the patient's skill improves, the assistance should be withdrawn. Once proficient in the parallel bars, the patient should progress to working outside of the bars with crutches. Before attempting to step with crutches, she should develop her dynamic balance skills in standing with these assistive devices.

Swing-Through Gait

A swing-through gait is faster than a four-point gait but requires more energy and entails a greater risk of falling. Tables 12–5 and 12–6 summarize the physical and skill prerequisites for independent ambulation using a swing-through gait pattern.

A person with a complete spinal cord injury about to walk with KAFOs should start in a balanced standing posture with her hips extended, pelvis forward, lumbar spine in lordosis, scapulae retracted, and head erect (Figure 12–7A). While in this posture she lifts both crutches and moves them forward (Figure 12–7B).

To take a step, the person leans on her crutches and lifts her pelvis (and legs) by extending her elbows, depressing and protracting her scapulae, and tucking her head (Figure 12–7C). Once the pelvis lifts enough for the feet to leave the ground, gravity will cause the torso and legs to swing forward as a pendulum suspended at the shoulders (Figure 12–7D).

When the person's heels strike (Figure 12–7E), she should move quickly to stabilize herself. By retracting her scapulae, moving her head and upper trunk posteriorly, and pushing on the crutches, she moves her pelvis forward to return to a stable standing posture (Figure 12–7F). Once in this posture, she balances on her feet while she repositions her crutches forward. She is then in position to take another step.

Swing-Through Gait—Therapeutic Strategies

Before practicing walking, a patient should have gained some skill in balanced standing. Gait training with a swing-through gait pattern should include practice lifting and moving two crutches at once, and taking a swing-through step. These skills can be practiced in combination, with the patient repositioning her crutches and stepping in sequence.

Lift and Move Two Crutches

Before attempting to reposition two crutches at once, a patient must be proficient in balanced standing with crutches. She should also be able to lift both hands simultaneously while maintaining a balanced standing posture.

Practice of this skill can begin with lifting and repositioning both hands in the parallel bars, and progress to maintaining balance while repositioning two crutches simultaneously. Practice should include moving the crutches forward, back, and to the side.

Swing-Through Step

Performing a swing-through step requires skillful use of the head–hips relationship, and skill in balanced standing, including moving in and out of the balanced posture. To practice stepping using a given assistive device (parallel bars or forearm crutches), the individual should be adept in standing using that assistive device.

Practice of swing-through stepping should start with the patient standing in a balanced posture in the parallel bars with her hands on the bars anterior to her hips. From this position, she should practice lifting her feet off of the floor by leaning forward onto her arms while extending her elbows, depressing and protracting her scapulae, and tucking her head. When her feet leave the ground, her trunk and legs will swing forward. During gait training, the therapist should stress the passive nature of the feet's motion: the crutch walker's task is to lift her feet; gravity will provide the force to move them forward. When the patient's heels strike, she should quickly regain the balanced standing posture by retracting her scapulae and throwing her head back, pushing her pelvis forward.

The therapist can help the patient learn the required motions by demonstrating, assisting with the motions, and providing verbal and tactile feedback during practice. The patient may use exaggerated motions when first practicing lifting her feet and regaining a balanced posture. As she develops a feel for the maneuver, she can reduce her head and upper body motions.

Practice should begin in the parallel bars, with the therapist guarding and assisting as needed. As the patient's skill improves, the assistance should be withdrawn. Once proficient in the parallel bars, the patient should progress to working outside of the bars with crutches. Before attempting to step with crutches, she should have developed her dynamic balance skills in standing with these assistive devices.

Swing-to and Drag-to Gait

Swing-to and drag-to gait patterns can be utilized by individuals who cannot safely walk using four-point or swing-through gaits. Tables 12–5 and 12–6 summarize the physical and skill prerequisites for independent ambulation using swing-to and drag-to gait patterns.

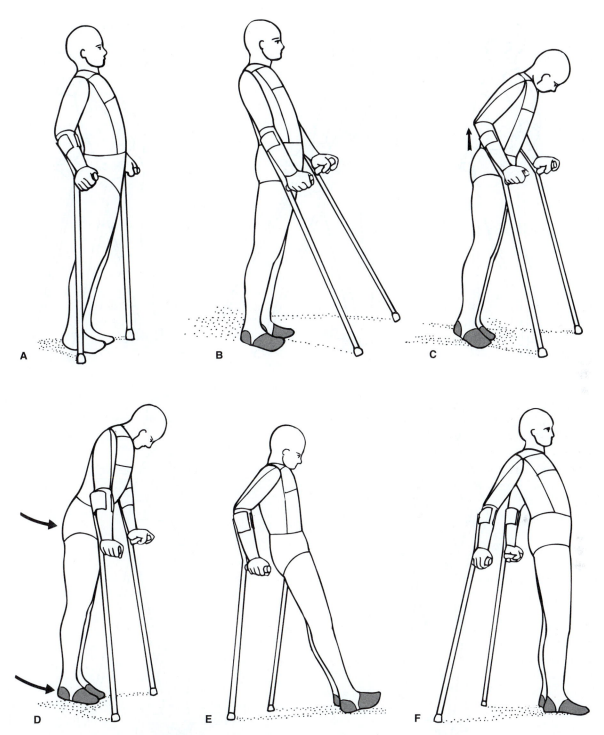

Figure 12–7   Swing-through gait. (A) Balanced standing posture. (B) Crutches advanced. (C) Lifting pelvis and legs by extending elbows, depressing and protracting scapulae, and tucking head. (D) Once lifted, torso and legs swing forward as a pendulum. (E) Heels strike. (F) Balanced standing posture regained by lifting head, retracting scapulae, and pushing on crutches to push pelvis forward.

Swing-to Gait

A swing-to gait is similar to a swing-through gait. The difference is that the person steps to, not past, her crutches (Figure 12–8). This gait pattern is slower than swing through, but it involves a smaller risk of falling.

The maneuvers used to perform a swing-to gait are the same as those used for a swing-through gait except that the person drops her feet before they swing past her crutches. At the end of the step, the feet and crutches are approximately collinear. This is an unstable position, as

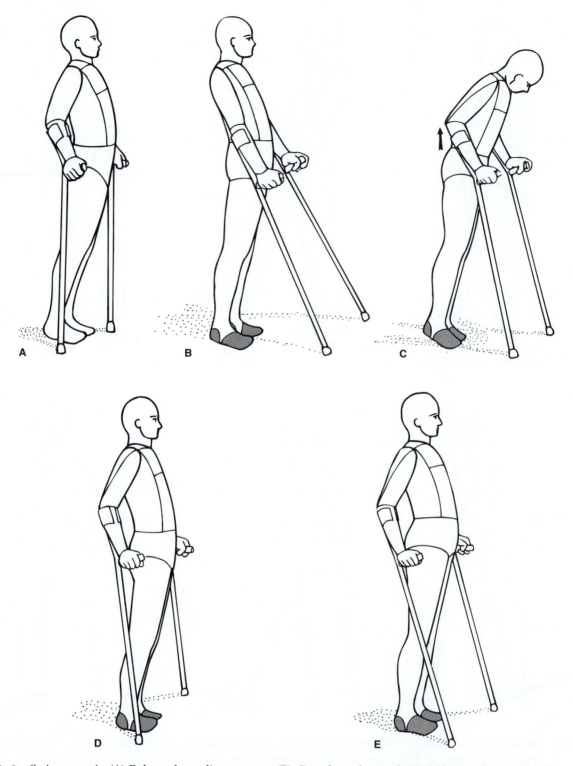

Figure 12–8   Swing-to gait. (A) Balanced standing posture. (B) Crutches advanced. (C) Lifting pelvis and legs by extending elbows, depressing and protracting scapulae, and tucking head. (D) Feet are advanced to, not past, crutches. Balanced standing posture resumed. (E) Crutches quickly repositioned anteriorly for greater stability.

the base of support is shallow in the anteroposterior di-mension. To maximize her stability while walking with a swing-to gait, the person should quickly reposition her crutches anteriorly once she has completed a step and re-gained a balanced standing posture.

Drag-to Gait

In the drag-to gait pattern, the feet remain on the floor as they are dragged to but not past the crutches. This is a slow, energy-consuming gait. It requires less strength than the other gait patterns, however, and thus may be the only option for a person with a relatively high lesion.

As is true with the other gait patterns, the person walking with a drag-to gait starts in the balanced standing posture and repositions her crutches anteriorly before taking a step. Depending on her stability in standing, she can reposition her crutches simultaneously or one at a time. After repositioning her crutches she leans forward, extends her elbows, and depresses her scapulae enough to unweight her legs and drag her feet toward the crutches.

After moving her feet, the person uses head and scapular motions to regain a balanced standing posture. As with a swing-to gait, she should quickly reposition her crutches at this point to increase her anteroposterior stability.

Swing-to and Drag-to Gait— Therapeutic Strategies

Before practicing walking, a patient should have gained some skill in balanced standing. Swing-to and drag-to gait patterns can be taught using the training strategies described for teaching a swing-through gait.

Stepping Backward or to the Side

Although walking primarily involves forward progression, functional ambulation also involves stepping backward or to the side. This skill is used to maneuver in small spaces and to position the feet in preparation for sitting down.

Stepping With One Foot

To step backward or to the side with one foot, the person lifts her leg using the same technique as is used in a four-point gait. She shifts her weight off of one leg and lifts it using active hip hiking, motions of her head and upper trunk, or a combination thereof to lift that half of her pelvis.

With her leg lifted, the person positions her foot by moving her pelvis. Using head and upper trunk motions to move her pelvis, she swings the leg as a pendulum. To step to the side, she moves her head and upper trunk back and forth laterally. This motion causes the unweighted leg to swing medially and laterally. To step backward, she moves her head and upper trunk up and down. This motion causes the unweighted leg to swing forward and back. Whether stepping forward, backward, or to the side, the person drops her pelvis (by lifting her head) to place her foot when it has swung to the desired position.

Stepping With Two Feet

To step backward or to the side with two feet, the person steps in a manner similar to a swing-to or drag-to gait. From a balanced standing position, she steps backward by placing her crutches posterior and lateral to her feet and then pushing down on the crutches. To step to the side, she first repositions her crutches a short distance in the direction toward which she plans to step. The crutches should not cross midline. The crutch toward which she plans to

step should be placed at a greater distance laterally. Once the crutches are positioned appropriately, the patient steps to the side by pushing down on the crutches. Whether stepping backward or to the side, the patient should quickly regain a balanced standing posture after each step.

Stepping Backward or to the Side— Therapeutic Strategies

The patient must be proficient in using the head–hips relationship, balanced standing, and weight shifting before attempting to step to the side or back. To practice stepping using a given assistive device (parallel bars or forearm crutches), the patient should be adept in standing and weight shifting using that assistive device. Prior practice in stepping forward should make learning to step back or to the side easier.

Stepping With One Foot

Starting in a balanced standing position, the patient practices shifting her weight off of one leg and lifting her pelvis on the unweighted side. With her leg lifted, the patient practices swinging it laterally or forward and back using head and upper trunk motions to move her pelvis. She may use exaggerated motions when first practicing. As she develops a feel for the maneuver, she can reduce her head and upper body motions. Once she has learned to swing her leg, the patient can practice placing her foot by lowering her pelvis when her foot has swung to the desired position.

Practice should begin in the parallel bars, with the therapist guarding and assisting as needed. As the patient's skill improves, the assistance should be withdrawn. Once proficient in the parallel bars, the patient should progress to working with crutches.

Stepping With Two Feet

Practice stepping backward with two feet can begin in the parallel bars, with the therapist guarding and assisting as needed. As the patient's skill improves, the assistance should be withdrawn. Once proficient in the parallel bars, the patient should progress to working outside of the bars with crutches. Before attempting to step with crutches, she should develop her dynamic balance skills in standing with these assistive devices.

Practice of lateral stepping is limited in the parallel bars, as the bars do not allow one hand to move toward the patient's midline while the other hand moves away. For this reason, lateral stepping with two feet should be practiced using forearm crutches.

Distance and Efficient Ambulation

Once a patient is able to walk with a given gait pattern, she will require practice to develop her endurance and perfect her skills. She should walk over increasing distances as her ability develops, and practice walking on surfaces (carpet, sidewalks, grass, etc.) on which she is likely to walk after discharge.

Negotiating Ramps

Ramp-negotiation skills are required for independent ambulation in the community. Tables 12–7 and 12–8 summarize the physical and skill prerequisites for independent ambulation over ramps.

The greatest challenge when walking up or down a ramp is avoiding being thrown down the slope. When a person wearing orthoses with immobile ankle joints stands on a slope, her orthoses, and therefore her hips, are thrown in the downhill direction.

TABLE 12–7 Ambulation Over Obstacles–Physical Prerequisites

		Ramps	Curbs	Stairs
Strength				
Trapezius		√	√	√
Deltoids		√	√	√
Biceps, brachialis, and/or brachioradialis		√	√	√
Serratus anterior		☑	☑	☑
Pectoralis major		☑	☑	☑
Latissimus dorsi		☑	☑	☑
Triceps		☑	☑	☑
Wrist and hand musculature		√	√	√
Abdominals		•	•	•
Quadratus lumborum		•	•	•
Iliopsoas		•	•	•
Range of Motion				
Scapular	Elevation	√	√	√
	Depression	√	√	√
	Abduction	√	√	√
	Adduction	√	√	√
	Downward rotation	√	√	√
Shoulder	Flexion	√	√	√
	Extension	√	√	√
Elbow	Extension	☑	☑	☑
Hip	Extension	☑	☑	☑
Knee	Extension	☑	☑	☑
Ankle	Dorsiflexion	√	√	√

√ Some strength is needed for this activity, or severe limitations in range will inhibit this activity.
☑ A large amount of strength or normal range is needed for this activity.
• Not required but helpful.

TABLE 12–8 Ambulation Over Obstacles–Skill Prerequisites

	Ascend Ramps	Descend Ramps	Ascend Curbs	Descend Curbs	Ascend Stairs	Descend Stairs
Swing-to ambulation over even surfaces (pp. 317–319)	√					
Swing-to ambulation up a slope (pp. 320, 321).	√					
Swing-through ambulation over even surfaces (p. 316).		√	√	√	√	√
Swing-through ambulation down a slope (pp. 320, 321).		√				
Balanced standing (p. 312).	√	√	√	√	√	√
Reposition crutches while standing (pp. 314, 316).	√	√	√	√	√	√
Step up curb or step (pp. 321, 322).			√		√	
Step down from curb or step (pp. 321, 322).				√		√

√ This prerequisite skill is required to perform this activity.

Ascend

When ascending a ramp, a person walking with KAFOs should keep her crutches well in front of her feet. To maximize hip stability, she should keep her body angled up the hill, with her pelvis well forward. She should use a step-to (or step-toward) gait, not a swing-through pattern.

Descend

When a person wearing KAFOs walks forward down a ramp, the slope tends to throw the hips toward a stable position. A swing-through gait pattern can be used.

Negotiating Ramps—Therapeutic Strategies

A patient must be proficient in ambulation over even surfaces before beginning practice on ramps. Even if she walks well on even surfaces, she is likely to be very unstable when first walking on slopes. This is especially true when ascending, because the inclined surface tends to throw the pelvis into an unstable position. The patient should be encouraged to keep her crutches well in front of her feet when ascending and to keep her body angled up the hill with her pelvis well forward. She should use a step-to (or step-toward) gait, not a swing-through pattern. When descending, she may step past her crutches.

Practice in ramp negotiation should not be limited to the gentle 1:12 grade of a standard public incline. Many if not most ramps in the community are far steeper than this. The patient who intends to walk in the community should develop the skills needed to ascend and descend ramps as steep as possible within her potential. Practice in ramp negotiation should start on gentle slopes, progressing to steeper inclines as the patient's skill allows. Close guarding will be required until the patient has mastered these techniques.

Negotiating Curbs

Curb negotiation skills are required for independent ambulation in the community. Although ramps have become common, they still are not universally present. Tables 12–7 and 12–8 summarize the physical and skill prerequisites for independent ambulation over curbs.

Ascend

To ascend a curb, the person approaches it face-on. She positions her feet with the toes at the edge of the curb (Figure 12–9A), regains a balanced standing posture, then places her crutch tips on the higher surface of the curb, a few inches from the edge (Figure 12–9B).

From the starting position, the person lifts her feet onto the curb. She does this by leaning forward on the crutches, tucking her head, extending her elbows, and depressing her scapulae (Figure 12–9C). As her feet lift, the toes will drag up the vertical surface of the curb. When the toes lift past the curb, her torso and legs will swing forward as a pendulum.

A person ascending a curb can step to or past her crutches. When her feet land, she quickly throws her head back and retracts her scapulae to push her pelvis forward and regain a balanced standing posture (Figure 12–9D).

Descend

When descending a curb, the person approaches it face-on. She assumes a balanced standing posture with her feet a few inches from the edge of the curb and places her crutch tips close to the edge of the curb (Figure 12–10A).

From the starting position, the person steps off the curb. She does this by leaning on the crutches, tucking her head, extending her elbows, and depressing her scapulae. When the feet lift, her torso and legs will swing forward as a pendulum (Figure 12–10B).

When the person's feet have swung past the edge of the curb, she drops them. (When "dropping" her legs, she

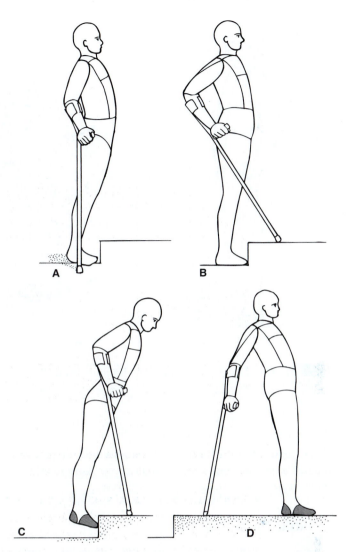

Figure 12–9   Ascending curb. (A) Balanced standing posture with toes at edge of curb. (B) Crutches onto curb. (C) Lifting feet onto curb by leaning on crutches, extending elbows, and depressing scapulae. (D) Pelvis pushed forward by throwing head back and retracting scapulae.

quickly lowers her torso/legs/feet with eccentrically controlled elbow and shoulder motions.) When her feet land, the person regains a balanced standing posture, pushing her pelvis forward by throwing her head back and retracting her scapulae (Figure 12–10C).

Negotiating Curbs—Therapeutic Strategies

Before trying to ambulate over curbs, the patient must be proficient in ambulation over even surfaces. During training, the therapist should emphasize maintaining control during ascent and descent, and rapid resumption of a balanced standing posture once the feet have landed. Close guarding

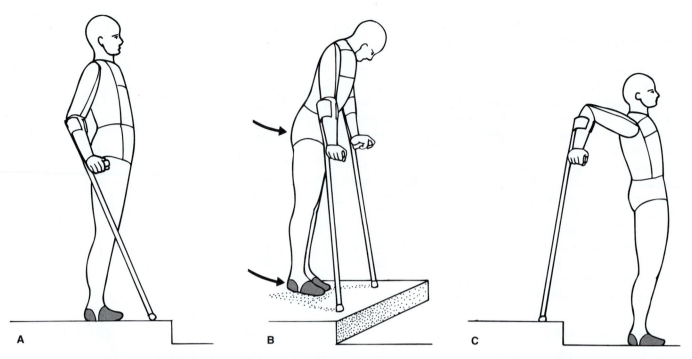

Figure 12–10   Descending curb. (A) Balanced standing posture with crutches close to edge of curb. (B) Swing-through step. (C) Pelvis pushed forward by throwing head back and retracting scapulae.

will be required until the patient has mastered these techniques. Practice should start on small curbs. As the patient's skill increases, the curb height can be increased.

Negotiating Stairs

Anyone who walks in the community inevitably comes across stairs. Many public and private buildings have stairs at their entrances. Within buildings, elevators are not always present and working. Patients who learn to climb stairs during gait training are less likely to discontinue ambulation after discharge.[11] In deciding whether to pursue ambulation on stairs as a functional goal, however, the therapist and patient should weigh the potential benefits of this skill against the risk of significant injury in the event of a fall on stairs.

In the following techniques for negotiating stairs, the person does not use a rail. The techniques are described in this way because rails are not always available in the community. The methods described can be adapted easily: when negotiating stairs using one crutch and one rail, the person holds the crutch not in use in the hand that holds the other crutch (Figure 12–11).

Ascend

Ascending stairs is similar to ascending a series of curbs. The curb negotiation techniques described above can be used to ascend stairs front-on (facing up the stairs).

In an alternative approach, the crutch walker can ascend stairs backward. In the starting position for this technique, the person stands facing away from the stairs. She should

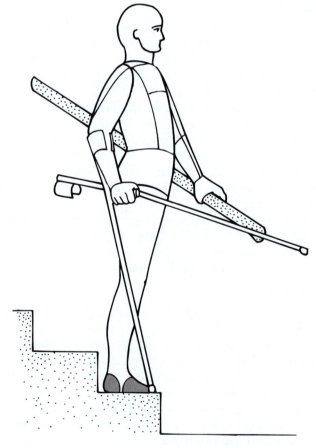

Figure 12–11   Descending stairs using a rail and one crutch, carrying second crutch.

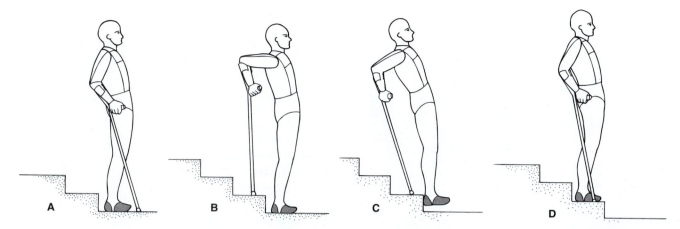

Figure 12–12   Ascending stairs backward. (A) Balanced standing posture with feet a few inches from lowest step. (B) Crutches placed on step. (C) Lifting feet onto step by leaning on crutches, extending elbows, and depressing scapulae. (D) Balanced standing posture regained.

stand in a balanced posture with her feet in front of the first stair and her crutches anterior to her feet (Figure 12–12A).

From the starting position, the person places her crutches on the lowest step (Figure 12–12B). She then leans on the crutches, extends her elbows, and depresses her scapulae to lift her feet onto the step (Figure 12–12C). When her feet lift past the step, her torso and legs will swing backward as a pendulum. When her feet land, she throws her head back and retracts her scapulae to push her pelvis forward and to regain a balanced standing posture (Figure 12–12D).

Descend

Descending stairs is much like descending a series of curbs. A technique similar to the method for negotiating curbs, described earlier, can be used to descend stairs. The person places her crutches close to the edge of the step on which she stands and lifts her feet; her torso and legs then swing forward as a pendulum.

The difference between descending a step and a curb is that when descending a step in a stairway, the crutch walker has a limited area on which her feet can land safely. Thus, when negotiating stairs, she must control the length of her step. If her feet land too far from their starting position, she will miss the next step. To avoid this problem, she should allow her feet to swing back over the step before she drops them.

Negotiating Stairs—Therapeutic Strategies

Practice in ascending and descending curbs should precede stair negotiation. As a patient masters the ability to negotiate curbs, she will develop the skills used on stairs: ascending and descending steps, quickly regaining a balanced standing position, and repositioning crutches from one step to another. Once a patient is skillful in negotiating step-high curbs, she can progress to practicing on stairs. Close guarding will be required until the patient has mastered these techniques.

Coming to Stand from a Wheelchair, Both Hands on Armrests

Functional ambulation requires the ability to get into a standing position. The techniques described below center on rising from a wheelchair. They can be adapted to surfaces other than wheelchairs.[u] Tables 12–9 and 12–10 summarize the physical and skill prerequisites for this activity.

In the most readily achievable method of coming to stand from a wheelchair, the person gets onto her feet while both hands remain on the wheelchair. Because both hands remain on a relatively stable surface, this method is easier, steadier, and requires less skill than the other techniques presented. Rising from a wheelchair using this method takes longer, however, because more steps are involved.

To rise from her wheelchair using this method, the person first locks the chair's brakes, places her crutches where she will be able to reach them once she is on her feet, and locks the orthotic knees. She then positions her buttocks so that she is sitting at the front edge of the seat, resting on the side of her pelvis. Once she is positioned appropriately on the seat, the person positions her legs in preparation to stand. The superior leg should rest on top of or slightly anterior to the other leg (Figure 12–13A).

In the next step the person turns and places her hands on the armrests (Figure 12–13B). She then gets onto her feet using the head–hips relationship: she presses forcefully down on the armrests, protracts her scapulae, and twists her head and upper trunk. Her head and upper trunk should move downward and rotate toward the side of the chair on which she sits (Figure 12–13C). This motion will cause her pelvis to lift up and over her feet. Once

---

[u] An individual who plans to walk in the community should practice getting up and down from other sitting surfaces such as car seats and standard chairs.

TABLE 12–9   Coming to Stand from Wheelchair–Physical Prerequisites

	Both Hands on Armrests	One Hand on Armrest and One on Crutch	Both Hands on Crutches
Strength			
Trapezius	√	√	√
Deltoids	☑	√	√
Biceps, brachialis, and/or brachioradialis	√	√	√
Serratus anterior	☑	☑	☑
Pectoralis major	☑	☑	☑
Latissimus dorsi	√	☑	☑
Triceps	☑	☑	☑
Wrist and hand musculature	√	√	√
Abdominals	•	•	•
Range of Motion			
Scapular Elevation	√	√	√
Depression	√	√	√
Abduction	√	√	√
Adduction	√	√	√
Upward rotation	√	√	√
Downward rotation		√	√
Shoulder Flexion	√	√	√
Extension	√	√	√
Internal rotation	√	☑	☑
Elbow Flexion	√	√	√
Extension	☑	☑	☑
Hip Flexion	√	√	√
Extension	☑	☑	☑
Knee Extension	☑	☑	☑
Ankle Dorsiflexion	√	√	√
Combined hip flexion and knee extension	☑	☑	☑

√ Some strength is needed for this activity, or severe limitations in range will inhibit this activity.
☑ A large amount of strength or normal range is needed for this activity.
• Not required but helpful.

TABLE 12–10   Coming to Stand from Wheelchair–Skill Prerequisites

	Both Hands on Armrests	One Hand on Armrest and One on Crutch	Both Hands on Crutches
Control pelvis using head–hips relationship.*	√	√	√
Position legs in preparation to stand (p. 326).	√	√	√
Hands on armrests, assume standing position from wheelchair (p. 326).	√		
Standing in front of wheelchair with hands on armrests, grasp crutch (p. 326).	√		
Standing with one hand on armrest and one on crutch, grasp second crutch (p. 326).	√	√	
Standing with crutches positioned forward, walk crutches back (pp. 326, 327).	√		
One hand on armrest and one on crutch, assume standing position from wheelchair (p. 327).		√	
Balanced standing (p. 312)	√	√	√
Both hands on crutches, assume standing position from wheelchair (pp. 328, 329).			√
While standing, lift and move both crutches (p. 316).			√

* Refer to Chapter 10 for a description of this skill and therapeutic strategies.
√ This prerequisite skill is required to perform this activity.

on her feet, the person uses the head–hips relationship to maintain balance.

The person now stands with her hands on the wheelchair's armrests (Figure 12–13D). Her next task is to substitute her crutches for the armrests. To grasp the first crutch, she shifts laterally to unweight one hand. While balancing on her feet and one hand, she grasps a crutch and positions it on her free arm (Figure 12–13E). She

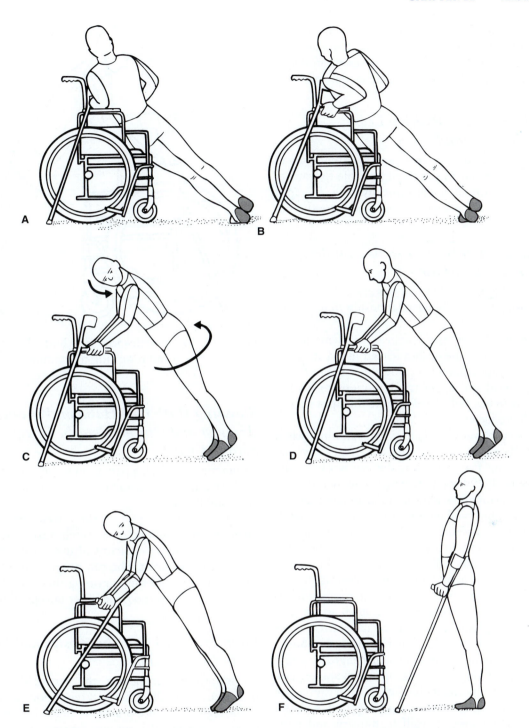

Figure 12–13   Coming to stand from a wheelchair, both hands on armrests. (A) Sitting at front edge of seat, resting on side of pelvis. (B) Hands on armrests. (C) Rising to feet using head–hips relationship. (D) Standing with hands on armrests. (E) Crutch positioned on arm. (F) Upright standing.

then places the crutch tip on the floor, lateral to the wheelchair. Shifting her weight onto the crutch, she un-weights her other hand and grasps the remaining crutch. After positioning the second crutch on her arm, she places the crutch tip on the floor, lateral to the wheelchair. From this position, she achieves an upright standing posture by walking her crutches back (Figure 12–13F).

Coming to Stand From a Wheelchair, Both Hands on Armrests—Therapeutic Strategies

Practice of this method of coming to stand from a wheelchair should begin after the patient has developed some skill in maintaining a balanced standing posture with forearm crutches. The patient should practice each of the component skills involved in coming to stand with two hands on the wheelchair, and combine these skills in series. Strategies for developing these skills are described in the following paragraphs.

Sitting in Wheelchair, Position Legs in Preparation to Stand

If an individual has the physical potential to come to standing from a wheelchair, she should be able to learn to position her legs without much difficulty. The therapist should demonstrate the maneuver and encourage the patient to practice.

With Hands on Armrests, Assume Standing Position From Wheelchair

Before a patient begins working on this skill, she must be proficient in using the head–hips relationship to move her pelvis.

During initial practice, the therapist can demonstrate and assist the patient as she pushes herself into a standing position. The therapist should encourage her to use forceful and abrupt head and upper trunk motions to lift her pelvis. As the patient's skill develops, the therapist's assistance should be reduced.

This maneuver is most difficult at its beginning, when the person lifts her buttocks from the seat. If an individual has difficulty lifting from the seat, she can work on the skill in reverse in the following manner. The therapist assists her to the starting position for practice: standing facing the chair with one hand on each armrest. The patient's feet should be in front of and slightly lateral to the casters, positioned so that when she pivots on her feet to move toward sitting, her buttocks will land on the seat. From this position, the patient turns and lowers her buttocks slightly toward the seat and then returns to the starting position (Figure 12–14). She should move over a small arc at first, lowering herself only as far as she can retain control of the motion and push back up. As her skill improves, she should increase the arc of motion. She should challenge her limits as she practices, working in a range in which she experiences difficulty but can maintain control. By pushing her limits in this manner, the patient gradually builds to the point where she can lower herself to the seat and push back up to standing.

Standing in Front of Wheelchair With Hands on Armrests, Grasp Crutch

Anyone who has the physical potential to assume a standing position from a wheelchair should achieve this prerequisite skill without much difficulty. The patient can start by practicing weight shifting while standing in front of a wheelchair with her hands on the armrests. She can progress to lifting a hand, then grasping a crutch. The therapist can assist the patient into position and guard her as she practices.

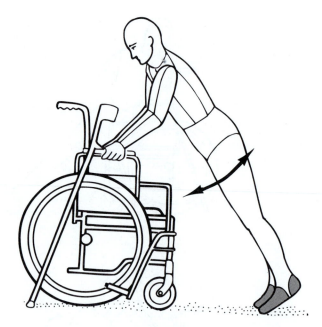

Figure 12–14   Practice lowering buttocks toward seat and returning to standing.

Standing With One Hand on Wheelchair Armrest and One on Crutch, Grasp Second Crutch

To practice this skill, a patient must be able to shift weight while standing with crutches, and balance in standing with one hand lifted.

The patient stands facing the wheelchair with one hand on an armrest and one on a crutch. From the starting position, the patient practices shifting her weight off of the hand on the armrest. She can progress to lifting the unweighted hand and then grasping the second crutch. The therapist can help the patient get into position and guard her as she practices.

Standing With Crutches Positioned Forward, Walk Crutches Back

To perform this maneuver, the person shifts her weight from one side to the other and repositions each crutch as it is unweighted. Before practicing this skill, a patient should be proficient in balanced upright standing and able to lift and reposition one crutch at a time while standing upright.

Walking the crutches back from a forward position is most difficult when the crutch tips are furthest from the feet. In this position, the person is furthest from upright and the greatest amount of weight is being borne through the crutches. As she walks her crutches toward her feet, she assumes a more upright posture. Her weight is increasingly borne through her legs, and the task becomes easier.

Practice of this skill will be easiest if the patient starts in the least challenging position and works toward the most difficult. She should start with her legs close to vertical, with the crutch tips a few inches in front of her feet.

From this position, she walks her crutches away from her feet and back again. As her skill improves, she walks her crutches over greater distances, walking the crutch tips as far forward as she can while maintaining control and retaining the ability to return to upright.

Coming to Stand From a Wheelchair With One Hand on Armrest, One on Crutch

When standing up from a wheelchair using this method, the person gets onto her feet with only one hand on the wheelchair. The other hand rests on a crutch, which provides a much less stable base of support. For this reason, this method requires more skill than does coming to stand with both hands on the wheelchair. The advantage of this method is that it is faster than coming to stand with both hands remaining on the chair. Tables 12–9 and 12–10 summarize the physical and skill prerequisites for this activity.

The person starts by locking the wheelchair's brakes and placing her crutches within easy reach. She then moves her buttocks to the front edge of the seat, locks the orthotic knees, and positions her legs and buttocks so that her legs extend diagonally from the seat.

After positioning her legs, the person grasps a crutch and places the cuff on her arm. The crutch should be held in the hand that is furthest from the chair. After grasping the crutch, the individual should place her free hand on the armrest that she faces (Figure 12–15A).

The person now sits diagonally at the front of her seat, with one hand on an armrest and one on a crutch. From this position she pushes down with both hands, keeping her head tucked. If she performs the maneuver correctly, her pelvis will lift and her feet will drag toward the chair (Figure 12–15B). When the legs reach a vertical or nearly vertical position, she pushes her pelvis forward to attain a balanced standing posture (Figure 12–15C).

Once on her feet in a balanced posture, the person shifts her weight laterally onto the crutch. She then lifts her free hand, grasps the second crutch (Figure 12–15D) and positions her arm in it, and places the crutch tip on the floor (Figure 12–15E). After repositioning her crutches as necessary, she is ready to walk.

Coming to Stand from a Wheelchair with One Hand on Armrest, One on Crutch— Therapeutic Strategies

Practice of this skill requires proficiency in using the head–hips relationship to move the pelvis. The patient must also be skillful in balanced standing with crutches, including moving in and out of a balanced standing posture. The patient should practice the component skills involved in coming to stand using this method: position the legs in preparation to stand, assume standing by pushing on one armrest and one crutch, balance in standing and grasp second crutch. Training strategies for developing

these prerequisite skills are described above and in the following paragraph. These skills can be combined in series during practice.

One Hand on Armrest And One on Crutch, Assume Standing Position From Wheelchair

During initial practice, the therapist can demonstrate and then assist the patient as she practices this maneuver. This skill does not lend itself to practicing in reverse, as the feet are dragged across the floor while the patient rises from sitting. The therapist should encourage the patient to push forcefully with her upper extremities to lift her pelvis and should provide assistance as needed. The assistance can be reduced as the patient's skill develops.

Coming to Stand from a Wheelchair With Both Hands on Crutches

This is the fastest method of rising to standing from a wheelchair using KAFOs. It also requires the most skill; rising from a chair while balancing on two crutches is a very challenging maneuver. Tables 12–9 and 12–10 summarize the physical and skill prerequisites for this activity.

The person starts by locking her wheelchair's brakes, moving her buttocks to the front edge of the seat, locking her orthotic knees, and positioning her legs so that they extend straight forward from the seat. She then grasps both crutches, positions them on her arms, and places the crutch tips lateral to the wheelchair (Figure 12–16A).

To rise to standing, the crutch walker pushes down forcefully on the crutches. As she first lifts from the chair, she should keep her trunk flexed forward at the hips (Figure 12–16B). As her legs move toward vertical, she extends her trunk toward and then past vertical by pushing on the crutches, lifting her head, and retracting her scapulae to push her pelvis forward (Figure 12–16C). As she reaches a vertical standing position, she quickly repositions her crutches forward. In this manner she assumes a balanced standing posture (Figure 12–16D).

Coming to Stand from a Wheelchair With Both Hands on Crutches—Therapeutic Strategies

Before attempting this maneuver, the patient must be proficient in using the head–hips relationship to move her pelvis. She must also be skillful in balanced standing with crutches, including moving in and out of a balanced standing posture. Once these skills are mastered, the patient can practice the prerequisite skills involved in coming to stand by pushing on two crutches: position the legs in preparation to stand, assume standing position from a wheelchair with both hands on crutches, and lift and move both crutches while standing. Training strategies for developing these

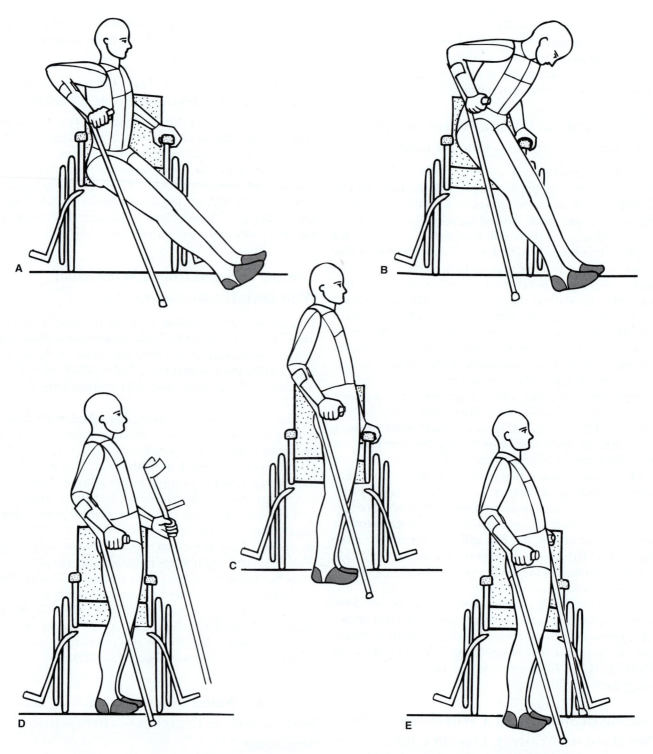

Figure 12–15   Coming to stand from a wheelchair, one hand on armrest and one on crutch. (A) Sitting at front edge of seat with one hand on armrest and one on crutch. (B) Lifting pelvis by tucking head while pushing on crutch and armrest. (C) Balanced standing posture. (D) Grasping second crutch. (E) Second crutch placed on floor.

skills are described above and in the following paragraph. The therapist can demonstrate the sequence of steps used to stand, and then assist the patient as she practices. As the patient's skill develops, the therapist can reduce the assistance given.

Both Hands on Crutches, Assume Standing Position From Wheelchair

Rising from sitting in this manner requires a forceful push to lift the body's weight. It also requires precise timing as the patient uses the head–hips relationship to achieve a

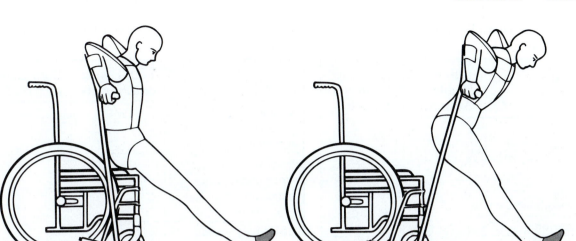
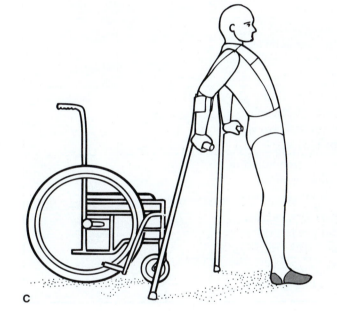
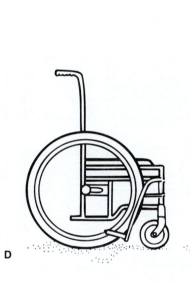
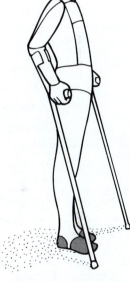

Figure 12–16   Coming to stand from a wheelchair, both hands on crutches. (A) Sitting at front edge of seat with both hands on crutches. (B) Rising from wheelchair. (C) Scapular retraction and head–hips relationship used to push pelvis forward. (D) Balanced standing posture with crutches repositioned anteriorly.

balanced standing posture while she lifts her body weight over her feet (Figure 12–16B and C). The therapist should encourage the patient to push forcefully and abruptly on her crutches and to keep her head tucked as her pelvis lifts. As the patient's legs move toward vertical, she must quickly push her pelvis forward to attain a balanced standing posture. During practice, the patient can work on perfecting her motions and timing. She can also experiment with different crutch positions to determine which position enables her to come to standing most easily; she may find that placing the crutch tips in a more posterior or anterior position on the floor makes the task easier.

Sitting Down From a Standing Position, Both Hands on Armrests

Functional ambulation requires the ability to sit down safely after walking. The following techniques center on sitting on a wheelchair. They can be adapted to surfaces other than wheelchairs. Tables 12–11 and 12–12 summarize the physical and skill prerequisites for sitting down from a standing position.

The challenge of rising from a chair is obvious: the person must lift herself onto her feet, maintaining her balance throughout the maneuver. Returning to the chair poses a

TABLE 12–11   Sitting Down From a Standing Position–Physical Prerequisites

	Both Hands on Armrests	Both Hands on Crutches
Strength		
Trapezius	√	√
Deltoids	√	√
Biceps, brachialis, and/or brachioradialis	√	√
Serratus anterior	☑	☑
Pectoralis major	☑	☑
Latissimus dorsi	√	☑
Triceps	☑	☑
Wrist and hand musculature	√	√
Abdominals	•	•
Range of Motion		
Scapular Elevation	√	√
Depression	√	√
Abduction	√	√
Adduction	√	√
Upward rotation	√	√
Downward rotation		√
Shoulder Flexion	√	√
Extension	√	√
Internal rotation	√	☑
Elbow Flexion	√	√
Extension	☑	☑
Hip Flexion	√	√
Extension	☑	☑
Knee Extension	☑	☑
Ankle Dorsiflexion	√	√
Combined hip flexion and knee extension	☑	☑

√ Some strength is needed for this activity, or severe limitations in range will inhibit this activity.
☑ A large amount of strength or normal range is needed for this activity.
• Not required but helpful.

less obvious challenge: the individual must lower herself into the chair without traumatizing her skin or tipping the chair. She does this by controlling her descent so that she lands squarely on the seat rather than on an armrest or on the backrest, and she lands without undue force.

TABLE 12–12   Sitting Down from A Standing Position–Skill Prerequisites

	Both Hands on Armrests	Both Hands on Crutches
Position self in preparation to sit in wheelchair (p. 331).	√	√
Standing facing wheelchair, place hands on armrests (pp. 331, 332).	√	
Move pelvis using head-hips relationship.*	√	√
Balanced standing (p. 312).	√	√
Facing wheelchair with hands on armrests, turn and lower self into chair (p. 332).	√	
Standing facing away from wheelchair, lower self into chair (p. 333).		√
While standing, lift and move both crutches (p. 316).	√	√
Step forward, back, and to the side (pp. 314–316, 319).	√	√
Weight shift in standing (p. 312).	√	

* Refer to Chapter 10 for a description of this skill and therapeutic strategies.
√ This prerequisite skill is required to perform this activity.

Sitting down from a standing position using this method is similar to coming to stand with both hands on the armrests, performed in reverse. While lowering herself to sitting, the person supports herself with both hands on the wheelchair. Because the wheelchair provides a relatively steady base of support, this method of sitting from a standing position requires the least skill to perform safely.

In the starting position the individual stands facing the wheelchair with her feet in front of and slightly lateral to the casters (Figure 12–17A). The appropriate foot position depends on the person's height. The feet should be placed so that when the crutch walker pivots on them, she will land squarely on the seat.

Standing in front of the wheelchair, the person shifts her weight onto one crutch and removes her unweighted hand and forearm from the other crutch. She then leans

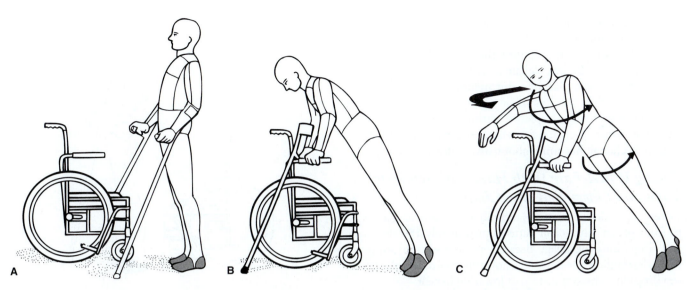

Figure 12–17   Sitting down from standing position, both hands on armrests. (A) Standing facing wheelchair. (B) Both hands placed on armrests. (C) Turning toward hand on armrest.

the unused crutch against the wheelchair and places her free hand on an armrest. Shifting her weight onto the armrest, she removes her other hand and forearm from its crutch, leans the crutch against the wheelchair, and places her hand on the other armrest (Figure 12–17B).

The person is now standing in front of the wheelchair supporting herself with a hand on each armrest. In the next step, she turns and lowers herself into the chair. The direction of the turn is determined by the position of her feet in relation to the wheelchair. The turn should be toward the feet: if the feet are to the left of the chair, the head and upper trunk should turn toward the left. As she turns, she releases one armrest. (If turning to the left, she releases the right armrest.) She can either throw her free arm in the direction of the turn (Figure 12–17C) to add momentum to the turn or place her hand on the rear of the seat, on the side toward which she is turning. After landing, she unlocks the orthotic knees and repositions her buttocks on the seat as needed.

Sitting Down From a Standing Position, Both Hands on Armrests—Therapeutic Strategies

To practice this maneuver, a patient must be proficient in using the head–hips relationship to move her pelvis, and in the following skills with crutches: moving in and out of a balanced standing posture, shifting weight, lifting a hand, repositioning the crutches, and stepping in all directions. Once she has mastered these basic skills, she can practice the component skills involved in this method of sitting from a standing position: she should learn to position herself in preparation to sit in a wheelchair, place her hands on the wheelchair's armrests, and turn and lower

herself onto the wheelchair seat. These skills, described in the following paragraphs, can be combined in series.

Position Self in Preparation to Sit in Wheelchair

When sitting down from a standing position, a person wearing KAFOs with the knees locked pivots on her feet as she descends. Thus, she must position her feet appropriately prior to sitting in order to land correctly in the wheelchair. If her feet are not properly positioned before she sits, her buttocks may hit the chair's backrest or armrest, or even miss the wheelchair altogether. For this reason, an important aspect of functional training involves helping the patient to learn where to position her feet before sitting down.

To find the optimal foot position, the therapist and patient can first make an educated guess, judging from the individual's leg length and predicting the path of her buttocks as she pivots on her feet. The patient can then position her feet and, with the therapist guarding closely, sit down in the chair. If she does not land appropriately on the seat, the patient and therapist should determine what was wrong with her initial foot position. (Were her feet too close to the chair? Too far away? Too far lateral to the chair's midline? Not lateral enough?) She can then try again with her feet in a different position. By this informed trial-and-error process and by learning from their mistakes, the patient and therapist can find an appropriate foot position for sitting down in the chair.

Standing Facing Wheelchair, Place Hands on Armrests

The patient should practice shifting her weight off one crutch, leaning the crutch on the wheelchair, and placing her unweighted hand on an armrest. She then repeats these actions with her other hand. During initial practice, the therapist provides guarding and assistance as needed. As the patient's skill improves, the assistance can be reduced.

The patient should get into the habit of leaning her crutches against the wheelchair where she can reach them. When crutches are placed in this manner instead of being tossed aside, they are less likely to be damaged. In addition, the crutch that is placed within reach remains retrievable. Once a crutch is tossed, the patient loses the option to change her mind about sitting down.

Facing Wheelchair With Hands on Armrests, Turn and Lower Self Into Chair

When sitting down using this technique, the person standing in front of her wheelchair turns approximately 180 degrees and drops into the chair. Because she releases an armrest while descending, the descent is not truly controlled: the person drops into the seat instead of lowering herself.

The therapist should encourage the patient to use head and upper trunk motions that are forceful enough to generate the momentum required to turn her torso and land on her buttocks. The therapist should guard closely at first. As the patient's skill develops, the guarding can be withdrawn.

Sitting Down from a Standing Position, Both Hands on Crutches

Using this method to sit down from a standing position, a person supports herself on two crutches while lowering herself into a wheelchair. This maneuver requires more skill than is needed if she supports herself on the armrests.

In the starting position for this maneuver, the crutch walker stands well in front of the wheelchair, facing away from it (Figure 12–18A). The appropriate foot position depends on her height. The person should place her feet so that when she pivots on them, she will land squarely on the seat. It is critical that she places her feet an appropriate distance from the chair. If she stands too far from the chair, she will miss the seat when she sits. If she stands too close to the chair, she will hit the backrest instead of the seat and may tip the chair over backward.

Standing facing away from the wheelchair, the crutch walker balances on her feet and repositions her crutches posteriorly (Figure 12–18B). The exact placement of the crutches will vary among individuals. The person should position the crutches so that she will be able to pivot on them and lower her buttocks onto the seat.

After positioning her crutches, the person supports her weight on the crutches and tucks her head forward. This causes her pelvis to move backward out of the position of stable standing, and she jackknifes at the hips (Figure 12–18C). She then lowers herself onto the seat. After landing, she unlocks the orthotic knees and repositions her buttocks on the seat as needed.

A person who has orthoses that have knee mechanisms with bail controls (described earlier in this chapter) can use a slightly different technique to sit down. She first stands

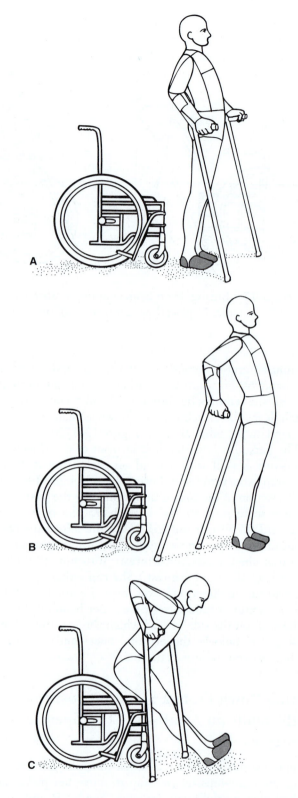

Figure 12–18   Sitting down from standing position, both hands on crutches. (A) Standing facing away from wheelchair. (B) Crutches repositioned posteriorly. (C) Lowering self onto wheelchair seat.

facing away from the chair with her legs against or close to the chair so that the bail controls are above the sitting surface. She then positions her crutches lateral to the chair (one on each side of the chair), and leans back on them. This motion will cause the bail controls to press against the sitting surface and unlock the knees. When this occurs, the knees will flex. The person should control her descent by supporting her weight and balancing on the crutches as she lowers her buttocks to the wheelchair seat. Because of the inherent instability of unlocking the knees while weight is being borne through the legs, this method of sitting down may require more practice than does sitting down with the knees locked.

Sitting Down From a Standing Position, Both Hands on Crutches—Therapeutic Strategies

To practice this maneuver, a patient must be proficient in using the head–hips relationship to move her pelvis and in the following skills with crutches: moving in and out of a balanced standing posture, repositioning the crutches, and stepping in all directions. Once she has mastered these basic skills, she can practice positioning herself and her crutches in preparation to sit in a wheelchair and lowering herself onto the wheelchair seat. These skills, described earlier and in the following paragraph, can be combined in series.

Standing Facing Away From Wheelchair, Lower Self Into Chair

During functional training, the therapist and patient work together to determine the best placement for the feet and crutches relative to the wheelchair.[v] The patient also practices the stand-to-sit maneuver, working to control her descent to the extent possible. Because the crutches do not provide a stable base of support, she is not likely to be in total control of the descent, able to stop or reverse her motion at will. She should, however, have enough control to land without excessive force and with her buttocks squarely in the seat. As the patient practices with guarding, the therapist should encourage her to control her motion as she lowers herself into the wheelchair. As her skill develops, the guarding can be withdrawn.

Falling Safely

Ambulation involves a risk of falling. Anyone who walks, especially if she has impaired motor and sensory function, is likely to fall eventually. Practice of falling techniques may minimize the risk of injury. Tables 12–13 and 12–14 summarize the physical and skill prerequisites for falling safely.

When falling, there are two things that a crutch walker can do to minimize her risk of injury. First, she can move her crutches out of the way so that she does not injure

---

[v] The strategies described in the earlier section, "Position self in preparation to sit in wheelchair," can be used for this determination.

TABLE 12–13 Falling Safely and Standing from the Floor–Physical Prerequisites

	Fall Safely	Stand From the Floor
Strength		
Trapezius		√
Deltoids	√	√
Biceps, brachialis, and/or brachioradialis	√	√
Serratus anterior	☑	☑
Pectoralis major	☑	☑
Triceps	☑	☑
Wrist and hand musculature	√	√
Abdominals		•
Range of Motion		
Scapular Elevation		√
Scapular Abduction	√	√
Scapular Adduction	√	√
Scapular Upward rotation	√	☑
Scapular Downward rotation		√
Shoulder Flexion	√	☑
Shoulder Extension		√
Shoulder Internal rotation		√
Shoulder Horizontal adduction		√
Shoulder Horizontal abduction	√	☑
Elbow Flexion	√	√
Elbow Extension	√	☑
Hip Flexion		√
Hip Extension		☑
Knee Extension		☑
Ankle Dorsiflexion		√
Combined hip flexion and knee extension		☑

√ Some strength is needed for this activity, or severe limitations in range will inhibit this activity.
☑ A large amount of strength or normal range is needed for this activity.
• Not required but helpful.

herself by landing on a crutch or by having a crutch exert excessive force on her arm. While falling, the person throws her crutches laterally (or laterally and posteriorly) away from the path of fall. She should aim to get the

TABLE 12–14 Falling Safely and Standing from the Floor–Skill Prerequisites

	Fall Safely	Stand From the Floor
Throw crutches (p. 334).	√	
Catch self on hands (p. 334).	√	
Position self in prone*		√
Position crutches in preparation to stand (p. 336).		√
Assume plantigrade posture from prone (p. 336).		√
Dynamic balance in plantigrade and modified plantigrade (pp. 336, 337).		√
In plantigrade, walk hands toward feet (p. 337).		√
In plantigrade, grasp and position crutch (p. 337).		√
In modified plantigrade with one hand on crutch, grasp and position second crutch (p. 338).		√
From modified plantigrade supported on two crutches, push torso to upright (p. 338).		√
Standing with crutches positioned forward, walk crutches back (pp. 326, 327).		√

* Refer to Chapter 9 for a description of this skill and therapeutic strategies.
√ This prerequisite skill is required to perform this activity.

crutch tips up off of the floor, so that the crutches do not act as fulcrums on her arms when she lands.

The second thing that a person can do when she falls is to break her fall with her arms. She should land on her palms and cushion the fall by allowing her elbows and shoulders to "give" when she lands. She must *not* hold her arms rigid as she falls onto them.

Falling Safely—Therapeutic Strategies

The two components of this maneuver, throwing the crutches and landing on the hands, can initially be practiced separately or in combination. Before training is complete, however, the patient must practice both together.

Throw Crutches

In throwing the crutches while falling, the aim is to position them so that they will not cause injury. The patient should be encouraged to throw her crutches out of her path of fall, swinging the crutch tips upward so that they do not catch on the ground. The throw should not be forceful. The goal is to position the crutches out of the way, but not to fling them out of reach. The forearm cuffs may remain on the arms.

To get a feel for the throw, the patient can practice throwing one crutch at a time while the therapist guards her. For added security while practicing throwing one crutch, the patient can stand outside of a set of parallel bars and hold the nearest bar.

Catch Self on Hands

When a patient practices falling and landing on her hands, the therapist should stress to the patient that she *must* allow her arms to "give" to absorb the shock. During initial practice, the force of the fall should be minimized. The therapist can accomplish this by having the person fall over a short distance onto a floor mat, and by lowering her instead of allowing her to fall unrestrained. As the patient's skill develops, she can progress to falling unrestrained over a short distance and gradually build the distance over which she falls.

Assume Standing Position from the Floor

After getting onto the floor, either by falling or by design, a person needs to be able to get back up. This task is challenging but feasible for people with intact upper extremity function. Tables 12–13 and 12–14 summarize the physical and skill prerequisites for assuming a standing position from the floor.

To prepare to rise from the floor, the person gets into a prone position with her hips adducted and externally rotated, and the orthotic knees locked in extension. She then places a crutch on either side of herself. The crutch tips should point away from her feet, and the grips should be at or caudal to the level of her greater trochanters. In this position, the crutches will be within reach when she is ready to use them.

After positioning her crutches and legs, the person places her palms on the floor next to her shoulders (Figure 12–19A). She then moves from prone to plantigrade by lifting her pelvis from the floor using the head–hips relationship, pushing down and forward (away from her feet) while tucking her head (Figure 12–19B). When she has lifted her pelvis as high as she can, she walks her hands toward her feet while keeping her head tucked. This maneuver will elevate the pelvis further (Figure 12–19C).

As the person walks her hands toward her feet, her legs become more vertical. By walking her hands back, she moves her legs as far as she can toward (not past) vertical. The remaining steps involved in coming to stand will be easier with more vertically oriented legs.

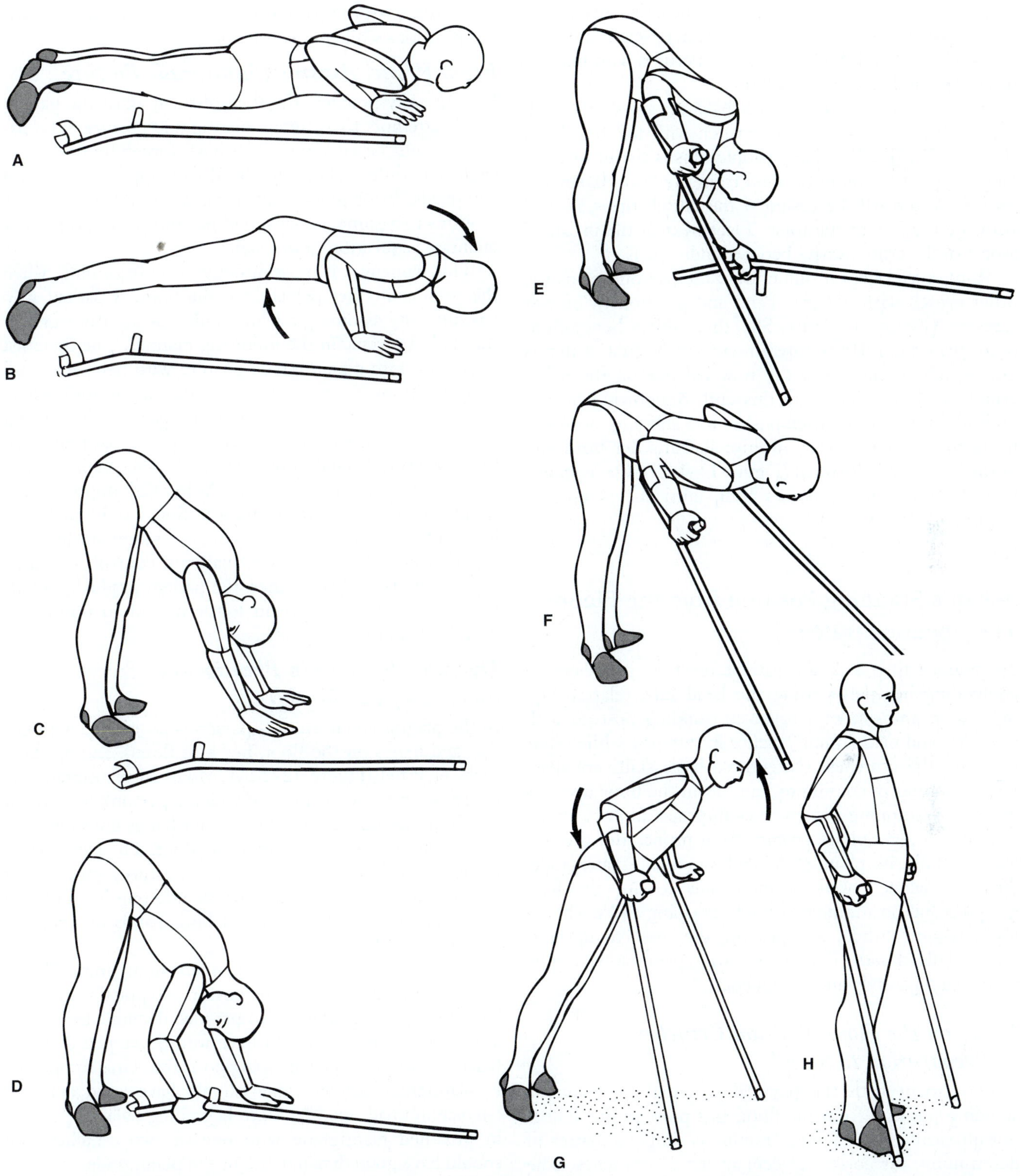

Figure 12–19   Assuming standing position from the floor. (A) Starting position: prone with legs and crutches positioned appropriately, palms on floor. (B) Lifting to plantigrade using head–hips relationship. (C) Pelvis elevated fully. (D) Grasping first crutch. (E) Balancing on one crutch while grasping second crutch. (F) Forearm cuffs positioned. (G) Pushing trunk upright. (H) Upright standing.

Once the individual has elevated her pelvis maximally by walking her hands back, she shifts her weight and balances on one hand. She then grasps a crutch with her unweighted hand (Figure 12–19D).

In the next step the person balances on one crutch while grasping the remaining crutch with her free hand (Figure 12–19E). For many people, this is the most challenging part of coming to stand from the floor. Balancing on one crutch will be easiest if the crutch tip is aligned with the midline of the torso. Placement of the proximal aspect of the crutch varies between individuals.

While propping on one crutch, the person grasps the other crutch with her free hand and positions it on her forearm (Figure 12–19F). She then shifts her weight onto this crutch. If the forearm cuff of the first crutch is not on her forearm, she can now balance on the other crutch while repositioning this cuff. Supporting herself on both crutches, she then pushes to a standing position: using the head–hips relationship, she lifts her head and pushes her pelvis forward (Figure 12–19G). Once standing, she walks her crutches back until she is upright (Figure 12–19H).

Assume Standing Position from the Floor—Therapeutic Strategies

To practice this skill, the patient must be proficient in controlling her pelvis using the head–hips relationship, moving in and out of a balanced standing posture with crutches, and maintaining balance in standing while repositioning the crutches. Once these basic skills are mastered, training in coming to stand from the floor involves practice positioning the crutches in preparation to stand, assuming a plantigrade posture from prone, and the following skills in plantigrade and modified plantigrade: dynamic balance, walking the hands toward the feet, grasping and positioning a crutch, grasping and positioning a second crutch, and pushing the torso to upright. These skills, described in the following paragraphs, can be practiced separately and in sequence.

Lying on the Floor, Position Crutches in Preparation to Stand

For a patient with the physical potential to assume a standing position from the floor, this prerequisite skill is not physically challenging. Training is simply a matter of determining the correct placement for the crutches. The person should position her crutches so that she will be able to reach them easily when the time comes. The appropriate position will depend on how far back she walks her hands in plantigrade as she comes to stand. The crutches' hand grips are likely to be reached easily if they are positioned at or caudal to the level of the greater trochanters. The therapist and patient can determine the optimal crutch position through problem solving and trial

and error, with the patient grasping the crutches in various positions while in plantigrade.

From Prone, Assume Plantigrade Posture

During early practice, the therapist can assist the patient as she attempts to assume a plantigrade posture. The patient should be encouraged to push forcefully down and cephalad while tucking her head and upper torso to lift her pelvis. Prior practice in using head and upper trunk motions to assume a quadruped position from prone may facilitate acquisition of this skill.

This maneuver is most difficult at its beginning, when the person lifts her pelvis from the floor. A patient who has difficulty assuming a plantigrade posture can work on the skill in reverse in the following manner. The therapist assists her into a plantigrade posture with her pelvis well off of the floor. From this position, the patient lowers herself slightly toward prone and pushes back to the starting position. She should move over a small arc of motion at first, lowering herself only as far as she can retain control of the motion and push back up. As her skill improves, she should increase the arc of motion. She should challenge her limits as she practices, working in a range in which she experiences difficulty but can maintain control. By pushing her limits in this manner, the patient gradually builds to the point where she can lower herself to prone and push back up to plantigrade.

Dynamic Balance in Plantigrade and Modified Plantigrade

In the plantigrade posture, a person is positioned with her feet and hands on the floor, her hips flexed, and her buttocks elevated (Figure 12–20A). Modified plantigrade includes a variety of postures in which a person's feet are on the floor, her hips are flexed, and her hands are supported by a surface that is higher than the floor. The hand placement in the modified plantigrade postures involved in coming to stand from the floor include one hand on the floor and one on a crutch, and both hands on crutches (Figure 12–20B and C).

A patient need not be independent in attaining plantigrade or modified plantigrade postures to practice dynamic balance in these positions. To practice dynamic balance in a given posture, she should have well-developed dynamic balance skills in less challenging postures. Thus to practice in plantigrade, an individual should have good dynamic balance in quadruped.[w] Before beginning balance practice in modified plantigrade with one or two crutches, she should have good dynamic balance in plantigrade.

To develop dynamic balance in plantigrade or modified plantigrade, the patient can start with practice maintaining the posture. The therapist can assist her into position and have her attempt to maintain the posture using head,

---

[w] Strategies for developing dynamic balance in quadruped are presented in Chapter 10.

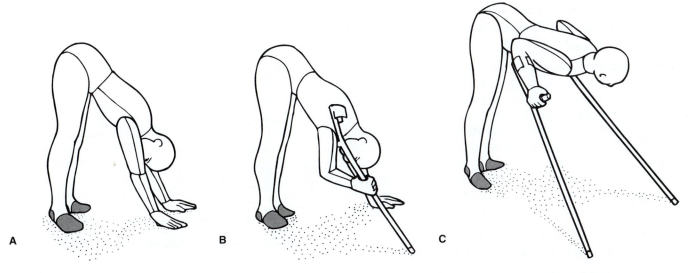

Figure 12–20 Plantigrade and modified plantigrade postures. (A) Plantigrade. (B and C) Modified plantigrade postures involved in coming to stand from the floor with KAFOs and forearm crutches.

scapular, and upper trunk motions to control her pelvis. The therapist helps at first, reducing the assistance as the patient's skill improves. The patient can progress to maintaining the position while the therapist applies resistance in various directions.

One task when practicing modified plantigrade with one hand on a crutch involves determining the crutch position that best suits the individual. Three crutch positions used in coming to stand from the floor are illustrated in Figure 12–21. While working on balance in modified plantigrade, the patient can try the different crutch positions to see which one affords her the best control.

Once an individual is able to stabilize herself in plantigrade or modified plantigrade, she can progress to shifting her weight in that posture, then weight shifting and lifting the unweighted hand, and finally maintaining her balance as she lifts a hand and reaches in different directions. All of these actions can be performed with and without resistance supplied by the therapist.

In Plantigrade, Walk Hands Toward Feet

To practice walking her hands back while in a plantigrade posture, a patient she does not have to be independent in assuming this posture. However, she should have well-developed dynamic balance skills in plantigrade. This will allow her to learn to walk her hands back with minimal practice. During early training, the therapist may help her control her pelvis as she attempts the maneuver. This assistance can be decreased as the patient's skill develops.

In Plantigrade, Grasp and Position Crutch

In this maneuver the person moves from plantigrade to modified plantigrade. In the end posture she supports her weight with one hand on the floor and one on a crutch. A patient need not be independent in assuming a plantigrade posture to practice this skill, but she should have well-developed dynamic balance skills in plantigrade. The therapist can help the patient maintain her balance during early practice. As her skill builds, this assistance can be decreased.

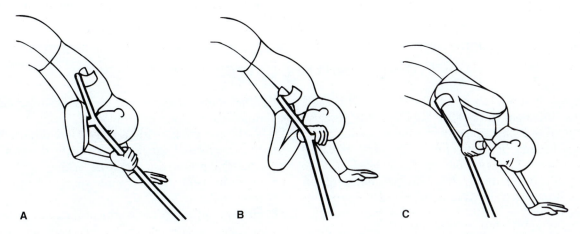

Figure 12–21 Three crutch-position options for coming to stand from the floor.

In Modified Plantigrade With One Hand on Crutch, Grasp and Position Second Crutch With Free Hand

In this maneuver, the patient moves from one modified plantigrade posture to another. In the end posture she supports her trunk with two crutches (Figure 12–19F). Before attempting this skill, she should have well-developed dynamic balance skills in modified plantigrade. Even a skillful patient is likely to require a moderate amount of practice to develop the ability to balance on one crutch while grasping another. The therapist can help the patient maintain her balance during early practice. As her skill builds, this assistance can be decreased.

From Modified Plantigrade Supported on Two Crutches, Push Torso to Upright

From the starting position for this maneuver (Figure 12–19F), the person lifts her trunk by pushing downward on the crutches. While raising her trunk, she pushes her buttocks forward by lifting her head.

    During early practice, the therapist can help the patient stabilize her pelvis as she lifts her torso. This assistance can be removed as the patient's skill improves.

Don and Doff Orthoses

A person can put on her orthoses while sitting in bed or in her wheelchair. The technique is essentially the same in either location. When donning an orthosis while sitting in a wheelchair, the person can prop the orthosis on furniture to support it with the knee in extension (Figure 12–22). Whether in bed or in a wheelchair, she first positions her orthosis and opens the shoe and all straps. She then lifts her leg and positions it over the orthosis, with her knee flexed. She slides her foot into the shoe, checks to make sure that her toes are positioned appropriately, then fastens the shoe and all straps.

    Removing an orthosis is generally easiest if the individual remains seated in her wheelchair. This task simply involves opening all straps and the shoe and lifting the leg out of the orthosis.

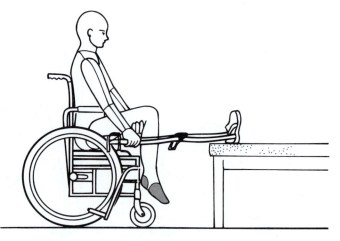

Figure 12–22   Donning orthosis while sitting in wheelchair.

Don and Doff Orthoses—Therapeutic Strategies

This skill should be readily achievable by anyone with the potential for independent ambulation. During early practice, the therapist can provide suggestions and assist the patient as needed. After a brief period of supervised practice with feedback, the patient should be able to practice this skill independently.

AMBULATION AND THERAPEUTIC STRATEGIES WITH ANKLE-FOOT ORTHOSES FOLLOWING COMPLETE SPINAL CORD INJURY

Standard AFOs

Standard AFOs (as opposed to floor-reaction AFOs) are typically recommended for individuals who have adequate quadriceps strength and proprioception to enable them to stabilize their knees during stance without KAFOs. This group includes people with complete

---

Problem-Solving Exercise 12–3

Your outpatient has L2 paraplegia, ASIA B. He is able to walk independently with KAFOs and forearm crutches over even surfaces for 200 feet, using either a swing-through or four-point gait pattern. His goal is to come to standing from the floor. He is able to assume a plantigrade position, but is unable to lift a hand and reach for a crutch without losing his balance.

- What range-of-motion or muscle flexibility limitations could cause this problem?
- What strength limitations could cause this problem?
- If strength and range are adequate for this task, what skill prerequisites may be lacking?
- Describe a functional training program to address this problem.
- How would you progress the program?

paraplegia with a neurological level of injury ranging from L3 through S1, and thus includes individuals with a wide range of lower extremity function. Table 12–4 includes information on the motor function present and the orthotic control typically required at different levels of complete paraplegia.

The ambulatory capabilities of people with complete paraplegia using AFOs are influenced by the motor function in their lower extremities. Those with higher lesions have less functioning musculature with which to stabilize their hips in the frontal and sagittal planes. As a result, they must rely more heavily on their upper extremities to compensate for this lack of muscular support. This reliance on the upper extremities necessitates the use of relatively supportive assistive devices such as forearm crutches or walkers. Walking remains a physically demanding activity, and thus may be less functional than wheelchair propulsion for long distances. People with lower lesions have more intact motor function around their hips, allowing them to walk with less (or no) reliance on their upper extremities. As a result, walking may be performed using less supportive assistive devices such as standard canes, or even without any assistive devices. Walking is also less physically demanding for people with lower lesions, making community ambulation more feasible.

Standard AFOs—Therapeutic Strategies

Gait training with standard AFOs should emphasize the development of as normal a gait pattern as possible. A more normal gait pattern is likely to be more energy-efficient than an abnormal pattern, and may place less stress on the patient's joints.

Gait training with standard AFOs should develop the capacity for controlled knee flexion during early stance, knee stability during stance, and toe clearance during swing. Additional areas on which to focus include minimization of weight bearing through the upper extremities; prevention of a strong knee extensor thrust during stance; and development of symmetry, upright posture, pelvic stability in the frontal plane, normal arm swing and trunk rotation, even cadence, and swing limb advancement without circumduction or scissoring. In addition to focusing on normalizing the gait pattern, gait training should address purely functional aspects of the patient's ambulatory ability. These functional aspects include the patient's ability to walk safely and independently for long distances, walk at speeds that are normal or near normal, and ambulate over various terrains and obstacles.

A variety of interventions can be provided to develop a more normal gait pattern and to enhance a patient's capacity for functional ambulation. Conventional gait training strategies presented in the discussion of incomplete injuries later in this chapter can also be used with people with complete injuries who are learning to walk with standard AFOs.

Floor-Reaction AFOs

Floor-reaction AFOs are occasionally recommended for individuals who have functioning hip flexors but lack the quadriceps strength needed to stabilize their knees during stance. This group includes people with complete L2 and L3 paraplegia. Ambulation is more frequently achieved using KAFOs when the neurological level of injury is this high.

Floor-reaction AFOs provide knee stability during stance by holding the ankles in a slightly plantarflexed position. This ankle position causes the floor reaction force vector to pass anterior to the knee during stance, creating an extension moment that stabilizes the knee in extension.[x]

Floor Reaction AFOs—Therapeutic Strategies

The knee stability provided by this type of AFO occurs only while the floor reaction force vector remains anterior to the knee.[41] Thus, to ensure knee stability, the person's center of gravity must remain relatively anterior. If the center of gravity is positioned posteriorly (as would occur if the person leaned back on crutches positioned behind her feet) or if the knee is positioned anteriorly (as could occur if the person did not fully extend her knee prior to stepping onto that leg), the ground reaction force is located posterior to the knee. A flexion moment at the knee results. Since the individual's quadriceps are not strong enough to stabilize the knee against this flexion moment, the knee will flex. During gait training with floor-reaction AFOs, the patient must learn to walk in such a way that the floor reaction force remains anterior to the knee whenever the knee is supporting weight.

FUNCTIONAL ELECTRICAL STIMULATION FOLLOWING COMPLETE SPINAL CORD INJURY

No chapter on ambulation after spinal cord injury would be complete without a mention of functional electrical stimulation (FES).[y] Since the midseventies, research has been done on eliciting contractions in paralyzed musculature for ambulation. Using FES and assistive devices, people with complete spinal cord lesions have been able to walk over even surfaces and negotiate mild inclines, curbs, and stairs.[45,68–72] FES has also been used to augment ambulation with mechanical orthoses.[44,45,47,73–75]

To date, the use of FES for functional ambulation following complete spinal cord injury remains limited. A variety of problems remain to be solved, including the development of fatigue in electrically stimulated muscles,

---

[x] One concern about this type of orthosis is the potential for the extension torque at the knees to cause ligamentous damage over time.
[y] FES is also called FNS, or functional neuromuscular stimulation.

the relative complexity of FES systems, the continued need for assistive devices, and the high cost of the equipment and training.[45,52,76–81] Moreover, like ambulation with mechanical orthoses, ambulation using FES is slow and has high energy requirements, making it a physically demanding activity.[15,45,81–83] For these reasons, FES is not a viable alternative to wheelchairs for functional mobility for people with complete lesions.[1,41,45,68,76,80,81,84–87] This is also true of hybrid systems that combine FES with RGOs.[13,44] Some individuals exercise by walking with FES.[81]

AMBULATION AND THERAPEUTIC STRATEGIES FOLLOWING INCOMPLETE SPINAL CORD INJURY

Walking requires the capacity to support the body's weight on a stable lower extremity during stance, advance the limb during swing, and progress the body's center of gravity in the direction of ambulation. Functional ambulation is more feasible for individuals who can perform these tasks safely with minimal or no bracing and with minimal or no weight bearing through their upper extremities. This capacity requires adequate strength and motor control in the lower extremities, trunk, and (if assistive devices are used) upper extremities.

The ambulatory capacity of an individual with an incomplete lesion depends largely on the voluntary motor function present below her neurologic level of injury; more intact motor function in the lower extremities is associated with higher levels of functional ambulation.[22,53,82,88–90] People who retain *or regain* only sensory function below their lesions (ASIA B) have ambulatory abilities similar to those with complete (ASIA A) injuries. Those who retain motor function below their lesions at the time of injury, and those who experience early motor return after their injuries, have a better prognosis for achieving functional ambulation.[53,91–94] Additional factors that have been associated with better ambulatory potential include younger age,[64,92,95,96] pattern of injury[82,95,97] (Brown-Séquard or central cord versus anterior cord syndrome), and sparing of pin prick sensation.[98,99] Table 12–15 presents research results that may be useful in predicting ambulatory outcome following spinal cord injury. Clinicians should keep in mind, however, that each patient's functional potential is influenced by a number of characteristics unique to that individual. Furthermore, future advances in therapeutic regimens are likely to lead to increases in ambulatory potential.

People with incomplete spinal cord injuries frequently experience neurological return for a year or more after they are injured, with the greatest return occurring early after injury. With this return comes the potential for greater levels of independence in ambulation. Individuals who experience return can benefit from therapeutic programs to take full advantage of their new motor and sensory capacities as they emerge. It is not practical, however, to continue rehabilitation uninterrupted throughout the time period during which neurological return may occur. A more efficient approach involves rehabilitation in stages. With this approach, patients undergo a series of inpatient, outpatient, or home health therapeutic programs. These programs are interspersed with periods of independent work at home. During the structured therapeutic intervention programs, patients work with therapists to maximize their level of independence within the constraints of their current impairments. They also develop functional skill techniques and home programs aimed at enabling them to continue to improve their motor abilities.[100]

The therapeutic program at each stage in the rehabilitation process should be based on a careful examination and evaluation of the individual's impairments and ambulatory abilities. The therapist should identify the factors that are contributing to the patient's inability or impaired ability to walk and perform related activities such as sit-to-stand. If the individual is unable to walk, the therapist should identify the factors causing this inability. If the patient is able to walk, the therapist should identify gait deviations, functional limitations, and factors causing these problems. There are multiple possible causes for any problem. For example, excessive knee flexion during stance could be caused by weakness in the quadriceps or plantarflexors, limited knee extension range of motion, elevated muscle tone in the hamstrings, impaired proprioception in the knee, or use of ineffective motor strategies. The therapist should examine the patient and analyze the findings to determine which of the possible factors are contributing to the patient's gait problems. The therapeutic program should then be based on this analysis.

Gait Training

Gait training following incomplete spinal cord injury should work toward the development of as normal a gait pattern as possible. Weight bearing on the upper extremities should be minimized to the extent possible without compromising safety. This normalization of gait pattern and minimization of upper extremity weight bearing will lead to a more energy-efficient gait, and may help prevent the development of upper extremity overuse injuries.

In addition to optimizing the patient's gait pattern, gait training should be directed at developing the capacity to walk independently, safely, over functional distances and at functional speeds. The patient should practice walking forward, backward, and to the side, because daily activities include walking in each of these directions. Over-ground walking practice can take place on even surfaces at first, with progression to ambulation over uneven surfaces and obstacles as the individual's skills develop.

There are currently two commonly employed general approaches to gait training following incomplete spinal cord injury: the conventional approach and locomotor training. Locomotor training, also called body weight–supported treadmill training (BWSTT), can be either

TABLE 12–15   Factors Associated with Future Ambulatory Potential

Factor	Subjects	Outcomes
Complete versus incomplete, and paraplegia versus tetraplegia	246 patients with complete paraplegia, incomplete paraplegia and tetraplegia[94]	Complete paraplegia: 5% community ambulators at 1 year. Incomplete paraplegia: 76% community ambulators at 1 year. Incomplete tetraplegia: 46% community ambulators at 1 year.
Initial ASIA classification	118 patients with tetraplegia[93]	Tetraplegia, ASIA A: 0% ambulatory at 1 year. Tetraplegia, ASIA B: 47% ambulatory at 1 year. Tetraplegia, motor incomplete (ASIA C & D): 87% ambulatory at 1 year.
Initial ASIA classification	41 patients with tetraplegia, all 50 years of age or older[91]	Tetraplegia, ASIA A: 0% ambulatory at follow-up. Tetraplegia, ASIA B: 20% ambulatory at follow-up. Tetraplegia, ASIA C: 85% ambulatory at follow-up. Tetraplegia, ASIA D: 90% ambulatory at follow-up. *Mean time of follow-up: 5.5 years after injury.*
Initial ASIA classification and age	105 patients with incomplete tetraplegia, ASIA C and D[92]	Tetraplegia, ASIA C, <50 years old: 91% ambulatory by discharge from inpatient rehabilitation. Tetraplegia, ASIA C, ≥50 years old: 42% ambulatory by discharge from inpatient rehabilitation. Tetraplegia, ASIA D: 100% ambulatory by discharge from inpatient rehabilitation regardless of age.
Lower Extremity Motor Score (LEMS)* at 1 month to 60 days after injury	54 patients with incomplete paraplegia due to trauma[5]	LEMS 0: 33% community ambulators at 1 year. LEMS 1–9: 70% community ambulators at 1 year. LEMS ≥ 10: 100% community ambulators at 1 year.
LEMS measured 0.5 to 0.7 years after injury	36 patients with complete and incomplete paraplegia and incomplete tetraplegia, *all with sufficient preserved lower extremity motor function to ambulate and adequate trunk extension strength to allow independent sitting without the use of the arms for support*[53]	Ambulatory performance at time of study (0.5 to 0.7 years after injury) LEMS ≤20: 100% household ambulators; most relied on two KAFOs and two crutches. LEMS ≥30: 100% community ambulators.

(Continued)

TABLE 12–15　(*Continued*)

Factor	Subjects	Outcomes
Preservation of hip flexor or quadriceps function at 30 to 60 days after injury	54 patients with incomplete paraplegia due to trauma[5]	All with ≥2/5 initial hip flexor *or* knee extensor strength were community ambulators at 1 year.
Quadriceps strength at 2 months after injury	17 patients with ASIA C injuries C4-T10[88]	≥3/5 in strongest quadriceps: 100% household or community ambulators at 1 year after injury. <3/5 in strongest quadriceps: 25% household or community ambulators at 1 year after injury.
Sparing of pin prick sensation below neurological level of injury, tested within 72 hours of injury	27 patients with ASIA B paraplegia and tetraplegia resulting from trauma[98]	Pin prick sensation spared: 88% recovered ability to walk independently ≥200 feet by discharge from rehabilitation. Light touch spared but pin prick sensation absent: 11% recovered ability to walk independently ≥200 feet by discharge from rehabilitation.
Sparing of pin prick sensation in lower extremities, tested within 72 hours of injury	97 patients with ASIA B paraplegia and tetraplegia resulting from trauma[99]	Pin prick sensation spared in ≥50% of L2-S1 dermatomes: 40% able to walk independently ≥150 feet 1 year after injury. Pin sensation spared in <50% of L2-S1 dermatomes: 16% able to walk independently ≥150 feet 1 year after injury
Pattern of injury	38 patients with cervical Brown-Séquard and Brown-Séquard-plus syndromes resulting from trauma[97]	"Pure" Brown-Sequard: 20% independent ambulators at time of discharge from rehabilitation. Brown-Sequard-plus: 85% independent ambulators at time of discharge from rehabilitation. Upper limb weaker than lower limb: more likely to walk at discharge.
Pattern of injury and age	32 patients with cervical central cord syndrome[95]	≤50 years old: all able to walk independently at discharge. 50–70 years old: 69% able to walk independently at discharge. ≥70 years old: 40% able to walk independently at discharge.

KAFOs, knee-ankle-foot orthoses.
* LEMS is explained in Chapter 7.

therapist-assisted or robotic-assisted. The best evidence available to date regarding the relative efficacy of conventional therapy versus BWSTT is provided by a single-blinded, parallel group, randomized multicenter clinical trial[z] that found therapist-assisted locomotor training and conventional therapy of comparable intensity to be equally

---

[z] This study directly compares two groups receiving different interventions. Other articles include case studies and reports of studies investigating interventions without providing comparison groups that receive alternative interventions. These articles do not allow a comparison of the efficacy of the different approaches to the restoration of ambulation.[21] See also references 24, 118, and 145 to 148.

effective in improving walking ability[aa] in patients with incomplete paraplegia and tetraplegia.[21,22] Both groups performed better than expected based on past studies of outcomes. The high outcomes were likely due to the intensive and task-oriented nature of both regimens, initiated relatively early (within 8 weeks) after injury and possibly also due to the large number of subjects with cervical central cord injuries.[21]

Conventional Approach to Gait Training

Traditionally, gait training following motor incomplete spinal cord injury has begun with standing and pre-gait activities (such as weight-shifts) as soon as the individual is able to tolerate an upright standing position, followed by progression to stepping and walking. Therapists use verbal cueing, manual facilitation, and structured practice of motor skills to develop ambulatory abilities. They provide physical assistance as needed with components of gait such as hip and knee stabilization during stance, swing limb advancement, and maintenance of an upright trunk. During early standing and walking, supportive assistive devices such as parallel bars or wheeled walkers are typically used to enhance stability, and orthoses are often used to provide stabilization at the ankles or knees.[bb] As a patient's ambulatory ability develops, therapists reduce the cueing, facilitation, physical assistance, and orthotic stabilization provided, and patients progress to walking with less supportive assistive devices.

The therapeutic interventions that have traditionally been used to restore ambulation following incomplete spinal cord injury are not unique to this population. Therapists can often employ strategies that they use with people who have similar impairments and functional limitations resulting from other pathologies. For example, a patient who has asymmetrical paralysis resulting from Brown-Séquard syndrome may have a clinical picture that resembles hemiplegia due to a stroke or head injury. Many therapeutic activities aimed at developing improved locomotor capability after a stroke or head injury could be employed with this individual.[cc]

In many instances, patients benefit from therapeutic activities that develop component skills used in ambulation. Examples of such activities include practice of the following skills: shifting weight while maintaining knee stability, shifting weight in a stride-stance position, maintaining knee stability in stance without hyperextending the knee, initiating swing from a stride-stance position, progressing the body's weight forward to step past the stance foot, stepping forward with proper placement of the foot, and maintaining an upright trunk and head posture while standing and stepping.[101-103] Emphasis is placed on developing postural

control, dynamic stability, symmetry, and limb and trunk kinematics approaching normal to the extent possible.

Some patients may benefit from therapeutic activities that develop more basic skills. Examples of such therapeutic activities include dynamic balance while standing with the feet in different positions or on various surfaces; practice stabilizing and moving in different postures such as standing, modified plantigrade, kneeling, quadruped, bridging and hooklying; and practice balancing and moving while supported on a therapeutic ball.[101,102,104] Each of these activities is intended to develop a foundation of balance and coordinated motor control to undergird the individual's capacity to walk.

Therapist-Assisted Locomotor Training

This approach involves step-training on a treadmill, using a suspension system to partially support the patient's body weight. Manual assistance is provided as needed to enable the patient to step.[105-111] Treadmill speed, amount of body weight-support, and manual assistance are tailored to the needs of each patient. Early training typically occurs at a slow speed, with a relatively large portion of the patient's weight supported by the suspension system, and with the assistance of one or more therapists[dd] to move the lower extremities through stepping patterns. Assistance may also be provided at the trunk and upper extremities to promote normal motions.[18,19] Training sessions consist of brief bouts of stepping, interspersed with periods of rest (in standing). As the patient's performance improves, each of these parameters is adjusted accordingly: treadmill speed is increased, body weight support and manual assistance are reduced, and the time spent stepping between rests is increased.[19] When the patient is able to stand with minimal upper extremity or orthotic support, over-ground gait training is added to the program. A therapeutic program that includes locomotor training both on a treadmill and over ground may enhance outcomes by providing the patient with both intensive step training and practice of walking under normal environmental conditions.[24,112]

Therapist-assisted locomotor training has been shown to improve the ambulatory capabilities of people with long-standing motor incomplete spinal cord injuries, as well as those with relatively recent injuries. A follow-up study done 6 months to 6.5 years after training revealed that the functional improvements (in non-treadmill walking) were maintained over time in most cases.[113] Although numerous research studies and case reports provide evidence for the efficacy of therapist-assisted locomotor training following motor incomplete spinal cord injury,[18,19,21,24,110] the protocols vary in their initial training parameters and progression. Table 12–16 provides an example of a therapist-assisted locomotor training program. Future research is likely to clarify the selection of initial parameters and their progression, in addition to identifying the optimal timing post-injury

---

[aa] Walking speed, distance, and level of independence.

[bb] Alternatively, a mobile support system can be used to provide partial unweighting during over-ground ambulation.

[cc] A comprehensive description of strategies for developing ambulation skills of people with neurological disabilities is beyond the scope of this book. The reader is encouraged to find additional information in the following references: 101, 102, 104, and 149 to 152.

[dd] Detailed descriptions of techniques for providing manual assistance are included in reference 18.

TABLE 12–16   Example of Therapist-Assisted Locomotor Training Program

Patient selection	Early after injury: ASIA C or D.
	≥6 months after injury: ASIA C or D, with some ability to walk over ground.
	All patients must have orthopedic, cardiovascular, and integumentary status allowing safe participation in training.
Initial parameters on treadmill	Body weight support: should allow maximal loading through the lower extremities, but provide enough support to allow knee stability (avoid excessive flexion) during the stance phase of gait, as well as an upright trunk posture and acceptable stepping kinematics.*
	Treadmill speed: maximal speed that is slow enough to allow coordinated stepping with acceptable kinematics.*
	Manual assistance: provided as needed to allow coordinated, symmetrical stepping with acceptable kinematics.* May be required for any of the following: one or both lower extremities, trunk, upper extremities.
	Duration of bouts of stepping: only as long as stepping is performed with acceptable kinematics.*
	Duration of stepping session (sum of bouts): 20 to 30 minutes total stepping practice, within limits of exercise-induced fatigue.
	Frequency: three to five times per week.
	Additional considerations: optimize gait pattern without upper extremity support or orthotic stabilization.
Progression on treadmill	Reduce body weight support or manual assistance; increase treadmill speed, duration of bouts of stepping, or duration of stepping session. These parameters should be progressed to the extent possible without compromising the patient's ability to perform coordinated, symmetrical stepping with acceptable kinematics.*
Initiation of over-ground training	Initiate over-ground training in conjunction with treadmill training when the patient exhibits the capacity to stand without excessive upper extremity weight bearing and with minimal orthotic support.
Characteristics of over-ground training	10 to 20 minutes of over-ground walking practice in each session. Minimize upper extremity weight bearing and orthotic stabilization to the extent possible. May begin with static and dynamic standing, emphasizing stability and upright posture, progressing to stepping. Manual assistance may be required. Emphasize coordinated, symmetrical stepping with acceptable kinematics.* Progress in the following areas as performance allows: walk with less supportive assistive devices and less orthotic stabilization, increase speed and distance, practice negotiating environmental obstacles, reduce assistance and guarding.
Duration of training	12 weeks.

Sources: References 18, 19, 21, 22, 25, 110, and 114 to 116.
* Acceptable kinematics = trunk and lower extremity motions that approximate normal. Weight shift and loading of stance limb, hip extension in late stance, and interlimb coordination of loading and unloading may be particularly important.

and the characteristics of patients who will be most likely to benefit from this approach.

Robotic-Assisted Locomotor Training

Robotic-assisted locomotor training (also called automated locomotor training[20,117]) involves body weight–supported training on a treadmill, using a motorized orthosis (also called a driven gait orthosis, or DGO) to move the hips and knees through sagittal plane motions similar to normal gait (Figure 12–23). Toe-drag during swing is prevented by either an elastic strap[20,89,118] or an AFO. The treadmill's speed and the amount of body weight support provided are adjusted to the patient's tolerance and to allow an optimal walking pattern. The speed is increased and the support is reduced as the patient's tolerance and performance improve.[20,118]

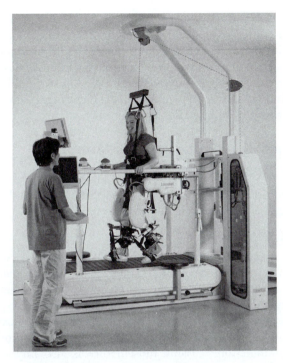

Figure 12–23   Robotic-assisted body weight–supported treadmill training. (Reproduced with permission from Hocoma.)

Robotic-assisted training can be provided by one therapist who sets up and monitors the session. In contrast, for patients with limited motor function, both therapist-assisted locomotor training and conventional gait training can involve up to four clinicians.[18,89] Thus robotic-assisted training can be a more efficient approach in terms of staffing requirements.[20,118] Moreover, it is less physically demanding for therapists,[ee] making it feasible to provide more prolonged practice sessions.[20,118,119] Finally, robotic-assisted locomotor training provides consistent lower extremity stepping practice resembling normal walking.[112]

Concerns about robotic-assisted locomotor training are that the current designs of motorized orthoses allow only slow walking and provide abnormal sensory input, patients' lower extremities are moved passively, and motions are restricted to the sagittal plane. Each of these constraints may limit the beneficial effects of training. Solutions to these problems include instructing patients to move actively with the orthoses, and transitioning to therapist-assisted locomotor training[89,118,120] and over-ground gait training as the patient's motor skills allow. Patients who are able to walk over ground faster than robotic systems allow may benefit more from therapist-assisted, as opposed to robotic-assisted, locomotor training.[20]

Robotic-assisted locomotor training has not been studied as extensively as therapist-assisted locomotor training. One small (N = 20) multicenter trial of individuals with chronic (2 to 17 years' duration) motor incomplete tetraplegia and paraplegia compared over-ground walking ability before and after 8 weeks of robotic-assisted locomotor training. Significant improvement occurred in gait speed and endurance as well as performance on the Timed Up and Go test.[ff] There were no significant improvements in subjects' gait patterns or their requirements for assistive devices, orthoses, or physical assistance. Subjects who were nonambulatory before the training remained unable to walk.[20,89]

Preliminary evidence regarding the relative efficacy of robotic-assisted versus therapist-assisted locomotor training comes from a small (N = 30) pilot study that compared robotic-assisted BWSTT, therapist-assisted BWSTT, and over-ground ambulation with a mobile suspension system. The subjects were individuals with motor incomplete spinal cord injuries sustained 14 to 180 days prior to enrollment in the study. All three training regimens resulted in significant improvements in functional walking ability,[gg] and the different regimens were equally effective.[89]

Functional Electrical Stimulation

FES can be utilized in several different ways to enhance ambulation following spinal cord injury. It can be used as a training device in combination with either body weight–supported treadmill training or over-ground gait training.[112,121–123] Alternatively, it can function as an orthosis for functional ambulation.[124–127] When serving as an orthosis, FES can elicit contraction of multiple muscles to enhance both stance and swing[15] or only to improve toe clearance during swing (Figure 12–24).[128] Finally, FES can be used in combination with mechanical orthoses.[45,47]

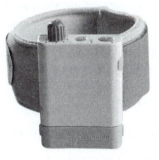

Figure 12–24   FES device used to elicit contraction of the dorsiflexors to enhance toe clearance during swing. (Reproduced with permission from Innovative Neurotronics.)

---

ee Therapist-assisted locomotor training can be uncomfortable[20] or injurious[89] for the clinicians involved because of the positions and motions of their lower backs when assisting the patient's lower extremity motions.

---

ff The Timed Up and Go test measures the time taken to stand from an armchair, walk 3 meters, turn, walk back to the chair, and sit down.

gg Walking ability was measured using the Functional Independence Measure (FIM) subscore and the Walking Index for Spinal Cord Injury II (WISCI).

Aquatic Therapy

Aquatic therapy can be a useful adjunct to "land therapy" in developing ambulation skills. The buoyant force that water exerts on people as they stand partially immersed in water supports a portion of their weight. The percentage of weight supported depends in part on the depth of water in which they stand; standing in deeper water increases the buoyant force, effectively reducing the weight borne through the lower extremities. Patients who have limited voluntary motor function in their trunk and lower extremities may be able to practice standing and walking in shoulder-high water. The support provided by the water at this depth makes walking possible for some people who are nonambulatory on land.[129] As their strength and walking ability improve, they can practice walking in progressively more shallow water, accepting more of their weight on their lower extremities.

Orthotic Considerations

Orthotic prescription should be based on a careful analysis of the patient's biomechanical needs. Orthoses are frequently designed to compensate for functional deficits such as the inability to support the body's weight during stance or the inability to clear the foot during swing. Alternatively or in addition, orthoses may be designed to provide joint protection. For example, people who habitually thrust their knees into extension with excessive force during stance (knee extension thrust) may damage their knees over time, leading to pain and diminished function. When a knee extension thrust persists despite therapeutic attempts to eliminate this gait deviation, orthotic stabilization may be indicated to protect the knee.

Because neurological return is likely to occur during the first year or more after an incomplete injury, an individual's needs for orthotic stabilization are likely to change with time. This change in biomechanical needs may be accommodated with orthotic changes such as conversion of a KAFO to an AFO or alteration of the control provided at the ankle joint. The prescription of orthoses that allow adjustment will maximize their continued usefulness as the patient's needs change.[1]

Assistive Device Considerations

The assistive device(s) selected for an individual should allow safe ambulation and negotiation of obstacles and conditions within the environment(s) in which she will function post-discharge. Assistive devices should allow maximal mobility to the extent that is possible without compromising safety. Canes are the least restrictive (and least supportive) assistive devices, followed by forearm crutches, with walkers being most restrictive of movement. A final consideration in assistive device selection is the potential for overuse injuries of the upper extremities. In this respect, wheeled walkers may be superior to forearm crutches; one small study of subjects with incomplete injuries found that wheeled walkers were associated with lower compressing and distracting forces on the upper extremities than were forearm crutches.[130] The selection of an assistive device should be based on a careful analysis in order to find the assistive device that is most suitable for the individual's unique physical characteristics, ambulatory abilities, and functional requirements.[131]

Muscle Strength, Range of Motion, and Muscle Tone

In addition to gait training, the therapeutic program should address muscle strength, range of motion, and muscle tone.

Muscle Strength

The strengthening program should address innervated muscles involved in walking. The therapist should analyze the patient's strength deficits in relation to her ambulatory ability and gait pattern, and develop a strengthening program accordingly. Strength in the hip extensors, flexors, and abductors may be particularly important for community ambulation.[90] Trunk musculature is also important for ambulation; adequate strength is required in the trunk to stabilize the upper body on the pelvis during gait. Patients who utilize assistive devices also require strength in their upper extremities, particularly in their triceps and shoulder girdle depressors.

Strength can be developed through progressive resistive exercises, proprioceptive neuromuscular facilitation techniques, isometric exercises, isokinetic exercise, and electrical stimulation.[132-137] The strengthening program will better prepare the patient for the demands of walking if it includes open- and closed-chain activities as well as exercises involving both concentric and eccentric contractions.

Range of Motion

As is true for all other functional skills, range of motion is critical for ambulation. The therapeutic program should restore or maintain normal joint range and muscle flexibility to enhance ambulation.

Muscle Tone

Elevated muscle tone is common among people with incomplete spinal cord injuries. When severe, it can interfere with ambulation in a variety of ways. Elevated tone in the hip extensors, hip adductors, quadriceps, or plantarflexors can impede swing limb advancement by preventing the normal sequence of motions that make it possible to clear the floor and progress the leg forward. During stance, hyperactivity in the quadriceps or plantarflexors can interfere with the knee and ankle motions that allow for a smooth transfer of weight onto the lower extremity, and can cause a knee extension thrust or genu recurvatum later in stance. Elevated muscle tone in the trunk or upper extremities can also interfere with ambulation. Involuntary spasms in the trunk musculature can interfere with balance, and elevated tone in the upper extremities can interfere with balance and utilization of assistive devices. Although elevated muscle tone often interferes with ambulation, at times it can help. For example, involuntary muscle contractions may augment the ability to stabilize the knees in standing when voluntary contractions do not provide adequate force.

Strategies for treating elevated muscle tone are presented in Chapter 3. In planning therapies to reduce muscle tone, the rehabilitation team should take into consideration its influence on function: will the individual be more or less functional if tone is reduced? It is not always possible to answer this question without actually reducing the patient's muscle tone and noting the effect that this change has on her ability to walk and perform other activities. Finding the optimal level of muscle tone reduction may require trial and evaluation of various medications and dosages.

Summary

- Walking is of high priority to many patients because of its psychological and social significance. The high energy costs of ambulation with orthoses and assistive devices, however, make ambulation following spinal cord injury prohibitively difficult for many people.

- A person with a complete spinal cord injury who wishes to walk functionally must utilize assistive devices, lower extremity orthoses, and compensatory strategies for this activity. This chapter presents descriptions of lower extremity orthoses commonly used for people with spinal cord injuries, principles of orthotic prescription, and compensatory techniques that can be used for ambulation.

- The orthotic requirements and methods of ambulation possible for a person with an incomplete spinal cord injury will depend largely on the extent of motor sparing or return below her lesion. If she has little or no voluntary motor function below her lesion, she is likely to walk using orthoses and gait patterns similar to those used by people with complete injuries. If she has more significant motor function in her trunk and lower extremities, she may be able to walk with less orthotic support and with a more normal gait pattern.

- During rehabilitation, the therapist and patient work together to discover the movement strategies that will enable the patient to walk and perform other ambulation-related skills. The therapeutic program then consists of activities directed at developing the strength, range of motion, and skill needed to perform these functional tasks. This chapter presents a variety of strategies for developing the skills involved.

- The therapist and patient should take appropriate precautions during gait training to prevent motion of unstable vertebrae, skin abrasions and pressure ulcers, and injury from falls.

Suggested Resources

ORGANIZATION

International Functional Electrical Stimulation Society: *http://home.ifess.org*

PUBLICATIONS

Handbooks published by the Los Amigos Research and Education Institute, available for purchase from *www.larei.org/books.htm*

- *Neuromuscular Electrical Stimulation–A Practical Guide*
- *Observational Gait Analysis*

WEB SITE

Spinal Cord Injury Rehabilitation Evidence, Chapter 6, Lower Limb Rehabilitation Following Spinal Cord Injury: *www.icord.org/scire/chapters.php*

13

Sexuality and Sexual Functioning

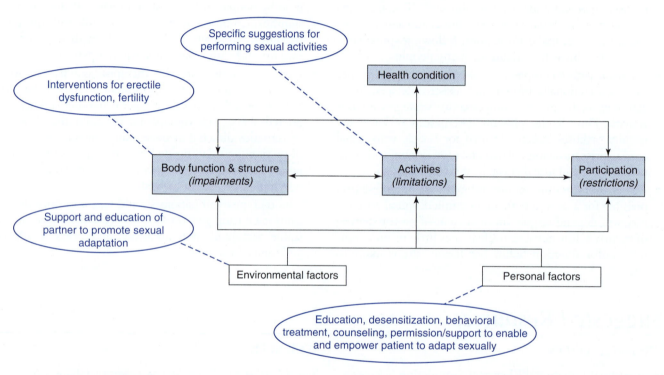

Chapter 13 presents information sexual function and fertility after spinal cord injury, and therapeutic strategies for facilitating adaptation.

Sexuality is a central aspect of our lives. From birth on, our gender influences how we define ourselves and how we are seen by others. (Imagine a birth announcement that does not specify the infant's gender!) Because sexuality is such a basic component of our physical and psychological makeup, it is an important ingredient of holistic health. Feelings of sexual inadequacy can have a strong effect on a person's sense of identity and self-esteem.[1] Sexuality is also important in our social relations. It is used to form and to maintain relationships, to wield power, to communicate with others,[2] and to bolster self-esteem.[3] Feelings of unattractiveness can lead to withdrawal from social and sexual relationships.[4]

"It is a tremendous core of who I am. Everything else comes out of that. How I think and feel about my body, my physical body. How I would define myself as a woman. How I am in all of my relationships, whether they are sexual or otherwise."

anonymous
SCI survivor[5]

We express our sexuality not only, not even mostly, through sexual intercourse. Our attire, interactions with others, the images we present, our flirtations, smiles, and reactions to others are expressions of our sexuality. And yes, we express our sexuality in a wide variety of "sexual acts," ranging from holding hands to more intimate sexual encounters.

The essence of a person's sexual nature is in his or her mind. Spinal cord injury does not alter this; people continue to desire sexual expression, and most remain sexually active.[4,6–16] Unfortunately, damage to the spinal cord brings on changes that can interfere with sexual expression and activity. Both sexual activity and sexual satisfaction decrease after injury. Although both areas subsequently increase, they remain at lower levels than before the injury.[17] In one survey, people with spinal cord injuries reported that decreased sexual function is one of the more difficult sequelae of cord injury to deal with, second only to decreased ability to walk or move.[18]

Perhaps the most obvious way in which a spinal cord injury affects sexuality is in its effect on the person's physical capacity to perform sexual acts. Changes in genital functioning, motor abilities, sensation, range of motion, and muscle tone may interfere with a person's accustomed modes of sexual expression. Spinal cord injury can also create logistical problems: altered body language, the potential for bowel and bladder accidents, decreased spontaneity resulting from the need to manage catheters, and the mechanics of undressing can complicate sexual encounters. In addition, a person with impaired mobility faces architectural and transportation barriers that can impede his or her ability to meet potential partners.

The social consequences of spinal cord injury add to the problem. People with disabilities are often viewed by others as asexual, devoid of sexual urges, and undeserving of sexual expression and pleasure. In a society that places a high premium on physical appearance, people with disabilities are often not seen as desirable partners. These societal attitudes can limit the opportunity for sexual expression.[2,6,19–24]

Attitudinal barriers to sexual expression also come from within. After spinal cord injury, a person may view himself or herself as asexual, undesirable, and undeserving of sexual gratification.[2,6]

> "No one was comfortable talking to me about sexuality except my former hospital roommate, and she thought the whole thing was a waste of time after paralysis. It all gave me the impression that paralyzed people were asexual and undesirable. I felt ugly and ashamed of my body, unable to explore my adolescence in a more positive light."
>
> Kris Ann Piazza
> writer, editor, community board member,
> public speaker,
> C5 SCI survivor[25]

Ignorance is an additional barrier to adjustment. Many people with spinal cord injuries lack knowledge about their own sexual functioning, potential for sexual expression, and strategies for finding sexual gratification.[2]

In the past the focus of both research and intervention in this area has been on the male, specifically on his genital functioning and fertility.[11,13,15,26,27] This may be due to the higher prevalence of males among people with spinal cord injuries, the fact that male genitals are more readily studied, or societal bias.[27–29] One assumption underlying the predominance of male-oriented research and intervention is that women with spinal cord injuries have an easier adjustment to make because their injuries do not impair their ability to perform in their accustomed role of passive participant in sexual activities.[30,31] This position, based on outdated notions of sex roles, is no longer defensible. Women now often take the initiative in sexual encounters instead of passively waiting to be approached. Additionally, like her male counterpart, a woman with a spinal cord injury may have difficulty with some of the positions and sexual activities to which she was accustomed prior to her injury. She will have the same potential for problems with bowel and bladder accidents interrupting intimate encounters and will be subject to society's discriminatory attitudes regarding sexuality and disability. She may feel unattractive and undesirable as a result of her injury.[8,9,32,33]

> "I used to feel that I really couldn't have real relationships because I thought that, as a disabled woman, I wasn't as desirable. I figured that there was really no reason for anyone to be interested in me if he could have a woman who could walk, totally discounting my whole self and my uniqueness as a person. I didn't feel really good about myself until I started feeling sexually attractive, feeling that I could function, not competitively, but on an equal footing with any other woman."
>
> Susan Schapiro
> computer programmer, marathoner, kayaker,
> T11-T12 SCI survivor[34]

Some aspects of a woman's sexuality will not be as profoundly affected by cord injury as a man's. The alterations in her genital functioning may not be as obvious and her fertility will not be affected. She may face more social difficulties, however, being more vulnerable than a man to being perceived as unattractive and therefore unacceptable as a sexual partner.[35] Health professionals should remember that spinal cord injury significantly affects sexuality, whether the person is male or female.

Sexuality and the potential for sexual expression are major concerns for most people who sustain spinal cord injuries.[36] This concern often surfaces very soon after injury.[1,36] Faced with bodily changes and social stigma, a person with a spinal cord injury may feel less of a man or woman. Depression and lowered self-esteem can result.[37] Because of the psychological and social importance of sexuality, it is critical that this area be addressed during rehabilitation.

"Being able to have sex with a woman was the way I defined my manhood. Without it, what would I be? The only answer I could think of was 'less than a man.'"

Mark Zupan
paralympic athlete, engineer, author,
C7 SCI survivor[38]

PHYSICAL ASPECTS OF SEXUAL FUNCTIONING

Although physical sexual responses are only a part of sexuality, they are certainly a significant part. Health professionals should be knowledgeable in this area so that they can educate their patients appropriately.

Neurological Control of Genital Function

Male

The male's genital functions during sexual activity consist of erection and ejaculation. Ejaculation occurs in two stages, seminal emission and propulsatile ejaculation.[39]

Erection

Erection is a vascular event, occurring when the erectile bodies of the penis (corpus cavernosa and corpus spongiosum) become distended with blood. This distention occurs when vasodilation of the arteries supplying the penis, combined with relaxation of the smooth muscle of the corpus cavernosum and corpus spongiosum, allows increased blood flow into the erectile bodies. Engorgement of the erectile bodies causes compression of the veins that drain them. The resulting reduction in venous outflow further contributes to the erection by entrapping blood in the erectile bodies.[40–43]

Both the sympathetic and parasympathetic divisions of the autonomic nervous system are involved in the control of erections. When autonomic input causes the rate of blood flow into the erectile bodies to exceed the rate of flow out, the penis becomes erect.[41,44,45] Continuing autonomic stimulation is required to maintain the erection.[45,46]

Neurological control of erection involves two regions in the spinal cord, as well as higher centers. Efferent pathways from supraspinal centers synapse in the thoracolumbar (sympathetic) and sacral (parasympathetic) erection centers of the spinal cord. The input from higher centers provides both facilitation and inhibition of erection.[42,47–49]

Erection can be initiated from two different sources: psychological arousal or sensory stimulation in the genital area or pelvic viscera. Psychogenic erections are brought on by psychological arousal. This arousal can be initiated by erotic thoughts or a variety of sensory experiences (smells, sounds, etc.). Erections brought on by sensory stimulation in the genital region or pelvic viscera are called reflex or reflexogenic erections. Normal functioning involves a combination of psychogenic and reflexogenic erection.[45] In fact, both are needed for an erection to be maintained.[50]

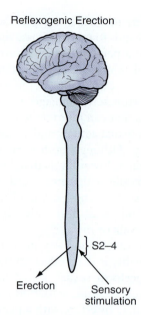

Figure 13–1   Neurological control of reflexive erection.

Reflex erections (Figure 13–1) are mediated by the sacral cord. Parasympathetic efferents from S2 through S4 cause vasodilation of the penile corporal arterioles when stimulated, as well as relaxation of the smooth muscle fibers in the corpus cavernosum and spongiosum. Erection is initiated when sensory stimulation from the penis, perineal area, rectum, or bladder travels to S2-S4. This stimulation causes firing of the parasympathetic efferents, resulting in erection.[42–44,50]

The neural control of psychogenic erection (Figure 13–2) is not as well understood as that of reflexive erection. Sympathetic efferents from T11 through L2[48,51–54] are known to be involved in psychogenic erections; both humans and experimental animals who lack sacral reflex functioning but have intact thoracolumbar erection centers

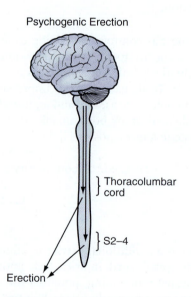

Figure 13–2   Neurological control of psychogenic erection.

in communication with their brains exhibit erections in response to psychogenic stimuli.[42,48,52] The mechanism by which thoracolumbar-mediated erections occur remains unknown.[42] Psychogenic erections may also be mediated in the sacral cord, occurring when facilitory impulses from higher centers cause the sacral efferents to fire.[41,45]

Seminal Emission

Emission is the process by which semen reaches the posterior urethra in preparation for ejaculation. In emission, peristaltic contraction of the smooth muscle of the vas deferens causes sperm to be transported from the epididymis to the end of the vas deferens (ampulla).[44,46] Secretions from the seminal vesicles and prostate are added to the sperm to form semen.[55] Contraction of the smooth muscle of the ampulla, seminal vesicles and prostate, and partial closure of the bladder neck causes the semen to enter the posterior urethra.[44,46,50] Figure 13–3 illustrates the structures involved.

Neurological control of emission involves supraspinal centers and both the sacral and thoracolumbar spinal cord (Figure 13–4). Afferents from the genitals enter the second through fourth segments of the sacral cord. From there, they ascend to the brain. Efferents from the brain travel via the anterolateral columns to the thoracolumbar cord. Sympathetic efferents from the thoracolumbar cord innervate the vas deferens, seminal vesicles, prostate, and base of the bladder. The sympathetic outflow from T10 through L2 to these structures causes emission.[39,41,44,49] Emission can also occur as a result of direct input from the sacral cord to the thoracolumbar cord without involvement of higher centers. Normally, emission is stimulated by input from both sources.[49]

Propulsatile Ejaculation

Propulsatile ejaculation is the process by which semen is propelled from the posterior urethra. It involves contraction

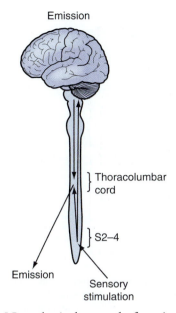

Figure 13–4   Neurological control of seminal emission.

of striated musculature: the bulbocavernosus, ischiocavernosus, and other pelvic floor musculature.[41,50,56] The rhythmic contraction of these muscles, combined with closure of the bladder neck, propels the semen forward[a] and out of the urethra.[44,46]

Propulsatile ejaculation occurs as a result of a somatic sacral reflex (Figure 13–5). Sensory afferents are activated when semen enters the posterior urethra as a result of emission. These afferents travel to S2-S4, where they synapse with somatic efferents. Reflexive contraction of the bulbocavernosus and ischiocavernosus muscles results,[44,49] causing propulsion of the semen. The efferents also stimulate reflexive contraction of the vesical sphincter, preventing retrograde ejaculation.[55]

Female

The genital responses exhibited by women during sexual acts include genital arousal[57] (vaginal lubrication, and vasocongestion of erectile tissue in the clitoris, vagina, labia minora, and labia majora); contraction of the smooth muscle of the fallopian tubes, uterus, and paraurethral Skene glands; and rhythmic contraction of the perineal musculature.

Vaginal Lubrication

Vaginal lubrication involves the secretion of mucus from the vaginal epithelium and Bartholin's glands into the vaginal opening. Neurological control of vaginal lubrication is thought to be similar to that of penile erection. Reflexive lubrication occurs as a result of parasympathetic stimulation that arises from S2-S4.[1,43,58–60] Both the thoracolumbar and sacral cord are thought to be involved in psychogenic lubrication.[43,46]

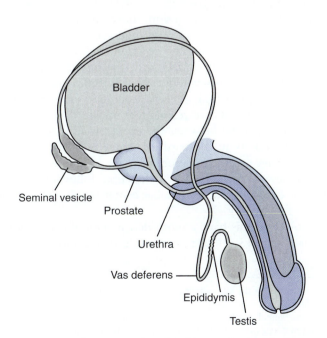

Figure 13–3   Structures involved in seminal emission.

---

[a] Normal ejaculation, in which the semen is propelled forward, is called antegrade ejaculation. In retrograde ejaculation, semen is propelled back into the bladder. This occurs when the bladder neck fails to close during ejaculation or when it has been resected surgically.[50]

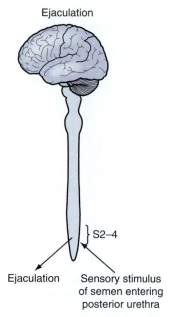

Ejaculation

S2–4

Ejaculation   Sensory stimulus
of semen entering
posterior urethra

Figure 13–5   Neurological control of propulsatile
ejaculation.

Vasocongestion

The engorgement of erectile tissue in the corpora cavernosa of the clitoris, vagina, labia minora, and labia majora
that occurs during sexual activity is the result of vascular dilation. Reflexive vasocongestion is the result of parasympathetic stimulation that arises from S2-S4.[1,59–61] Psychogenic
vasocongestion appears to depend primarily on sympathetic
outflow from the thoracolumbar cord.[62]

Smooth Muscle Contractions in the Fallopian Tubes, Uterus, and Skene Glands

In the female equivalent of seminal emission, the smooth
musculature of the fallopian tubes, uterus, and paraurethral Skene glands contracts. The neurological control
of these events is similar to the control of emission in the
male.[46] These reactions are caused by sympathetic outflow
from the thoracolumbar cord.[1,43,46,58]

Striated Muscle Contractions

The female analogue of propulsatile ejaculation involves
rhythmic contraction of the bulbospongiosus (vaginal
sphincter) and ischiocavernosus, pelvic floor, and anal
sphincter. This muscular response is controlled by a somatic reflex involving S2-S4.[1,58]

Genital Function Following Injury

The impact that a spinal cord injury has on genital functioning is not completely understood. Much of the data has
been gathered using retrospective surveys rather than
observation, and there has been inadequate control of variables such as time since injury, etiology, spasticity, and the
influence of medication, surgery, and medical conditions.[26]
Moreover, after spinal cord injury in humans, it can be

difficult to determine with certainty whether any neurological connections remain between the brain and the centers
in the spinal cord that are involved in sexual function.[42]

Despite these limitations, research has shown that the
level and completeness of a spinal cord lesion affect its
impact on genital functioning. However, there are exceptions to any "rule of thumb" that one attempts to impose.
It is important to keep this in mind when counseling
patients.

Male

The preservation of erection, seminal emission, and
propulsatile ejaculation capabilities after spinal cord injury
varies with the level and completeness of lesion. Additional factors that can influence genital function after cord
injury include medical status, bladder infections, pressure
ulcers, medications,[39,63] and psychological factors.[39,41,52,64]

In discussions of sexual functioning, cord lesions are
often classified as upper motor neuron (UMN) or lower
motor neuron (LMN) lesions. So-called UMN lesions
leave the functioning of the sacral cord intact. People with
these lesions display intact bulbocavernosus reflexes[b] and
anal sphincter tone. Most such lesions are above T12.[44] So-
called LMN lesions disrupt the functioning of the sacral
cord. People with this level of lesion have a lax anal sphincter and absent bulbocavernosus reflex. Usually, the lesion is
below T12 in these cases.[44] Table 13–1 presents statistics on
male genital functioning using this classification of lesions.

Erection

Erection is the most likely of the genital functions to be
preserved[c] after spinal cord injury; most men retain the
capacity to have erections.[12,43,51,64] This is due to the presence of erectile centers in two areas of the cord; a man
with a spinal cord injury is likely to have either his thoracolumbar or sacral erection center functional.

The neurological basis of the erection capabilities of a
person with a complete lesion above the thoracolumbar
erection center are illustrated in Figure 13–6. With a complete lesion above T11, the erection centers in the cord
will no longer be in contact with the brain. As a result,
psychogenic erections will not occur.[65] Reflex erections are
likely to be preserved, however, because the sacral segments of the spinal cord remain functional.[10,45,50,52,65]

Lesions that lie between the thoracolumbar and sacral
erection centers in the cord can spare both psychogenic
and reflexive erectile function.[52] Figure 13–7 illustrates the
neurological basis of erectile function following lesions
that lie below the thoracolumbar center but do not disrupt
sacral functioning.

Lower lesions have a more detrimental effect on erections. Figure 13–8 illustrates the effects of complete lesions

---

[b] Contraction of the bulbocavernosus muscle elicited by tapping the penis
or clitoris.
[c] During spinal shock, erections are absent. Resumption of erectile function can occur within a few days or can be delayed for over a year.[43]

TABLE 13–1   Statistics on Male Genital Functioning Following Spinal Cord Injury

	UMN Lesions		LMN Lesions	
	Complete (%)	**Incomplete (%)**	**Complete (%)**	**Incomplete (%)**
Psychogenic erections	0	25	25–40	80–85
Reflexogenic erections	> 90	95–100	0–25	90
Ejaculation*	~1	~25	14–35	≤70

*These statistics are based on studies that do not distinguish between emission and propulsatile ejaculation and therefore are inflated.
Sources: References 10, 26, 44, 45, 50, and 55.

that extend low enough to disrupt the sacral reflex arc. This disruption of sacral functioning can occur with lesions as high as T12.[52] A complete lesion that falls within the thoracolumbar erection center (Figure 13–8B) is likely to lead to the inability to have psychogenic erections.[53,66] In contrast, a lesion below this level will leave all of the thoracolumbar erection center in communication with the brain (Figure 13–8A). As a result, psychogenic erections will be possible.[66] Reflex erections are not likely to be preserved in people with low lesions, since these lesions are likely to disrupt the functioning of the sacral cord.[10,44,48,65] Men with incomplete lesions are more likely to retain the capacity to have erections.[10]

In summary, most men with spinal cord injuries retain the capacity for penile erection. Men with high lesions are likely to exhibit reflexogenic erections, and those with low lesions may have psychogenic or reflexogenic erections. Incomplete lesions are most likely to result in sparing of erection.

Although most men with spinal cord injuries retain the capacity to have erections, many who have erections are unable to use them in intercourse.[26,43,49,67] This makes sense when one recalls that the erections exhibited by neurologically intact men during sexual activity are sustained by input from both the thoracolumbar and sacral erection centers. Loss of input from either center may alter the quality (rigidity) of erection, the ability to sustain an erection, or both.

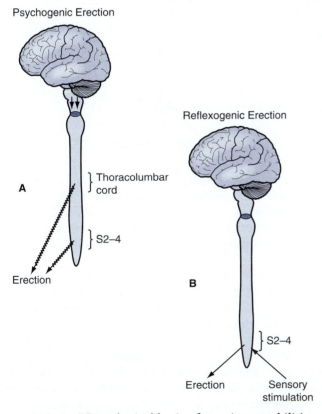

Figure 13–6   Neurological basis of erection capabilities after complete spinal cord injury rostral to thoracolumbar erection center. (A) Psychogenic erection impaired due to loss of input from brain to erection centers. (B) Reflexogenic erection spared due to preservation of sacral reflex arc.

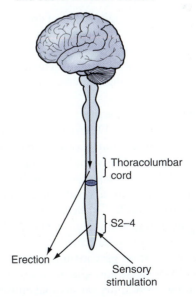

Figure 13–7   Neurological basis of erection capabilities after complete spinal cord injury that is caudal to thoracolumbar erection center but leaves sacral reflex arc intact.

Complete Lesion Extending Caudally Enough to Disrupt the Sacral Reflex Arc

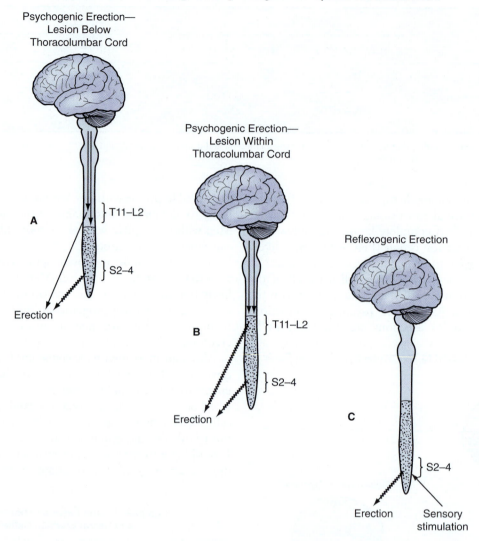

Figure 13–8   Neurological basis of erection capabilities after complete spinal cord injury that extends low enough to disrupt the sacral reflex arc. (A) With lesion below thoracolumbar erection center, psychogenic erection may be spared due to preserved input from brain to thoracolumbar erection center. (B) With lesion within thoracolumbar erection center, psychogenic erection impaired due to loss of input from brain to both sacral and thoracolumbar erection centers. (C) Reflexogenic erection impaired due to disruption of sacral reflex arc.

Emission and Ejaculation

The information available on emission and propulsatile ejaculation following spinal cord injury is not as complete as that on erection. Many studies lump the two functions together, and data are lacking on emission itself.

Emission occurs as a result of sympathetic outflow from T10 through L2.[1,39,68] Because this outflow is caused primarily by input from higher centers,[44,55] one would expect the effect of spinal cord injury on emission to be similar to its effect on psychogenic erection.

Figure 13–9 illustrates the neurological basis of the effect of a low cord injury on seminal emission. If some or all of T10 – L2 remains in contact with the brain, outflow from this area could cause emission. Higher lesions that interrupt supraspinal input to the thoracolumbar cord would be expected to impair emission (Figure 13–10).

Propulsatile ejaculation is the most neurologically vulnerable of the genital functions.[d] For propulsatile ejaculation to occur, emission must occur. Emission is brought on by outflow from the thoracolumbar cord, in turn stimulated primarily by input from higher centers. An intact sacral arc is also required for propulsatile ejaculation, since it occurs as the result of a sacral reflex. Thus propulsatile ejaculation involves both the thoracolumbar and sacral regions of the spinal cord, as well as supraspinal centers.

Figure 13–11 illustrates the effect of a complete low lesion on propulsatile ejaculation. A lesion that is low enough to

---

[d] The following discussion of ejaculatory function following spinal cord injury refers to ejaculation that occurs without the use of a vibrator or electrical stimulation. Ejaculation induced using these types of augmentation is addressed later in the chapter.

Impact of Complete Low Lesion
on Emission

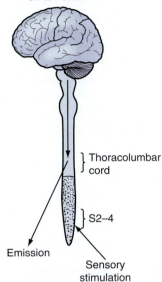

Figure 13–9   Neurological basis of impact of complete low spinal cord injury on seminal emission. Emission may be spared due to preserved input from brain to thoracolumbar cord.

preserve the thoracolumbar outflow required for emission is likely to interrupt the functioning of the sacral cord. Thus, propulsatile ejaculation is not likely to occur with a complete low lesion. The incidence of ejaculation is greater with incomplete lesions. Since many studies do not distinguish

Impact of Complete High Lesion
on Emission

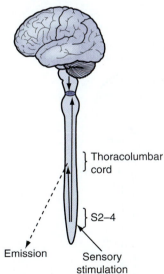

Figure 13–10   Neurological basis of impact of complete high spinal cord injury on seminal emission. Emission impaired due to loss of input from brain to thoracolumbar cord. A small minority of individuals may exhibit emission due to input from the sacral cord to the thoracolumbar cord.

Impact of Complete Low Lesion
on Ejaculation

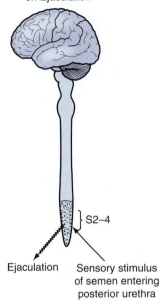

Figure 13–11   Neurological basis of impact of complete low spinal cord injury on ejaculation. Ejaculation impaired due to disruption of sacral reflex arc.

between emission and propulsatile ejaculation, the figures on the incidence of ejaculation (Table 13–1) are inflated. In many instances, what is reported as ejaculation may actually be dribbling of semen due to emission.

A complete lesion that is high enough to allow preservation of the sacral cord is likely to interrupt the thoracolumbar cord's communication with higher centers (Figure 13–12). As a result, emission and, therefore, ejaculation are quite uncommon following these lesions.

In summary, few men with spinal cord injuries exhibit both stages of ejaculation. For propulsatile ejaculation to occur, emission must occur, and these two functions combined involve supraspinal centers and both the thoracolumbar and sacral areas of the cord. Men with incomplete lesions are more likely to ejaculate than are those with complete lesions. In contrast to erectile capabilities, men with low lesions are more likely to ejaculate than are men with high lesions.[44] Research flaws make the validity of these trends questionable.

Female

The neurological control of genital arousal (vaginal lubrication and vasocongestion of the genitalia) is comparable to the control of penile erection in men. Based on what is known about the genital functioning of men after spinal cord injury, one would expect most women with spinal cord injuries to retain the capacity for genital arousal. This expectation has been supported by laboratory research, focusing primarily on vasocongestion.

If neurological control of genital functioning is comparable in women and men with spinal cord injuries, women

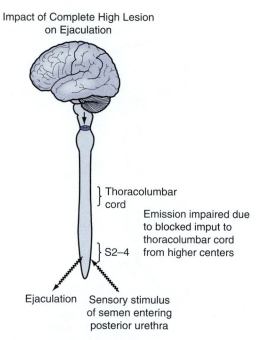

Impact of Complete High Lesion
on Ejaculation

} Thoracolumbar cord

Emission impaired due
to blocked imput to
thoracolumbar cord
from higher centers

} S2–4

Ejaculation   Sensory stimulus
of semen entering
posterior urethra

Figure 13–12   Neurological basis of impact of complete high spinal cord injury on propulsatile ejaculation. Propulsatile ejaculation impaired due to impaired emission, which results from loss of input from brain to thoracolumbar cord.

with complete lesions above the thoracolumbar cord would be expected to exhibit reflexive, but not psychogenic, genital arousal (Figure 13–13). A laboratory study supported these expectations: women with complete spinal cord injuries above T6 exhibited vaginal vasocongestion in response to manual stimulation in the clitoral region, but not in response to audiovisual erotic stimuli.[69]

Lesions that lie below the thoracolumbar portion of the cord but leave the sacral reflex arc intact would be expected to spare both psychogenic and reflexive genital arousal (Figure 13–14). Complete lesions that leave the thoracolumbar cord intact and in communication with the brain, but disrupt sacral cord function, would be expected to spare psychogenic genital arousal and disrupt reflexive arousal (Figure 13–15A). A small study that gathered information through interviews supported this assumption.[70] Additional evidence of sparing of psychogenic genital responses in individuals with lesions below the thoracolumbar cord was provided by a laboratory study in which sensory preservation in the T11 through L2 dermatomes correlated with genital vasocongestion in response to audiovisual erotic stimuli.[62]

Contraction of smooth musculature in the fallopian tubes, uterus, and paraurethral Skene glands is caused by outflow from the thoracolumbar cord, as is emission in men. Although data is lacking, one can draw tentative conclusions about the effects of cord injury based on neuroanatomy. A

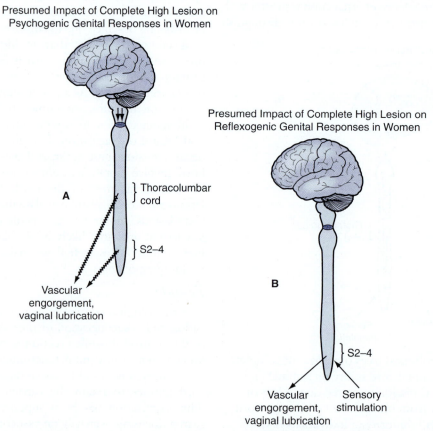

Presumed Impact of Complete High Lesion on
Psychogenic Genital Responses in Women

A

} Thoracolumbar cord

} S2–4

Vascular
engorgement,
vaginal lubrication

Presumed Impact of Complete High Lesion on
Reflexogenic Genital Responses in Women

B

} S2–4

Vascular   Sensory
engorgement,   stimulation
vaginal lubrication

Figure 13–13   Impact of complete high spinal cord injury on genital arousal in women. (A) Psychogenic genital arousal impaired due to loss of input from brain to thoracolumbar and sacral cord. (B) Reflexogenic genital arousal spared due to preservation of sacral reflex arc.

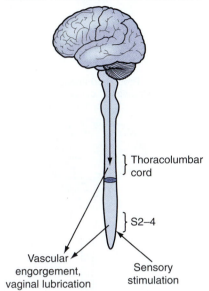

Presumed Impact of Complete Lesion
Between Thoracolumbar and Sacral Cord

} Thoracolumbar
cord

} S2–4

Vascular
engorgement,
vaginal lubrication

Sensory
stimulation

Figure 13–14   Presumed impact of complete spinal cord injury that is caudal to thoracolumbar erection center but leaves sacral reflex arc intact.

complete lesion above the thoracolumbar region of the cord would be likely to disrupt these physical responses; a lesion below this level should leave them intact in most instances.

Rhythmic contraction of striated pelvic musculature, the analogue of propulsatile ejaculation, is a sacral reflex. If the impact of spinal cord injury is equivalent in both sexes, one would expect few women with spinal cord injuries to exhibit this motor response. The statistics on ejaculation in males following cord injury are highly questionable, however, because studies tend to report emission as ejaculation. Thus it is unknown how many people with spinal cord injuries exhibit the rhythmic contraction of striated pelvic musculature associated with propulsatile ejaculation in men and its analogue in women.

Extragenital Sexual Responses

Physical responses to sexual excitation are not limited to the genitals. Both males and females exhibit nipple erection, engorgement of breast tissue, a light rash ("sex flush") on the face and upper chest, pupil dilation, and increases in heart rate, respiratory rate, and blood pressure.[3,50,61,62] These responses are controlled by supraspinal centers, and thus are not altered[e] by spinal cord injury.

Orgasm

Orgasm is an intensely pleasurable subjective experience, usually associated with ejaculation in the male and its physical equivalent in the female. However, it does not

---

[e] Systolic blood pressure responses are an exception.[69]

have to be associated with these physical responses,[50,67,71] and is not totally dependent upon genital sensation. Some men and women with complete spinal cord injuries still experience orgasm.[39,62,67,71,72] In the absence of pelvic innervation, climax can be achieved through fantasy and erotic imagery, or through stimulation of innervated areas above the level of injury.[5,9,39,58,70] Others experience orgasm following genital stimulation, despite complete spinal cord injury.[39,62,72,73] The orgasms experienced by people with spinal cord injuries are typically reported as satisfying, often followed by a resolution of sexual tension similar to that experienced by people without cord injuries.[72] In women, the duration of stimulation required to achieve climax may be longer than in noninjured individuals.[33,62] This increased time to orgasm is not present in men with spinal cord injury.[71]

The incidence of orgasm appears to vary with the integrity of the sacral reflex arc: both men and women are more likely to achieve orgasm if their S2-S5 cord segments remain functional.[39,71] The effect of lesion completeness appears to vary with gender. Males with incomplete injuries are more likely to achieve orgasm than those with complete injuries.[71] Women do not show this difference.[29,72] A few people with high lesions report severe spasticity just before and during orgasm.[55,70] Following orgasm, some individuals (both genders) report that their spasticity is reduced or eliminated for a period of time.[58,70]

Fertility

Spinal cord injury occurs most frequently between the ages of 16 and 30,[74,75] prime childbearing years. As a result, fertility is likely to be a significant concern for many who sustain spinal cord injuries.

Male

Few men with spinal cord injuries father children without medical intervention. Most estimates of the incidence of spontaneous paternity following injury are 5% or lower.[26,44,53,76,77]

Impaired erection and ejaculation are obvious sources of infertility after spinal cord injury. Techniques now exist that can be used to elicit ejaculation in men with spinal cord injuries. In one method of harvesting sperm, vibroejaculation, a vibrator is applied to the penis.[41,76–79] Ejaculation can be elicited in this manner in 67%[80] to over 80% of men with lesions above T10[76,77,81] and in 12% of men with lesions at or below T10.[77] Vibroejaculation and self-insemination can be performed at home.[56,67,76,80–83] Autonomic dysreflexia can occur during vibroejaculation, as can bruising and superficial skin damage to the penis.[28,41,56,80,84]

Electroejaculation, an alternative means of eliciting ejaculation, involves applying electric stimulation using a rectal probe.[41,76,79,82] Successful semen retrieval through electroejaculation is possible in 85% to 100% of men with spinal cord injury.[76,81,82,85] Electroejaculation must be performed in a hospital or clinic. Potential complications include autonomic dysreflexia, pain, heart arrhythmias,

Complete Lesion Extending Caudally Enough to Disrupt the Sacral Reflex Arc

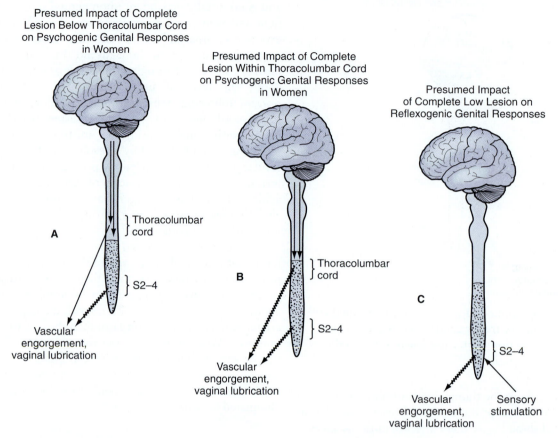

Figure 13–15   Presumed impact of complete lesion extending low enough to disrupt sacral reflex arc. (A) With lesion below thoracolumbar cord, psychogenic vasocongestion and vaginal lubrication may be spared due to preserved input from brain to thoracolumbar cord. (B) With lesion affecting thoracolumbar cord, psychogenic vasocongestion and vaginal lubrication impaired due to loss of input from brain to sacral and thoracolumbar cord. (C) Reflexogenic vasocongestion and vaginal lubrication impaired due to disruption of sacral reflex arc.

and burns.[28,41,67,80] Electroejaculation is most appropriately used in patients for whom vibroejaculation is not successful.[76,80,83,86–88]

Unfortunately there is more to the problem of infertility than the inability to place semen in a partner's vagina. Even among men who are able to achieve ejaculation, "naturally" or through technological means, impregnation remains problematic. Men with spinal cord injuries tend to have low sperm counts, and their sperm tend to have decreased viability, low motility, decreased ability to penetrate cervical mucus, and an abnormally high incidence of malformation.[26,41,53,76,89–94] Sperm quality does not appear to be related to time since injury.[67,95]

The cause of inferior sperm quality after spinal cord injury is unknown. Suggested reasons include infection, medications, stasis of seminal and prostatic fluid, a lower state of overall health, abnormal hormone levels, stress, abnormalities in the seminal plasma, antisperm antibodies, and impaired autonomic regulation of semen production.[41,56,76,78,80,84,91,95,96] With repeated ejaculations over

time, the quality of sperm may improve.[78,85,91,94,95,97,98] Urologic management techniques also have an impact on fertility; men who empty their bladders through intermittent catheterization are more likely to produce motile sperm than are men using other bladder-emptying techniques.[56,97,99] Sperm harvested using vibratory stimulation is of higher quality than that harvested using electroejaculation.[41,56,67,76,82,86,87,94]

Recent advances in reproductive technology have benefited men with spinal cord injuries. Sperm can now be harvested using vibroejaculation, electroejaculation, or surgical removal of the sperm directly from the vas deferens, epididymis, or testicle. Fertilization can be achieved through vaginal, cervical, intrauterine, or intrafallopian insemination; in vitro fertilization (IVF); gamete intrafallopian transfer (GIFT); or intracytoplasmic sperm injection combined with IVF or GIFT.[41,76,78–83,86,100–103] The overall estimated live birth rate using assisted reproductive techniques is 40%.[94] Unfortunately any of these approaches can be both financially and emotionally taxing.[41,80,104]

Female

Although it is thought that spinal cord injury does not change a woman's fertility[1,7,9,53] research comparing the fertility of women with spinal cord injuries to that of non-injured women is lacking.[94] The menstrual cycle typically stops at the time of injury but resumes an average of 4.3 months later.[105] Women with spinal cord injuries can become pregnant and carry their babies to full term.[31] Most women with spinal cord injuries who become pregnant deliver healthy babies vaginally.[26,106–108]

Although a woman remains fertile after spinal cord injury and can deliver normally, pregnancy has its risks. Most women with lesions above T7 exhibit autonomic dysreflexia during labor contractions.[106] Women with lesions above T10[70,109] can go into labor without realizing it.[f] Other hazards of pregnancy for women with spinal cord injuries include increased risk of anemia, urinary tract infections, pressure ulcers, deep venous thrombosis, respiratory compromise, and constipation.[7,9,26,70,106, 107,109,110] Lasting changes in the postural orientation of the pelvis may develop. Premature labor and low birth weight are more common than in the general population.[110] Delivery using forceps or cesarean section may occur more frequently than in the general population.[9,28,106]

Because of the complications of pregnancy unique to women with spinal cord injuries, it is advisable for their obstetricians to consult with rehabilitation specialists. With proper management, the increased risks of pregnancy and labor should not pose a major threat to the health of the mother or child. Pressure ulcers, urinary tract infections, respiratory complications, and constipation can be prevented with proper care. A physician aware of the risks of early and undetected labor can monitor the patient closely toward the end of pregnancy and take appropriate precautions when dilation begins. During labor, blood pressure should be monitored continuously. Autonomic dysreflexia can be stopped or prevented with general anesthesia, epidural anesthesia, or various antihypertensive medications.[106,108–111]

Since women remain fertile following spinal cord injury, contraceptives are an important concern. The physiological and functional sequelae of spinal cord injury may complicate the selection between contraceptive options. Oral contraceptives increase the already elevated risk of deep vein thrombosis.[7,112] Intrauterine devices (IUDs) have been associated with pelvic inflammatory disease[65] and can perforate the uterus. A woman with a spinal cord injury may not detect these problems because of sensory deficits.[53,112] Impaired upper extremity function can make the use of barrier methods of contraception (male or female condoms, diaphragms, cervical caps, spermicides) problematic unless the partner is able to assist.[112] Diaphragms increase the

risk of urinary tract infection[112] and can be dislodged when a woman performs a Credé maneuver[g] to empty her bladder.[113] Levonorgestrel implants may be an option, but they have not been studied in women with spinal cord injury.[65] As is true for women without spinal cord injuries, surgical sterilization is an option for individuals who do not wish to bear children at any time in the future.

Because of the risks and logistical problems associated with the different methods of contraception, the choice may be difficult. The rehabilitation team, in consultation with a gynecologist, should assist the patient in finding the solution that is most suitable for her.

THERAPEUTIC INTERVENTION

The physical and social effects of spinal cord injury have a profound impact on sexuality and sexual functioning. People can, however, adjust. No matter what the level of lesion, motor ability, sensation, or genital functioning, people can adapt. They can once again come to see themselves as sexual beings, forming and maintaining relationships, giving and receiving pleasure.

Goals of Intervention

The overall goals of the sexual component of a rehabilitation program after spinal cord injury should be for the person to become comfortable with himself or herself as a sexual being and to learn whatever is needed to make sexual expression and fulfillment possible.

The rehabilitation team should affirm the sexuality of the person with a spinal cord injury. The patient and family should receive the message that sexuality and sexual functioning are common and legitimate concerns, and that a fulfilling sex life is a reasonable goal.

People with spinal cord injury also need to gain a basic understanding of how they can function sexually. This understanding should include physical and psychological sexual responses before and after injury, fertility, techniques for giving and receiving pleasure, and strategies for dealing with spinal cord injury–related issues such as spasticity or incontinence.

Knowledge in the area of sexuality and sexual functioning is important, but this information will be all but worthless to the person who does not feel worthy or capable of sexual gratification. In a rehabilitation program, a patient should work to regain his or her sense of self-worth, sexuality, and attractiveness as a sexual partner.[32]

Communication is a critical ingredient in all sexual encounters. Perhaps it becomes even more important following spinal cord injury. Patients may need to develop skills in meeting people, putting them at ease, developing relationship, dealing with misunderstandings or misgivings, initiating and declining sexual activities, communicating

---

[f] Although it is possible for labor to go undetected, most women with spinal cord injuries are able to sense the onset of labor. The sensations may be different from those experienced by able-bodied women.[106]

[g] The Credé maneuver is described in Chapter 14.

what does and does not pleasure them, and letting partners know what they can expect in a sexual encounter.[30,113–115]

> "I verbalized a lot of things: You know I'm paralyzed, you know I don't have much sensation, or if you don't know this, I'm gonna tell you. And I'm gonna show you. And I'm gonna reach out and touch you, and I'm gonna hold you because that's something I need to do and I want to do. And it's worked."
>
> Mark Johnson
> rehabilitation counselor, activist,
> C5-C6 SCI survivor[34]

Knowledge, comfort with self, and communication skills are essential, but these are just the beginning. Ultimately, the goal is for the person to be able to put these things into practice. Patients should be encouraged to explore and experiment, learning how their bodies respond and what is now pleasurable. Alone or with their partners,[h] they can try different positions and sexual activities. The rehabilitation team can assist in this process by providing a private room for intimate encounters and offering support when needed.

Strategies

There are a variety of approaches to sexual rehabilitation following spinal cord injury. Several basic strategies are presented in this section. Most programs incorporate more than one of these strategies. Perhaps the perfect program would include elements of all of them.

Psychosexual and Physical Evaluation

Ideally, sexual rehabilitation begins with an evaluation. One or more members of the rehabilitation team assess the patient's sexual functioning in much the same way that they evaluate other areas of function. This evaluation includes obtaining a history and performing a physical examination.

In taking a psychosexual history, a health professional investigates psychosocial issues that can affect a person's sexual adjustment. Areas of investigation can include the patient's past and present sexual attitudes, values and behavior; level of understanding of his or her sexual functioning; communication skills; past and present relationships; feelings about himself or herself as a sexual being; and present sexual desires and concerns.[1,36] If the patient has a partner, both the patient's and partner's level of adjustment to the injury should also be addressed.[43]

A sexual evaluation also includes a history of the patient's pre- and postinjury sexual function and medical status. The health professional investigates the patient's current medications,[43,46] history of erectile and ejaculatory functioning or menstruation and pregnancy, urinary tract and bowel

functioning and complications, genitourinary surgery, venereal disease, and contraceptive use.[1,46]

A thorough sexual evaluation entails an examination that investigates the patient's physical potential for sexual functioning. This examination should address the functioning of both the thoracolumbar and sacral portions of the spinal cord, including genital sensation and responses, sacral reflexes, bladder function,[i] and sensation in the thoracolumbar dermatomes.[52,57] The evaluation can also include sperm count studies or a pelvic examination, depending on the patient's gender.[1,36,116] Finally, the examination can include the patient's strength, range of motion, muscle tone, pain, and functional status, as these areas are relevant to the individual's potential for participating in various sexual activities.[36]

An evaluation of psychosocial and physical sexual functioning is a valuable part of a rehabilitation program. It provides the rehabilitation team and patient with an understanding of the patient's functioning and enables them to set goals and design a program accordingly. The evaluation itself can also be therapeutic, as it demonstrates to the person that the rehabilitation team considers his or her sexuality and sexual functioning to be an important area of concern.

Education

In sexual rehabilitation, education is a must and a minimum. Patients should learn about their physical sexual responses and those of their partners: how the body responds to sexual stimuli, how and why a spinal cord injury affects this function, how these sexual responses can be elicited, and how they can be utilized in sexual encounters. People with spinal cord injuries need to know about their fertility and about options in contraception and assisted reproduction as indicated. They should learn that sexual pleasure and even orgasm are still possible, whether or not they can experience sensations from their genitals. And they should know how to deal with logistical problems such as urinary devices or altered genital functioning. Without this knowledge, a person with a spinal cord injury may be at a loss regarding how to go about pursuing sexual gratification. Worse, he or she may be unaware that sexual gratification is even possible.

The educational component of sexual rehabilitation can take many forms. The information can be presented in lectures, films, slides, group discussions, or question-and-answer sessions.[116,117] Romano and Lassiter[117] emphasized that education regarding sexuality should begin with a review of the physical and emotional aspects of "normal" sexual functioning. Like the general public, people with spinal cord injuries are likely to be ignorant in this area but reluctant to admit to this ignorance.

People vary in the timing of their readiness to receive information on sexual functioning and fertility after spinal

---

[h] Not all patients have sexual partners available. Options in these cases include encouraging patients to explore their bodies on their own and emphasizing strategies for finding partners.

[i] Bladder function can provide insight into the functioning of the sacral and thoracolumbar portions of the spinal cord.[52]

cord injury. Moreover, an individual's needs and priorities may change with time.[114,118,119] For this reason, the educational component of a sexual rehabilitation program should include information on resources that will be available after discharge. These resources can include professionals, peer mentors, and organizations in the patient's community, as well as web-based sources of information and support.[39,114,119]

Desensitization and Attitude

Sexual activities are emotionally charged and value-laden; sexual behavior is immersed in taboos and imperatives. People come to rehabilitation with compelling, deep-seated feelings about what they should and should not do in a sexual encounter, what is desirable, and what is wrong or unappealing. These preexisting attitudes can be a formidable barrier to sexual adjustment after spinal cord injury. They can prevent a person from experimenting comfortably with his or her sexual expression. Attitudes can even inhibit a person's ability to absorb the information presented in an educational program. To achieve sexual fulfillment following spinal cord injury, a person may need to reassess his or her attitudes regarding sexual behavior. The challenge for health professionals is to help patients in this process and at the same time remain respectful of each individual's values, preferences, and readiness to deal with sexual issues.

Elements of desensitization and attitude change are incorporated in many sexual rehabilitation programs. Sexual issues can be addressed over time, with the presentations and discussions gradually becoming more explicit. Contact with others who have adapted well sexually after injury can also assist with attitude change.

Behavioral Treatment

Knowledge and attitude change can pave the way for sexual adjustment, but they may not be sufficient. Even armed with an understanding and acceptance of his or her potential for sexual functioning, a person with a spinal cord injury faces social barriers to sexual gratification. The injury may have brought about role changes, conflict, and communication difficulties in preexisting relationships. Meeting people and initiating sexual relations may be problematic because of the social stigma associated with disability. Moreover, the person with a spinal cord injury may have motor or sensory deficits that interfere with nonverbal communication techniques that he or she had previously used to express desires and test the waters with potential partners.

A variety of communication skills may be helpful to the person with a spinal cord injury (or anyone) in developing and maintaining sexual relations. These skills include verbal and nonverbal expression of affection,[120] desires, and needs; assertiveness; and techniques for meeting and attracting potential partners.[117,121] Someone who learns to project confidence in himself or herself as a sexual being and knows how to put a partner at ease is more likely to be successful in this arena.

"Those of us with spinal cord injuries need to regain a positive sense of self, a positive self-image, then project that to the people around us so that they will have reason to find us interesting, attractive and – the bottom line – sexual.

Of course, disability may set you apart from some people you encounter. Most folks will have some discomfort with your disability at first, but are usually able to overcome this if you help them to get to know 'you,' the person. Take responsibility for putting others at ease."

Jack Dahlberg
rehabilitation consultant, husband, father,
SCI survivor[122]

Various approaches can be used to develop communication skills for sexual encounters. Patients can role play, rehearse behaviors, and receive feedback on their communication. They can also practice expressing desires and giving feedback, both verbally and nonverbally.[115,117]

In addition to developing new communication skills, a person with a spinal cord injury needs to learn how his or her body now functions sexually. If the patient is in a relationship, the partner must also learn and adapt if the relationship is to continue. Couples frequently develop new means of sexual expression after spinal cord injury and find these alternative sexual activities to be enjoyable and satisfying.[4,12,20] To enhance sexual adjustment, the rehabilitation team should give the couple both the permission and the opportunity to explore their bodies and relearn how to give and receive pleasure. To facilitate this exploration, patients can be instructed in sensory exercises and the use of fantasy. A couple[j] may be given "homework assignments" involving various sexual activities tailored to their needs.[113,115] In addition to experimenting with giving and receiving pleasure, patients and their partners can practice eliciting genital responses through fantasy or physical stimulation, depending on whether they have retained psychogenic or reflexive genital responses.[52] For inpatients, private rooms can be made available to enable couples or individuals to explore and redevelop their sexual potentials.[36] These rooms may also be used to provide much-needed private time for couples and families.[21]

Counseling

Sexual adjustment following spinal cord injury requires some major adaptations. A person may be faced with altered functioning and loss of sensation in the genitals, a body that no longer looks or works the same as it used to, urinary appliances and the threat of incontinence during sex, loss of fertility, and altered social relations with others. Counseling can help him or her come to terms with these changes and regain a sense of sexual self-worth.

---

[j] If a partner is not available, the patient can be encouraged to experiment on his or her own.

Group therapy can provide a nonthreatening atmosphere for discussing sexual concerns. Many find it helpful to get together with other people with spinal cord injuries to discuss their feelings and the problems that they anticipate or have already faced. Participants often find comfort in learning that others are facing problems similar to theirs.[116,117] Group counseling sessions can also provide opportunities for problem solving and mutual support.

More individualized counseling can also be helpful in sexual adjustment after spinal cord injury. One approach involves seeing both the patient and partner, as both have adjustments to make. The two can be seen individually and as a couple. In joint sessions the couple can develop their communication skills and discuss their expectations and emotions with each other.[10,116]

Specific Suggestions

Specific suggestions can be an invaluable aid to sexual adjustment after spinal cord injury. An individual who is simply told to "experiment" and then is turned loose to find his or her own way may have difficulty finding that way. He or she may be reluctant to experiment without at least some initial guidance. Unanswered questions such as "What do I do with this catheter?" or "How exactly can I have intercourse?" may leave the individual reluctant to try sexual activities. Specific suggestions about the logistics of sexual encounters can pave the way for more comfortable and confident exploration.

People with impaired genital sensation may benefit from suggestions for maximizing their pleasure during sexual encounters. They should be encouraged to explore their bodies and find what areas give pleasure when stimulated. People with spinal cord injuries often find that their lowest innervated dermatomes are more sensitive to touch. Many find stimulation of the earlobes, neck, and mouth to be extremely pleasurable. By concentrating on pleasurable sensations, using fantasy, and reassigning pleasurable sensations to the genitals, people with cord injuries can maximize their pleasure, even to the point of orgasm.[5,39,58,113,115] Vibrators can also be useful for enhancing pleasure.[20,39]

Suggestions regarding pleasuring techniques for the partner can also be helpful. Patients can be encouraged to try oral or manual stimulation of the partner's genitals. People with impaired hand function may find that vibrators are useful for stimulating their partners.[113,115]

Another area to address is dysfunctional vaginal lubrication or penile erection during intercourse. Men and women with intact sensation in the T11 to L2 dermatomes (associated with psychogenic arousal) may be able to enhance their genital responses through fantasy and foreplay.[123] Those with intact sacral reflex arcs may require more physical stimulation of their genitals,[123] possibly using a vibrator or manual stimulation.[10,70,113,124] When vaginal lubrication or erection remains inadequate despite the strategies just described, additional compensatory strategies can be effective. Women who do not produce adequate vaginal lubrication for intercourse can use a lubricant. Men have several options for achieving erections, described in a separate section that follows.

Health professionals can also make suggestions regarding positions for intercourse. A male with a spinal cord injury may prefer his partner to be in a superior position ("on top"), side lying, or sitting in his lap in a chair or wheelchair, facing toward or away from him. A woman may prefer her partner to be in a superior position or side lying. If she has severe adductor spasticity, a rear approach may be best. Alternatively, she may have intercourse sitting in a wheelchair, sitting at the edge of the seat with her partner kneeling in front of her.[115,125,126]

People who use indwelling catheters are often concerned about managing this equipment during intercourse. They may fear that they will injure themselves during intercourse or that the catheters will get in the way. Patients should be assured that they can remove catheters prior to sexual intercourse if they prefer or they can safely leave them in place. A man can fold his urethral catheter back along the side of his penis, either cover it with a condom or leave it uncovered, and lubricate well.[31,125] A woman who wishes to leave her urethral catheter in place should lubricate it to avoid problems from friction during intercourse,[70] and tape the catheter to her abdomen[127] or thigh[31] so that it remains out of the way. A suprapubic catheter should be taped to the abdomen, and an ileal conduit bag should be positioned out of the way.[31,117]

People who manage their bladder incontinence without indwelling catheters may have urinary accidents during sexual activities. This is especially true for people who have reflexively functioning bladders; stimulation of the thighs, genitals, or other pelvic structures may initiate the voiding reflex. This risk can be reduced by emptying the bladder immediately prior to sexual activity[70,113] and, possibly, by avoiding drinking large amounts of fluid beforehand.[119] In addition, individuals may wish to note which sexual stimuli tend to induce voiding and then avoid these stimuli during sexual encounters. It may also be wise to keep a towel handy and to inform partners of the possibility of bladder accidents.[31,117] These steps can reduce the embarrassment and inconvenience of any accidents that occur.

Bowel accidents during sexual activity are another area of concern. Patients should be reassured that a regular bowel program can minimize the possibility of having a bowel accident during sex.[113] It may also be helpful to coordinate the timing of sexual activity with the bowel regimen so that sexual activity occurs when accidents are least likely.[119]

A common concern expressed by many patients is that the partner may contract a urinary tract infection during intercourse. Both parties should be assured that this is unlikely[k] if standard hygiene practices are used.[31]

---

[k] Sexually transmitted diseases should be a concern, however, just as they are in the general population. Because of the health risks associated with sexual activity, the rehabilitation program should include education on sexually transmitted diseases.

Problem-Solving Exercise 13-1

Your patient recently sustained a spinal cord injury classified as T5, ASIA A. He wants to know whether he will ever be able to have sex again. He makes it clear that he is interested in learning about sexual intercourse in particular.

- What should you tell him?

Patients who are subject to autonomic dysreflexia (people with lesions above T6) should be informed that it can be triggered by sexual activity but need not pose a major threat if handled correctly. If a headache occurs during genital stimulation, the couple should stop the stimulation briefly. The headache should then resolve quickly.[1] When it does, the couple can resume their sexual activity, avoiding the particular stimulation that appeared to bring on the headache.[125]

People who require assistance in preparation for sexual activities (undressing, transfers, positioning, management of catheters) may find that having a sexual partner provide this assistance creates problems. Both parties may find it difficult to shift from nurse–patient to lover–lover roles. Moreover, the caretaker/lover may spend so much energy on the preparation that he or she has little left over for the sexual activity. When problems such as these arise, an attendant can be of help.[10]

Suggestions for maximizing pleasure for both partners and suggestions about the mechanics and logistics of sexual activity can be of great assistance to a newly injured person. Ultimately, however, each person still must find his or her own way sexually. He or she will need to experiment, discovering what positions and activities yield the most pleasure and satisfaction.[m]

Interventions for Erectile Dysfunction

Various physical aids are available for men with erectile dysfunction who wish to include penetration in their sexual activity but are unable to obtain or sustain erections using the strategies described earlier. Noninvasive options include the use of a firm casing that is worn over the penis or an artificial penis that can either be strapped above the anatomical penis or held in the hand.[116,126,128] One option for men who have reflex erections is a constricting band that is placed around the base of the erect penis to trap blood within the erectile bodies and prolong the erection. Alternatively, a vacuum pump may be used to achieve an erection, which is then maintained with a constricting band at the base of the penis.[65,67,129,130] When vacuum pumps and constricting bands are used according to manufacturers' specifications, complications are uncommon and mild.[131]

Many men use oral medication to enhance their erectile capabilities. Sildenafil, vardenafil, and tadalafil have all been shown to be safe and effective for men with spinal cord injuries.[123] Alternatively, such men can safely achieve erection by injecting vasoactive drugs (papaverine, phentolamine, prostaglandin E1, or a combination of these) into the corpus cavernosum.[131]

Most men are able to achieve satisfactory erections using one of the methods just described.[131] Implanted penile prostheses are an option for those who cannot do so or who find these methods unacceptable.[131] There are two classes of penile prostheses: inflatable and rod type. Inflatable prostheses include a pump and reservoir and can be inflated or deflated as needed.[126] Rod-type prostheses provide a permanent erection. In addition to providing erection for intercourse, penile prostheses can aid in intermittent catheterization[132] or in the fit of condom catheters.[126,131] Because of the high rate of serious complications, all other treatments for erectile dysfunction should be tried before resorting to these devices.[67,133]

A variety of options are available for achieving erections. The rehabilitation team should keep in mind, however, that erection and vaginal penetration are not prerequisites for a satisfying sex life.

> "[There's a prevalent belief that] if your neurology is such that you do not get an erection physiologically, then you must have an erection prosthetically. I have no objection to this procedure, but I do object to the procedure being offered to newly injured people who have not had an adequate trial at living an integrated life as a para or a quad, who have not learned to like themselves again, who still see themselves as some kind of abomination, who think the big thing in sex is genital activity."
>
> George Hohmann
> psychologist, husband, father,
> T9-T10 SCI survivor[34]

Sexuality as Part of the Overall Rehabilitation Program

Coming to terms with one's sexuality and sexual functioning is an important component of adjustment after spinal cord injury. Seen in this light, sexual rehabilitation is clearly a key ingredient of rehabilitation after cord injury.

---

[1] Additional information on autonomic dysreflexia is presented in Chapters 2 and 3.
[m] The following sources provide additional specific suggestions for sexual activity after spinal cord injury: references 122, 126, and 141

Problem-Solving Exercise 13–2

Your patient has a spinal cord injury classified as T8, ASIA B. After a home visit, she confides that she and her husband "messed around" while she was at home. She then laughs and tells you that she wet the bed "just when things were starting to get interesting."

- How should you respond?

Despite the importance of sexuality, it is often neglected by the rehabilitation team.[5,114,134] Because of both poorly defined roles and feelings of discomfort, each team member may avoid the topic, hoping that other team members will deal with it. Individual health professionals or the team as a whole may limit their intervention to discussion of fertility or even avoid the issue altogether.[114,118] This problem appears to be more common when the patient is female; women are less likely than men to receive information on sexuality and sexual functioning after spinal cord injury.[11,13,15]

When the rehabilitation team does not address sexual functioning, patients are often reluctant to bring up the topic.[114,127] They may find the subject too embarrassing, or may interpret the team's silence as an indication that sex is no longer an appropriate area of concern for them.[135] Even when patients take the initiative to bring up the topic, health professionals may dodge questions and avoid discussions on sexual functioning. This behavior is likely to increase patients' anxiety about their sexuality and sexual functioning.[3]

To ensure that sexuality is addressed adequately with every patient, sexual rehabilitation (with defined roles and goals) should be an official component of the program. It should not be left to chance, with each team member hoping or assuming that someone else is taking care of it.

Sexuality should be addressed with all patients who have spinal cord injuries, regardless of their gender, age,[123,136,137] or sexual orientation. Sexual rehabilitation should be comprehensive and tailored to the needs of each patient. This includes providing information and services appropriate for the individual's gender,[n] age,[o] physical functioning, sexual orientation, psychosocial status, and state of readiness. Sexual rehabilitation should begin early,[15,114] with continuing access to services for a prolonged period post-discharge.[17] If a patient has a sexual partner, that person should be involved in the process,[p] since he or she will also have adjustments to make,[3,118] and the partner's sexual adjustment can have an impact on the psychosocial well-being of the individual with a spinal cord injury.[120]

Team Approach

Successful sexual rehabilitation requires a team approach. The various members of the rehabilitation team should be comfortable affirming patients' sexuality, answering questions about sexual concerns, and supporting the sexual component of the rehabilitation program.[116] Patients will then be able to discuss their concerns with whomever they feel the most comfortable.

Being an effective team member requires more than knowledge in the area of sexual functioning. Values and attitudes are also important. A health professional who is uncomfortable discussing sexual issues, who sees people with disabilities as sexless, or who is repelled by the sexual options open to people with spinal cord injuries will not be an effective participant in sexual rehabilitation. In fact, he or she is likely to have a detrimental effect on patients. Overtly or covertly, the health professional may convey negative attitudes that undermine the patient's progress.[3,37]

All members of the rehabilitation team should have the knowledge and attitudes needed to support patients in their sexual rehabilitation. Specialized training may be required to prepare team members for their roles in sexual rehabilitation. Workshops on sexuality and sexual functioning can improve health professionals' knowledge and communication skills, increase their comfort with sexual issues, and make them more likely to address these issues with their patients.[134,138]

PLISSIT Model

Although the entire rehabilitation team should be able to support the sexual component of the program, not all health professionals must (or even can) provide intensive sexual therapy to their patients. Different professionals will provide different input, depending on their comfort, experience, interest, and expertise.

The PLISSIT model of intervention can be useful for the team approach to sexual rehabilitation.[134,138] PLISSIT is an acronym representing the levels of intervention described in the approach: *Permission, Limited Information, Specific Suggestions,* and *Intensive Therapy.*[127] Using this model, health professionals can supply varying levels of intervention. The level that a given person provides can be determined by both the patient's need and the professional's expertise and comfort.

---

[n] Women with spinal cord injuries have reported that the quality of their sexual rehabilitation has suffered because the focus tends to be on male functioning and perspectives.[114,142]

[o] Children and adolescents with spinal cord injuries should receive age-appropriate sexual education that addresses both normal functioning and the impact of spinal cord injury. Their parents should also be provided with education on sexuality, sexual functioning, and fertility after spinal cord injury.[123,136,143]

[p] *With the patient's permission,* the partner should be included.

Permission giving is the most basic level of intervention in the PLISSIT model. At this level the health professional gives the patient "permission" to be sexual; through verbal or nonverbal behavior, the health professional affirms the patient's sexuality and encourages him or her to explore its expression.[139,140] This is the minimal level of intervention, which all members of the team should be able to provide. The "permission" from various health professionals will provide much-needed support to the patient.

At the next level of intervention, the health professional provides limited information: the patient is educated about his or her sexual functioning.[10,127,139,140] For patients with spinal cord injury, the education can cover anatomy and physiology, genital functioning following injury, fertility, and birth control.

At the third level of intervention, the health professional provides the patient with specific suggestions.[127,139] Suggestions can cover the logistics and mechanics of sexual acts, meeting and seducing people, and giving and receiving pleasure. A variety of health professionals may provide this level of intervention, addressing issues most pertinent to their fields. For example, a nurse may discuss options for managing a catheter during sexual encounters, and a physical therapist may make suggestions regarding positioning during intercourse.

Intensive therapy is the highest level of intervention, provided by health professionals with specialized training.[127,139] Counseling, behavioral treatment, and attitude reassessment fall into this category of intervention.

Summary

- Spinal cord injury has profound effects on sexuality and sexual functioning. Changes in genital functioning, sensation, and musculoskeletal functioning may make a person's accustomed modes of sexual expression difficult or impossible. In addition, the physical and social sequelae of a cord injury are likely to disrupt a person's sense of self, including his or her sense of self as a sexual being. Logistical problems such as incontinence or difficulty in meeting people can further complicate the picture.
- Male genital functions during sexual activity include erection, seminal emission, and propulsatile ejaculation. Female genital functions during sexual activity include vaginal lubrication, vasocongestion of the genitals, and muscle contractions in both smooth and striated musculature. Neurological control of these functions involves the sacral and thoracolumbar spinal cord as well as supraspinal centers. The impact of spinal cord injury on the various genital functions depends on the lesion's level and degree of completeness.
- Spinal cord injury profoundly impairs male fertility. Recent advances in reproductive technology, however, have made biological fatherhood a reasonable goal.
- Spinal cord injury does not alter a woman's fertility. Because of certain risks involved in pregnancy and childbirth, however, obstetricians caring for women with cord injuries should consult with rehabilitation specialists.
- Sexual rehabilitation is an important component of rehabilitation after spinal cord injury. Different rehabilitation centers take a variety of approaches in addressing sexuality. Some or all of the following elements can be included in a sexual rehabilitation program: psychosexual and physical evaluation, education, desensitization, attitude reassessment, behavioral treatment, counseling, specific suggestions, and interventions for erectile dysfunction.

Suggested Resources

PUBLICATIONS

Karp, G. *Disability & the Art of Kissing: Questions and Answers on the True Nature of Intimacy*, 2006. Self-published, available for purchase from *www.lifeonwheels.net*

Kaufman M, Silverberg S, Odette F. *The Ultimate Guide to Sex and Disability: For All of us Who Live with Disabilities, Chronic Pain and Illness*, 2007. San Francisco, CA: Cleis Press.

Sexuality and Reproductive Health in Adults with Spinal Cord Injury: A Clinical Practice Guideline for Health-Care Providers, 2009. Published by the Paralyzed Veterans of America. Available for free download from *www.pva.org*

WEB SITES

Sexual Health Network: *www.sexualhealth.com*

Spinal Cord Injury Rehabilitation Evidence, Chapter 11, Sexual Health Following Spinal Cord Injury: *www.icord.org/scire/chapters.php*

14

Bladder and Bowel Management

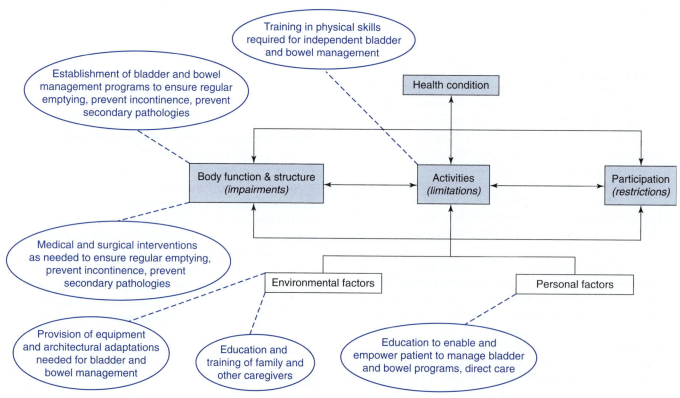

Chapter 14 presents information on bladder and bowel function and management practices after spinal cord injury.

Most people with spinal cord injuries lose volitional control of their bladders and bowels; since the bladder and lower bowel are innervated by sacral cord segments, all complete lesions and many incomplete lesions result in urinary and fecal incontinence. Because of the profound impact that incontinence can have on a person's health and lifestyle, bladder and bowel management are critical concerns following spinal cord injury.

COMPLICATIONS RELATED TO BLADDER AND BOWEL DYSFUNCTION

Bladder and bowel dysfunction following spinal cord injury can cause life-threatening complications if not managed appropriately. Kidney damage can occur when excessive

pressure in the bladder (high intravesical pressure) causes urine to reflux into the ureters (vesicoureteral reflux).[1,2] Hydronephrosis and eventual renal failure can result. Kidney function is also threatened by urinary tract infection, a common sequela of bladder dysfunction after spinal cord injury.[1,3–5] Factors that contribute to urinary tract infections include high intravesical pressures, large volumes of urine left in the bladder after emptying (high residual volumes), vesicoureteral reflux, prolonged time intervals between emptyings, and contamination from catheters.[1,6] Spinal cord injury is also associated with a high incidence of kidney and bladder stones and an elevated risk of bladder cancer.[1,7,8]

Altered bowel function can also lead to serious complications. Decreased bowel motility and impaired evacuation can lead to colonic stasis, constipation, fecal impaction, and megacolon.[9–12] Additional common complications include ileus, abdominal pain, appetite loss, diarrhea, hemorrhoids, and diverticulosis.[3,10–12]

Impaired bladder and bowel function can pose a more immediate threat to people with cervical or high thoracic lesions. Bladder distention or fecal impaction can trigger autonomic dysreflexia, a heightened autonomic response that can progress rapidly to death.[a]

Incontinence can also cause skin breakdown. Feces or urine that remains in contact with the skin for prolonged periods can damage the skin. Once breakdown occurs, the person may have to restrict her activities while the skin heals, and the healed area will remain vulnerable to subsequent pressure ulcers. She may face prolonged hospitalization, sepsis, amputations, and even death.[b]

In addition to the impact on physical health, bladder and bowel dysfunction can have profound psychosocial consequences. Involuntary voiding and bowel movements (bowel and bladder "accidents") can cause embarrassment and social isolation. They can hinder return to home after rehabilitation and interfere with participation in social activities, employment, sexual relationships, and other life situations.[13–16] Incontinence may be associated with lower quality of life and life satisfaction,[17] and a higher prevalence of depression.[18]

Bladder Function

Urine flows from the kidneys to the bladder through the ureters, and exits through the urethra. In normal functioning, urine can voluntarily be stored in the bladder or voided. Figure 14–1 illustrates the urinary tract and musculature involved in bladder control.

Normal Bladder Function

Several muscles are involved in bladder control. The bladder wall contains the detrusor, which is composed of smooth muscle. At the bladder neck (the portion of the bladder that surrounds the urethral opening), the detrusor encircles the point of juncture of the urethra with the bladder. Smooth muscle fibers also extend down the urethra. Elastic tissue in the proximal urethra adds to this functional[c] sphincter.[19] The external urethral sphincter and the periurethral skeletal muscles of the pelvic floor surround the urethra.

Innervation

Normal bladder function depends upon the neurological control of the detrusor, urethral smooth muscle, external

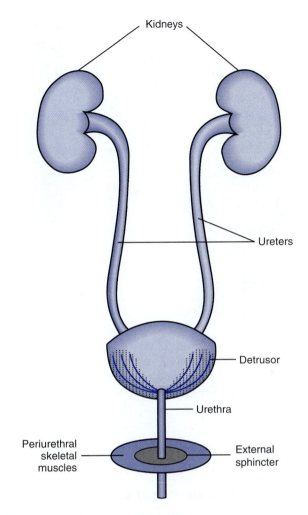

Figure 14–1   Schematic drawing of urinary tract and musculature involved in bladder control.

sphincter, and periurethral pelvic floor muscles (Figure 14–2). This control occurs at three levels: the sacral spinal cord, the pons, and several extrapontine regions of the brain. The sacral micturition center is the site of spinal reflexes involved in urination. The pontine micturition center integrates input from other areas of the brain and coordinates bladder emptying through efferent pathways projecting to parasympathetic, sympathetic, and somatic motor neurons in the spinal cord.[1]

Parasympathetic innervation arises from sacral cord segments 2, 3, and 4. Parasympathetic stimulation causes contraction of the detrusor and relaxation of the urethral smooth muscle.[1,20]

Sympathetic innervation arises from the 11th thoracic through the 2nd lumbar segments of the cord. Sympathetic stimulation causes relaxation of the detrusor in the body of the bladder, and contraction in the bladder neck and urethral smooth muscle.[1,19,20]

Somatic innervation from sacral segments 2 through 4 supplies the external urethral sphincter and the periurethral

---

[a] Autonomic dysreflexia is discussed in more detail in Chapters 2 and 3.
[b] Skin breakdown and its treatment and prevention are presented in Chapter 5.
[c] Although the literature contains references to an internal sphincter between the bladder and the urethra, there is no true sphincter at this junction.[19]

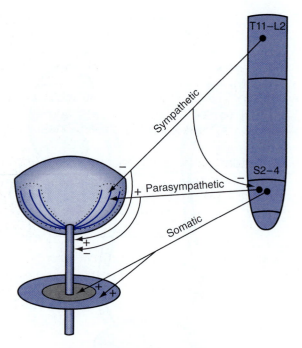

Figure 14–2   Innervation of the muscles involved bladder storage and emptying. Descending input from the pontine micturition center not shown.

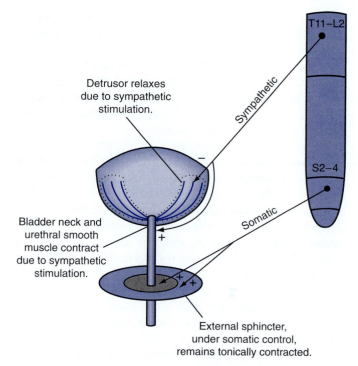

Figure 14–3   Urine storage: relaxation of the detrusor in the body of the bladder, contraction of smooth muscle in the bladder neck and urethra, tonic contraction of the external sphincter.

pelvic floor musculature. The sphincter and pelvic floor musculature can be contracted voluntarily.[19]

Storage and Elimination of Urine

During urine storage, sympathetic efferents cause relaxation in the body of the bladder as well as contraction in the bladder neck and urethral smooth muscle. The external sphincter (under somatic control) remains tonically contracted (Figure 14–3). Mild bladder distention triggers these sympathetic and somatic responses, which are mediated by spinal reflexes and descending input from the pons. The resulting combination of bladder relaxation and contraction at its outlet allows urine to be stored at low pressures.[1,21]

During urination, parasympathetic efferents cause contraction in the body of the bladder and relaxation in the bladder neck and urethral smooth muscle. The external sphincter also relaxes (Figure 14–4). The combination of bladder contraction and relaxation at its outlet allows urine to be expelled from the bladder. These actions occur as a result of sacral spinal reflexive responses to bladder distention (at volumes approaching the bladder's capacity), modulated by supraspinal centers.[1,19]

The pontine micturition center coordinates the parasympathetic, sympathetic, and somatic impulses to the muscles involved in voiding. This coordination of detrusor contraction with relaxation at the bladder outlet is necessary for effective bladder emptying.[1]

The cerebral cortex is involved in the voluntary control of urination. This control occurs primarily through inhibition of the sacral micturition center[19] and voluntary contraction of the external sphincter[1,21] to delay voiding until circumstances are appropriate for urination.

Bladder Function Following Spinal Cord Injury

Complete spinal cord injury results in the loss of voluntary bladder control and sensory awareness of bladder fullness or urination. It also disrupts communication between the pontine micturition center and the spinal cord, leading to a loss of coordination among the muscles involved in urinary storage and voiding. Depending on the lesion, sacral reflexes may or may not remain functional.

The following descriptions refer to bladder function after complete injuries. After an *incomplete* spinal cord injury, the bladder's function will depend on the extent and location of the lesion; both the integrity of the sacral reflex arc and its connection to the brain will determine the bladder's functioning and control.

Bladder Function During Spinal Shock

During spinal shock the bladder remains flaccid, with no reflex activity. It usually remains flaccid for 6 to 8 weeks after injury.[19,21] The functional sphincter at the bladder's outlet remains closed, causing urinary retention.[22] After spinal shock has resolved, the level of lesion will influence whether the bladder functions areflexively or reflexively.

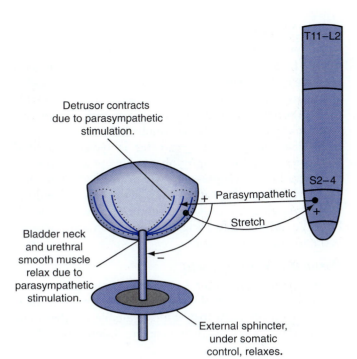

Figure 14–4   Urination: contraction of the detrusor in the body of the bladder, relaxation of the external sphincter and smooth muscle in the bladder neck and urethra.

Areflexive Bladder

If the sacral reflex arc is disrupted, the bladder remains areflexive after spinal shock resolves. This occurs either when a cord lesion disrupts the functioning of the second through fourth segments of the sacral cord or when the cauda equina is injured. People with injuries at or below T12[d] tend to have areflexive bladders.[22]

Without input from the sacral cord, the bladder does not receive parasympathetic stimulation. As a result, the detrusor remains flaccid. The external sphincter may have normal or low tone.[1] The absence of sacral voiding reflexes results in urinary retention (Figure 14–5).

The incontinence that occurs with an areflexive bladder is called overflow, or dribbling, incontinence. When enough pressure builds in the bladder, small amounts of urine are forced out through the urethra. A large volume of urine remains in the bladder. If it is not drained artificially, the bladder can become severely distended. The large residual volume also increases the risk of urinary tract infection.[4]

Reflexive Bladder

People with cervical and thoracic injuries tend to have reflexively functioning bladders.[22] In these individuals, the S2-S4 reflex arc remains intact but the descending input

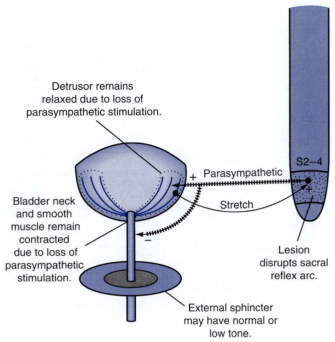

Figure 14–5   Areflexive bladder. Disruption of the sacral reflex arc causes loss of parasympathetic input to the bladder, leading to urinary retention.

to these segments has been disrupted. As a result, the bladder empties reflexively once filling causes sufficient stretch of its wall (Figure 14–6).[1,19] Reflexive emptying can also be triggered by increasing intraabdominal pressure or sensory stimuli in the sacral dermatomes.

Detrusor–Sphincter Dyssynergia

Many people with reflexive bladders exhibit detrusor–sphincter dyssynergia. In those who exhibit this condition, involuntary external sphincter contraction occurs concurrently with detrusor contraction (Figure 14–7).[e] High intravesical pressures and high postvoid residuals result.[1] Complications associated with detrusor–sphincter dyssynergia include recurrent urinary tract infections, sepsis, autonomic dysreflexia, vesicoureteral reflux, urinary stones, hydronephrosis, and renal damage.[23–26]

Bladder Management

Bladder management after spinal cord injury is aimed at ensuring complete (or near complete) emptying of the bladder at appropriate times, low-pressure voiding and storage of urine, and prevention of urinary incontinence between planned voidings. When these outcomes are achieved, morbidity and mortality from urinary tract–related complications are greatly reduced. Moreover, prevention of urinary incontinence can enhance psychosocial adaptation: return to social and sexual activities, school, and work will be easier

---

[d] Although one might expect S2 to be the "dividing line" between reflexive and areflexive bladders, T12 or lower neurological level of injury is typically associated with areflexia in the bladder, genitals, anus and lower extremities.

[e] Dyssynergia can also occur in the smooth muscle "sphincter" at the base of the bladder.[21]

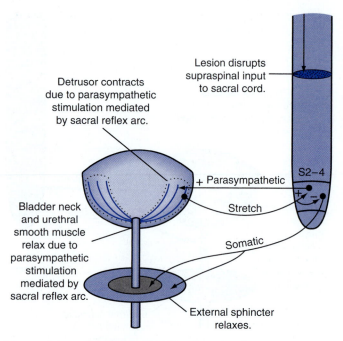

Figure 14–6   Reflexive bladder. Sacral reflexes remain intact but descending input is lost. Voluntary control is lost; bladder empties reflexively when full.

for the person who does not experience urinary accidents at inopportune times.

Bladder emptying at appropriate intervals is the primary focus of urinary management following cord injury. This emptying is particularly critical when the person has either an areflexive bladder or a reflexive bladder with detrusor–sphincter dyssynergia. In these cases, proper management is required to prevent high intravesical pressure and its sequelae.

Whether the bladder functions reflexively or areflexively, it may not empty itself completely. A urinary management program after cord injury ensures that the bladder is emptied periodically, thus eliminating stagnant urine and reducing the risk of infection.[f]

---

[f] Urinary tract infections can also result from bladder management practices. Strategies to reduce infection include hand washing, use of clean technique for catheterization, and washing catheters after using them.[19]

Early Management

Since the bladder will not empty itself during spinal shock, it must be emptied artificially to prevent high intravesical pressure and its sequelae. Overdistention can cause reflux and damage the bladder wall,[27] leaving it more vulnerable to infection[28] and inhibiting its resumption of reflexive functioning when spinal shock resolves.[29]

An indwelling urethral catheter is typically utilized during the initial postinjury phase. This practice ensures that high intravesical pressures will be avoided. Soon after injury, the indwelling catheter is usually removed and the bladder is emptied using intermittent catheterization.[27] Intermittent and indwelling catheterization are discussed in the following paragraphs.

Postacute Management

As the acute phase after injury passes, the patient and health care team establish a more permanent bladder management program that is most suitable for that individual. Many people with incomplete lesions are able to

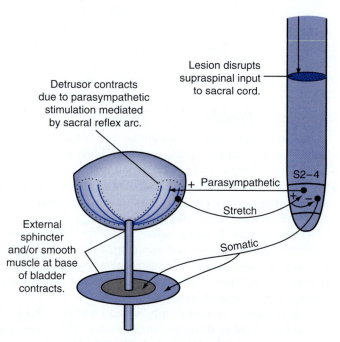

Figure 14–7   Detrusor–sphincter dyssynergia. Detrusor contraction combined with contraction at the outlet of the bladder results in high intravesical pressures and high postvoid residuals.

Problem-Solving Exercise 14–1

Your patient, who has L5 paraplegia (ASIA A), tells you that he drinks large quantities of beer on the weekends. He reports that when he gets home (often after several hours of drinking) he catheterizes himself. "You wouldn't believe how much comes out of me!"

- Why does this patient's bladder store large volumes of urine without voiding spontaneously?
- What harm could come from the patient's habit of drinking excessive amounts of fluid between voidings?

void normally, through voluntary sphincter control.[3,30] People with complete lesions, and those who have incomplete lesions but lack bladder control, must use alternative techniques to manage their bladders. The choice of management strategies will be influenced by the manner in which the patient's bladder functions,[g] the patient's capacity to perform self-catheterization, the availability of caregiver support (if needed), gender, the patient's preference, and the requirements of the patient's lifestyle.[19,31–33]

Intermittent Catheterization

Intermittent catheterization involves inserting a catheter into the bladder to empty it and then removing the catheter. This procedure, repeated every 4 to 6 hours,[h] can be initiated during spinal shock.[19]

Intermittent catheterization allows effective bladder emptying with a lower risk of complications than that posed by the use of indwelling catheters. It also allows the individual to remain catheter-free between voidings.

Disadvantages of intermittent catheterization include the need to limit fluid intake and to adhere to a schedule of catheterization at regular intervals. These measures are required to avoid bladder overdistention.[19] Intermittent catheterization also poses the risk of urethral trauma[19] and epididymo-orchitis.[34]

Intermittent catheterization is the most commonly used method for long-term bladder management.[13,32,35] It is most appropriate for individuals who are motivated, willing and able to adhere to a regular catheterization schedule, and either have the capacity (upper extremity function and cognitive ability) to self-catheterize or have access to reliable assistance.[19] It is not appropriate for individuals who are prone to autonomic dysreflexia despite treatment or who have abnormal urethral anatomy, a bladder capacity less than 200 milliliters, or a high fluid intake regimen.[19]

Indwelling Catheterization

Indwelling catheterization involves inserting a catheter into the bladder and leaving it in place for an extended period of time (up to 30 days).[19] Catheters can either be inserted through the urethra or surgically placed through the abdominal wall (suprapubically).

Indwelling catheters are used by many individuals who are unable to manage their bladders satisfactorily by other methods. Daily care requirements are minimal: cleansing the urine collecting bags and the area of insertion, and emptying the bags as needed. Thus indwelling catheters can be advantageous for people who are unable to catheterize themselves and cannot obtain reliable attendant care. Because the bladder is drained continuously, indwelling

catheters are also appropriate for individuals who have a high fluid intake, are prone to high detrusor pressures or autonomic dysreflexia, or have lifestyles that interfere with regular bladder emptying by other means.[19,32] Many females use indwelling catheters because of the lack of effective external collecting devices.[19,35]

Indwelling catheters have significant disadvantages. Recurrent urinary tract infection is common, and the risks of kidney and bladder stones, bladder cancer, and pyelonephritis are increased.[1,7,8,19,22,25,28,36] Individuals with indwelling catheters are encouraged to drink at least 2 liters of fluid daily to reduce the risk[i] of urinary stones.[19] The bladder's capacity and compliance typically decrease over time when indwelling catheters are used.[19] Indwelling *urethral* catheters can cause urethral erosion, periurethral abscesses, urethrocutaneous fistulas, and epididymitis.[37–39] Urethral catheters can also complicate sexual encounters.[19] The insertion of a *suprapubic* catheter creates a new orifice, which may be experienced as mutilating.[40] Because of the problems associated with the chronic use of indwelling catheters, other management regimens are preferable when possible.[4,24,28]

Credé and Valsalva Maneuvers

The Credé maneuver involves applying pressure to the abdomen, starting at the umbilicus and pressing downward. The Valsalva maneuver involves closing the glottis and contracting the abdominals as if to exhale forcefully. These techniques can be used either to force urine from a flaccid bladder or to stimulate and augment voiding in a reflexively functioning bladder.[19]

Credé and Valsalva maneuvers are most appropriately used by individuals with flaccid bladders, but even in these individuals these techniques may not be optimal. High intravesical pressures occur during the maneuvers, and sphincter contraction or other obstruction at the bladder outlet will inhibit emptying. Chronic use of the Credé maneuver frequently causes complications, including inguinal hernias, rectal prolapse, hemorrhoids, vesicoureteral reflux, and hydronephrosis.[19,41]

Reflex Voiding

Individuals with reflexively functioning bladders can stimulate reflex emptying by tapping their lower abdomens, performing a Credé or Valsalva maneuver, stroking their inner thighs, or pulling their pubic hair.[30,42,43] Because reflex voiding is also triggered by bladder filling, urination will occur between planned voidings.

When detrusor–sphincter dyssynergia is present, sphincter contraction impedes reflexive emptying. Because the sphincter contraction is intermittent rather than continuous, voiding occurs despite the dyssynergia. Intravesical pressures are high, however, and the bladder is not completely emptied.[19]

---

[g] Urodynamic studies provide information about the functioning of the bladder and sphincter, including the presence or absence of bladder contractions and detrusor–sphincter dyssynergia, and intravesical pressures during storage and voiding.[31]

[h] More frequent catheterization will be required if the bladder becomes full before 4 hours have passed or if bacteriuria is present.[30]

[i] Fluid intake may not be associated with stone development.[7]

Reflex voiding is most appropriate for males[j] with reflexively functioning bladders that empty effectively (have small postvoid residual volumes), without high intravesical pressure during voiding. Individuals who void reflexively need to be able to wear condom catheters (described in the following section) and have either adequate upper extremity function to manage these devices or have access to assistance.[19] Reflex voiding is not an appropriate bladder management strategy for individuals who are prone to autonomic dysreflexia despite treatment, or who have detrusor–sphincter dyssynergia that cannot be managed adequately with treatment.[19]

Because the bladder empties automatically, fluid restriction is not necessary. Daily management includes application of the condom catheter (preceded by washing and drying the penis), cleansing the urine collecting bags, and emptying them as needed. This care is far less burdensome than intermittent catheterization multiple times a day on a strict schedule. Thus reflexive voiding may be a viable management strategy for individuals who are either unwilling or unable to comply with the rigid requirements of intermittent catheterization. Complications include penile damage from condom catheters, as well as the sequelae of high intravesical pressures and high residual volumes.[19,44] A gradual reduction in bladder capacity will occur.[19]

Management of Incontinent Episodes

If urination or leakage occurs between planned voidings or catheterizations, measures need to be taken to keep the skin dry and to prevent embarrassing "accidents." For males, these goals are accomplished using a condom catheter,[k] attached via tubing to a collecting bag. During the day, the urine can be collected in a leg bag, which is easily concealed under clothing. Complications of condom catheters include breakdown of the penile skin and (rarely) urethral fistulas.[19] Although properly fitted and applied condom catheters are usually effective, urine can leak if the drainage tubing becomes kinked or blocked.

The problem of maintaining dry skin is more difficult for females, as they lack a point of attachment for an external catheter. To date, no satisfactory external catheter has been developed for females. Women who are unable to remain dry between planned voidings can use incontinence pads or indwelling catheters.[19] Incontinence pads can lead to skin breakdown.[19]

Urinary Diversion Surgery

When an individual is unable to achieve satisfactory bladder management using other methods, an ileal or colon conduit can be constructed.[l] In this surgery, the ureters are connected to a segment of the intestine. The intestinal segment is routed through the abdominal wall to drain into a urine collecting device,[l] or a stoma is created that can be catheterized intermittently.[19,28] Alternatively, a section of the appendix or other tubular structure can be anastomosed to the bladder and abdominal wall. This conduit can be constructed either to drain into an external collecting device[19] or be catheterized intermittently.[45]

Functional electrical stimulation

Functional electrical stimulation (FES) is an option for people with complete injuries and intact sacral reflexes.[46,47] The electrodes of neurostimulation devices are surgically implanted on the S2 through S4 anterior nerve roots.[47–51] Stimulation causes contraction of both the detrusor and external sphincter. Because detrusor contraction lasts longer than external sphincter contraction, voiding can be accomplished by providing the electric stimulation in a series of bursts.[49,51] Benefits of FES include effective emptying, improved continence, catheter-free management, fewer urinary tract infections, reduced use of anticholinergic medication, and improved quality of life.[51–54]

Surgical ablation of the sacral dorsal nerve roots (dorsal rhizotomy) is typically performed in conjunction with the implantation of a neurostimulation device.[47,49,55] Dorsal rhizotomy can enhance the bladder's compliance and storage capacity, eliminate incontinence due to reflexive detrusor contraction, reduce the occurrence of autonomic dysreflexia, and prevent the problem of external sphincter contraction impeding bladder emptying.[19,49,50] Dorsal rhizotomies also have significant drawbacks: they eliminate sensation and reflexive responses of the genitals, eliminate reflexive urination, impair reflexive defecation, and can cause stress incontinence.[19,47,49]

Adjunct Interventions

Frequently, the functioning of an individual's lower urinary tract interferes with effective management using one or more of the methods just described. Problems such as limited bladder compliance and capacity, an overactive detrusor, detrusor–sphincter dyssynergia, or an incompetent sphincter can lead to high intravesical pressure during storage or voiding, incomplete emptying, and urinary accidents and leaking. These problems must be addressed to achieve optimal outcomes.

Limited Bladder Compliance and Capacity

When limited bladder compliance and capacity restrict the volume of urine that can be stored at low pressure, surgical augmentation of the bladder may be indicated. Bladder augmentation surgery involves expansion of the bladder using a segment of the ileum, colon, or stomach.[1,19,32,56,57]

---

[j] Females do not have an effective external collecting device available to manage the incontinence that will occur between planned voidings.[1,19,32]
[k] A condom catheter, or penile sheath, attaches to the shaft of the penis. An external device that attaches to the glans of the penis may be used by males who cannot use condom catheters.[78]

[l] In deciding on this and other surgical options for urinary management, consideration should be given to the irreversible nature of the procedures and the need for assistance during the recovery period.

TABLE 14–1   Common Medications for Bladder Management

Therapeutic Objective	Medications (Examples)	Common Side Effects
Inhibit detrusor hyperactivity to reduce intravesical pressures and increase bladder compliance and capacity	Anticholinergic agents (oxybutynin, propantheline, tolterodine)	Dry mouth, constipation, blurred vision
Lower bladder outlet resistance	Alpha-adrenergic blockers (tamsulosin, terazosin, doxazosin, prazosin)	Hypotension
	Botulinum toxin injections into sphincter	Autonomic dysreflexia and hematuria during injection. Mild generalized weakness lasting 2–3 weeks.
Improve bladder storage by increasing outlet resistance	Alpha adrenergics (ephedrine, pseudoephedrine)	Agitation, insomnia, anxiety

Sources: References 1, 19, 22, and 58.

Overactive Detrusor

Hyperreflexive detrusor activity can cause both high pressures within the bladder and incontinence between planned voidings. Pharmacological management (Table 14–1) can often control these problems. When it cannot, surgical augmentation of the bladder may increase the capacity for low-pressure storage.[19,56,57]

Detrusor–Sphincter Dyssynergia

Detrusor–sphincter dyssynergia causes elevated intravesical pressure during both storage and voiding of urine, as well as incomplete emptying. Bladder emptying techniques that involve an increase in intravesical pressure (suprapubic percussion or the Credé maneuver, for example) should be avoided.[24,25] Bladder emptying can be achieved through intermittent catheterization or use of an indwelling catheter. Reflexive emptying may be appropriate if pharmacological or surgical interventions allow effective voiding and low intravesical pressures.[33]

Management of detrusor–sphincter dyssynergia involves interventions to allow low-pressure storage and voiding. Pharmaceutical treatment may be adequate to achieve these outcomes by inhibiting detrusor activity or lowering bladder outlet resistance (see Table 14–1). If medical management is not adequate, a variety of surgical options are available. The external sphincter's capacity to impede the flow of urine can be reduced by external sphincterotomy, intraurethral balloon dilation, or placement of a urethral stent.[1,19,23–25,28,59,60] Bladder augmentation may be performed to allow low-pressure storage.[31,56] Combined dorsal rhizotomy and implantation of a functional electrical stimulation device can enhance both storage and voiding.

Incompetent Sphincter

When the sphincter mechanism at the proximal urethra is ineffective, storage and continence can be improved using periurethral collagen injections.[46,61] Alternatively, males may benefit from insertion of an artificial urinary sphincter,

although this procedure has a high rate of complications and subsequent removal.[46]

BOWEL FUNCTION

To understand the nature of bowel function after spinal cord injury, one must understand normal bowel functioning. Figure 14–8 illustrates the large intestine, rectum, internal and external anal sphincters, and puborectalis.

Normal Bowel Function

A normally functioning bowel can store or expel feces, depending on whether circumstances are appropriate for

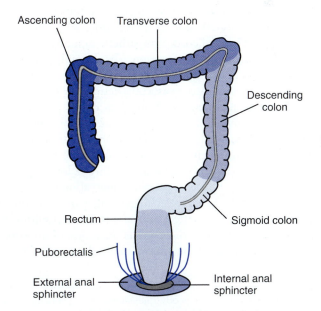

Figure 14–8   Schematic drawing of large intestine, rectum, internal and external sphincters, and puborectalis.

defecation. Normal bowel function involves the control of the smooth muscle of the intestinal wall, the internal and external anal sphincters, and the pelvic floor musculature. This control is provided by the intrinsic, autonomic, and somatic nervous systems.

Intrinsic System

The gastrointestinal (GI) tract has its own intrinsic nervous system, also called the enteric nervous system. It extends from the esophagus to the anus and is responsible for coordinating the GI tract's actions. Of the three sources of neurological control of the gut, the intrinsic system is the most basic. In fact, even if all central nervous system (CNS) input is eliminated, the intrinsic system enables the intestinal tract to continue its usual functions of digestion, absorption, and propulsion of the food mass.[11,21]

Peristaltic contractions are initiated and maintained by reflexes of the intrinsic system. Distention of a section of the intestine initiates reflexive contraction of the smooth muscle rostral to the distention and relaxation of the smooth muscle caudal to this point, propelling the intestinal contents toward the anus.[10,62,63] As the mass is propelled caudally, the next section of the intestine is distended and the peristaltic reflex is again stimulated.

The intrinsic system may also be involved in the gastrocolic reflex.[m] In this reflex, ingestion of food or drink causes increased propulsion in the small bowel and colon.[11]

Autonomic System

Autonomic control is important in the regulation of colonic peristalsis and defecation.[21,62] The autonomic system also coordinates the GI tract's actions with the rest of the body; sympathetic and parasympathetic input alters GI function in response to emotions and exercise. This control is achieved primarily through the autonomic system's influence on the intrinsic nervous system.[62]

Sympathetic innervation of the GI tract arises from the thoracolumbar[n] spinal cord. Sympathetic input has a dampening effect on digestive functions. In general, it inhibits peristalsis, increases sphincter tone, reduces the secretion of digestive juices, and causes vasoconstriction.[21,62,64]

Both the cranial and sacral divisions of the parasympathetic system innervate the GI tract. The cephalad portions of the digestive tract, from the esophagus through the transverse colon, receive innervation from the hypothalamus via the vagus nerve. The descending colon, sigmoid, and rectum receive parasympathetic innervation from sacral cord segments 2 through 4. In general, parasympathetic input has an excitatory effect on the intestines, resulting in an increase in peristaltic movements, secretion of intestinal juices and relaxation of the internal anal sphincter.[21,62,64]

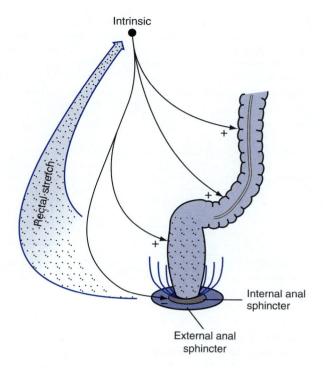

Figure 14–9   Intrinsic defecation reflex. Rectal stretch causes peristalsis and relaxation of the internal anal sphincter.

Somatic System

The external anal sphincter and pelvic floor muscles are composed of striated muscle fibers. They receive somatic innervation from sacral cord segments 2 through 4.

Reflexes Involved in Defecation

The intrinsic defecation reflex, mediated by the intrinsic system, is an important component of defecation. This reflex, elicited when feces enter the rectum, causes relaxation of the internal anal sphincter and peristalsis in the descending colon, sigmoid, and rectum (Figure 14–9). The intrinsic defecation reflex is not usually strong enough, however, to cause defecation.[65]

Normal defecation requires the parasympathetic defecation reflex. This sacral spinal reflex is stimulated by rectal filling. The parasympathetic defecation reflex causes relaxation of the internal anal sphincter and an intensification of peristalsis in the descending colon, sigmoid, and rectum (Figure 14–10).[62,65]

Continence and Defecation

The internal anal sphincter helps to maintain continence through tonic contraction.[11,31] The external anal sphincter and other muscles of the pelvic floor also play a key role in continence, remaining active even at rest. The puborectalis is particularly important in maintaining continence. This striated muscle forms a sling around the rectoanal junction. Tonic contraction of the puborectalis creates a sharp angle between the rectum and the anal canal, preventing the passage of feces.[31]

---

[m] The gastrocolic reflex is poorly understood. The parasympathetic system may also be involved.[11,62]

[n] There is inconsistency in the literature regarding the location of the sympathetic nervous system in the spinal cord. Reports describe it as extending as high as T5[11] and as low as L5.[62]

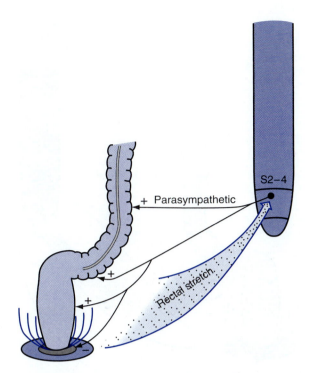

Figure 14–10   Parasympathetic defecation reflex. Rectal stretch causes intensification of peristalsis and relaxation of the internal anal sphincter.

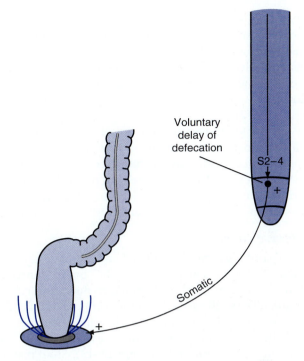

Figure 14–11   Voluntary delay of defecation through contraction of external anal sphincter and pelvic floor musculature.

When feces enter the rectum and the internal sphincter relaxes, contraction of the external anal sphincter and puborectalis prevents unwanted defecation. The contraction of these muscles is under both reflexive and voluntary control.[11] Voluntary control involves descending input from the cerebral cortex, pons, and several other regions of the brain. Defecation at unwanted times is prevented by maintained contraction of the external anal sphincter and pelvic floor musculature (Figure 14–11).[21] If feces enter the rectum at a time when defecation is appropriate, voluntary control involves relaxation of the external anal sphincter and pelvic floor musculature. In addition, defecation can be initiated voluntarily by closing the glottis and contracting the abdominals. The resulting increase in intraabdominal pressure forces feces into the rectum, stimulating the defecation reflexes.[21]

Bowel Function Following Spinal Cord Injury

Complete spinal cord injury results in the loss of both voluntary bowel control and sensory awareness° of rectal fullness or defecation. It also disrupts communication between the autonomic and intrinsic nervous systems,

leading to reduced colonic motility and ineffective defecation. Moreover, the portions of the intestines that are innervated below the lesion will no longer alter their functions with emotions and exercise. Depending on the lesion, the parasympathetic defecation reflex may or may not remain functional.

The following descriptions refer to bowel function after complete injuries. After an *incomplete* spinal cord injury, the bowel's function will depend on the extent and location of the lesion; both the integrity of the sacral reflex arc and its connection to the brain will determine the bowel's functioning and control.

Bowel Function During Spinal Shock

During spinal shock, peristalsis may be reduced and defecation reflexes may be diminished or absent.[10] After spinal shock has resolved, the level of lesion will influence whether the bowel functions areflexively or reflexively.

Many patients exhibit paralytic ileus during the acute phase after injury. This condition is characterized by atonia and an absence of peristalsis in the intestines. When ileus occurs, it usually appears within 24 hours of the injury and lasts about a week[42] but can last for several weeks.[9] Intestinal function returns spontaneously as paralytic ileus resolves. Peristalsis resumes, pushing the products of digestion through the intestines, and the gastrocolic reflex returns. This resumption of intestinal function is possible because the intrinsic system remains intact following spinal cord lesions.

° Nonspecific sensory awareness is retained in some cases, possibly conducted by autonomic afferents.

Areflexive Bowel

When the sacral reflex arc is interrupted, either from spinal cord or peripheral nerve damage, the bowel functions areflexively. The intrinsic defecation reflex remains intact, but the stronger parasympathetic defecation reflex is lost. As a result, the bowel will not empty reflexively (Figure 14–12).

With an areflexive (flaccid) bowel, the internal anal sphincter remains active although its tone is low. A large amount of feces can become impacted in the rectum.[11] Because the external anal sphincter and pelvic floor musculature remain flaccid, incontinence can occur when stool passes unhindered from the rectum.[10,11,31,62,63]

Reflexive Bowel

If sacral cord segments 2 through 4 and the corresponding peripheral nerves remain intact, the bowel functions reflexively. The internal anal sphincter maintains resting tone and relaxes reflexively when the rectum is distended.[62]

Because both the intrinsic and parasympathetic defecation reflexes remain functional, reflex defecation can occur when the rectum fills (Figure 14–13). Stool may be retained, however, due to poorly coordinated peristalsis, dyssynergia of the internal anal sphincter (failure to relax

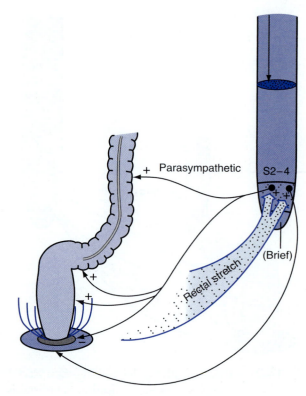

Figure 14–13   Reflexive bowel. Sacral reflexes remain intact, but descending input is lost. Reflexive defecation occurs when the rectum fills.

during rectal contraction), spasticity in the external anal sphincter and pelvic floor musculature, loss of descending input to the external anal sphincter and puborectalis (loss of voluntary relaxation for defecation), or a combination of these factors.[10–12,62,63]

Bowel Management

After spinal cord injury, a bowel program is required to induce bowel movements at regularly scheduled intervals. Periodic emptying of stool will help prevent constipation, overdistention and impaction, thus helping to prevent autonomic dysreflexia and other complications.

Bowel programs are also aimed at minimizing the occurrence of bowel accidents. This goal can be achieved by evacuating the bowels on a regular schedule.[66] Prevention of incontinence is particularly important for psychosocial and sexual adjustment, facilitating participation in social, sexual, vocational, and educational activities.[10,11,31,67,68]

Reducing the occurrence of bowel accidents has the added benefit of making it easier to keep the skin clean. (If someone has a bowel movement at the wrong time or place, it may be impossible to clean the skin immediately.) Better skin hygiene will reduce the risk of skin breakdown.

Early Management

During the period of spinal shock, peristalsis is reduced and defecation reflexes are absent. The rectum should be evacuated manually during this time.[10,11,63]

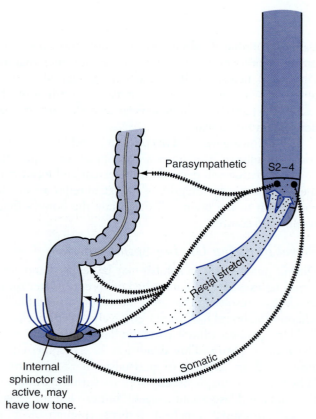

Figure 14–12   Areflexive bowel. Disruption of the sacral reflex arc causes loss of parasympathetic defecation reflex. Internal anal sphincter remains active; external sphincter is flaccid.

In the acute period following injury, the patient is monitored for paralytic ileus. If this condition develops, the loss of peristalsis can result in abdominal distention. Severe distention can cause vomiting, aspiration, dehydration, and electrolyte imbalance. It can interfere with breathing by impeding the diaphragm's motions.[29,43] Distention can also damage the walls of the bowel, impairing future functioning.

If paralytic ileus develops, measures are taken to prevent distention. The gastric contents are aspirated via nasogastric or orogastric tube, and the patient is not allowed to take any solids or liquids by mouth until her bowel sounds resume.[29,42] In some cases when paralytic ileus does not resolve spontaneously, gastric motility is increased using medications.[9] Surface electrical stimulation has also been used to increase gastrointestinal motility in patients exhibiting paralytic ileus.[67]

Bowel Retraining

After paralytic ileus resolves, a bowel training program can be initiated. The general pattern of a bowel training program is the same regardless of the level of lesion: the bowel is conditioned to empty at scheduled intervals.

At the outset of a bowel training program, a bowel movement is elicited at the same time every day[p] or every other day.[9,10,69] This can be done in the morning or evening, depending on the patient's preferences. Because a bowel program can be time-consuming, patients need to decide whether morning or evening schedules will be most suitable to their lifestyles.[31,32,66,70]

The techniques employed to elicit bowel movements depend on the manner in which the person's bowel functions. If the individual has an *areflexive bowel*, stool is manually removed from the rectum.[62,70] Inserting a suppository several minutes before the manual evacuation can facilitate the process.[42] Contraction of the abdominal musculature can help move feces into the rectum.[11,63]

If the individual has a *reflexive bowel*, a bowel movement is elicited by stimulation of reflexive defecation. This is accomplished through digital stimulation of the rectum, use of a suppository, or both.[11,62,71] Prior to stimulation of reflexive defecation, hard stool may need to be removed from the rectum manually.[10,42,71]

Regardless of whether an individual has a flaccid or reflexive bowel, there are several factors that she can exploit to aid in her bowel program. Eating or drinking before the bowel program can promote bowel movements by eliciting the gastrocolic reflex.[11,63,70,71] Physical activity can enhance bowel motility.[10,67] Abdominal massage can promote the movement of feces toward the rectum. The

pressure of the massage strokes should follow the pattern of the large intestine, moving in a clockwise direction.[10,72]

Performing the bowel program while sitting upright or leaning forward is preferable when possible, as this positioning can assist in the movement of feces. Orthostatic hypotension or pressure ulcers may preclude sitting, however.[10,33,66] If the bowel program is performed in bed, the person should lie on her left side. (Bedpans should *not* be used, as they are likely to cause skin breakdown.)[71]

A bowel program can be enhanced by ensuring that the stools are of a consistency that is most suited to the method of evacuation employed. The optimal stool consistency for people with reflexive bowels is formed and soft. For people with areflexive bowels, optimal stool consistency is formed and firm but not hard.[10,31,62,71] People with spinal cord injuries can control their stool consistency by drinking adequate amounts of fluid[q] and consuming a diet with appropriate amounts[r] of fiber.[11,31,62] Individuals can note the effects of different foods, and modify their diets as indicated.[10]

Many use medications to soften their stools or enhance their colonic motility (see Table 14–2). Typically, as time passes and a regular pattern of bowel emptying is established, individuals who utilize these agents can reduce or discontinue their use gradually.[9]

Colostomy or Ileostomy

When acceptable outcomes cannot be achieved using standard bowel management practices, colostomy or ileostomy may be performed. Indications include severe and intractable constipation, incontinence, or perianal pressure ulcers.[10,11] Advantages include less manual dexterity needed for daily care, a reduction in the time required for bowel care, and elimination of fecal incontinence.[11,31,62,74]

Functional Electrical Stimulation

Sacral nerve stimulators used for voiding, described earlier in this chapter, often also improve bowel function. Reported benefits of sacral nerve stimulators include reductions of all of the following: incontinence, constipation, time required for bowel programs, and medications used to enhance bowel function.[49,51,52] Many individuals are able to use the stimulator to defecate, using a different stimulation pattern than the one used to void.[49]

A different method of FES involves enhancing defecation by stimulating the abdominal musculature using surface electrodes. In a small study, this intervention effectively reduced the time required for the bowel programs of subjects with tetraplegia.[75]

---

[p] There is disagreement in the literature regarding the frequency with which bowel movements should be elicited initially. The Consortium for Spinal Cord Medicine[10] recommends a daily schedule at first. Some individuals subsequently reduce the frequency of their bowel programs, but evacuation at least every other day may be advisable to prevent overdistention of the colon and rectum.[10]

[q] Some *bladder* management programs include restricted fluid intake to prevent bladder distention or incontinence between planned voidings. For this reason, an individual's fluid intake may represent a compromise between the different intake levels that would be optimal for her bladder and bowel programs.

[r] A diet *high* in fiber may not be indicated.[10]

TABLE 14–2   Common Medications for Bowel Management

Therapeutic Objective	Medications (Examples)	Common Side Effects
Optimize stool consistency	Bulking agents (calcium polycarbophil, methylcellulose, psyllium)	Bloating and flatulence, impaction, diarrhea.
	Stool softeners (ducosate sodium)	Loose stools, incontinence.
Induce and augment peristalsis to enhance colon transit	Stimulant laxatives (bisacodyl, senna)	Abdominal cramps, bowel accidents, diarrhea, dehydration, electrolyte imbalance. Prolonged use can lead to an atonic, nonfunctioning colon.
Stimulate peristalsis, adjust consistency of hard stool	Osmotic laxatives (magnesium salts, lactulose)	Liquid stool, abdominal cramps, incontinence.
Stimulate evacuation	Contact irritants, suppository (bisacodyl or glycerine)	Local irritation.
	Contact irritants, enema (saline, water, or docusate sodium)	Local irritation, rectal trauma, autonomic dysreflexia. Long-term use can cause dependence.

Sources: References 11, 31, 32, 58, 62, 66, 70, and 73.

Problem-Solving Exercise 14–2

Two weeks ago, your patient sustained a C5 spinal cord injury (ASIA C). She confides that her loss of bowel control concerns her more than anything else. "How can I go anywhere or do anything if I know I could mess myself at any time?"

- What can you tell her about her capacity to avoid bowel accidents in the future?

INCONTINENCE MANAGEMENT TRAINING PROGRAM

During rehabilitation, the patient and health professionals work together to establish bladder and bowel management programs. This involves determining the most appropriate management strategies for that individual, implementing the strategies, and adjusting the programs as needed. It also involves education and training that will enable the individual to manage her bladder and bowel after discharge.

In incontinence management training programs, people with spinal cord injuries should gain the knowledge required for them to carry out or direct their own care. They should acquire an understanding of their bladder and bowel function, the management strategies that they should use, and the consequences of improper management. They should also learn how to avoid complications, how to detect them if they occur, and what to do if they develop.

When possible, patients undergoing rehabilitation should learn the physical skills involved in carrying out their bladder and bowel routines. In some cases, independence is possible even without innervation of the hand musculature. A variety of devices are available to enhance independence in bladder and bowel care.

When physical impairments or other constraints are such that patients are not expected to be fully independent in their self-care after discharge, training programs should include the family members or attendants who will be providing assistance after discharge. In addition, patients should develop the ability to instruct others in the management techniques. This ability will free them from dependence on family members or attendants who have been trained by the hospital staff.

Whether the individual will perform bladder and bowel management independently or with assistance after discharge, she is likely to require bathroom equipment such as a raised and padded toilet seat[s] or a shower/commode chair. Architectural adaptation of the home may

---

[s] Because a bowel program can take an hour or more, the seat should be padded to reduce the risk of pressure ulcers from prolonged sitting.

also be necessary to permit access to the bathroom. The rehabilitation team should work with patients to obtain the equipment and home modifications that are needed to carry out their incontinence management programs.

During rehabilitation, patients should be encouraged to participate in their bladder and bowel management. As they practice the physical techniques, their skills will improve. If they are involved in decision making and problem solving, they will be better prepared to direct their programs after discharge. As active participants, they may also come to value their programs more and carry them out consistently after discharge.

ADL Training and Implications for Therapy

The nursing staff is responsible for the bulk of a patient's incontinence management training program, including education and establishing bladder and bowel management regimens. Physical and occupational therapists work with the patient to select equipment, recommend architectural adaptations, and develop the necessary physical skills. These skills include gross activities such as sitting upright, toilet transfers, leg management, and maintaining an upright sitting position while reaching around to the anus. In therapy, the patient also acquires the manipulation skills used in self-catheterization, the application and removal of urinary collecting devices, dressing and undressing, and hygiene.

Understandably, incontinence can be an emotionally charged area of concern. Episodes of incontinence that occur in therapy should be handled in a matter-of-fact, tactful manner. The therapist should model comfort with the issue.

If a bowel or bladder accident occurs in therapy, it must be dealt with quickly. This expeditious management serves two purposes. First, it ensures that the individual's skin does not remain in contact with urine or feces for a prolonged period of time. As importantly, it helps to develop the habit of cleaning quickly following an accident. A therapist who ignores accidents that occur at inconvenient times (such as during group classes) models a lack of concern for hygiene. This can undermine the team's efforts to teach the patient to maintain clean, dry skin.

FOLLOW-UP

Unless neurological return occurs, bladder and bowel management programs must continue for the duration of the individual's life. The management strategies used are likely to change over time, however, as a result of changes in bladder and bowel function or life circumstances.[12,31,35,76] Because of the impact that bladder and bowel functioning and management have on both physical health and participation in life situations, they are an important focus of postdischarge follow-up.

Follow-up during the first year after discharge from inpatient rehabilitation may be particularly critical in today's health care environment. Because of shortened inpatient stays, recently injured individuals are likely to be discharged before they have reached their functional potential, and before their bladder and bowel functioning has stabilized. Moreover, the practitioners who provide their care in the community may be unfamiliar with the unique needs of people with spinal cord injuries. Rehabilitation specialists may be able to promote better management practices and reduce complications by providing education, outreach, and support to patients and their community health professionals after discharge.[76]

In addition to the initial postdischarge follow-up, annual evaluations can investigate the presence of complications, efficacy of bladder and bowel management techniques, and changes in urinary tract and gastrointestinal function.[3,4,10,28] These follow-up evaluations will make it possible to adjust the management programs as indicated and either prevent complications or detect and treat them early. Evaluations should be performed more frequently for individuals who experience problems or change their management practices.[19]

Long-term follow-up can also include education on bladder and bowel management. Reviewing management practices may encourage better self-care habits.[12] One small study found that an educational program (provided to individuals who were 1 to 29 years postdischarge) was associated with a reduction in urinary tract infections.[77]

Problem-Solving Exercise 14–3

Your patient, who has T9 paraplegia (ASIA A), has expressed interest in performing his bowel program on a toilet when he returns home after inpatient rehabilitation.

- What safety issues are important to consider for this task?

- What equipment might be appropriate for this individual to enhance his safety and independence in this activity?
- What therapeutic activities in physical therapy could help this patient achieve his goal?

Summary

- Any spinal cord injury that disrupts the functioning of the sacral cord or interrupts its communication with the brain will result in incontinence. A variety of physical and psychosocial problems can result.
- Normal bladder control involves coordinated action of the autonomic and somatic nervous systems. Normal bowel control involves the coordinated action of the autonomic and somatic nervous systems as well as the gastrointestinal tract's intrinsic nervous system.
- The manner in which the bladder and bowel function after spinal cord injury depends on the status of the sacral reflex arc and its communication with higher centers.
- During rehabilitation, the health care team and the patient work together to establish satisfactory bladder and bowel management programs. By emptying the bladder and bowel at planned intervals and preventing incontinent episodes between times, these programs help to prevent the serious physical and psychosocial problems that can result from incontinence.
- In addition to establishing bladder and bowel management programs, the rehabilitation team works with the patient (and prospective caregivers) to develop the knowledge, problem-solving abilities, and skills needed to continue their programs after discharge.
- Postdischarge follow-up is necessary to ensure that the individual's bladder and bowel management programs continue to be effective and to prevent, detect, and treat any complications that may occur.

Suggested Resources

ORGANIZATION

National Association for Continence: *www.nafc.org*

PUBLICATIONS

Clinical practice guidelines published by Paralyzed Veterans of America, available for free download from *www.pva.org*

- *Bladder Management for Adults with Spinal Cord Injury: A Clinical Practice Guideline for Health-Care Providers, 2005.*
- *Neurogenic Bowel Management in Adults with Spinal Cord Injury, 1998.*

WEB SITE

Spinal Cord Injury Rehabilitation Evidence, Chapter 12, Neurogenic Bowel Following Spinal Cord Injury; Chapter 13, Bladder Health and Function Following Spinal Cord Injury: *www.icord.org/scire/chapters.php*

15

Architectural Adaptations

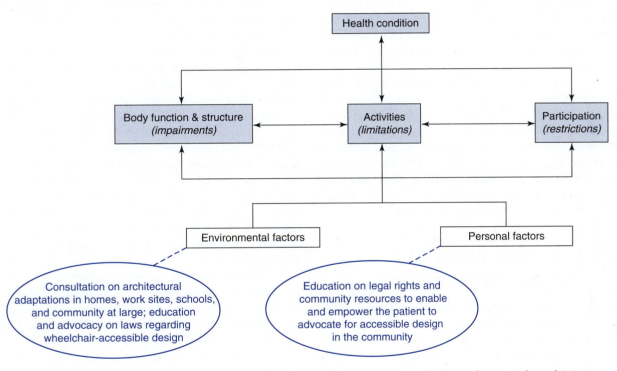

Chapter 15 presents information wheelchair-accessible design relevant to rehabilitation after spinal cord injury.

Much of rehabilitation focuses on maximizing the potential to participate in home and community life after discharge. This participation may be impeded, however, when people leave rehabilitation centers and encounter barriers in the physical environment. Features such as curbs, stairs, narrow doorways, and appliances or controls that are positioned out of reach can prevent people from functioning independently at home and in the community. Thus inaccessible architecture can disable people as profoundly as can physical impairments themselves.

Because architectural accessibility can have such a strong impact on participation, this area should be addressed during rehabilitation. The team's involvement can include home evaluations, education and advocacy on architectural barriers and adaptations, problem solving and recommendations regarding home modification, and education about legal rights. The rehabilitation team can also consult with employers, school systems, and others in the community regarding architectural accessibility.

This chapter presents typical design features that make homes accessible both to people who use wheelchairs and to those whose ability to grasp is impaired. In general, these same features are required to make a nonresidential environment accessible. Rehabilitation professionals who are involved in architectural adaptations in work sites, school environments, or in the community at large should become familiar with additional guidelines that apply to certain features (stadium seating, food service lines, etc.) that are unique to nonresidential environments.[1–3]

It is important to remember that no single design will be perfectly suited to all people with spinal cord injuries. The ideal physical environment for a given individual will depend on his functional capacities. Such features as the optimal height of controls, appliances, and plumbing fixtures and the required width of doorways will depend on whether the person is ambulatory, uses a wheelchair for all activities, or uses a wheelchair only for certain activities. If a wheelchair is used, both the person's skill in its use and chair's overall length and width will dictate the minimal doorway widths and turning spaces that must be present. The individual's reaching capacity will depend on whether he walks or uses a wheelchair and will also be influenced by his body build, range of motion, and motor abilities. Motor function will also determine his capacity for grasping and manipulating controls and doorknobs.

Because people with spinal cord injuries vary in body build, ambulatory status, equipment use, reach capacity, and ability to grasp and manipulate, an adapted home that is ideal for one individual may be totally unsuitable for another. When a home is being designed or modified for a particular person, the environment should be tailored to suit his needs and preferences. Rather than providing "standard" accessible features, the home's design should reflect the specific individual's requirements.[4]

U.S. LAWS REGARDING ARCHITECTURAL ACCESSIBILITY

The Architectural Barriers Act[5] mandates that virtually any[a] newly constructed, *federally owned or federally funded* public buildings, as well as federally funded alterations on existing buildings, must be accessible to people with physical disabilities. Of relevance to this chapter, at least 5% of all units and common areas in residential facilities (hotels, motels, apartment buildings, etc.) must be accessible.

The Fair Housing Act, as amended in 1988, expanded protection from discrimination in housing to *include structures that do not receive federal funds*. This law prohibits discrimination against people with disabilities in the area of rental, sale, or financing of housing. It also gives tenants with disabilities the right to modify rental property *at their own expense*. The tenant may be required to restore the property to its original condition (within reason) when the lease expires. Newly constructed multifamily dwellings with at least four units must be accessible.[4,6]

The Americans with Disabilities Act (ADA) mandates that all newly constructed or renovated restaurants, stores, and other businesses open to the general public must be accessible[b] to people with disabilities. Moreover, physical barriers in existing structures must be removed if this removal can be achieved readily. The Americans with Disabilities Act differs from the Architectural Barriers Act in that it applies to *privately owned facilities* as well as state and local government facilities. It also expands the protection provided by the Fair Housing Act (FHA). Whereas the FHA mandates an accessible route to all of the public and common areas in a multifamily housing complex, it does not state that the facilities in these areas must be accessible. For example, a public area containing laundry facilities must be reachable through an accessible route, but the laundry machines themselves do not have to be usable from a wheelchair. In contrast, the ADA requires that all of the features of the complex are accessible to and usable by people with disabilities.[7]

The laws just mentioned mandate accessibility. But what architectural features make a building accessible? Three widely used sets of standards and guidelines are available that specify in detail the design features required to make a facility accessible to people with disabilities. These include the *Uniform Federal Accessibility Standards* (UFAS),[1] the *American National Standard Accessible and Usable Buildings and Facilities* (ICC/ANSI standards),[3] and the *Americans with Disabilities Act and Architectural Barriers Act Accessibility Guidelines* (ADA-ABA guidelines).[2] The design requirements specified in these documents are very similar.[c] It should be noted that different states and localities have their own laws (building codes) regarding accessible construction.[4,7,8]

Unfortunately, laws regarding architectural accessibility are not always followed.[9–14] People who feel that their rights have been violated can contact the Department of Housing and Urban Development (HUD),[d] the U.S. Access Board,[e] or the U.S. Department of Justice.[f]

The published standards mentioned above are *minimal standards*.[4,7] They do not apply to privately owned single-family homes, but they can provide a *starting place* for planning.[4,7] Private homes should be modified to suit the needs and preferences of the individuals who will be living in them, not modified to meet a set of standards.

---

[b] In addition to architectural access to public accommodations, the ADA prohibits discrimination in employment, state and local government, transportation, and telecommunication services.[6]

[c] This chapter presents some of the design features described in these standards and guidelines. A complete description of the technical details in these documents is beyond the scope of this text.

[d] To obtain information or file a complaint regarding the Fair Housing Act: (800) 669-9777.

[e] To obtain technical assistance regarding the Architectural Barriers Act: ta@access-board.gov. To file a complaint: enforce@access-board.gov.

[f] To obtain information or file a complaint regarding the Americans with Disabilities Act: (800) 514-0301. Private lawsuits can also be used to enforce the law.

Access to Health Care and Fitness Facilities

Architectural barriers can have a significant impact on wellness and fitness. Structural barriers are common in facilities that provide primary preventive services (physicians' offices, for example). These barriers interfere with access to routine preventive and medical services[15] and thus are likely to be detrimental to the health and wellness of individuals with impaired mobility. Physical barriers are also common in fitness and recreational facilities and in public areas (sidewalks and natural environments, for example) in which nondisabled people typically exercise by walking.[9–12,16] These barriers can interfere with exercise and active lifestyles and thus affect fitness.[17]

Many of the barriers in health care facilities, fitness centers, and recreational facilities exist in violation of federal laws.[11,15,16] Rehabilitation professionals may have a positive impact by educating patients about their rights; advocating for accessibility in the community; and providing education and consultation to community planners, owners of fitness clubs and recreational facilities, and health professionals involved in primary care.

DESIGN FEATURES

For an apartment or house to be truly wheelchair-accessible, it must have more than wide doorways and a ramp at the front door. An accessible environment allows a person to propel a wheelchair from the parking area or public transportation site to the home's entrance and to enter and move throughout the home. Within and around the home, the environment is structured so that a person with physical impairments can perform everyday functions such as getting the mail, cooking, operating lights, doing laundry, using the toilet, and bathing. Appliances, lighting and environmental controls, plumbing fixtures, work surfaces, and storage are designed and arranged for use from a wheelchair.

General Features

Certain features are common to all wheelchair-accessible environments: provision for negotiating any changes in floor or ground level, adequate width in doorways and halls to allow passage of a wheelchair, floors that do not provide excessive resistance to wheelchair propulsion, clear floor and knee space to allow maneuvering the wheelchair and access to various features of the home, and design and location of these features allowing their access and use.

Paths and Ramps

A home must have at least one accessible route leading to it. This route should connect the home with an accessible parking area as well as with the sidewalk and public transportation stops when present. Paths should be smooth, level, and at least 36 inches wide.[1–3] If the home's entrance is not level with the ground, provision must be made for the difference in level. Usually, a ramp is the most practical solution for wheelchair users.

A ramp meeting ADA-ABA,[2] ICC/ANSI,[3] and UFAS[1] specifications for accessibility has a maximum slope of 1:12, or 1 foot of rise for every 12 feet of horizontal distance. The minimum width is 36 inches. Some individuals find it difficult to negotiate a ramp of this width. For this reason, a 48-inch width may be more appropriate.[8]

Horizontal landings must be provided at the top and bottom of the ramp and at 30-foot intervals in the ramp. These landings must be at least as wide as the ramp and at least 60 inches long. When a ramp changes direction at a landing, the landing must be at least 60 inches square. Ramps with a rise greater than 6 inches should have a handrail on each side, between 34 and 38[g] inches above the surface of the ramp. If a cross slope (slope perpendicular to

---

[g] UFAS standards specify a rail height between 30 and 34 inches high.[1]

Problem-Solving Exercise 15–1

Your friend lives in an apartment building (owned by a private corporation) that was recently renovated. All of the mailboxes in the building are too high to reach from a wheelchair, and your friend cannot get her mail.

- Is there a law that is applicable in this situation?
- What should your friend do about her problem?

the direction of the ramp) is present, it must not exceed a 1:48 incline. Ramps and landings that are elevated above ground level must be constructed in a way that prevents people from falling off. Protection at the edges of such ramps and landings can be provided by extending the ramp surface at least 12 inches beyond the handrail, or constructing a curb or barrier close to the surface of the ramp. All ramp surfaces must be slip-resistant.[1–3]

A ramp built according to the standards just presented will be safe and negotiable by most people using wheelchairs. Private homes, however, do not have to meet the exact specifications listed. Considerations relevant to the individual concerned may make it most practical to deviate from these specifications. For example, a ramp with a 1:12 slope can take up a great deal of space, and an incline this gradual may not be necessary for the person using it. On the other hand, some individuals require a more gradual slope. Before a ramp is built for a particular person, it should be determined how gradual a slope he will require.[h]

Three additional features can enhance the function and safety of a home ramp. Lighting will make it safer to negotiate at night. A roof over the ramp will protect both the ramp and the user from the weather. This may be particularly helpful in regions that have ice and snow in the winter. Finally, when a ramp leads to a door, a platform at the top of the ramp will make it easier and safer to get in and out of the door.[18,19] Such a platform will make it possible to unlock the door and open or close it without having to stabilize the wheelchair on the ramp while doing so. The platform should be large enough to allow the person to maneuver his wheelchair and operate the door. The exact size and shape of platform needed will depend on the door (size and direction of opening) and the direction of approach.[i]

People needing ramps can purchase them prefabricated or can have them custom built of concrete, wood, or brick. Prefabricated ramps should come with nonslip surfaces. To create a nonslip surface on a concrete ramp, its surface can be brushed or grooved perpendicular to the path of travel.[18,19] A variety of options are available for creating a nonslip surface on a wooden ramp. These include firmly attaching commercially available grit tape, indoor–outdoor carpeting, or ribbed rubber matting; painting the ramp with paint mixed with sand; or applying a commercially available nonslip coating.[18]

Ramps are considered by some to be necessary evils for an adapted home because they can be unattractive. When attention is paid to design and landscaping, however, a ramp need not detract from a home's beauty.[19]

Ramps can also be constructed to accommodate elevation changes within a home. Interior ramps are feasible only when the vertical distance between the levels is small–a few inches at most.

Lifts and Elevators

When the vertical distance between levels is too great or when space limitations make a ramp impractical, a platform lift or an elevator can be used to move between levels in a wheelchair. Both types of device can be installed indoors or outdoors.

Inclined platform lifts move up and down over a slanted path rather than moving vertically. This type of lift can be installed over existing stairs. Some models have the advantage of leaving the stairs available for use when the platform is positioned out of the way. They can, however, cause people walking over them to trip and fall.[7]

Vertical platform lifts move vertically from one level to another rather than following an inclined path. Unlike an elevator, a vertical lift is not enclosed within a shaft.[7]

Elevator or lift selection should include consideration of the available space, the size of the wheelchair, and the safety of both the user and others in the home. Controls should be selected that are designed and positioned so that the wheelchair user can safely and easily operate them.[7] Additional safety features include mechanisms that prevent lifts from descending on people standing below, and safety rails for those riding the lifts.

Individuals who can walk but are not able to negotiate stairs safely can often utilize chair lifts to move between levels in their homes. A chair lift (also called a stairway lift, stair lift, or seat lift) consists of a seat that runs up and down a staircase on a track. These devices can be installed in straight stairways as well as on stairways with curves or landings. Most models allow the chair component to swivel at the top and bottom of the stairway to make transfers easier. Like inclined platform lifts, chair lifts can create obstacles to other members of the household.[7] It is possible for people who use wheelchairs to use chair lifts, but to do so they must be able to transfer in and out of the lift seat. They must also have access to a wheelchair both at the top and the bottom of the lift. For these reasons, chair lifts are not as practical for people who use wheelchairs as are platform lifts or elevators.

Doorways and Doors

Perhaps the most critical feature of an accessible doorway is its width. To be accessible, a doorway must have adequate clear space when the door is open to allow a wheelchair user to propel through without contacting the door, door frame, or hardware. An ideal doorway is a few inches wider than the wheelchair, to allow easy and comfortable passage through the space.[8] Clear space in a doorway is the actual unobstructed space available for passage, measured when the door is opened 90 degrees. Most doors are hinged so that even when open they partially block the doorway (Figure 15–1). As a result, the clear space is narrower than the doorway itself.

ADA-ABA,[2] ICC/ANSI,[3] and UFAS[1] standards specify that an accessible doorway must provide a clear space that

---

[h] The therapist can assess the wheelchair user's ability to negotiate ramps with a variety of slopes. This assessment can be done on different ramps in and around the rehabilitation facility. If a variety of ramps are not available, ramp negotiation can be assessed during community outings.
[i] ICC/ANSI[3] and ADA-ABA[2] provide detailed specifications for maneuvering clearances at doors.

Problem-Solving Exercise 15–2

Your patient, who uses a wheelchair, will return to live in his single-story home when he leaves the inpatient rehabilitation facility. He plans to have a ramp built to allow access to his home, and is deciding on the ramp's location. The house's front door is 3 feet above the level of the ground. A side door opens to the carport and is 2 feet above the carport's cement floor.

- Assuming a 1:12 ratio, how long (horizontal distance) should a ramp at each of these doors be?

- Would ramps at these doors need platforms? If so, where?
- What other considerations can you think of that would be relevant to the choice of ramp location (front versus side door)?
- What are some possible alternative solutions to the problem of providing access to this house?

is at least 32 inches wide. Private homes do not always need doorways this wide. For many chairs, a doorway that has 30 inches of clear space will provide adequate clearance if the door can be approached directly. A door that must be approached at an angle may need to be wider. The minimal doorway width required by an individual is determined primarily by the overall width of his chair. As a rule, power wheelchairs are significantly wider than manual chairs. Additional factors determining a wheelchair's overall width include the seat width, wheelchair brand, type of tire, canting of the wheels, and handrim style. In making decisions about home modification, the wheelchair user and rehabilitation team should determine the minimal doorway width that the individual can negotiate in *his* wheelchair.

If one or more doorways in a home are too narrow, several options are available. Installing swing-clear hinges (also called offset hinges) will allow the door to swing completely out of the doorway, adding 1½ to 2 inches to the clear space.[18,19] Removing the lowest 36 inches of the door stop molding (the trim that protrudes furthest into the opening) can widen the clear space up to ½ inch on each side.[18] Alternatively, the door can be removed and replaced with a curtain.[19] When a door must be widened more than a couple of inches, the doorway itself must be rebuilt and a wider door installed.

An accessible doorway must also have adequate clear floor space on both sides (push side and pull side) of the door to allow the wheelchair user to open and close the door. The door width, location of the hinges, direction of approach, and direction of the door's swing will determine the size and location of the clear floor space requirements.[1–4,8] Figure 15–2 provides examples of ADA-ABA requirements. When floor space on the pull side of an existing door is limited, the hinges may need to be repositioned to allow the door to swing in the opposite direction.[8,19]

The threshold is another feature of a doorway influencing its accessibility. Thresholds, or sills, lie at the base of doorways. A doorway that either has no threshold or has one that is flush with the floor will be the easiest to negotiate.[8] If a threshold is present, it should be as low as possible and shaped to allow easy passage of a wheelchair. An accessible door can have a threshold of up to one-fourth inch in height without beveling. Thresholds between one-fourth and one-half inch high must be beveled. A small ramp is required when a threshold is greater than ½ inch tall.[1–3] Thresholds of *interior* doorways can be removed to allow easier passage through doors. The thresholds of *exterior* doors should not be removed, as they generally are needed to seal against rain and drafts. If a threshold of an exterior

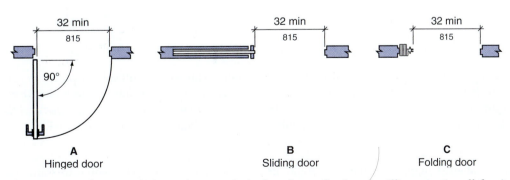

Figure 15–1   Clear space in doorway. Dimensions are in inches (large font) and millimeters (small font). (Redrawn from *Americans With Disabilities Act and Architectural Barriers Act Accessibility Guidelines* (2004 updated guidelines), United States Access Board, 2004.)

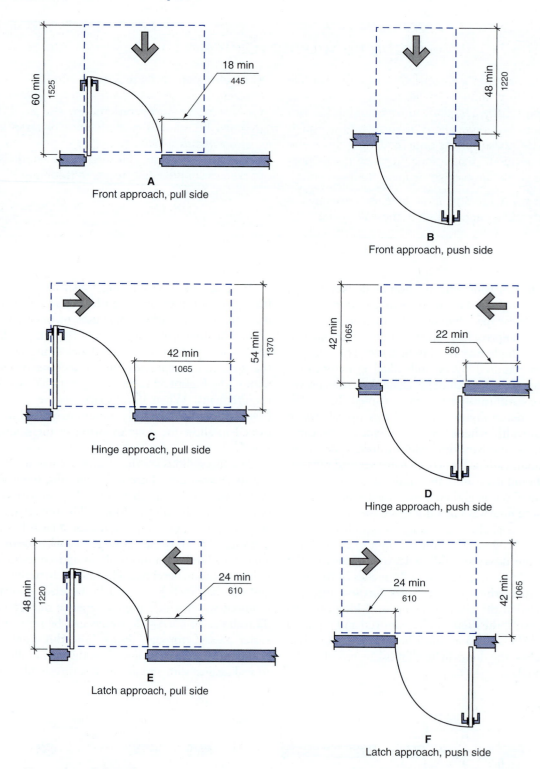

Figure 15–2   Examples of clear floor space allowing access to door from either pull side or push side, approaching the door front-on or from either side (hinge side or latch side). Dimensions are in inches (large font) and millimeters (small font). (Redrawn from *Americans With Disabilities Act and Architectural Barriers Act Accessibility Guidelines* (2004 updated guidelines), United States Access Board, 2004.)

door is too tall or shaped inappropriately, it should be modified (shortened, beveled, or both) or replaced with beveled thresholds. Weather stripping attached to the base of the door itself can help to seal out the weather.[7,19]

For a door to be accessible to someone with impaired grasp, adaptation of the knob may be required. Adapters can be placed on knobs that allow them to be operated as levers (Figure 15–3), or the doorknobs can be replaced

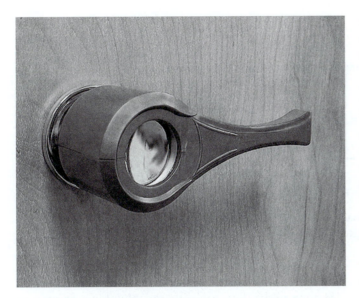

Figure 15–3   Doorknob adapter, used to make standard doorknob usable with impaired grasp. (Reproduced with permission from Dynamic-Living.com.)

with lever-type door handles. Alternatively, interior doorknobs can be eliminated altogether and replaced with catches that allow doors to be operated without manipulating any knobs or handles. This type of door catch, commonly used with kitchen cabinets, makes it possible to open and close the door by applying pressure against the door's surface.[8,20] When this type of door catch is used, a pull bar or loop should be installed on the pull side of the door to allow opening from this side.[8]

When a lock is present, it must be accessible. If the user has good grasping and manipulating abilities or can function with an adapted key or key holder, the lock need only be placed within reach. Someone who cannot operate a standard lock may require a keyless entry system.[7,18]

Finally, an accessible door is one that the individual can open and close independently. Doors should open with 5 pounds or less of force, using one hand. For most people, the modifications described above are sufficient; given door handles and locks that they can operate, most are able to open and close standard doors. Power operators for opening and closing doors are alternatives for those who are unable to do so.[8,19] This option can be useful either when impaired grasp interferes with door management or when there is not enough clear floor space to allow a person to reach and operate the door from a wheelchair.[19]

Hallways

Although a 32-inch-wide clear space will allow passage through a doorway, a hallway of this width is too narrow for wheelchair users. A hallway 36 inches wide will allow propulsion of a wheelchair.[1-3] For access to rooms opening onto the hallway from the side, provision must be made for turning the chair. This can be accomplished with a wider hallway or wide doorways.

Clear Floor Space

For a room to be accessible to wheelchair users, it must have adequate clear floor space to allow maneuvering. To allow for turning 180 degrees in a wheelchair, the floor should be unobstructed in an area large enough to enclose either a circle of at least 60 inches in diameter (Figure 15–4A) or a T-shaped area with dimensions as shown in Figure 15–4B.[1-3] A circular clear floor space is preferable because it allows easier maneuvering than does a T-shaped area.

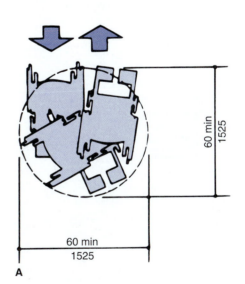

A

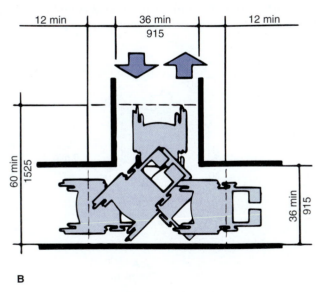

B

Figure 15–4   Wheelchair turning space. (A) Circular. (B) T-shaped. Dimensions are in inches (above the lines) and millimeters (below the lines). (Reproduced from *Uniform Federal Accessibility Standards*. U.S. Government Printing Office, 1988.)

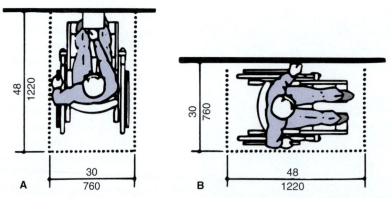

Figure 15–5   Clear floor space. (A) Front or forward approach. (B) Parallel approach. Dimensions are in inches (above the lines) and millimeters (below the lines). (Reproduced from *Uniform Federal Accessibility Standards.* U.S. Government Printing Office, 1988.)

Clear floor space is also required in front of the home's appliances, light switches, electric outlets, environmental controls, plumbing fixtures, windows, work spaces, and storage areas. This clear floor space allows access to these features from a wheelchair. An unobstructed rectangular floor space measuring 30 by 48 inches will accommodate a stationary wheelchair.[1–3] The orientation of the clear floor space will determine whether the person must approach the object head-on (front or forward approach) or from the side (parallel approach; Figure 15–5).

A private home may not need to meet the exact clear floor space specifications described above. Depending on his wheelchair's dimensions and his skill, a given person may be able to function in a slightly smaller space. On the other hand, a larger space will allow easier maneuvering. When adapting an existing home for a particular individual, that person's preferences and requirements for clear floor space should be taken into account.

Clear floor space does not imply that the area is unobstructed from floor to ceiling. Where there is adequate clearance under low cabinets and plumbing fixtures to allow free passage of the feet or the feet and knees,[j] this floor space can be used for maneuvering.

Clear Knee Space

Certain features such as sinks and kitchen work spaces are most readily used from a wheelchair if they can be approached closely front-on. This close access requires the presence of unobstructed space (clear knee space) to allow the wheelchair user to place his knees under the object. Because a wheelchair user's feet are typically lower than his knees and protrude further forward, the clear space can be lower toward the back. Clear knee space should be at least 30 inches wide, and extend at least 11 inches deep at 9 inches above the floor, and at least 8 inches deep at 27 inches above the floor (Figure 15–6).[2,3] It must be part

---

[j] A space 9 inches high will allow the feet to pass. A 27-inch-high space will permit passage of the knees.[2,3]

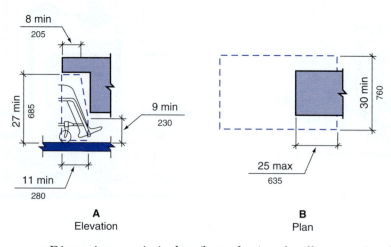

Figure 15–6   Clear knee space. Dimensions are in inches (large font) and millimeters (small font). (Reproduced from *Americans With Disabilities Act and Architectural Barriers Act Accessibility Guidelines* (2004 updated guidelines), United States Access Board, 2004.)

of or contiguous with a 30- by 48-inch clear floor space.[1] The surface above the clear knee space (the underside of a counter, for example) should be free of any hazards such as abrasive surfaces or high heat.[2]

Reach Range

The height that a person can reach from his wheelchair will depend on whether he reaches forward or to the side. A forward reach is more limited; the person cannot reach as high or as low. The arrangement of the clear floor space in front of an object will determine whether a side reach (parallel approach) or forward reach (front approach) can be used. Reach range is reduced when an obstruction prevents close access, such as when a switch is positioned at the back of a kitchen counter (Figure 15–7). Forward- and side-reach ranges are also influenced by body build, range of motion, and motor abilities. When adapting an existing home for a particular individual, his capacities in forward and side reach should be considered.

The ADA-ABA guidelines and ICC/ANSI standards specify that accessible elements such as thermostats, appliance controls, and electric outlets can be no higher than 48 inches and no lower than 15 inches above the floor when an unobstructed forward approach will be used (Figure 15–8). The same dimensions apply when an unobstructed parallel approach is possible, except that a maximum of 54 inches in height is allowed in certain circumstances.[2,3]

Controls and Outlets

Electric outlets and all controls, including thermostats, light switches, appliance controls, and door hardware should be located within the allowable reach range.[2,3] Controls should also be designed so that they can be used

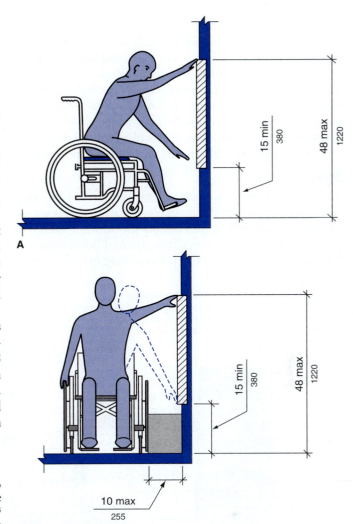

A

B

Figure 15–8   Reach ranges. Dimensions are in inches (large font) and millimeters (small font). (A) Forward reach. (B) Side reach. (Redrawn from *Americans With Disabilities Act and Architectural Barriers Act Accessibility Guidelines* (2004 updated guidelines), United States Access Board, 2004.)

with one hand and should not require a twisting motion or a strong grasp or pinch. The force required for operation must not exceed 5 pounds.[1–3]

Floors

Floors should not offer excessive resistance to wheelchair propulsion. Surfaces such as wood, linoleum, laminate, cork, or tile provide the easiest surfaces for propulsion and are easy to care for. Carpeting significantly increases the difficulty of propulsion, and padding under the carpet adds to this problem.[2] If carpeting is used, it should be securely attached to the floor and have a very short pile.[2,3] If a cushion or pad is used under carpeting, it should be firm.[2,3]

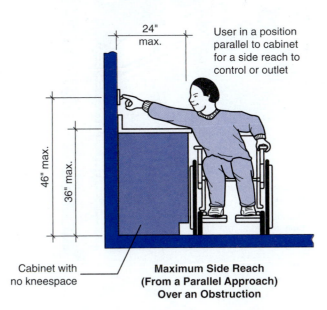

Figure 15–7   Side reach limited by obstruction. (Reproduced from *Fair Housing Act Design Manual* (1998 revision), U.S. Department of Housing and Urban Development.)

Windows

Windows accessible to people with impaired grasp are operable with 5 pounds or less of force and have hardware (locks, levers, and cranks) that meets all of the specifications for controls given previously.[2,3] A variety of window styles and hardware options are available. If a new home is being built or if an addition is being added, windows and hardware should be selected that will be most suitable for the individuals' physical capacity and esthetic preferences.

Storage Space

An accessible home has storage areas that can be used from a wheelchair. To be accessible, a storage area must be within reach and adjacent to adequate clear floor space.[1–3]

Much of the storage space in a standard home does not fall within the reach range of a person sitting in a wheelchair.

However, numerous commercially available products such as closet organizers and kitchen cabinet accessories can be used to maximize accessible storage in an existing home. In addition, new shelving can be added, and existing shelves that are within reach can be enlarged. Hardware on doors and drawers can be adapted or replaced to accommodate impaired grasp.[18,19,21]

Esthetics

A wheelchair-accessible home need not (and should not) look like an institution. With attention to color, furniture arrangement, lighting, accessories, wall decorations, window treatments, and landscaping, the accessible environment can be attractive and homey and reflect the tastes of the people who live there (Figure 15–9).[4,19,21–23]

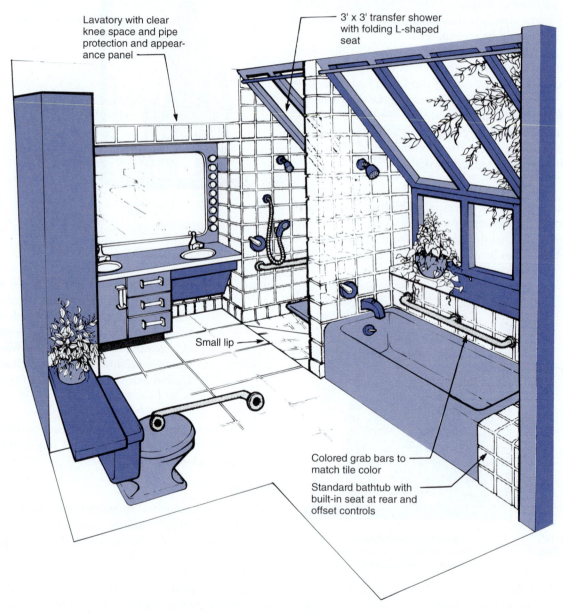

Figure 15–9   Accessible bathroom without institutional look. (Redrawn from Bostrom, Mace, and Long. *Adaptable Housing: A Technical Manual for Implementing Adaptable Dwelling Unit Specifications.* Department of Housing and Urban Development, 1987.)

Application in Kitchens and Bathrooms

In a fully accessible home, the features described in the first half of this chapter are present throughout. All rooms have accessible doorways, adequate clear floor space, and floors that can be traversed in a wheelchair. Controls, storage areas, and electric outlets are within reach. When needed, all controls and hardware are adapted for use with impaired grasp.

Kitchens and bathrooms require special attention because of the nature of their use. Suggestions for accessible design in these areas are presented in the following sections.

Kitchen

An accessible kitchen has features that allow meal preparation and cleanup by a person using a wheelchair (Figure 15–10). Ideally, the various appliances and work surfaces will be arranged for the most efficient use of the kitchen and able to accommodate multiple people in the kitchen at once.[k]

Work Surfaces

An accessible kitchen must have *at least* one work surface on which to perform such tasks as cutting and mixing. A standard countertop is too high to be used from a wheelchair. Moreover, the cabinets and drawers beneath the counters in most kitchens make it impossible to approach the counters face-on in a wheelchair.[24]

Perhaps the ideal work surface for a wheelchair user is a lowered countertop with adequate clear knee space underneath and clear floor space allowing a front approach. This design makes counter space accessible, and makes it possible to reach items stored in overhead cabinets (lowest shelves) and on the back of the counter. Lowered countertops should be at least 30 inches wide.[2] When funds allow, adjustable-height countertops are useful.[18]

Pullout boards (breadboards) can also be used to provide accessible work surfaces (Figure 15–11). These boards allow access from three sides, and can be installed throughout the kitchen.[18] Alternatively, a table can serve as a work surface when financial constraints preclude remodeling.[19,20]

Whether lowered counters, pullout boards, or tables are used, most lowered work surfaces should be between 30 and 32 inches high. Some people find that they can perform certain activities, such as beating and mixing, most easily on a work surface that is even lower. A pullout board may be the best means of addressing this need.

Cooking Appliances

An accessible kitchen has adequate clear floor space in front of the cooking appliances, the appliances and their controls are within the appropriate reach range, and all controls are located so that they can be manipulated without reaching across burners. A cook with impaired grasp will also require suitable controls on the appliances. Where knee spaces are available beneath cooking appliances, there must be adequate insulation present to prevent burns.[1,3]

Among conventional ovens, side-opening wall ovens are most convenient for people using wheelchairs, as this type of oven allows the cook to get close. The door should be hinged so that it opens toward a countertop. The oven can be installed lower than standard to allow access. Microwave ovens should also be placed within reach. Pullout shelves in front of the oven and microwave will make it easier and safer to use these appliances.[18,19] When an existing oven is inaccessible and funding for remodeling is limited, a toaster oven can be used instead of a wall oven. It can be placed on a low countertop, table, trolley, or sturdy pullout shelf.[20,25]

A cooktop built into a low counter with clear knee space underneath (Figure 15–12) is convenient and accessible but may increase the risk of burns from spills.[19] A cooktop that is 32 inches above the floor will allow access by both seated and standing cooks.[7] Burners that are incorporated into a large, flat surface are easily cleaned and allow pots to be slid on and off readily. To reduce the danger of reaching over hot burners to reach pots in the rear, the burners can be arranged either in a line parallel to the counter edge or in a staggered pattern. The controls should be placed to the side or in front of the burners. An angled mirror hung behind and above the cooktop will make it easier for a seated cook to see into the pots while cooking.[4,7] When funding for remodeling is limited, portable burners on a low countertop, table, trolley, or sturdy pullout board can be used in place of a built-in stove. These options require more lifting.[20,25]

Sink

A wheelchair-accessible sink is low (up to 34 inches high),[2,3,19] shallow (6½ inches deep or less), and has adequate clear knee and floor space to allow a forward approach (Figure 15–13). The sink, drain, and hot water pipes must be insulated to prevent burns, and the area under the sink must be free of sharp or abrasive surfaces. The faucet controls should be within easy reach. If the sink is to be used by someone with impaired grasp, the controls must be designed appropriately.[1–4,25] A retractable spray hose is an additional convenient feature. It makes rinsing food and dishes easier and can be used to fill pots on an adjacent counter so that they do not have to be lifted from the sink after being filled.[19,20,25]

Dishwasher

To be accessible, a dishwasher must have controls within reach, and adjacent clear floor space that is not blocked when the dishwasher is open.[3] The dishwasher will be easiest to use if it is adjacent to a sink that has clear knee space underneath.[19] Dishwashers can be mounted at standard height or raised above the floor for easier access.[18]

Storage Space

Much of the space that is used for storage in standard kitchens is either out of reach from a wheelchair or has to

---

[k] Meal preparation, serving, and cleanup are frequently performed by multiple members of a family. Moreover, a number of other activities such as socializing and homework often occur in the kitchen.[7]

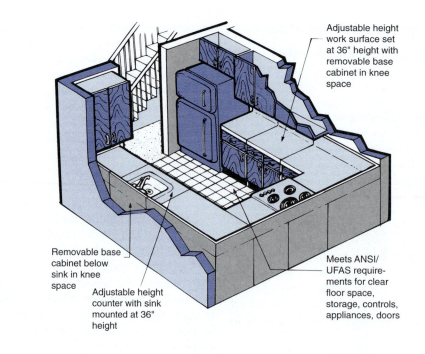

Adjustable height work surface set at 36" height with removable base cabinet in knee space

Removable base cabinet below sink in knee space

Adjustable height counter with sink mounted at 36" height

Meets ANSI/ UFAS requirements for clear floor space, storage, controls, appliances, doors

A

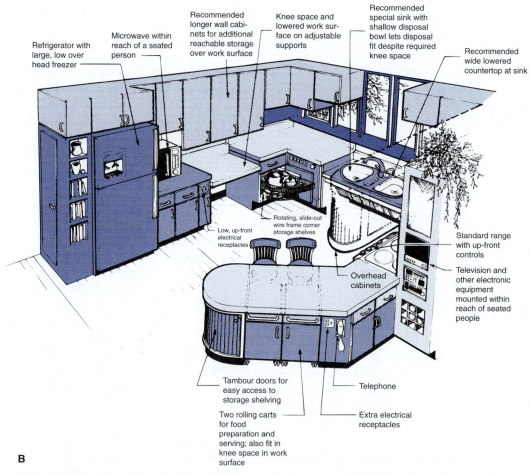

Refrigerator with large, low over head freezer

Microwave within reach of a seated person

Recommended longer wall cabinets for additional reachable storage over work surface

Knee space and lowered work surface on adjustable supports

Recommended special sink with shallow disposal bowl lets disposal fit despite required knee space

Recommended wide lowered countertop at sink

Low, up-front electrical receptacles

Rotating, slide-out wire frame corner storage shelves

Overhead cabinets

Standard range with up-front controls

Television and other electronic equipment mounted within reach of seated people

Tambour doors for easy access to storage shelving

Two rolling carts for food preparation and serving; also fit in knee space in work surface

Telephone

Extra electrical receptacles

B

Figure 15–10   Accessible kitchens. (A) Small kitchen with minimal modifications. (B) Elaborate kitchen. (Adapted from Bostrom, Mace, and Long. *Adaptable Housing: A Technical Manual for Implementing Adaptable Dwelling Unit Specifications.* Department of Housing and Urban Development, 1987.)

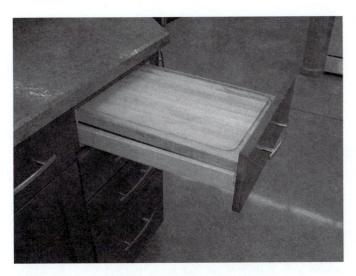

Figure 15–11   Pullout board provides accessible work surface.

be eliminated to provide clear knee space. For this reason, provision of adequate storage space can be particularly challenging in an accessible kitchen.

Some storage space can be gained by constructing shelves at the back of low counters that have clear knee space underneath. Deep full-extension drawers,[1] slide-out

---

[1] Full-extension drawers are mounted on special slides that allow the drawers to be pulled completely out from under the countertop to fully expose their contents.[8]

bins, lazy susans, and sliding shelves can increase the area available for storage in base cabinets and pantries. Handles on the cabinet doors should be within reach, and operable with minimal force and manipulation.[8,19,21]

Refrigerator/Freezer

A side-by-side refrigerator/freezer or a refrigerator with a bottom freezer will allow access to both compartments.[18,19] Shelves that slide out make foods stored at the back easier to reach. The temperature controls must be within reach, and both the controls and the door catch should be designed so that they can be worked with minimal force and manipulation.[2] The refrigerator should be located so that its doors can be opened fully, allowing closer access from a wheelchair.[8]

Planning Kitchen Modifications

People differ in the exact features of a kitchen that are most suitable to them. For example, the optimal counter height varies between people, and some individuals require different levels of work surface for different activities. Others who have difficulty lifting may function best in kitchens where the counters are all at the same height so that they can slide objects from place to place.[25,26] People also vary in their requirements for other kitchen features, such as appliance and sink controls, sink height and depth, and reach range for storage. Moreover, physical abilities may change with the passage of time. When building or remodeling a kitchen for a particular person, care should be taken to design the kitchen in such a way that it is most suitable for that individual's current and (projected) future needs. When a kitchen is being designed to be used by a number

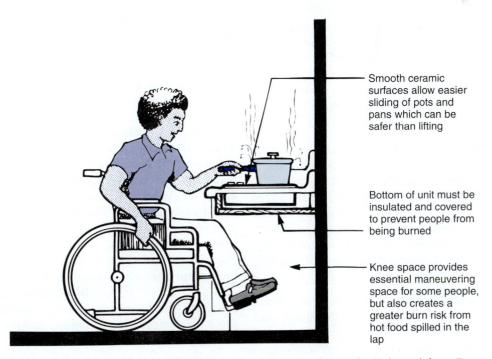

Figure 15–12   Cooktop built into low counter with clear knee space underneath. (Adapted from Bostrom, Mace, and Long. *Adaptable Housing: A Technical Manual for Implementing Adaptable Dwelling Unit Specifications.* Department of Housing and Urban Development, 1987.)

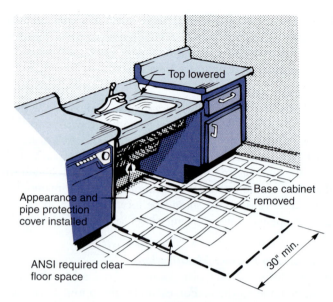

Sink in Minimum Width Adjustable Counter Segment

Figure 15–13   Accessible sink. (Adapted from Bostrom, Mace, and Long. *Adaptable Housing: A Technical Manual for Implementing Adaptable Dwelling Unit Specifications.* Department of Housing and Urban Development, 1987.)

of different family members, the design should allow for the safe, comfortable, and efficient functioning of a variety of people with different body builds and physical abilities. For example, including both low and standard-height work surfaces will allow family members to work in the kitchen in either a seated or standing position.[7,19] Adjustable features will make it possible to adapt the kitchen as needed either to accommodate new residents (in a rental unit, for example) or to allow for continued use of the kitchen as the people in the home age and their abilities change.

Bathroom

An accessible bathroom must have a doorway, clear floor space, and plumbing fixtures that allow a person using a wheelchair to maneuver and use the facilities (Figures 15–9 and 15–15B). Additional features include grab bars where needed, storage areas and electrical outlets within reach, and a mirror that can be viewed from a wheelchair. The latter is made possible by mounting the mirror with its lowest edge no higher than 40 inches above the floor[1–3] or by tilting it.[21]

Door

The bathroom door should have the features of any accessible door: adequate width, small or no threshold, and hardware that can be worked with minimal force and manipulation. Additional privacy and safety considerations are unique to bathroom doors. The wheelchair user should be able to close the door once inside the bathroom. If the door opens into the bathroom, closure from within

requires additional clear floor space. Folding doors do not require as much added clear floor space but have the disadvantage of significantly reducing the width of the clear space in the doorway.[20] Sliding doors and standard doors that swing outward do not require any added clear floor space in order to be closed from within the bathroom. These doors also have a safety advantage: they are not blocked when someone falls against them in the bathroom.[25] As a final alternative, a bathroom's door can be removed and replaced with a curtain. This solves the problems of closure and blocking from within but does not provide the level of privacy afforded by a door.

Toilet

The toilet in an accessible bathroom must have adequate clear floor space on one side, and the seat at a height that allows safe transfers to and from the wheelchair. ADA-ABA,[2] ICC/ANSI,[3] and UFAS[1] standards specify that the top of a toilet seat should fall between 17 and 19 inches above the floor. Transfers will be easiest if the toilet seat and the wheelchair sitting surface[m] are the same height. A removable raised toilet seat is often the most practical solution; these seats are relatively inexpensive, do not require renovation, and can be removed for traveling. Additional features that make a toilet accessible include grab bars when needed and a toilet paper dispenser within reach. A cabinet beside the toilet can be convenient both for aiding balance and for storing equipment and supplies for bowel and bladder management.[25]

Tub or Shower

An accessible bathtub should be next to clear floor space that allows the wheelchair to be positioned for transfers. Faucet controls should be within reach of a person sitting in the tub; if they are to be used by someone with impaired grasp, they should be designed accordingly. Many individuals require grab bars, and many also require either a tub bench or a built-in tub seat. A hand-held shower spray unit is convenient in any accessible tub and is required if a tub bench or built-in seat is used.

In general, a shower is more convenient than a tub. There are two types of accessible showers: roll-in showers and those with built-in seats. Either type must be bordered by adequate clear floor space to allow access. The shower enclosure must not obstruct entrance into the shower, and the controls must be within reach.[1–3]

A roll-in shower is designed to be used while sitting in a wheelchair.[n] Federal and industry standards[1–3] specify that this type of shower must measure at least 30 by 60 inches and must either have no threshold[1] or a threshold no higher than ½ inch.[2,3] If the shower is built without a threshold, the floor of the shower is available as clear floor space for maneuvering within the bathroom.

---

[m] If a wheelchair cushion is used, the top of the cushion rather than the wheelchair seat is the sitting surface.

[n] The bather uses a "shower chair," not a standard wheelchair.

The standards for showers with seats (as opposed to roll-in showers) specify that the stall measures 36 inches square, and the controls must be positioned opposite the shower seat. The seat can be folding or nonfolding and must be positioned between 17 and 19 inches above the floor.[1–3]

Tubs and showers can be equipped with scald-proof thermostatically controlled valves as an additional safety feature.[3,4,7,8] These valves are particularly beneficial for people who have impaired sensation.

Grab Bars

Wherever grab bars are installed, their placement should meet the needs of the individual using them. The bars must be affixed to either the floor, wall studs, or wood that has been attached to the studs; standard wall board is not strong enough to anchor grab bars. Similarly, towel racks and soap dishes cannot be used to substitute for grab bars.

Lavatory

An accessible bathroom lavatory has the same basic requirements as a kitchen sink: no more than 6½ inches deep, insulated hot water and drain pipes, an underside free of sharp or abrasive surfaces, and faucet and drain controls that are easily operated and within reach. The accessible basin must also be relatively low; the upper surface must be no higher than 34 inches. Adequate clear floor and knee space must be present to allow forward approach in a wheelchair.[1–3]

Planning Bathroom Modifications

Depending on the individual's requirements and resources, and the layout of the existing structure, adapting a bathroom can be as simple as adding a tub bench and modifying cabinets under a sink, and as complex as building a new room. Whether the modifications will be simple or complex, they should be appropriate for the person for whom the modifications are being made. For example, the ideal toilet seat height for a given individual will depend on the level of his wheelchair's seat and cushion height. His transfer techniques will influence the clear floor space requirements by the toilet; if he is skillful, he may be able to transfer with his wheelchair positioned diagonally in front of the toilet instead of beside it. In like manner, people vary in their requirements for other bathroom features, such as the type of tub or shower and the position of clear floor space needed for its access.

Adaptable Design

Certain features of accessible housing are considered to be unacceptable by some individuals who do not need these features. Grab bars in the bathroom may be seen as esthetically unappealing, and free knee space under sinks reduces the available storage space. Some owners of rental housing have found that wheelchair-accessible units are difficult to rent.[27]

Adaptable housing is an option that may appeal to owners of rental units who wish to minimize their vacancy rates by renting their accessible units to able-bodied people.

It is also of interest to homeowners who wish to make their homes accessible but who are concerned about the resale value of their homes.

An adaptable home has permanent accessible features such as wide doors and hallways, a ground-level entrance, and controls mounted low enough to be reached from a wheelchair. In addition, the home has features (Figure 15–14) such as removable base cabinets and adjustable-height counters and sinks that can be altered to suit residents with and without disabilities. Bathroom walls are reinforced in appropriate places to accommodate grab bars. The bars themselves can be removed or installed as needed. An adaptable home looks like any other home when adjusted for an able-bodied resident but can be made fully accessible without major structural changes. The needed changes can be made *with minimal time and expense, and using unskilled labor* (Figure 15–15).[4,8,24,27]

Universal Design

In recent years, there has been increasing awareness that "standard" building designs best meet the needs of a fairly small portion of the population: nonelderly able-bodied adults of average (male) height.[7,23] People who do not fit these specifications are less functional, comfortable, and safe in standard environments. In response to this problem, a growing number of people in the design and construction industry have begun to employ and promote universal design principles.

Homes built or remodeled according to universal design principles are meant to meet the diverse needs of a variety of individuals: short or tall, young or old, with or without physical impairments.[4,22,27] For example, the kitchen may have work surfaces of various heights to allow comfortable function while standing or sitting in a wheelchair.

Many of the features that make a universally designed home wheelchair-accessible also make it more comfortable, safe, and convenient for nondisabled residents. For example, a lever-style door handle makes it easier to open the door while carrying a bag of groceries, an accessible route at the front door is safer when wet or icy, and adjustable-height closet rods make clothing more accessible to children.[28]

Universal design makes sense for *all* homes, not just the homes of people with physical impairments. Universally designed environments remain suitable for their inhabitants when they acquire temporary or permanent physical impairments as a result of accident, illness, or aging.

STRATEGIES

No standard set of specifications can be used to create an environment that would be perfect for all people. An ideal home is one designed to match the current and future needs and preferences that are unique to the person or people living there. When a home is being built or remodeled for a person with physical impairments, this outcome is possible

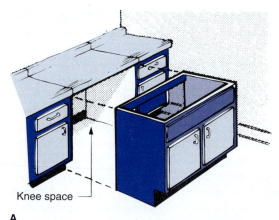

Knee space

A

Element # 1: Removable Base Cabinets

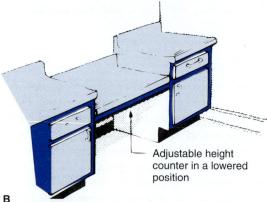

Adjustable height counter in a lowered position

B

Element # 2: Adjustable Counters

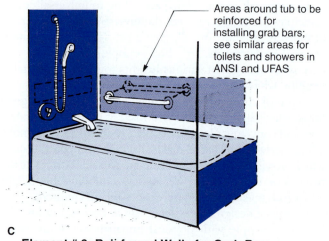

Areas around tub to be reinforced for installing grab bars; see similar areas for toilets and showers in ANSI and UFAS

C

Element # 3: Reinforced Walls for Grab Bars

Figure 15–14 Adaptable features. (A) Removable base cabinets. (B) Adjustable-height counters. Sinks also adjustable. (C) Reinforced walls for grab bars. (Reproduced from Bostrom, Mace, and Long. *Adaptable Housing: A Technical Manual for Implementing Adaptable Dwelling Unit Specifications.* Department of Housing and Urban Development, 1987.)

only with careful analysis and planning. The person with the disabling condition, other members of the household, and the rehabilitation team must work closely together.

The first issue to be addressed is where the person will live after discharge. Will he or his family own or rent the property? Will he live alone or with friends or relatives? How permanent will his living arrangement be? Modification of a rented home will require the approval of the owner. A child or adolescent returning to his parent's home may not need the kitchen and laundry facilities to be accessible, particularly if he was not responsible for kitchen or laundry chores prior to his injury. And if a person's immediate post-discharge living arrangement will be temporary, the modifications to that environment should be kept to a minimum.

Once it has been determined where an individual will live following discharge, modifications should be made only after careful planning. The first step in planning involves determination of the person's unique requirements. The rehabilitation team and the person with a spinal cord injury should work together to discover his requirements in the following areas: slope of ramp that he can negotiate, door width and threshold requirements, clear floor- and knee-space dimensions needed, maximal and comfortable forward and side reach ranges, capabilities in manipulating controls, and optimal heights for counters, appliances, and plumbing fixtures. Planning based on the individual's requirements will make it possible to minimize home modifications, thus minimizing expense. It may be found that many of the home's features, though not accessible by federal or industry standards, are accessible to the individual concerned.

Before planning home modifications, the patient and the rehabilitation team should determine which features of the home need to be changed. Perhaps the best way to make this determination is for the individual to spend some time at home. It will then become apparent, for example, which doorways need to be widened and what appliances are out of reach. It should be kept in mind, however, that the person's exact accessibility requirements are likely to change as rehabilitation progresses. His needs will change as he grows stronger and more skillful, and when his permanent wheelchair arrives. Thus it is important to avoid making major modifications to the home prematurely.

To supplement the information gathered in the informal home assessment just described, a health professional or family member should perform a detailed evaluation of the home. Ideally, the patient will be present during the home evaluation. The evaluation should involve assessment of all relevant features of the home: layout of the entrance paths and immediate area surrounding the home; height of entrances above the ground; dimensions of structures and available space surrounding entrances; changes in floor and ground level within and around the home; thresholds and clear space within all doorways; force and manipulation required to work all controls and hardware (cabinet handles, door knobs and locks, etc.); height of these controls and hardware; clear floor space available for maneuvering in hallways and rooms and for access to plumbing fixtures, appliances, storage areas, windows, and thermostat controls; height of and clear knee space under counters, appliances, and plumbing fixtures; and height of all electrical outlets and light switches.

Whether the evaluation is performed by a health professional or by a family member, the evaluator should first receive guidance regarding what to measure, how to measure it, and how to record the evaluation findings.

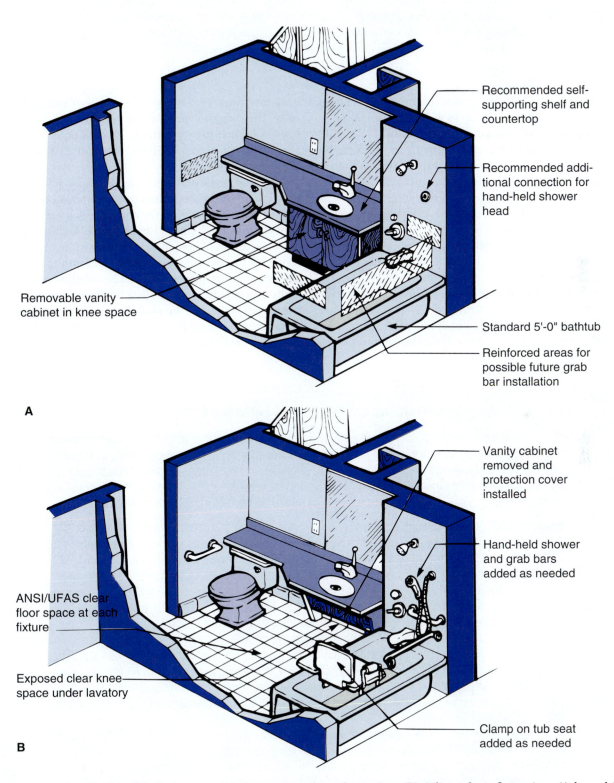

Recommended self-supporting shelf and countertop

Recommended additional connection for hand-held shower head

Removable vanity cabinet in knee space

Standard 5'-0" bathtub

Reinforced areas for possible future grab bar installation

A

Vanity cabinet removed and protection cover installed

Hand-held shower and grab bars added as needed

ANSI/UFAS clear floor space at each fixture

Exposed clear knee space under lavatory

Clamp on tub seat added as needed

B

Figure 15–15   Small adaptable bathroom. (A) Conventional configuration. (B) Adjusted configuration. (Adapted from Bostrom, Mace, and Long. *Adaptable Housing: A Technical Manual for Implementing Adaptable Dwelling Unit Specifications.* Department of Housing and Urban Development, 1987.)

Architectural Adaptation and Upper Extremity Preservation

Architectural adaptation can allow wheelchair users to function in their environments with less damaging stress on their upper extremities. For example, appropriate-height storage, environmental controls, and work spaces minimize the amount of overhead reaching required to function, and hard and smooth floor surfaces allow wheelchair propulsion with reduced strain on the upper extremities. Environments built or adapted to meet ADA standards may help prevent overuse injuries of the upper extremities.[29]

The evaluation results will be most useful if the findings are recorded in a detailed sketch as well as in a checklist.

Based on a careful assessment of the individual's abilities, equipment, and home environment, the patient, his family, and the rehabilitation team can work together to plan home modifications. Unfortunately, funding is another factor that must be taken into account. Certainly all possible funding sources should be investigated. When funds are limited, expense must be a major consideration when choosing between options. Home modifications may have to be prioritized, with remodeling being done in stages as finances allow.

The rehabilitation team's role in home modification takes on another dimension with patients who plan to live in rental units after discharge. These individuals should be educated regarding their housing rights and should know how to ensure that these rights are not violated. Specifically, they should learn about federal and local housing laws relevant to accessibility and should be informed about the recourses available to them in the event that their rights are violated.

Although accessible housing is likely to be the most pressing architecture-related concern during rehabilitation, structural barriers within the community are also important contributors to disability. Inaccessible architecture in the workplace, school, and in the community at large will interfere with the individual's reintegration into the community and resumption of social roles. The rehabilitation team can address problems in these areas by educating patients about their legal rights and by consulting with employers, school systems, and others in the community regarding architectural accessibility.

Home Modifications and Training in Activities of Daily Living

Abilities in ADLs (activities of daily living) and IADLs (instrumental activities of daily living) are explored and developed during functional training. These capabilities reflect an interplay between the individual's body function and structure, skills in compensatory strategies when needed, equipment characteristics, and the physical environment. Because all of these factors are interrelated, functional training, equipment selection, and planning for home modifications should be intertwined during rehabilitation.

Example: Bathing. During rehabilitation, physical and occupational therapists work with patients to develop their capacity to bathe independently when possible, or with assistance if needed. One component of this task involves training in transfers to and from the bathing facilities, often a bathtub. To the extent possible, transfer practice should occur in conditions similar to those that the patient will encounter after discharge. For example, the wheelchair should be positioned in clear floor space that is available in the home's bathroom. Based on information gathered in the home evaluation, practice in therapy can occur using movable barriers or tape on the floor to indicate floor space that will be available for maneuvering and transfers. Training is also likely to involve trials of one or more tub benches, and selection this equipment. This selection will be influenced by the patient's transfer abilities as well as the clear floor space in the bathroom. (If the bench extends outside of the tub, it will encroach on the clear floor space and can affect the options available for positioning the wheelchair.) Functional training also involves practice of the bathing skills themselves, and selection and use of equipment such as hand-held shower spray units.

Throughout the process of functional training and equipment selection, the layout of the home's bathroom is considered. The patient and rehabilitation team work together to determine what modifications will be required in the bathroom to allow safe use of the facilities. Whether the patient will function independently or with assistance, decisions regarding transfer techniques, equipment selection, and environmental adaptation are intertwined.

Summary

- Architectural accessibility has a great impact on a person's ability to function and participate in life situations; inaccessible environments can disable people as profoundly as can physical impairments themselves.

- The United States has a number of laws relevant to wheelchair-accessible architectural design, and three sets of standards that specify the characteristics of an accessible environment. These standards do not apply to privately owned single-family homes, but can provide a starting point for planning.

- Certain design features are required for a building to be accessible. These features include provision for negotiating any changes in floor or ground level, adequate width in doorways and halls for a wheelchair, floors that do not provide excessive resistance to wheelchair propulsion, clear floor space and knee space to allow maneuvering the wheelchair and gaining access to various features of the home (appliances, storage areas, work surfaces, etc.), and location and design of these features allowing their access and use.

- *Adaptable design* refers to housing design that can be easily altered to accommodate residents with physical impairments. To be truly adaptable, the house or apartment must be designed so that it can be made fully wheelchair-accessible with minimal time and expense, and using unskilled labor.

- *Universal design* refers to housing that is equally usable by most people, regardless of age, body build, or physical ability. Homes built or remodeled using universal design principles make it possible for family members with different physical characteristics and functional abilities to function safely and comfortably in the same environment.

- When homes are built or remodeled for people undergoing rehabilitation, the new home environments should be designed to match the preferences, current and future needs, and available funds of the individuals who will live there. The design should be based on an analysis of the individual's physical abilities and (if remodeling) the home's current structure. Individuals who plan to live in rental housing should participate in the same process. In addition, they should receive education about their legal rights in the area of rental housing.

- To promote community reintegration and the resumption of social roles after spinal cord injury, the rehabilitation team should address architectural accessibility in work places and schools, and in the community at large.

Suggested Resources

PUBLICATIONS

A Guide to Disability Rights Laws. (2005) Published by the U.S. Department of Justice. Available free from *www.ada.gov/cguide.htm*

Accessible Home Design: Architectural Solutions for the Wheelchair User (2nd edition). Published by Paralyzed Veterans of America. Available for purchase from *www.pva.org*

Americans With Disabilities Act and Architectural Barriers Act Accessibility Guidelines. (2004 updated guidelines) Published by United States Access Board. Available free from *www.access-board.gov*

Practical Guide to Universal Home Design. (2004) Published by the Iowa Program for Assistive Technology, Center for Disabilities and Development, University of Iowa Hospitals and Clinics. Available free from *www.uiowa.edu/infotech/universalhomedesign.htm*

The Assist Guidebook to the Accessible Home: Practical Designs for Home Modifications and New Construction. (2005). Published by ASSIST Inc. Available free from *www.assistutah.org*

ORGANIZATIONS

Center for Universal Design, North Carolina State University: *www.design.ncsu.edu/cud/index.htm*

U.S. Government

- Department of Justice, ADA Homepage: *www.ada.gov*
- Access Board: *www.access-board.gov/contact.htm*
- Department of Housing and Urban Development: *www.hud.gov/offices/fheo/FHLaws/index.cfm*

Appendix
Solutions to Problem-Solving Exercises

CHAPTER 1

Problem-Solving Exercise 1–1

IMPAIRMENTS: lower extremity paralysis, limited range of motion

ACTIVITY LIMITATIONS: unable to walk, transfer independently, negotiate obstacles (uneven terrain, ramps, curbs) in a wheelchair

PARTICIPATION RESTRICTIONS: unable to return to work, take care of son, live at home with husband and son

ENVIRONMENTAL BARRIERS: step at home's entrance, narrow bathroom doorway. (Uneven terrain, ramps, and curbs are also environmental barriers. The *inability to negotiate these obstacles*, however, would be classified as activity limitation.)

CHAPTER 2

Problem-Solving Exercise 2–1

ASIA CLASSIFICATION: This patient's neurological level of injury is right T11, left T12. (If identifying only one level, it is T11.) He has complete (ASIA A) paraplegia.

MOTOR RETURN: Based on his initial presentation (ASIA A and no sparing of pinprick sensation in the lower extremities), this patient is not likely to regain significant motor functioning in his lower extremities. HOWEVER, although motor return is not likely, it *is* possible. Thus it would not be accurate to tell him that he definitely will not regain the use of his legs.

Problem-Solving Exercise 2–2

The following table presents the ASIA Impairment Scale, clinical syndrome, and neuroanatomical basis for the clinical presentation of each patient.

All of the patients have incomplete injuries. Because of this, the term *zone of partial preservation* does not apply to any of them.

CHAPTER 3

Problem-Solving Exercise 3–1

Your first priority is to correct the orientation of the orthosis. With the patient supine, you can safely remove

Patient	ASIA Impairment Scale (AIS)	Clinical Syndrome	Neuroanatomical Basis for Clinical Presentation
#1	B	Anterior cord	Damage to the anterior and anterolateral aspects of the cord results in bilateral loss of voluntary motor function because all of the descending tracts are located in these areas. Pain and temperature sensations are lost due to interruption of the anterolateral system. The dorsal columns remain intact, resulting in preserved proprioception. The patient's ability to detect pressure during the rectal examination may reflect preservation of deep touch, another sensory modality that travels in the dorsal columns.
#2	D	Central cord	The clinical picture typical of central cord syndrome is due to the spatial orientation of the fiber tracts in the cord: fibers innervating the cervical segments are located more centrally within the cord. Thus, damage in the central region of the cord affects the tracts that innervate the upper extremities. Fibers innervating thoracic, lumbar, and sacral segments are located progressively more peripherally in the cord and are spared if the peripheral area of the cord is undamaged.

(Continued)

Patient	ASIA Impairment Scale (AIS)	Clinical Syndrome	Neuroanatomical Basis for Clinical Presentation
#3	D	Brown–Séquard	The clinical presentation of Brown–Séquard syndrome makes sense when one recalls the course of the motor and sensory pathways. The descending fibers of the lateral corticospinal, rubrospinal, and reticulospinal tracts travel in the spinal cord on the same side of the body as the motor neurons that they innervate. The sensory fibers in the dorsal columns also travel in the cord on the same side as they innervate. A lesion on one side of the spinal cord, then, disrupts motor functioning, proprioception, vibratory sense, and two-point discrimination on the side of the lesion. Fibers carrying pain and temperature information cross soon after entry into the spinal cord, before ascending in the anterolateral system. As a result, they travel in the opposite side of the spinal cord as the side of the body that they innervate. Because of this, a lesion of one side of the cord results in a contralateral loss of pain and temperature sensitivity.

the front of the orthosis and replace it in its correct position.

To prevent the problem from reoccurring, you need to educate the patient and others who are involved in donning the orthosis. This group may include the family or attendants if the patient is living at home or staff members if the patient is in a hospital, rehabilitation facility, or extended care facility.

Education in this area should address proper orientation and donning techniques for the orthosis. Written instructions and photographs or clear drawings of the orthosis in its correct position can help with clarification and carryover. Posting these illustrations by the orthotic wearer's bed may be helpful in an inpatient setting, where a number of different staff members are likely to assist with orthotic donning. Clear and easily seen labels on the orthosis may also be helpful, particularly if the orthotic wearer and/or those providing assistance have difficulty determining the correct orientation of the orthosis.

In addition to *informing* the patient and those who assist him about proper orthotic orientation, you should work to *convince* them that it is important. Doing so may enhance the likelihood of the patient following the instructions.

Problem-Solving Exercise 3–2

You should suspect autonomic dysreflexia. In response to these signs and symptoms, you should immediately take the patient's blood pressure. If it is elevated, you should position her in short sitting and loosen any constricting clothing or assistive devices. The underlying source of the noxious sensation causing the dysreflexia should be investigated and eliminated as quickly as possible. (Refer to the chapter for a

full description of the interventions that are appropriate in response to autonomic dysreflexia.) If the underlying problem cannot be identified and remedied quickly in therapy (the urinary catheter was kinked, for example), proper response involves obtaining the assistance of appropriate medical professionals. If the patient is an inpatient (or an outpatient in a setting that has ready access to nursing care), communicate rapidly with the nursing staff to involve them in managing the dysreflexia. If you are seeing the patient in an outpatient setting or in the home and are unable to identify and resolve the source of the patient's dysreflexia quickly, she should be transported to an emergency room.

Problem-Solving Exercise 3–3

You should suspect deep vein thrombosis. In response to these signs, you should stop the therapy session and obtain assistance from appropriate medical professionals. If in an inpatient setting, you should transport the patient to his room and communicate with the nursing/medical staff regarding the suspected DVT. If the patient is being seen in an outpatient setting or in the home, arrange for him to be evaluated by a physician on an emergency basis. Therapy should remain suspended until either a DVT is ruled out or anticoagulant therapy has been initiated and the patient has been cleared by his physician to resume activity.

CHAPTER 4

Problem-Solving Exercise 4–1

Many nondisabled people (including health professionals) feel that their quality of life would be poor after a spinal cord injury and that they would not feel worthy. Many also report that they would rather die than have to utilize a ventilator. In contrast, most people with spinal cord injuries (after a period of adjustment) report that they have a good quality of life and feel that they are worthy. Moreover, the majority of people with high cord injuries who use ventilators report that they are glad to be alive.[a]

One question remains: What do your responses tell you about your perceptions of life after a spinal cord injury? If you feel that your quality of life would be poor, that you would not feel worthy, or that you would be better off dead than on a ventilator, your view of life after spinal cord injury is more pessimistic than that held by the majority of people who have survived such injuries. This does not mean that you are a bad person or that you should never work with people who have spinal cord injuries. You should, however, be aware of your biases and your potential for conveying an overly pessimistic view *to* and *about* your patients.

Problem-Solving Exercise 4–2

A wheelchair selection process that involves the patient in decision making would reinforce his sense of independence and autonomy. The patient should be provided with information about the different equipment options and should be given the opportunity to try out a variety of wheelchairs with different features. Together with his physical and occupational therapist, he can discuss the pros and cons of various brands and features as they relate to his unique requirements (physical characteristics, abilities, accustomed activities and roles, home and community physical environment, financial resources, etc.) and personal preferences. The wheelchair prescription should reflect a true collaboration between the therapists and patient.

In addition to empowering the patient, a collaborative selection process is likely to result in the purchase of a wheelchair that best matches the individual's preferences, values, priorities, and functional and physical requirements.

Problem-Solving Exercise 4–3

A lap blanket, the prize for the winner in the wheelchair division, is an object that is associated with infirmity and inactivity. In contrast, the prizes awarded to the able-bodied runners (athletic equipment and gift certificates from athletic stores) affirmed their athleticism. The message conveyed by these contrasting prizes was that the able-bodied runners were the *real* athletes in this event, and the participants using wheelchairs were not truly athletes. In fact, they were "*invalids.*"

On the surface, a race involving athletes both with and without disabilities would seem to be an event that could

work to enhance the image of the participants with disabilities. One seemingly minor detail in the event, the nature of the awards, however, could cause the opposite to occur. Anyone present (athletes, their friends and families, other spectators) would receive a clear message that the athletes using wheelchairs were infirm or ill. This message could be generalized to include everyone with disabling conditions. *Thus the event would reinforce the stigma associated with disability.*

The organizers of the race could have conveyed a more positive message to and about the athletes using wheelchairs by awarding them the same types of prizes that they awarded the other athletes: athletic equipment and gift certificates from athletic stores.

The reader could understandably assume that nobody would make such a blatant error when including athletes with disabilities in a race; however, the incident described actually occurred. It is an example of how well-meaning rehabilitation professionals (the organizers of the race) can inadvertently perpetuate negative attitudes about people with disabling conditions.

CHAPTER 5
Problem-Solving Exercise 5–1

Factors that make this patient highly susceptible to pressure ulcers:

- Complete spinal cord injury (ASIA A)
- Advanced age
- Cardiovascular disease
- Pulmonary disease
- Level of activity (in bed only)
- Low level of independence (requires assistance to move in bed)
- Male gender

The following interventions are indicated to prevent pressure ulcers while the patient remains in bed:

- Pressure-relieving support surface
- Turning in bed *at least* every 2 hours
- Positioning in bed to minimize pressure on bony prominences
- Avoidance of elevation of head of bed above 30 degrees
- Skin inspection every time the patient is turned

As soon as possible, the patient should begin spending time sitting in a wheelchair. Time spent in sitting (with appropriate precautions taken) will reduce his risk of developing pressure ulcers and may enhance his pulmonary status. The following interventions are indicated to prevent pressure ulcers while the patient sits in a wheelchair:

- Proper positioning in a wheelchair that has appropriate dimensions, components, and adjustment

[a] Source: Gerhart, K. Quality of life: the danger of differing perceptions. *Top Spinal Cord Inj Rehabil.* 1997, 2(3):78–84.

- Use of an appropriate pressure-relieving wheelchair cushion
- Pressure reliefs every 15 minutes
- Limited time in sitting at first, with gradual increase as skin tolerance allows
- Skin inspection after each sitting session

Education of the patient and family members should begin immediately, and the patient should be included as an active participant in all aspects of his preventive skin care program. As soon as possible and within his medical limitations, the patient should begin training in techniques for independent bed positioning, pressure reliefs, and skin inspection. A program for the prevention of pressure ulcers must also include optimization of the patient's medical and nutritional status.

Problem-Solving Exercise 5–2

The fact that the redness blanches indicates that the patient does not have a pressure ulcer. However, the increased time that the redness takes to resolve warrants concern.

Any of the following problems with the new wheelchair could cause an increase in pressure over both of the patient's ischial tuberosities, with increased skin redness resulting.

- Seat too short in the anteroposterior dimension (too shallow)
- Footrests adjusted too high
- Armrests absent from wheelchair

The following problems with the new wheelchair could cause an increase in shear forces over the patient's ischial tuberosities, with increased skin redness resulting.

- Seat too long in the anteroposterior dimension
- Footrests too low
- Seat or backrest upholstery that is stretched out
- Power recline feature (if previous wheelchair allowed pressure reliefs using power tilt)

Because the redness appears over both ischial tuberosities, wheelchair problems that cause a laterally leaning posture (seat too wide, armrests too low or uneven) are not likely sources of this patient's skin redness.

It would be advisable to assess the patient's capacity to perform pressure reliefs in the current wheelchair; the new chair may have components that make it more difficult for the patient to perform pressure reliefs effectively.

To prevent the development of a pressure ulcer over the ischial tuberosities, you should evaluate the new wheelchair and make adjustments as indicated. If the wheelchair is inappropriate and cannot be adjusted to make it appropriate (for example, if the seat is too shallow from front to back), you should provide the patient with a different wheelchair that has the appropriate dimensions and components.

Because the patient's skin did not show signs of actual breakdown, she should be able to resume sitting. It would be prudent, however, to monitor her skin's status very closely when she does so.

CHAPTER 6

Problem-Solving Exercise 6–1

Innervation of muscles of inspiration and forced expiration with complete C8 tetraplegia.

Muscles used in inhalation:

- Fully innervated: diaphragm, scalenes, sternocleidomastoid, serratus anterior, trapezius, levator scapulae, and rhomboid major and minor.
- Partially innervated: pectoralis minor, pectoralis major, and erector spinae.
- Not innervated: intercostals, levatores costorum, serratus posterior superior, and abdominals.

Muscles used in forced exhalation:

- Fully innervated: clavicular portion of the pectoralis major.
- Partially innervated: none.
- Not innervated: intercostals, abdominals, serratus posterior inferior, and quadratus lumborum.

The most likely explanation for this patient's increased respiratory rate and shortness of breath is that his diaphragm moves into a less advantageous position when his trunk is elevated from horizontal, as occurs when the head of the bed is elevated. Because his abdominal musculature is not innervated, it does not support the abdominal viscera. This lack of support allows gravity to pull the abdominal contents caudally when the patient sits with his trunk elevated. The diaphragm descends and flattens, placing its fibers in a mechanically disadvantageous position and making it more difficult for the patient to breathe.

Problem-Solving Exercise 6–2

The treatment program for this patient should be designed to develop a diaphragmatic breathing pattern and to increase the strength and endurance in the diaphragm.

BREATHING PATTERN: Early practice of diaphragmatic breathing may begin in supine, as the diaphragm will be placed on a slight stretch and will be better able to function effectively in this position. If the cervical spine is stable, the patient's neck can be positioned in flexion to place the sternocleidomastoid and scalenes in a shortened position. In this manner, positioning can be used to encourage diaphragmatic breathing and discourage use of the accessory muscles. The therapist can also use verbal and visual cues to encourage deep breathing with protrusion of the abdomen during inspiration, and can provide a quick stretch to the diaphragm to facilitate its contraction. As the patient's breathing pattern improves, the patient can practice diaphragmatic breathing with her trunk in more upright positions and with the neck in neutral alignment. The patient can also practice diaphragmatic breathing with less reliance on input from the therapist.

STRENGTH AND ENDURANCE: The patient can develop the strength and endurance of her diaphragm through resisted inspiratory exercises. Initial exercises can be performed with manual resistance provided by the therapist. The patient can progress to breathing exercises with resistance provided either by weights placed on her abdomen or a resistive inspiratory muscle trainer. Whichever method of exercise is selected, the resistance should be low enough that the patient is able to maintain a diaphragmatic breathing pattern during the exercises. Positioning the patient as described above will encourage the use of the diaphragm rather than the accessory muscles during these exercises.

Problem-Solving Exercise 6–3

EXAMINATION: Observe the patient's attempt to cough and note the effectiveness of his performance during each phase of the cough (maximal inhalation, glottis closure, contraction of the muscles of forced exhalation with the glottis closed, and continued forced exhalation with the glottis open). Note whether his posture and body motions while coughing are appropriate for effective inhalation and forced exhalation. A measure of vital capacity or peak expiratory flow will provide information on his ability to exhale forcefully. Finally, you should assess the strength in the patient's trunk, upper extremities, and muscles of ventilation.

TREATMENT PROGRAM: The treatment program should include instruction in and practice of the sequence of effective coughing: maximal inhalation, brief hold (glottis closure), and cough. The technique that the patient uses will be determined by the motor function in his abdominals. If his abdominal musculature is innervated, he may learn to cough effectively without using his arms for self-coughing. If his abdominals lack innervation, he will need to use his arms to assist his own coughing. Whichever technique is utilized, the patient should learn to maximize his inhalation and forced exhalation by performing appropriate motions. (If possible, he should combine inhalation with trunk and neck extension, shoulder flexion, and scapular adduction. He should combine forced exhalation with trunk and neck flexion, shoulder extension, and scapular abduction.) In addition to practicing the actions involved in coughing, the patient may benefit from a strengthening program. Increased strength in the muscles used for inhalation and forced exhalation may increase cough effectiveness. The abdominals in particular should be strengthened if they are innervated. The patient is also likely to benefit from a strengthening program for any upper extremity or trunk muscles that will be used to perform the motions involved in effective coughing.

CHAPTER 7

Problem-Solving Exercise 7–1

You should test all key muscles on both sides of the body. Even though the patient's diagnosis is complete tetraplegia, there may be some previously undetected motor function below the level of the lesion.

The key muscles are the elbow flexors, wrist extensors, elbow extensors, finger flexors to the middle finger, small finger abductors, hip flexors, knee extensors, ankle dorsiflexors, long toe extensors, and ankle plantarflexors. You should also test additional muscles that are functionally relevant but are not ASIA key muscles. For patients with complete C6 tetraplegia, these additional muscles include the deltoids, serratus anterior, and clavicular portion of the pectoralis major.

To prevent muscle substitution while you test finger flexion, hold the patient's wrist in either 0 degrees of extension or slight flexion and do not allow *any* wrist motion while she attempts to flex her fingers. With her wrist immobilized, she will be unable to utilize a tenodesis grasp. Any finger flexion motion that the patient exhibits while her wrist is immobile can be attributed to activity in her finger flexors.

Problem-Solving Exercise 7–2

To determine whether it is deltoid or serratus weakness that allows you to push the patient's arm down from the test position, palpate and/or observe the patient's scapula while performing a standard manual muscle test for the anterior deltoid. If the deltoid is stronger than the serratus anterior, a downward force applied to the arm will result in scapular winging and downward rotation. If the serratus is stronger than the deltoid, the scapula will remain stable while the arm is forced down from the test position.

To test the anterior deltoid in isolation from the serratus, the therapist should manually stabilize the scapula in a position of abduction and upward rotation while performing the standard anterior deltoid muscle test. An inability to maintain shoulder flexion against resistance with the scapula stabilized in this position is an indication of anterior deltoid weakness.

Because the deltoid receives innervation from higher levels of the spinal cord (C5 and C6) than does the serratus anterior (primarily C6 and 7, with some C5), a person with tetraplegia is likely to have greater strength in his deltoids than in his serratus anterior. When this is the case, and the deltoids are strong enough, the serratus can be tested using the arm as a lever. When the deltoids are too weak to perform the standard serratus muscle test, the therapist can apply forces directly to the scapula rather than using the arm as a lever while testing the serratus.

Problem-Solving Exercise 7–3

The first patient described is likely to achieve functional outcomes at *or below* those listed in Table 7-2. Factors that may impact positively on his functional outcome include strong musculature through the C7 myotome, normal range of motion, a lack of spasticity severe enough to impact significantly on function, good overall health, and cooperation in therapy. Possible limiting factors include his age, previous sedentary lifestyle, and lack of initiative in therapy.

Expected outcomes:

- Bed skills: independent to some assist
- Transfers: independent even, some assist with uneven
- Wheelchair skills: independent propelling manual wheelchair indoors and on level outdoor terrain, some assist with uneven terrain
- Ambulation: no functional ambulation

The second patient described may achieve exceptional outcomes, as presented in Table 7-3. Factors that may affect his functional outcome positively include his age, strong musculature through the C7 myotome, normal range of motion, a lack of spasticity severe enough to affect function significantly, good overall health, and a high level of motivation in therapy. In addition, the fact that he was a star athlete prior to his injury suggests that he is likely to acquire motor skills readily.

Expected outcomes:

- Bed skills: independent
- Transfers: independent even and uneven, including transfers between wheelchair and floor
- Wheelchair skills: independent propelling manual wheelchair indoors and on slightly uneven outdoor terrain, negotiating 4-inch curbs and ramps with 1:12 or steeper grade
- Ambulation: no functional ambulation

Problem-Solving Exercise 7–4

Your patient's stated goal of walking is not realistic. With C5 tetraplegia, ASIA A, she is unlikely to experience adequate motor return to walk functionally.

There is no easy answer for how to respond to this patient. It is still relatively early postinjury. Although adequate motor return for functional ambulation is unlikely, it is not impossible. Moreover, the patient is still early in the process of adapting to, even comprehending, her injury. Her stated goal of ambulation might be an expression of hope, lack of understanding, or denial. On the other hand, it might be a way of asking you for your opinion about her potential for ambulation.

Not only is there no easy answer, there is no one way to respond that would be appropriate for all patients in this situation. You will need to use your judgment about her readiness to discuss this topic and the manner of addressing it that will be most likely to be helpful at this time. Possible responses might include any of the following:

- Clarify her understanding of her prognosis–what she has been told and what she understands about her potential for motor return and walking.
- Discuss her prognosis with her. It may be most appropriate to talk in terms of likely outcomes rather than speaking in absolutes. (See the discussion of hope and truth in Chapter 4.)
- Speak with the patient about pursuing outcomes that can be achieved with her current motor function, with the reassurance that goals can be added if motor return makes this possible.
- Present realistic options in a positive light, emphasizing her potential to return to participation in life situations.

Whatever your response to this patient's stated goal of walking, it is important to remain empathetic and constructive and respond in a way that is both honest and respectful of the patient's current state of readiness to deal with her prognosis.

Problem-Solving Exercise 7–5

Here's the problem in a nutshell: your patient's funding for inpatient rehabilitation will run out before she is physically ready to participate significantly in her rehabilitation. The best solution may be for her to leave the rehabilitation facility as soon as that can be arranged, and return once she has been cleared by her orthopedist for full weight bearing on her extremities.

Ideally, the patient will spend the interim period at home. That will be possible only if she has an adequate support system (family, friends, attendants, and/or home health professionals) to provide the assistance that she will require to remain healthy and somewhat functional. Additionally, discharge home will require that the patient has an appropriate seating system (wheelchair and cushion) and other needed equipment and a home environment in which she can function during her stay at home. A fully accessible home environment will not be absolutely necessary for the interim period as long as the patient has adequate assistance and equipment to "get by" temporarily. For example, she may need to use a bedside commode if her bathroom is not wheelchair-accessible, and her family may need to assist her in and out of the house if the entrance is not accessible.

This solution, discharging the patient and readmitting her when she is ready to participate in rehabilitation, will take the coordinated efforts of the rehabilitation team.

TASKS OF THE CASE MANAGER: Communicate with the insurance company to ensure that they are in agreement with the plan for postponement of inpatient rehabilitation. Make arrangements for the patient to receive the needed services (nursing care, attendant care, and therapies) during the interim period. Arrange follow-up so that the rehabilitation team can (1) monitor the patient's status, (2) intervene if needed, and (3) arrange for the patient's return to the rehabilitation facility once the orthopedic restrictions for the extremities have been discontinued.

TASKS OF THE NURSING STAFF AND THERAPISTS: Determine the appropriate discharge destination for the interim period between inpatient rehabilitation stays. Provide the needed family and patient education and training to ensure that the patient will remain healthy and will remain as functional as possible during the interim. Obtain the equipment and supplies that the patient will require during the time between her inpatient rehabilitation stays.

PHYSICAL THERAPY GOALS: If a discharge to the patient's home is planned, the goals will focus primarily on family and patient education and training. Because the patient will be dependent in virtually all activities at this time, the family (or an attendant) will need to learn safe techniques for transfers, assisting the patient with bed positioning, and wheelchair management. The patient should learn how to direct these activities. The patient and family should also be instructed in health maintenance activities such as skin care, as well as a program of exercises and activities to maintain or improve (as indicated to prepare for functional independence, and as allowed by the orthopedic restrictions) the patient's strength, range of motion, endurance, and tolerance to upright positioning. In addition to providing training and education, the therapist will need to ensure that the patient has the equipment that she will need to stay healthy and as functional as possible during the interim phase.

The exact physical therapy goals will depend on the patient's physical and functional status, her discharge destination, and the capabilities of the people who will be assisting her during the interim period. The following is a *partial* list of *possible* goals for this patient to be achieved by discharge:

- The family will independently demonstrate safe techniques in transferring the patient from wheelchair to bed, bed to wheelchair, wheelchair to car, and car to wheelchair using good body mechanics.
- The patient will instruct others in safe techniques for assisting in transfers between the wheelchair and a bed and between the wheelchair and a car.
- The patient will state the purpose and frequency of pressure reliefs in a wheelchair, and will instruct others in safe techniques for assisting with pressure reliefs. (Alternatively, if the patient will have the use of a

power wheelchair with power tilt or recline, the goal should include independence in pressure reliefs using this equipment.)

- The patient will be provided with an appropriate wheelchair and cushion. (Ideally, this will include a power tilt or recline feature in the wheelchair to allow independent pressure reliefs.)

CHAPTER 8

Problem-Solving Exercise 8–1

The patient will use the head–hips relationship to lift his buttocks onto the wheelchair seat. To move his buttocks up and to the right, he should throw his head down and to the left. The motion should be rapid, to impart adequate momentum to the buttocks. He will not utilize muscle substitution to maintain left elbow extension, as his triceps are fully innervated.

Problem-Solving Exercise 8–2

To enable your patient to practice rolling, make the task easier. This can be accomplished by any combination of the following "aids to rolling":

- Have the patient practice rolling from side lying or from a position between supine and side lying. Place a pillow or bolster behind her pelvis to prevent her from rolling back into supine.
- Cross the patient's legs. If the right leg is on top, have her roll to the left, and reverse this if the left leg is on top.
- Place a 1-pound wrist weight around one or both of the patient's distal forearms. (If she is in a side-lying position, she will only be able to throw the superior arm. In this case, only this arm should be weighted.)

Whatever combination of the above strategies is used, the task should be structured so that the patient can roll, but only with effort.

As the patient's ability to roll improves, you can make the task more challenging by removing or reducing the "aids to rolling" mentioned above.

- If the patient has been practicing rolling from a side-lying or semi–side-lying position, alter her starting position so that she rolls from a more supine position. (Tilt her back to a slightly more horizontal starting position.)
- Uncross the patient's legs.
- Remove the weight(s) from the patient's forearm(s).

If the patient has been practicing with a combination of "aids to rolling," remove one of these "aids" at a time as she progresses. Removing more than one at a time may make the task prohibitively difficult.

CHAPTER 9

Problem-Solving Exercise 9–1

Rolling without equipment is a reasonable goal for this patient unless comorbidities such as severe arthritis in his shoulders interfere. He should be able to achieve this goal during inpatient rehabilitation unless his progress is limited by secondary medical conditions or comorbidities, or his rehabilitation stay is significantly shortened by funding or other constraints.

Because he has intact upper extremity function, the patient may be able to roll with minimal practice after being shown the movement strategies involved. On the other hand, he may need to build his skill more gradually if his mild obesity makes rolling difficult. If this is the case, functional training strategies just described for Problem-Solving Exercise 8-2 can be employed.

Problem-Solving Exercise 9–2

This person's motor levels are left C7 and right C6.

The method of coming to sitting that the patient is likely to achieve most readily is the "walking on elbows" method. Her limited deltoid strength (on the right) and shoulder and elbow range are likely to interfere with the other methods of coming to sitting.

PHYSICAL PREREQUISITES: The strength and range prerequisites are presented in Table 9-7: To assume a sitting posture using this method, a person with a spinal cord injury needs adequate strength in her deltoids, elbow flexors, and shoulder internal and external rotators. She must also possess adequate range in elbow flexion and extension; shoulder flexion, abduction, internal rotation, and horizontal abduction; and in combined hip flexion and knee extension (hamstring flexibility).

STRENGTHENING PROGRAM: The patient could benefit from strengthening of her deltoids, shoulder internal and external rotators, elbow flexors, and triceps. Although she has 4/5 to 5/5 strength in most of these muscles, stronger musculature will enable her to come to sitting with greater ease. Greater strength in the triceps (currently 3/5 on the left and 2/5 on the right) in particular should make coming to sitting easier.

RANGE-OF-MOTION PROGRAM: The patient's limited hamstring flexibility will interfere with her performance of this activity; therefore hamstring stretching should have high priority in the therapeutic program. The limited range in elbow extension should also be addressed. Although full elbow extension range is not required to perform this skill, it will enable the patient to come to sitting more easily. Increasing shoulder extension range may be helpful for other activities, but will not be necessary to attain this goal. The long finger flexors should be allowed to remain slightly shortened, as this tightness will enable this individual to utilize a tenodesis grasp during other functional activities. All other joints have normal range of motion. The therapeutic program should be designed to maintain this range, to prevent future functional problems.

SKILL PREREQUISITES: The skill prerequisites for this functional task are presented in Table 9-8: To come to sitting using this method, the patient must be able to assume a prone-on-elbows position, shift weight and walk her elbows to the side in this position, move into forearm-supported side lying, walk her supporting elbow toward her legs in this position, push-pull into a sitting position, push with her arms to lift her trunk from a forward lean in sitting, and tolerate an upright sitting posture. Because this patient lacks adequate strength in her triceps, she must be able to use muscle substitution to aid in elbow extension.

FUNCTIONAL TRAINING PROGRAM: Because the patient has none of the needed skill prerequisites, functional training should start with the most basic skills: ability to extend the elbows using muscle substitution, tolerate an upright sitting position, and shift weight in the prone-on-elbows position once placed in that posture. When she has developed these abilities, she can work on more challenging skills, such as assuming the prone-on-elbows position, walking her elbows to the side in prone on elbows, moving from this position to forearm-supported side lying, and lifting her trunk from a forward lean in sitting. As her strength and skill develop, she can work on walking her elbow in forearm-supported side lying and moving from this position to a sitting posture. (Suggested techniques for teaching the patient each of these prerequisite skills are presented in Chapter 9.) As the patient masters the various prerequisite skills, she can practice them in combination. By building her skill in this manner, the patient progresses to independence in coming to sitting without equipment by walking on her elbows.

Problem-Solving Exercise 9–3

This patient has C4 tetraplegia, ASIA C.

POSSIBLE MOVEMENT STRATEGIES FOR ROLLING: For the purposes of this discussion, "superior hip" refers to the hip that is non–weight-bearing in side lying. For example, when a person is lying on his right side, the left hip will be referred to as "superior." Other joints will be labeled in the same manner.

Rolling from side lying toward prone: this individual may be able to roll toward prone by flexing his superior hip and rotating his trunk toward prone. Cervical rotation and flexion of the superior shoulder may be used to assist with the roll, but these motions will make only a minor contribution to the task. The patient is likely to be more successful in rolling if he moves slowly. By moving slowly, he may avoid eliciting involuntary extension in his trunk and extremities, which could interfere with rolling toward prone.

Rolling from side lying toward supine: the patient may be able to roll toward supine by extending his superior hip and rotating his trunk toward supine. He should also retract his superior scapula, extend this shoulder, and rotate his neck in the direction of the roll. The patient may find that by moving rapidly he can elicit involuntary trunk and lower extremity extension, and that this extension assists with the roll toward supine. On the other hand, the involuntary muscle contractions may interfere with rolling.

STRENGTHENING PROGRAM: The patient could benefit from strengthening of all of his innervated musculature; but for the purposes of achieving rolling from side lying, the following muscles may be prioritized: bilateral external and internal obliques, hip flexors, deltoids, and serratus anterior.

RANGE-OF-MOTION PROGRAM: The patient has adequate range of motion and muscle flexibility for rolling. Exercises should be aimed at preventing a loss of range and flexibility.

FUNCTIONAL TRAINING PROGRAM: During initial rolling practice, the therapist can demonstrate the actions involved in rolling (described above), assist the patient to a side-lying position, and ask him to attempt to roll. Alternatively, the therapist may assist the patient into side lying and then, without any suggestions as to the technique he should use, ask him to attempt to roll. With either approach, the patient and therapist can analyze the patient's success or failure in his attempt to roll. They can then make adjustments in his technique as necessary. The patient should practice rolling forward and back from side lying, moving through larger arcs of motion as his skill and strength develop.

CHAPTER 10

Problem-Solving Exercise 10–1

This patient could be having difficulty leaning forward because he is not throwing his arm and head forcefully enough to create adequate momentum to cause his trunk to lean forward. To help him improve his performance, you could encourage him to throw his arm and head more forcefully. Verbal cuing and demonstration might help him gain a better understanding of the motions involved.

A possible alternative source of the patient's problem is that he could be holding the chair too tightly with his stabilizing arm. You should encourage him to relax this arm while he attempts a forward lean, thus enabling his trunk to move. The patient might benefit from verbal and tactile cuing to show him the muscles that he needs to relax in order to allow his trunk to fall forward. If he is fearful of

relaxing his hold on the chair, he can practice letting go (relaxing the stabilizing arm) and catching himself with the stabilizing arm while you move his trunk into a forward lean. Once he has developed some confidence in his ability to catch himself in this manner, he can practice letting go and catching while he leans his trunk forward using momentum from motions of his head and other arm.

Problem-Solving Exercise 10–2

According to the ASIA classification system, this patient has a motor level of C6 bilaterally. She has a sensory level of C8 on the left and C7 on the right. The neurological level of injury is C6.

PHYSICAL PREREQUISITES: Because this patient lacks functional triceps strength, she will need to lock her elbows to hold them in extension during the transfer. **Strength:** The strength and range prerequisites are presented in Table 10-5: To perform an even transfer without equipment, a person with a complete spinal cord injury needs adequate strength in her deltoids and shoulder external rotators. Strength in the triceps, serratus anterior, pectoralis major and latissimus dorsi will make this transfer easier to achieve. **Range of motion:** Full range of motion is required in shoulder external rotation, elbow extension, forearm supination, and wrist extension. Severe limitation in shoulder flexion range will interfere with even transfers, but full range is not required.

SKILL PREREQUISITES: The skill prerequisites for this functional task are presented in Table 10-6: To perform an even transfer without equipment, the patient must be able to tolerate an upright sitting position, perform all related wheelchair skills (position the wheelchair, engage and disengage the wheel locks, stabilize and move her body in the wheelchair, move her feet on and off of the chair's footrests, and reposition the chair's footrests and armrests), prop forward on one extended arm, prop forward on two extended arms, unweight her buttocks by leaning forward on two extended arms, control her pelvis using head and shoulder motions, lift her buttocks by pivoting forward on extended arms, lift her buttocks and move laterally, and lift her feet on and off of the bed. Because of her limited triceps strength (1/5 on the right, 2/5 on the left), she will need to be able to extend and lock her elbows using muscle substitution.

FUNCTIONAL TRAINING PROGRAM: Because the patient is unable to tolerate an upright sitting position, functional training at this point is limited to activities that can be performed with the patient in a horizontal or reclined position. In either position, the patient can practice extending and locking her elbows. If she can tolerate sitting in a recliner wheelchair, she can practice stabilizing her trunk and moving it laterally in the chair. The program should also address the development of upright sitting tolerance. (Upright sitting tolerance is addressed in Chapter 11.)

PROGRESSION OF FUNCTIONAL TRAINING PROGRAM: Once the patient can tolerate upright sitting, she can practice the following skills while sitting in a wheelchair: positioning the chair, engaging and disengaging the chair's wheel locks, moving her feet on and off of the chair's footrests, removing and replacing the armrests, and moving the trunk and buttocks in the wheelchair. She can practice the following skills, while short sitting on a mat: propping forward on one and two arms with the elbows extended, and leaning forward on two arms to unweight the buttocks. She can progress to lifting her buttocks by pivoting on her arms, and then practice lifting her buttocks and moving laterally on the mat. She can then progress to practicing transfers between a wheelchair and a mat. Once she can transfer between a wheelchair and a mat fairly well, she can practice transfers between a wheelchair and a bed. The patient should also practice lifting her feet onto a mat, and then onto a bed.

Problem-Solving Exercise 10–3

This person has T12 paraplegia, ASIA B.

The method of floor-to-wheelchair transfer that he is likely to achieve most readily is a front-approach transfer. Limited shoulder extension will interfere with a back-approach transfer, and limited hamstring flexibility will interfere with a side-approach transfer.

STRENGTHENING PROGRAM: This patient could benefit from a strengthening program for his anterior deltoids, serratus anterior, triceps, pectoralis major, and latissimus dorsi.

RANGE-OF-MOTION PROGRAM: This patient has adequate joint range of motion and muscle flexibility to perform front-approach floor-to-wheelchair transfers. Exercises should be aimed at preventing a loss of range and flexibility. Increased hamstring and shoulder flexibility may be beneficial for other functional goals.

FUNCTIONAL TRAINING: Because the patient is already independent in even and slightly uneven transfers without equipment, he is ready to work on the more advanced skills required to transfer from the floor. He may benefit from practice in stabilizing and shifting weight in the quadruped position so as to enhance his ability to control his pelvis using the head–hips relationship. With guarding and assistance as needed, he can practice the following skills: positioning himself in side sitting in front of the chair, moving into a modified quadruped position (with one hand on the floor and one on the wheelchair seat), moving into a kneeling position in front of the chair, lifting himself from the floor, and turning to land on the wheelchair seat.

Problem-Solving Exercise 10–4

Patient #1: This patient's voluntary motor function is significantly more intact in her lower extremities than in her upper extremities. Although it is possible that she could learn to extend her elbows and hold them in extension using her anterior deltoids (strength information is not provided), she is likely to transfer most successfully using her lower extremities. This could be done using a stand–pivot or squat–pivot technique.

Functional training, stand–pivot transfer: The patient can practice coming to stand and sitting back down. If sit ↔ stand is prohibitively difficult from a standard-height mat or wheelchair, the patient can practice from an elevated mat. As her ability improves, she can practice with the mat positioned at progressively lower heights. Emphasis should be placed on developing the capacity to move sit ↔ stand safely and with good balance and control. The patient can also practice static and dynamic standing balance, progressing to taking small steps and turning right and left while in the standing position to prepare for the pivot portion of the transfer. In addition to practicing the components of the transfer, the patient can practice putting these skills together while transferring with assistance. During transfers, the patient should be encouraged to use the movement strategies that she has been developing in the sit ↔ stand and dynamic standing practice, and contribute to the transfers as much as she can. As her skill develops, the assistance provided can be reduced.

Functional training, squat–pivot transfer: The patient can practice lifting her buttocks and moving laterally (scooting) from a short-sitting position on a mat. If these maneuvers are prohibitively difficult from a standard-height mat or wheelchair, the patient can practice from an elevated mat. As her ability improves, she can practice lifting and scooting with the mat at progressively lower heights. Emphasis should be placed on developing the capacity to perform these maneuvers safely and with good balance and control. In addition to practicing the components of the transfer, the patient can practice incorporating these skills into transfers with assistance. The patient should be encouraged to use the movement strategies that she has been developing while practice lifting her buttocks and scooting, and contribute to the transfer as much as she can. As her skill develops, the assistance provided can be reduced.

Whether the patient is working on stand–pivot or squat–pivot transfers, she should progress to practicing transfers between her wheelchair and a bed. If space limitations at home restrict the available options for positioning the wheelchair, transfers should be practiced with the chair oriented by the bed in a position that will be possible in the home environment. If possible, transfer practice should involve a bed that is similar in height to the patient's bed at home.

In addition to practice of the transfers themselves, functional training should involve practice setting up for the transfer (position the wheelchair, lock the wheels, move the buttocks forward on the seat, etc.), moving the lower extremities on and off of the mat/bed, and preparing to leave in the wheelchair (position the buttocks appropriately on the seat, unlock the wheels, etc.). This patient is likely to use her lower extremity and trunk musculature to lift her lower extremities on and off of the mat/bed and to position herself in the wheelchair. Skills that require manipulation (locking the wheelchair, for example) are likely to be performed using compensatory strategies that were described earlier in the chapter. During functional training, the therapist and patient should work together to find the movement strategies that will be most effective for this patient. The therapist can provide assistance at first, and reduce this assistance as the patient's performance improves.

Patient #2: This patient's voluntary motor function is significantly more intact in his right extremities than in his left extremities. He is likely to transfer most successfully using his right extremities to perform most of the work of the transfer. (The left extremities should also be incorporated, but with 3/5 strength at this point, their contribution will be limited.) This patient may transfer using a stand–pivot or squat–pivot technique. Functional training can involve strategies similar to those just described for Patient #1. The main difference will be greater reliance on the right upper extremity to assist with balance during the transfer and to manipulate the wheelchair components.

CHAPTER 11

Problem-Solving Exercise 11–1

Moving the rear wheel axles forward relative to the seat will make it easier to lift the casters from the floor.

CHAIR STABILITY: Moving the axles forward will make the chair less stable in the posterior direction. (It will be easier to tip the wheelchair over backward.)

SAFETY: Antitipping devices can be added to the chair to reduce the likelihood that the wheelchair user will accidentally tip her chair over backward. The antitipping devices will also limit the height of curb that she can negotiate.

IMPACT OF AXLE POSITION ON PROPULSION: Moving the axles forward will make propulsion easier by reducing the chair's rolling resistance, reducing its downhill turning tendency, increasing its propulsion efficiency, and making the chair easier to turn. In addition to enhancing function, these effects may reduce the risk of upper extremity overuse injuries.

IMPACT OF AXLE POSITION ON TRANSFERS: Moving the axles forward will place the wheels in a more anterior position relative to the seat. The portion of the wheels that extend higher than the wheelchair seat might now interfere with lateral transfers. The wheelchair user might also find that the increased "tippiness" of the chair makes transfers more difficult.

TO MOVE OR NOT TO MOVE (That is the question): You should probably discuss the pros and cons of moving the axle with your patient, and (with her approval) try several axle positions. She can try out each position by propelling her chair, working on curb negotiation skills, performing transfers, and performing the other activities that are a part of her typical day. Together you can determine which axle position results in the best function, safety, and comfort.

Problem-Solving Exercise 11–2

This patient is unable to maintain his hand on the joystick while he tilts the chair through its full excursion because his shoulder and elbow flexors are too weak to overcome the pull of gravity as his body's position and the joystick move relative to gravity. As he tilts back, motions that were performed in a horizontal plane (essentially in a gravity-reduced position) must be performed in an increasingly vertical direction (against gravity).

POSSIBLE EQUIPMENT CHANGES: One approach to this problem is to add an extension to the wheelchair's armrest or backrest. It should be positioned so that it blocks shoulder extension and, in doing so, prevents the hand from falling off of the joystick. A disadvantage of this approach is that it will also limit the individual's capacity to utilize shoulder extension while upright. Moreover, it will not solve the problem of his inability to push the joystick upward against gravity when he is in a reclined position.

An alternative solution to the problem is to change the joystick's position. This position change might enhance the patient's ability in this activity. Moving the joystick posteriorly from its current position may make it easier to access during a tilt because less shoulder flexion will be required to push it forward. Another equipment change to consider is the use of an alternative input device such as a toggle switch or proximity switch to perform pressure reliefs.

STRENGTHENING PROGRAM: The patient may benefit from a strengthening program for his deltoids (particularly the anterior deltoid), elbow flexors, and serratus anterior.

FUNCTIONAL TRAINING ACTIVITY: The patient can practice tilting and returning to upright over increasing arcs of motion. As his strength and skill increase, he can increase the excursion of the chair's tilt. This practice can be done in conjunction with trials in equipment changes.

Problem-Solving Exercise 11–3

SAFE TECHNIQUE FOR DESCENDING STEEP CURB CUTS: This individual should be able to learn to descend curb cuts in a wheelie.

PHYSICAL PREREQUISITES: The strength and range prerequisites are presented in Table 11-12: Adequate strength and range of motion in finger flexion, elbow flexion and extension, and shoulder and scapular motions.

STRENGTH AND RANGE-OF-MOTION PROGRAM: Because this individual has normal strength and range in his upper extremities, he will not need a therapeutic exercise program to develop physical prerequisites for this skill. (Neither large amounts of strength nor a greater than normal range are needed.)

FUNCTIONAL TRAINING PROGRAM: The skill prerequisites for this functional task are presented in Table 11-13: To descend curb cuts in a wheelie position, the patient must be able to assume a wheelie position, maintain his balance point, glide forward, and control his wheelchair as it descends a slope in a wheelie. The functional training program should be tailored to the individual's needs, addressing areas of deficit in prerequisite skills. If the patient has none of the skill prerequisites, functional training should start with the most basic: assuming and maintaining a balanced wheelie position. When the patient is able to perform these maneuvers, he can practice gliding in a wheelie. After he has mastered that skill, he can work on descending ramps in a wheelie. This practice on ramps should start with mild inclines and progress to steep inclines as the patient's skill develops. Once he has developed some skill in descending steep inclines in a wheelie, he can practice outside on real curb cuts. In all activities, the therapist should guard the patient until he has developed his skill to the point where he can perform safely without guarding. Specific suggestions for each prerequisite skill are included in Chapter 11.

Problem-Solving Exercise 11–4

ADVANTAGES OF POWER-ASSIST WHEELS

For this individual, they

- Will allow propulsion with less strain on the upper extremities, resulting in more comfortable propulsion and possibly reducing the risk of overuse injuries.
- May enable her to negotiate long distances, uneven surfaces, inclines, and other mild obstacles in the community without assistance.
- May enable her to utilize public transportation.
- May enhance community reintegration by allowing independent mobility in a wheelchair and independent use of public transportation.

DISADVANTAGES OF POWER-ASSIST WHEELS

For this individual, they

- Add to the wheelchair's width, which would increase the dimension of clear space that this patient will require in doorways and narrow passages.
- Add weight to the wheelchair. (Because this individual uses public transportation, the weight of the wheels is less of a consideration than it would be for a person who uses a car.)
- Increase cost.
- Increase the difficulty of propulsion in the event of battery failure.

OBTAINING TRIAL EQUIPMENT: A wheelchair vendor or manufacturer's representative may provide power-assist wheels to trial. These individuals could also provide you with instruction in their use (adjustment of pushrim sensitivity and power assist, battery charging, etc.) if you are not already familiar with the equipment.

FUNCTIONAL TRAINING: Starting in a relatively large area free of obstacles, the patient can practice propelling with close supervision. As her skill develops, she can practice propelling in more confined spaces and negotiating obstacles. If possible (depending on the equipment), the therapist should adjust the pushrims' sensitivity and the power that the wheels deliver with each push. This adjustment should be tailored to the individual's needs and preferences to optimize her performance and satisfaction with the equipment.

In addition to practicing propulsion, the patient should practice manipulating the wheels' controls (on/off, power level). If she will be unable to remove and replace the wheels from the chair and manage the battery and charger, she should learn how to instruct others in these tasks.

OTHER EQUIPMENT OPTION TO DISCUSS: A power wheelchair could also enable the patient to be mobile in her community and avoid upper extremity strain.

CHAPTER 12

Problem-Solving Exercise 12–1

MOST LIKELY CAUSE OF THIS PATIENT'S KNEE INSTABILITY: This patient's knee instability during late stance is most likely the result of plantarflexor weakness. With 2/5 strength, the plantarflexors of the stance leg are unable to stabilize the tibia as the patient's center of gravity passes anterior to the ankle. The resulting forward collapse of the tibia (excessive dorsiflexion) causes the knee to flex.

AFOs OR KAFOs? AFOs would be most beneficial for this patient. Even though the gait deviation that is most evident is excessive *knee* flexion, the most likely cause of this problem is his inability to stabilize his *ankles* during late stance. AFOs could provide the needed stabilization at the ankles, which in turn would prevent the excessive knee flexion during late stance. KAFOs are not indicated because they are heavier than AFOs and would unnecessarily restrict knee motion.

ORTHOTIC CONTROL: The AFOs should stop dorsiflexion in about 5 to 10 degrees of dorsiflexion. The dorsiflexion stop will prevent excessive dorsiflexion during late stance, and in doing so will prevent tibial collapse and excessive knee flexion. Allowing some dorsiflexion will allow a more normal progression of the body's weight past the ankle. Plantar flexion should be left free. Because the dorsiflexors are strong, neither a plantar flexion stop nor a dorsiflexion assist is indicated. Leaving plantar flexion unrestricted will allow a more normal gait pattern.

Ideally, the stop will be adjustable. This will allow the position of the stop to be fine-tuned to optimize the individual's gait pattern.

Problem-Solving Exercise 12–2

This patient is jackknifing. This uncontrolled flexion at the hips occurs when her center of gravity falls anterior to her hips. This position of the center of gravity causes the ground reaction force to pass anterior to the hips, creating a flexion moment at these joints. Because the patient's hip extensors are not innervated, the hips flex.

MOVEMENT STRATEGY FOR BALANCED STANDING: The patient should stand with her pelvis forward and her shoulders back. She can use scapular motions and the head–hips relationship to achieve and maintain this posture: standing in the parallel bars, she can push her pelvis forward by retracting her scapulae and moving her head posteriorly.

POSSIBLE RANGE-OF-MOTION LIMITATION: Limited hip extension could contribute to this problem. Hip flexion contractures would make it impossible for the patient to stand in the position of stability: hips forward, shoulders back. Ankle plantarflexion contractures could also contribute to this problem. (The following paragraph explains how inadequate dorsiflexion can cause jackknifing.)

ORTHOTIC ADJUSTMENT: The patient is jackknifing because she is not maintaining her pelvis in a forward position. One possible cause of this problem is that the ankles of her orthoses are not positioned in enough dorsiflexion. If the ankles are not dorsiflexed enough, the pelvis will be positioned too posteriorly, making it difficult or impossible to assume or maintain a stable standing posture. To place an ankle in a more dorsiflexed position, you should:

1. Turn the set screws in the orthotic ankles' *anterior* channels counterclockwise. Each ankle has two

anterior channels, one medial and one lateral. When you make the adjustment, be sure to turn the set screws in the medial and lateral channels of each ankle the same amount. (Turn each screw one full turn counterclockwise, for example.) Turn the screws counterclockwise enough to allow the ankle to dorsiflex to the desired position.

2. Reposition the ankle to the more dorsiflexed position.

3. Turn the set screws in the *posterior* channels clockwise to hold the ankle in the new position. To avoid placing unnecessary stress on the orthotic ankle joint, turn the set screws in the medial and lateral posterior channels equally, and with the same number of turns that were performed on the screws of the anterior channels.

4. Repeat the process with the other orthosis. Be sure to adjust the right and left orthoses to the same degree of dorsiflexion.

GUARDING: To guard the patient, you should stand behind her in the parallel bars with one hand on her pelvis and one on her shoulder. When she starts to jackknife, you should push her pelvis forward and pull her upper trunk back. These forces will return her to a balanced standing posture.

Problem-Solving Exercise 12–3

POSSIBLE RANGE-OF-MOTION AND MUSCLE FLEXIBILITY LIMITATIONS: It is possible that the patient lacks adequate range of motion in scapular abduction, shoulder flexion and horizontal adduction, elbow extension, or hip flexion. A more likely cause of this patient's difficulty is inadequate hamstring flexibility. Hamstring tightness will limit hip flexion while the knees are locked in extension. This limitation will make it impossible for this individual to elevate his pelvis fully (Figure 12-19C) to a position in which his weight is supported more on his legs than on his arms. If he must support a large portion of his weight on his arms, the patient will have difficulty lifting one arm and balancing on the other arm.

POSSIBLE STRENGTH LIMITATIONS: Coming to stand from the floor requires adequate strength in scapular protraction, shoulder flexion and horizontal adduction, and elbow extension. This musculature must also be strong for ambulation with KAFOs and Lofstrand crutches. Because this patient walks independently, it is unlikely that he is weak in any of this musculature.

SKILL PREREQUISITES: To lift a hand and grasp a crutch while in plantigrade, the patient must have the following skills in plantigrade: weight shifting (dynamic balance), balance with one hand on the floor, walk hands toward the feet, grasp a crutch.

FUNCTIONAL TRAINING: The program design will depend on the individual's performance of the task.

- If the patient is attempting to lift a hand and grasp a crutch without first lifting his pelvis high enough to shift weight off of his hands, he should be instructed to walk his hands back further before attempting to grasp the crutch. He can then practice this skill.
- If the patient lifts his pelvis to an appropriate position but loses his balance when he lifts a hand, he may benefit from practice shifting his weight and maintaining dynamic balance in this position. Once he has developed the capacity to shift his weight, he can practice maintaining his balance while he lifts a hand and reaches in various directions.

PROGRAM PROGRESSION: Once the patient has learned to position his pelvis properly in plantigrade and has developed dynamic balance while lifting one hand in this position, he can practice grasping and positioning his crutch. He can also practice the other prerequisite skills for coming to stand from the floor, separately or in combination.

CHAPTER 13

Problem-Solving Exercise 13–1

The patient is asking about his capacity to have erections and use them in intercourse. Your response should address several issues:

- The typical impact of a complete T5 spinal cord injury on erectile function. (Psychogenic erections are likely to be absent, reflexive erections are likely to occur. Erections may or may not be rigid enough or last long enough for intercourse.)
- The variability between individuals in their erectile function after spinal cord injury.
- The potential for the individual to increase his capacity for erections by discovering and utilizing stimuli that cause, enhance, and prolong his erections.
- The availability of treatments for erectile dysfunction after spinal cord injury.

Your explanations should be provided in language that is both comprehensible and comfortable for the patient. You should be flexible in your choice of words and presentation style. For some individuals, a formal discussion using clinical terms will be most appropriate. Other individuals will be more receptive to, and better able to understand, an informal discussion using casual language.

If your patient is not already involved in a sexual rehabilitation program, you should refer him to the appropriate clinicians. Your involvement in the various components of the program will depend on your level of comfort and expertise, as well as the role expectations in your facility.

Problem-Solving Exercise 13–2

Your patient laughed when telling you that she urinated during sexual activity with her husband. The laughter might have been the result of nervousness or embarrassment about the topic, or your patient could be one of those amazingly resilient people who can find humor in any situation. Whatever the reason for the laughter, you can assume that your patient and her husband are concerned about the incident.

Your patient could benefit from specific suggestions for avoiding urinary accidents during sex. To reduce the risk of urinary accidents, she can empty her bladder immediately prior to engaging in sexual activity. She may also wish to avoid drinking large volumes of liquid when she knows that she might soon be engaging in sexual activity. If urinary accidents occur despite these precautions, she should note whether certain stimuli appear to be most likely to elicit bladder emptying and should avoid these particular stimuli.

If your patient and her husband are not already involved in a sexual rehabilitation program, you should refer them to the appropriate clinicians. Your involvement in the various components of the program will depend on your level of comfort and expertise as well as the role expectations in your facility.

CHAPTER 14

Problem-Solving Exercise 14–1

Considering the level of this patient's paraplegia, his bladder is most likely areflexive: the micturition reflex is absent. The detrusor remains flaccid and does not contract in response to filling. As a result, large volumes of urine are retained.

This individual's habit of allowing large volumes of urine to build in his bladder could cause overdistention, with resulting damage to the bladder wall. It could also cause urinary tract infections, reflux into the ureters, hydronephrosis, and kidney damage.

Problem-Solving Exercise 14–2

Because her spinal cord injury is incomplete (ASIA C) and recent, this patient might regain voluntary control of defecation. On the other hand, she might not. If she does not regain voluntary control, however, she should be able to minimize the likelihood of incontinent episodes through a regular bowel program. Your response to the patient's concerns should include an explanation of both of these possible outcomes (return of voluntary control or prevention of incontinence through a bowel program).

Problem-Solving Exercise 14–3

SAFETY ISSUES: Potential for skin damage from prolonged sitting on toilet seat, injury from fall during transfers to and from toilet or while performing bowel care.

EQUIPMENT: A padded toilet seat will help prevent skin breakdown. If the seat is level with the top of the wheelchair cushion, transfers will be easier. In addition, grab bars may enhance the patient's safety. If the patient's bathroom at home will have a roll-in shower, he may want to consider a shower/commode chair.

THERAPEUTIC ACTIVITIES IN PHYSICAL THERAPY: Functional training in support of this patient's goal includes toilet transfers (or shower/commode chair transfers), leg management, static sitting balance, and dynamic sitting balance while reaching in various directions including reaching around to the anus. Dressing and undressing are likely to be practiced in occupational therapy. In physical therapy, the patient can practice static and dynamic balance activities in support of this ADL training.

CHAPTER 15

Problem-Solving Exercise 15–1

APPLICABLE LAW: The Americans with Disabilities Act applies in this situation. This law states that any new renovations must be accessible to people with disabilities. The Fair Housing Amendments Act *does not* apply. This law states that all of the public and common areas in the building (in this case, the mail room or lobby) must be along an accessible route, but it does not require all of the facilities themselves to be accessible.

TO OBTAIN A MAILBOX WITHIN REACH: Probably the most appropriate first step for your friend to take would be to inform the building management about the problem. If they refuse to provide an accessible mailbox, your friend can contact the U.S. Department of Justice.

Problem-Solving Exercise 15–2

RAMP LENGTHS:

- Front door: The ramp's horizontal distance should be 36 feet.
- Carport door: The ramp's horizontal distance should be 24 feet.

PLATFORMS: A ramp at either location would require a platform (landing) at the top and bottom. Because a ramp at the front door would be over 30 feet long, it should also have a landing partway down.

CONSIDERATIONS RELEVANT TO CHOICE OF RAMP LOCATION include available space, esthetics, presence or absence of an accessible route to and from the potential ramp site, proximity to the vehicle parking spot, characteristics of the doors (width, threshold, hardware, etc.), presence or absence of an accessible route within the home from each of the doors.

POSSIBLE ALTERNATIVES:

- Earth berm with asphalt or concrete surface (An earth berm is a mound of dirt. It can be placed in an appropriate location and constructed to serve as a ramp.)
- Platform lift or elevator
- Alternate doorway (Another door may be closer to the ground.)

References

CHAPTER 1

1. Jette AM. Toward a common language for function, disability, and health. *Phys Ther*. 2006, 86(5):726–734.
2. World Health Organization. International Classification of Functioning, Disability and Health: ICF. Geneva, Switzerland: World Health Organization, 2001.
3. World Health Organization. Towards a Common Language for Functioning, Disability and Health: ICF. 2002, http://www.who.int/classifications/icf/training/icfbeginnersguide.pdf. Accessed 9/9/08.
4. Stucki G. International classification of functioning, disability, and health (ICF): a promising framework and classification for rehabilitation medicine. *Am J Phys Med Rehabil*. 2005, 84(10): 733–740.
5. Stucki G, Ewert T, Cieza A. Value and application of the ICF in rehabilitation medicine. *Disabil Rehabil*. 2003, 25(11/12): 628–634.
6. Guccione AA. Physical therapy diagnosis and the relationship between impairments and function. *Phys Ther*. 1991, 71(7): 499–503.
7. Jette AM. Physical disablement concepts for physical therapy research and practice. *Phys Ther*. 1994, 74(5):380–386.
8. Nagi S. Disability concepts revisited: implications for prevention. In: Pope A, Tarlov A, eds. *Disability in America: Toward a National Agenda for Prevention*. Washington, DC: National Academy Press, 1991:309–327.
9. Pope A, Tarlov A, eds. *Disability in America: Toward a National Agenda for Prevention*. Washington, DC: National Academy Press, 1991.
10. Rothstein J, ed. Guide to physical therapist practice: second edition. *Phys Ther*. 2001, 81(1):S6–765.
11. Dahl TH. International classification of functioning, disability and health: an introduction and discussion of its potential impact on rehabilitation services and research. *J Rehabil Med*. 2002, 34(5):201–204.
12. World Health Organization. ICF Checklist, Version 2.1a, Clinician Form for International Classification of Functioning, Disability and Health. 2003, http://www.who.int/classifications/icf/training/icfchecklist.pdf. Accessed 9/23/08.
13. Steiner WA, Ryser L, Huber E, Uebelhart D, Aeschlimann A, Stucki G. Use of the ICF model as a clinical problem-solving tool in physical therapy and rehabilitation medicine. *Phys Ther*. 2002, 82(11):1098–1107.
14. Donovan WH, Carter RE, Bedbrook GM, Young JS, Griffiths ER. Incidence of medical complications in spinal cord injury: patients in specialised, compared with non-specialised centres. *Paraplegia*. 1984, 22(5):282–290.
15. Oakes DD, Wilmot CB, Hall KM, Sherck JP. Benefits of early admission to a comprehensive trauma center for patients with spinal cord injury. *Arch Phys Med Rehabil*. 1990, 71(9):637–643.
16. Scivoletto G, Morganti B, Molinari M. Early versus delayed inpatient spinal cord injury rehabilitation: an Italian study. *Arch Phys Med Rehabil*. 2005, 86(3):512–516.
17. Tator CH, Duncan EG, Edmonds VE, Lapczak LI, Andrews DF. Neurological recovery, mortality and length of stay after acute spinal cord injury associated with changes in management. *Paraplegia*. 1995, 33(5):254–262.
18. Post MWM, Dallmeijer AJ, Angenot ELD, van Asbeck FWA, van der Woude LHV. Duration and functional outcome of spinal cord injury rehabilitation in the Netherlands. *J Rehabil Res Dev*. 2005, 42(3 Suppl 1):75–86.
19. Atrice M, Morrison S, McDowell S, Ackerman P, Foy T. Traumatic spinal cord injury. In: Umphred D, ed. *Neurological Rehabilitation*. 3rd ed. St. Louis: Mosby, 2007:484–532.
20. Durán FS, Lugo L, Ramírez L, Eusse E. Effects of an exercise program on the rehabilitation of patients with spinal cord injury. *Arch Phys Med Rehabil*. 2001, 82(10):1349–1354.
21. Hicks AL, Martin KA, Ditor DS, et al. Long-term exercise training in persons with spinal cord injury: effects on strength, arm ergometry performance and psychological well-being. *Spinal Cord*. 2003, 41(1):34–43.

CHAPTER 2

1. National Spinal Cord Injury Statistical Center. Spinal Cord Injury: Facts and Figures at a Glance. 2008, http://www.spinalcord.uab.edu. Accessed 12/15/08.
2. Jackson AB, Dijkers M, Devivo MJ, Poczatek RB. A demographic profile of new traumatic spinal cord injuries: change and stability over 30 years. *Arch Phys Med Rehabil*. 2004, 85(11): 1740–1748.
3. National Spinal Cord Injury Statistical Center. Annual Report for the Model Spinal Cord Injury Care Systems. http://www.spinalcord.uab.edu. Accessed 12/15/08.
4. Rosse C, Gaddum-Rosse P. *Hollinshead's Textbook of Anatomy*. 5th ed. Philadelphia: Lippincott-Raven, 1997.
5. Yashon D. *Spinal Injury*. 2nd ed. Norwalk, CT: Appleton Century Crofts, 1986.
6. de Groot J, Chusid J. *Correlative Neuroanatomy*. 20th ed. East Norwalk, CT: Appleton & Lange, 1988.

7. Denis F. The three column spine and its significance in the classification of acute thoracolumbar spinal injuries. *Spine*. 1983, 8(8):817–831.

8. Haines D, Mihailoff G, Yezierski R. The spinal cord. In: Haines D, ed. *Fundamental Neuroscience for Basic and Clinical Applications*. 3rd ed. Philadelphia: Churchill Livingstone Elsevier, 2006:142–157.

9. Gilman S, Newman S. *Manter and Gatz's Essentials of Clinical Neuroanatomy and Neurophysiology*. Philadelphia: F. A. Davis, 2003.

10. Burt A. *Textbook of Neuroanatomy*. Philadelphia: Saunders, 1993.

11. Marieb E. *Human Anatomy and Physiology*. 3rd ed. Redwood City, CA: Benjamin/Cummings, 1995.

12. Wynsberghe D, Noback C, Carola R. *Human Anatomy and Physiology*. 3rd ed. New York: McGraw-Hill, 1995.

13. Tator CH, Koyanagi I. Vascular mechanisms in the pathophysiology of human spinal cord injury. *J Neurosurg*. 1997, 86(3):483–492.

14. Brust J. Circulation of the brain. In: Kandel ER, Schwartz JH, Jessell TM, eds. *Principles of Neural Science*. 4th ed. New York: McGraw-Hill, 2000:1302–1316.

15. Kakulas BA. Neuropathology: the foundation for new treatments in spinal cord injury. *Spinal Cord*. 2004, 42(10):549–563.

16. Schmitt K, Niederer P, Walz F. *Trauma Biomechanics: Introduction to Accidental Injury*. New York: Springer, 2004.

17. Aflatoon K, Carbone J. Lower cervical spine injury. In: Frymoyer JW, Wiesel SW, eds. *The Adult and Pediatric Spine*. Vol 2. Philadelphia: Lippincott Williams & Wilkins, 2004:659–669.

18. Sheerin F. Spinal cord injury: causation and pathophysiology. *Emerg Nurse*. 2005, 12(9):29–38.

19. Okonkwo DO, Stone JR. Basic science of closed head injuries and spinal cord injuries. *Clin Sports Med*. 2003, 22(3):467–481.

20. Beric A, Dimitrijevic MR, Light JK. A clinical syndrome of rostral and caudal spinal injury: neurological, neurophysiological and urodynamic evidence for occult sacral lesion. *J Neurol Neurosurg Psychiatry*. 1987, 50(5):600–606.

21. Hendey GW, Wolfson AB, Mower WR, Hoffman JR. Spinal cord injury without radiographic abnormality: results of the National Emergency X-Radiography Utilization Study in blunt cervical trauma. *J Trauma*. 2002, 53(1):1–4.

22. Cook P. Radiology of the spine and spinal cord injury. In: Illis L, ed. *Spinal Cord Dysfunction: Assessment*. New York: Oxford University Press, 1988:41–103.

23. Launay F, Leet AI, Sponseller PD. Pediatric spinal cord injury without radiographic abnormality: a meta-analysis. *Clin Orthop*. 2005, 433:166–170.

24. Pang D, Pollack IF. Spinal cord injury without radiographic abnormality in children—the SCIWORA syndrome. *J Trauma*. 1989, 29(5):654–664.

25. Smith JA, Siegel JH, Siddiqi SQ. Spine and spinal cord injury in motor vehicle crashes: a function of change in velocity and energy dissipation on impact with respect to the direction of crash. *J Trauma*. 2005, 59(1):117–131.

26. Fine PR, Kuhlemeier KV, DeVivo MJ, Stover SL. Spinal cord injury: an epidemiologic perspective. *Paraplegia*. 1979, 17(2): 237–250.

27. Meyer P, ed. *Surgery of Spine Trauma*. New York: Churchill Livingstone, 1989.

28. Kennedy E, Stover SL, Fine PR. *Spinal Cord Injury: The Facts and Figures*. Birmingham, AL: The University of Alabama Spinal Cord Injury Statistical Center, 1986.

29. Waters RL, Sie IH, Adkins RH, Yakura JS. The neuropathology of violence-induced spinal cord injury. *Top Spinal Cord Inj Rehabil*. 1999, 4(3):23–28.

30. Ditunno JF, Cohen ME, Formal C, Whiteneck GG. Functional outcomes. In: Stover SL, DeLisa JA, Whiteneck GG, eds. *Spinal Cord Injury: Clinical Outcomes from the Model Systems*. Gaithersburg, MD: Aspen, 1995:170–184.

31. Galli RL, Spaite DW, Simon RR. *Emergency Orthopedics: The Spine*. Norwalk, CT: Appleton & Lange, 1989.

32. Rieser T, Mudiyam R, Waters R. Orthopedic evaluation of spinal cord injury and management of vertebral fractures. In: Adkins H, ed. *Spinal Cord Injury*. New York: Churchill Livingstone, 1985:1–35.

33. Aflatoon K, Carbone JJ. Cauda equina syndrome with acute lumbar burst fracture. *Top Spinal Cord Inj Rehabil*. 2002, 8(2):1–8.

34. Lewandroski K, McLain R. Thoracolumbar fractures: evaluation, classification, and treatment. In: Frymoyer JW, Wiesel SW, eds. *The Adult and Pediatric Spine*. Vol 2. 3rd ed. Philadelphia: Lippincott Williams & Wilkins, 2004:817–843.

35. Go BK, DeVivo MJ, Richards JS. The epidemiology of spinal cord injury. In: Stover SL, DeLisa JA, Whiteneck GG, eds. *Spinal Cord Injury: Clinical Outcomes from the Model Systems*. Gaithersburg, MD: Aspen, 1995:21–55.

36. Freedman M, Vaccaro A, Daffner S, Fried G. Rehabilitation of the patient with tetraplegia and paraplegia. In: Frymoyer JW, Wiesel SW, eds. *The Adult and Pediatric Spine*. Philadelphia: Lippincott Williams & Wilkins, 2004:619–632.

37. Waters RL, Sie I, Adkins RH, Yakura JS. Injury pattern effect on motor recovery after traumatic spinal cord injury. *Arch Phys Med Rehabil*. 1995, 76(5):440–443.

38. Rossignol S, Schwab M, Schwartz M, Fehlings MG. Spinal cord injury: time to move? *J Neurosci*. 2007, 27(44):11782–11792.

39. Tator CH, Fehlings MG. Review of the secondary injury theory of acute spinal cord trauma with emphasis on vascular mechanisms. *J Neurosurg*. 1991, 75(1):15–26.

40. Hughes J. Pathological changes after spinal cord injury. In: Illis L, ed. *Spinal Cord Dysfunction: Assessment*. New York: Oxford University Press, 1988:34–40.

41. Iizuka H, Yamamoto H, Iwasaki Y, et al. Evolution of tissue damage in compressive spinal cord injury in rats. *J Neurosurg*. 1987, 66(4):595–603.

42. Springer JE, Azbill RD, Mark RJ, et al. 4–hydroxynonenal, a lipid peroxidation product, rapidly accumulates following traumatic spinal cord injury and inhibits glutamate uptake. *J Neurochem*. 1997, 68(6):2469–2476.

43. Fleming JC, Norenberg MD, Ramsay DA, et al. The cellular inflammatory response in human spinal cords after injury. *Brain*. 2006, 129(Pt 12):3249–3269.

44. Hausmann ON. Post-traumatic inflammation following spinal cord injury. *Spinal Cord*. 2003, 41(7):369–378.

45. Waxman SG. Demyelination in spinal cord injury. *J Neurol Sci*. 1989, 91(1–2):1–14.

46. O'Brien MF, Lenke LG, Lou J, et al. Astrocyte response and transforming growth factor-beta localization in acute spinal cord injury. *Spine*. 1994, 19(20):2321–2329, discussion 2330.

47. Young W. Secondary injury mechanisms in acute spinal cord injury. *J Emerg Med*. 1993, 11(Suppl 1):13–22.

48. Zhang Z, Krebs CJ, Guth L. Experimental analysis of progressive necrosis after spinal cord trauma in the rat: etiological role of the inflammatory response. *Exp Neurol*. 1997, 143(1):141–152.

49. Demediuk P, Daly MP, Faden AI. Effect of impact trauma on neurotransmitter and nonneurotransmitter amino acids in rat spinal cord. *J Neurochem*. 1989, 52(5):1529–1536.

50. Cotman CW, Nieto-Sampedro M. Progress in facilitating the recovery of function after central nervous system trauma. *Ann N Y Acad Sci*. 1985, 457:83–104.

51. Fredericks C. Disorders of the spinal cord. In: Fredericks C, Saladin L, eds. *Pathophysiology of the Motor Systems: Principles and Clinical Presentations*. Philadelphia: F. A. Davis, 1996: 394–423.

52. Young W, Ranshhoff J. Acute spinal cord injuries: experimental therapy, pathophysiological mechanisms, and recovery of function. In: Sherk H, Dunn E, Eismont F, eds. *The Cervical Spine*. 2nd ed. Philadelphia: Lippincott, 1989:464–495.

53. Anthes DL, Theriault E, Tator CH. Ultrastructural evidence for arteriolar vasospasm after spinal cord trauma. *Neurosurgery.* 1996, 39(4):804–814.

54. Northrup B, Alderman J. Nonsurgical treatment. In: Sherk H, Dunn E, Eismont F, eds. *The Cervical Spine.* 2nd ed. Philadelphia: Lippincott, 1989.

55. Zhang Z, Guth L. Experimental spinal cord injury: Wallerian degeneration in the dorsal column is followed by revascularization, glial proliferation, and nerve regeneration. *Exp Neurol.* 1997, 147(1):159–171.

56. Stys PK. Anoxic and ischemic injury of myelinated axons in CNS white matter: from mechanistic concepts to therapeutics. *J Cereb Blood Flow Metab.* 1998, 18(1):2–25.

57. Carlson SL, Parrish ME, Springer JE, et al. Acute inflammatory response in spinal cord following impact injury. *Exp Neurol.* 1998, 151(1):77–88.

58. Bethea JR, Castro M, Keane RW, et al. Traumatic spinal cord injury induces nuclear factor-kappaB activation. *J Neurosci.* 1998, 18(9):3251–3260.

59. Choi DW, Rothman SM. The role of glutamate neurotoxicity in hypoxic–ischemic neuronal death. *Annu Rev Neurosci.* 1990, 13:171–182.

60. Faden AI, Simon RP. A potential role for excitotoxins in the pathophysiology of spinal cord injury. *Ann Neurol.* 1988, 23(6):623–626.

61. Tator CH. Biology of neurological recovery and functional restoration after spinal cord injury. *Neurosurgery.* 1998, 42(4):696–707, discussion 707–698.

62. Yanase M, Sakou T, Fukuda T. Role of N-methyl-D-aspartate receptor in acute spinal cord injury. *J Neurosurg.* 1995, 83(5):884–888.

63. Isaac L, Pejic L. Secondary mechanisms of spinal cord injury. *Surg Neurol.* 1995, 43(5):484–485.

64. Leybaert L, de Hemptinne A. Changes of intracellular free calcium following mechanical injury in a spinal cord slice preparation. *Exp Brain Res.* 1996, 112(3):392–402.

65. Balentine JD. Spinal cord trauma: in search of the meaning of granular axoplasm and vesicular myelin. *J Neuropathol Exp Neurol.* 1988, 47(2):77–92.

66. Banik NL, Matzelle DC, Gantt-Wilford G, Osborne A, Hogan EL. Increased calpain content and progressive degradation of neurofilament protein in spinal cord injury. *Brain Res.* 1997, 752(1–2):301–306.

67. Banik NL, Shields DC, Ray S, et al. Role of calpain in spinal cord injury: effects of calpain and free radical inhibitors. *Ann N Y Acad Sci.* 1998, 844:131–137.

68. Emery E, Aldana P, Bunge MB, et al. Apoptosis after traumatic human spinal cord injury. *J Neurosurg.* 1998, 89(6):911–920.

69. Lou J, Lenke LG, Ludwig FJ, O'Brien MF. Apoptosis as a mechanism of neuronal cell death following acute experimental spinal cord injury. *Spinal Cord.* 1998, 36(10):683–690.

70. Shuman SL, Bresnahan JC, Beattie MS. Apoptosis of microglia and oligodendrocytes after spinal cord contusion in rats. *J Neurosci Res.* 1997, 50(5):798–808.

71. Bohlman H, Boada E. Fractures and dislocations of the lower cervical spine. In: Sherk H, Dunn F, Eismont J, eds. *The Cervical Spine.* 2nd ed. Philadelphia: J. B. Lippincott, 1989.

72. Ditunno JF, Little JW, Tessler A, Burns AS. Spinal shock revisited: a four-phase model. *Spinal Cord.* 2004, 42(7):383–395.

73. Silver JR. Early autonomic dysreflexia. *Spinal Cord.* 2000, 38(4):229–233.

74. Little JW, Ditunno JF Jr, Stiens SA, Harris RM. Incomplete spinal cord injury: neuronal mechanisms of motor recovery and hyperreflexia *Arch Phys Med Rehabil.* 1999, 80(5):587–599.

75. Jankowska E, Hammar I. Spinal interneurones, how can studies in animals contribute to the understanding of spinal interneuronal systems in man? *Brain Res Rev.* 2002, 40(1–3):19–28.

76. Lapointe NP, Ung RV, Guertin PA. Plasticity in sublesionally located neurons following spinal cord injury. *J Neurophysiol.* 2007, 98(5):2497–2500.

77. Carro-Juarez M, Rodriguez-Manzo G. The spinal pattern generator for ejaculation. *Brain Res Rev.* 2008, 58(1):106–120.

78. Burns AS, Ditunno JF. Establishing prognosis and maximizing functional outcomes after spinal cord injury: a review of current and future directions in rehabilitation management. *Spine.* 2001, 26(Suppl 24):S137–S145.

79. Kirshblum S, Millis S, McKinley W, Tulsky D. Late neurologic recovery after traumatic spinal cord injury. *Arch Phys Med Rehabil.* 2004, 85(11):1811–1817.

80. Kirshblum SC, O'Connor KC. Predicting neurologic recovery in traumatic cervical spinal cord injury. *Arch Phys Med Rehabil.* 1998, 79(11):1456–1466.

81. Pollard ME, Apple DF. Factors associated with improved neurologic outcomes in patients with incomplete tetraplegia. *Spine.* 2003, 28(1):33–39.

82. Waters RL, Adkins RH, Yakura JS, Sie I. Motor and sensory recovery following complete tetraplegia. *Arch Phys Med Rehabil.* 1993, 74(3):242–247.

83. Waters RL, Yakura JS, Adkins RH, Sie I. Recovery following complete paraplegia. *Arch Phys Med Rehabil.* 1992, 73(9):784–789.

84. Ditunno JF Jr, Stover SL, Freed MM, Ahn JH. Motor recovery of the upper extremities in traumatic quadriplegia: a multicenter study. *Arch Phys Med Rehabil.* 1992, 73(5):431–436.

85. Waters RL, Adkins RH, Yakura JS, Sie I. Motor and sensory recovery following incomplete paraplegia. *Arch Phys Med Rehabil.* 1994, 75(1):67–72.

86. Waters RL, Adkins RH, Yakura JS, Sie I. Motor and sensory recovery following incomplete tetraplegia. *Arch Phys Med Rehabil.* 1994, 75(3):306–311.

87. Piepmeier JM, Jenkins NR. Late neurological changes following traumatic spinal cord injury. *J Neurosurg.* 1988, 69(3):399–402.

88. Mange KC, Ditunno JF Jr, Herbison GJ, Jaweed MM. Recovery of strength at the zone of injury in motor complete and motor incomplete cervical spinal cord injured patients. *Arch Phys Med Rehabil.* 1990, 71(8):562–565.

89. Little JW, Burns SP, James JJ, Stiens SA. Neurologic recovery and neurologic decline after spinal cord injury. *Phys Med Rehabil Clin N Am.* 2000, 11(1):73–89.

90. Mange KC, Marino RJ, Gregory PC, et al. Course of motor recovery in the zone of partial preservation in spinal cord injury. *Arch Phys Med Rehabil.* 1992, 73(5):437–441.

91. Wu L, Marino RJ, Herbison GJ, Ditunno JF Jr. Recovery of zero-grade muscles in the zone of partial preservation in motor complete quadriplegia. *Arch Phys Med Rehabil.* 1992, 73(1):40–43.

92. Blaustein DM, Zafonte R, Thomas D, et al. Predicting recovery of motor complete quadriplegic patients. 24 hour v 72 hour motor index scores. *Am J Phys Med Rehabil.* 1993, 72(5):306–311.

93. Consortium for Spinal Cord Medicine. *Outcomes Following Traumatic Spinal Cord Injury: Clinical Practice Guidelines for Health-Care Professionals.* Washington, DC: Paralyzed Veterans of America, 1999.

94. Consortium for Spinal Cord Medicine. *Early Acute Management in Adults with Spinal Cord Injury: A Clinical Practice Guideline for Health-Care Providers* Washington, DC: Paralyzed Veterans of America, 2008.

95. Marino RJ, Ditunno JF Jr, Donovan WH, Maynard F Jr. Neurologic recovery after traumatic spinal cord injury: data from the Model Spinal Cord Injury Systems. *Arch Phys Med Rehabil.* 1999, 80(11):1391–1396.

96. Poynton AR, O'Farrell DA, Shannon F, et al. Sparing of sensation to pin prick predicts recovery of a motor segment after injury to the spinal cord. *J Bone Joint Surg Br.* 1997, 79(6):952–954.

97. American Spinal Injury Association. *Standards for Neurological Classification of Spinal Injury Patients*. Atlanta: American Spinal Injury Association, 1989.

98. Ditunno JF Jr, Cohen ME, Hauck WW, et al. Recovery of upper-extremity strength in complete and incomplete tetraplegia: a multicenter study. *Arch Phys Med Rehabil*. 2000, 81(4):389–393.

99. Geisler FH, Coleman WP, Grieco G, Poonian D. Measurements and recovery patterns in a multicenter study of acute spinal cord injury. *Spine*. 2001, 26(Suppl 24):S68–86.

100. Pagliacci MC, Celani MG, Zampolini M, et al. An Italian survey of traumatic spinal cord injury. The Gruppo Italiano Studio Epidemiologico Mielolesioni study. *Arch Phys Med Rehabil*. 2003, 84(9):1266–1275.

101. Poynton AR, O'Farrell DA, Shannon F, Murray P, McManus F, Walsh MG. An evaluation of the factors affecting neurological recovery following spinal cord injury. *Injury*. 1997, 28(8): 545–548.

102. Scivoletto G, Morganti B, Molinari M. Neurologic recovery of spinal cord injury patients in Italy. *Arch Phys Med Rehabil*. 2004, 85(3):485–489.

103. Browne BJ, Jacobs SR, Herbison GJ, Ditunno JF Jr. Pin sensation as a predictor of extensor carpi radialis recovery in spinal cord injury. *Arch Phys Med Rehabil*. 1993, 74(1):14–18.

104. Katoh S, el Masry WS. Motor recovery of patients presenting with motor paralysis and sensory sparing following cervical spinal cord injuries. *Paraplegia*. 1995, 33(9):506–509.

105. Kirshblum SC, O'Connor KC. Levels of spinal cord injury and predictors of neurologic recovery. *Phys Med Rehabil Clin N Am*. 2000, 11(1):1–27, vii.

106. Ishida Y, Tominaga T. Predictors of neurologic recovery in acute central cervical cord injury with only upper extremity impairment. *Spine*. 2002, 27(15):1652–1658, discussion 1658.

107. McKinley W, Cifu D, Seel R, et al. Age-related outcomes in persons with spinal cord injury: a summary paper. *NeuroRehabilitation*. 2003, 18(1):83–90.

108. Cifu DX, Seel RT, Kreutzer JS, McKinley WO. A multicenter investigation of age-related differences in lengths of stay, hospitalization charges, and outcomes for a matched tetraplegia sample. *Arch Phys Med Rehabil*. 1999, 80(7):733–740.

109. Farmer J, Vaccaro A, Albert TJ, et al. Neurologic deterioration after cervical spinal cord injury. *J Spinal Disord*. 1998, 11(3): 192–196.

110. Ditunno JF Jr, Formal CS. Chronic spinal cord injury. *N Engl J Med*. 1994, 330(8):550–556.

111. Dunlop SA. Activity-dependent plasticity: implications for recovery after spinal cord injury. *Trends Neurosci*. 2008, 31(8): 410–418.

112. Lynskey JV, Belanger A, Jung R. Activity-dependent plasticity in spinal cord injury. *J Rehabil Res Dev*. 2008, 45(2):229–240.

113. Wolpaw JR. Spinal cord plasticity in acquisition and maintenance of motor skills. *Acta Physiol (Oxf)*. 2007, 189(2):155–169.

114. Blesch A, Tuszynski MH. Spinal cord injury: plasticity, regeneration and the challenge of translational drug development. *Trends Neurosci*. 2008.

115. Anderson KD, Borisoff JF, Johnson RD, et al. Long-term effects of spinal cord injury on sexual function in men: implications for neuroplasticity. *Spinal Cord*. 2007, 45(5):338–348.

116. Harkema SJ. Plasticity of interneuronal networks of the functionally isolated human spinal cord. *Brain Res Rev*. 2008, 57(1): 255–264.

117. Cohen ME, Sheehan TP, Herbison GJ. Content validity and reliability of the International Standards for Neurological Classification of Spinal Cord Injury. *Top Spinal Cord Inj Rehabil*. 1996, 1(4):15–31.

118. American Spinal Injury Association. *International Standards for Neurological Classification of Spinal Cord Injury*. Atlanta: American Spinal Injury Association, 2000, reprinted 2008.

119. Roth EJ, Lawler MH, Yarkony GM. Traumatic central cord syndrome: clinical features and functional outcomes. *Arch Phys Med Rehabil*. 1990, 71(1):18–23.

120. McLeod J, Lance J. *Introductory Neurology*. 3rd ed. Boston: Blackwell, 1989.

121. Roth EJ, Park T, Pang T, et al. Traumatic cervical Brown-Sequard and Brown-Sequard-plus syndromes: the spectrum of presentations and outcomes. *Paraplegia*. 1991, 29(9):582–589.

122. Rogers L. Radiologic assessment of acute neurologic and vertebral injuries. In: Meyer P, ed. *Surgery of Spine Trauma*. New York: Churchill Livingstone, 1989:185–263.

123. Harris JH Jr, Edeiken-Monroe B, Kopaniky DR. A practical classification of acute cervical spine injuries. *Orthop Clin North Am*. 1986, 17(1):15–30.

124. Chase T. Physical fitness strategies. In: Lanig I, ed. *A Practical Guide to Health Promotion After Spinal Cord Injury*. Gaithersburg, MD: Aspen, 1996:243–291.

125. Illis L. Clinical evaluation and pathophysiology of the spinal cord in the chronic stage. In: Illis L, ed. *Spinal Cord Dysfunction: Assessment*. New York: Oxford University Press, 1988:107–128.

126. Fried GW, Fried KM. Spinal cord injury and use of botulinum toxin in reducing spasticity. *Phys Med Rehabil Clin N Am*. 2003, 14(4):901–910.

127. Little JW, Micklesen P, Umlauf R, Britell C. Lower extremity manifestations of spasticity in chronic spinal cord injury. *Am J Phys Med Rehabil*. 1989, 68(1):32–36.

128. Maynard FM, Karunas RS, Waring WP III. Epidemiology of spasticity following traumatic spinal cord injury. *Arch Phys Med Rehabil*. 1990, 71(8):566–569.

129. Robinson CJ, Kett NA, Bolam JM. Spasticity in spinal cord injured patients: 2. Initial measures and long-term effects of surface electrical stimulation. *Arch Phys Med Rehabil*. 1988, 69(10):862–868.

130. Maynard FM, Karunas RS, Adkins RH, et al. Management of the neuromusculoskeletal systems. In: Stover SL, DeLisa JA, Whiteneck GG, eds. *Spinal Cord Injury: Clinical Outcomes from the Model Systems*. Gaithersburg, MD: Aspen, 1995:145–169.

131. Fredericks C. Clinical presentations in disorders of motor function. In: Fredericks C, Saladin L, eds. *Pathophysiology of the Motor Systems: Principles and Clinical Presentations*. Philadelphia: F.A. Davis, 1996:257–288.

132. Mayer NH. Clinicophysiologic concepts of spasticity and motor dysfunction in adults with an upper motoneuron lesion. *Muscle Nerve Suppl*. 1997, 6:S1–S13.

133. Priebe MM. Assessment of spinal cord injury spasticity in clinical trials. *Top Spinal Cord Inj Rehabil*. 2006, 11(3):69–77.

134. Moore DP. Helping your patients with spasticity reach maximal function. *Postgrad Med*. 1998, 104(2):123–126, 129–131, 135.

135. Adams MM, Hicks AL. Spasticity after spinal cord injury. *Spinal Cord*. 2005, 43(10):577–586.

136. Burchiel KJ, Hsu FP. Pain and spasticity after spinal cord injury: mechanisms and treatment. *Spine*. 2001, 26(Suppl 24): S146–S160.

137. Stein AB, Pomerantz F, Schechtman J. Evaluation and management of spasticity in spinal cord injury. *Top Spinal Cord Inj Rehabil*. 1997, 2(4):70–83.

138. Berman SA, Young RR, Sarkarati M, Shefner JM. Injury zone denervation in traumatic quadriplegia in humans. *Muscle Nerve*. 1996, 19(6):701–706.

139. Glenn MB, Bergman SB. Cardiovascular changes following spinal cord injury. *Top Spinal Cord Inj Rehabil*. 1997, 2(4):47–53.

140. Iversen S, Iversen L, Saper CB. The autonomic nervous system and the hypothalamus. In: Kandel ER, Schwartz JH, Jessell TM, eds. *Principles of Neural Science*. 4th ed. New York: McGraw-Hill, 2000:960–981.

141. Naftel J, Hardy S. Visceral motor pathways. In: Haines D, ed. *Fundamental Neuroscience for Basic and Clinical Applications*. 3rd ed. Philadelphia: Churchill Livingstone Elsevier, 2006:472–485.

142. Martini FH. *Fundamentals of Anatomy and Physiology*. 4th ed. Upper Saddle River, NJ: Prentice Hall, 1998.

143. Lehmann KG, Lane JG, Piepmeier JM, Batsford WP. Cardiovascular abnormalities accompanying acute spinal cord injury in humans: incidence, time course and severity. *J Am Coll Cardiol*. 1987, 10(1):46–52.

144. Claydon VE, Steeves JD, Krassioukov A. Orthostatic hypotension following spinal cord injury: understanding clinical pathophysiology. *Spinal Cord*. 2006, 44(6):341–351.

145. Cole J. The pathophysiology of the autonomic nervous system in spinal cord injury. In: Illis L, ed. *Spinal Cord Dysfunction: Assessment*. New York: Oxford University Press, 1988:201–235.

146. Nobunaga AI. Orthostatic hypotension in spinal cord injury. *Top Spinal Cord Inj Rehabil*. 1997, 4(1):73–80.

147. Naso F. Cardiovascular problems in patients with spinal cord injury. *Phys Med Rehabil Clin N Am*. 1992, 3(4):741–749.

148. Phillips WT, Kiratli BJ, Sarkarati M, et al. Effect of spinal cord injury on the heart and cardiovascular fitness. *Curr Probl Cardiol*. 1998, 23(11):641–716.

149. Grimm DR, De Meersman RE, Almenoff PL, et al. Sympathovagal balance of the heart in subjects with spinal cord injury. *Am J Physiol*. 1997, 272(2 Pt 2):H835–H842.

150. Davis GM. Exercise capacity of individuals with paraplegia. *Med Sci Sports Exerc*. 1993, 25(4):423–432.

151. Figoni SF. Exercise responses and quadriplegia. *Med Sci Sports Exerc*. 1993, 25(4):433–441.

152. Hopman MT, Oeseburg B, Binkhorst RA. Cardiovascular responses in paraplegic subjects during arm exercise. *Eur J Appl Physiol Occup Physiol*. 1992, 65(1):73–78.

153. King ML, Lichtman SW, Pellicone JT, et al. Exertional hypotension in spinal cord injury. *Chest*. 1994, 106(4):1166–1171.

154. Nash MS. Exercise reconditioning of the heart and peripheral circulation after spinal cord injury. *Top Spinal Cord Inj Rehabil*. 1998, 3(3):1–15.

155. Kessler KM, Pina I, Green B, et al. Cardiovascular findings in quadriplegic and paraplegic patients and in normal subjects. *Am J Cardiol*. 1986, 58(6):525–530.

156. Hooker SP, Wells CL. Effects of low- and moderate-intensity training in spinal cord-injured persons. *Med Sci Sports Exerc*. 1989, 21(1):18–22.

157. Jacobs PL, Nash MS. Exercise recommendations for individuals with spinal cord injury. *Sports Med*. 2004, 34(11):727–751.

158. Warburton D, Eng JJ, Krassioukov A, Sproule S. Cardiovascular health and exercise rehabilitation in spinal cord injury. *Top Spinal Cord Inj Rehabil*. 2007, 13(1):98–122.

159. Washburn RA, Figoni SF. Physical activity and chronic cardiovascular disease prevention in spinal cord injury: a comprehensive literature review. *Top Spinal Cord Inj Rehabil*. 1998, 3(3):16–32.

160. Rimmer JH. Exercise and physical activity in persons aging with a physical disability. *Phys Med Rehabil Clin N Am*. 2005, 16(1):41–56.

161. Bloch R. Autonomic dysfunction. In: Bloch R, Basbaum M, eds. *Management of Spinal Cord Injuries*. Baltimore: Williams & Wilkins, 1986:149–163.

162. Price MJ, Campbell IG. Effects of spinal cord lesion level upon thermoregulation during exercise in the heat. *Med Sci Sports Exerc*. 2003, 35(7):1100–1107.

163. da Paz AC, Beraldo PS, Almeida MC, et al. Traumatic injury to the spinal cord. Prevalence in Brazilian hospitals. *Paraplegia*. 1992, 30(9):636–640.

164. Knutsdottir S. Spinal cord injuries in Iceland 1973–1989. A follow up study. *Paraplegia*. 1993, 31(1):68–72.

165. Nakajima A, Honda S, Yoshimura S, Ono Y, Kawamura J, Moriai N. The disease pattern and causes of death of spinal cord injured patients in Japan. *Paraplegia*. 1989, 27(3):163–171.

166. Yarkony G, Heinemann AW. Pressure ulcers. In: Stover SL, DeLisa JA, Whiteneck GG, eds. *Spinal Cord Injury: Clinical Outcomes from the Model Systems*. Gaithersburg, MD: Aspen, 1995:100–119.

167. Sipski ML, Richards JS. Spinal cord injury rehabilitation: state of the science. *Am J Phys Med Rehabil*. 2006, 85(4):310–342.

168. DeVivo MJ, Black KJ, Stover SL. Causes of death during the first 12 years after spinal cord injury. *Arch Phys Med Rehabil*. 1993, 74(3):248–254.

169. DeVivo MJ. Long-term survival and causes of death. In: Stover SL, DeLisa JA, Whiteneck GG, eds. *Spinal Cord Injury: Clinical Outcomes from the Model Systems*. Gaithersburg, MD: Aspen, 1995:289–316.

170. Kiwerski JE. Factors contributing to the increased threat to life following spinal cord injury. *Paraplegia*. 1993, 31(12):793–799.

171. Derenne JP, Macklem PT, Roussos C. The respiratory muscles: mechanics, control, and pathophysiology. *Am Rev Respir Dis*. 1978, 118(1):119–133.

172. Wang AY, Jaeger RJ, Yarkony GM, Turba RM. Cough in spinal cord injured patients: the relationship between motor level and peak expiratory flow. *Spinal Cord*. 1997, 35(5):299–302.

173. Dalyan M, Sherman A, Cardenas DD. Factors associated with contractures in acute spinal cord injury. *Spinal Cord*. 1998, 36(6):405–408.

174. van Kuijk AA, Geurts AC, van Kuppevelt HJ. Neurogenic heterotopic ossification in spinal cord injury. *Spinal Cord*. 2002, 40(7):313–326.

175. Freebourn TM, Barber DB, Able AC. The treatment of immature heterotopic ossification in spinal cord injury with combination surgery, radiation therapy and NSAID. *Spinal Cord*. 1999, 37(1):50–53.

176. Frost FS. Role of rehabilitation after spinal cord injury. *Urol Clin North Am*. 1993, 20(3):549–559.

177. Lal S, Hamilton BB, Heinemann A, Betts HB. Risk factors for heterotopic ossification in spinal cord injury. *Arch Phys Med Rehabil*. 1989, 70(5):387–390.

178. Maimoun L, Fattal C, Micallef JP, et al. Bone loss in spinal cord-injured patients: from physiopathology to therapy. *Spinal Cord*. 2006, 44(4):203–210.

179. Kannisto M, Alaranta H, Merikanto J, et al. Bone mineral status after pediatric spinal cord injury. *Spinal Cord*. 1998, 36(9):641–646.

180. Szollar SM, Martin EM, Sartoris DJ, et al. Bone mineral density and indexes of bone metabolism in spinal cord injury. *Am J Phys Med Rehabil*. 1998, 77(1):28–35.

181. Rodriguez GP, Claus-Walker J, Kent MC, Garza HM. Collagen metabolite excretion as a predictor of bone- and skin-related complications in spinal cord injury. *Arch Phys Med Rehabil*. 1989, 70(6):442–444.

182. Chen B, Stein A. Osteoporosis in acute spinal cord injury. *Top Spinal Cord Inj Rehabil*. 2003, 9(1):26–35.

183. Kocina P. Body composition of spinal cord injured adults. *Sports Med*. 1997, 23(1):48–60.

184. Demirel G, Yilmaz H, Paker N, Onel S. Osteoporosis after spinal cord injury. *Spinal Cord*. 1998, 36(12):822–825.

185. Roberts D, Lee W, Cuneo RC, et al. Longitudinal study of bone turnover after acute spinal cord injury. *J Clin Endocrinol Metab*. 1998, 83(2):415–422.

186. Capoor J, Stein AB. Aging with spinal cord injury. *Phys Med Rehabil Clin N Am*. 2005, 16(1):129–161.

187. Bauman WA, Garland DE, Schwartz E. Calcium metabolism and osteoporosis in individuals with spinal cord injury. *Top Spinal Cord Inj Rehabil*. 1997, 2(4):84–95.

188. Levi R, Hultling C, Seiger A. The Stockholm spinal cord injury study: 2. Associations between clinical patient characteristics and post-acute medical problems. *Paraplegia*. 1995, 33(10):585–594.

189. Barrett H, McClelland JM, Rutkowski SB, Siddall PJ. Pain characteristics in patients admitted to hospital with complications

after spinal cord injury. *Arch Phys Med Rehabil.* 2003, 84(6): 789–795.

190. Cardenas DD, Bryce TN, Shem K, et al. Gender and minority differences in the pain experience of people with spinal cord injury. *Arch Phys Med Rehabil.* 2004, 85(11):1774–1781.

191. Donnelly C, Eng JJ. Pain following spinal cord injury: the impact on community reintegration. *Spinal Cord.* 2005, 43(5): 278–282.

192. Rintala DH, Holmes SA, Fiess RN. Prevalence and characteristics of chronic pain in veterans with spinal cord injury. *J Rehabil Res Dev.* 2005, 42(5):573–584.

193. Siddall PJ, Loeser JD. Pain following spinal cord injury. *Spinal Cord.* 2001, 39(2):63–73.

194. Siddall PJ, McClelland JM, Rutkowski SB, Cousins MJ. A longitudinal study of the prevalence and characteristics of pain in the first 5 years following spinal cord injury. *Pain.* 2003, 103(3): 249–257.

195. Finnerup NB, Jensen TS. Spinal cord injury pain—mechanisms and treatment. *Eur J Neurol.* 2004, 11(2):73–82.

196. Siddall PJ, Middleton JW. A proposed algorithm for the management of pain following spinal cord injury. *Spinal Cord.* 2006, 44(2):67–77.

197. Apple D. Pain above the injury level. *Top Spinal Cord Inj Rehabil.* 2001, 7(2):18–29.

198. van Drongelen S, de Groot S, Veeger HE, et al. Upper extremity musculoskeletal pain during and after rehabilitation in wheelchair-using persons with a spinal cord injury. *Spinal Cord.* 2006, 44(3):152–159.

199. Silfverskiold J, Waters RL. Shoulder pain and functional disability in spinal cord injury patients. *Clin Orthop.* 1991, (272):141–145.

200. Consortium for Spinal Cord Medicine. *Preservation of Upper Limb Function Following Spinal Cord Injury: A Clinical Practice Guideline for Health-Care Professionals.* Washington, DC: Paralyzed Veterans of America, 2005.

201. Nyland J, Quigley P, Huang C, et al. Preserving transfer independence among individuals with spinal cord injury. *Spinal Cord.* 2000, 38(11):649–657.

202. Waters RL, Sie IH. Upper extremity changes with SCI contrasted to common aging in the musculoskeletal system. *Top Spinal Cord Inj Rehabil.* 2001, 6(3):61–68.

203. Gellman H, Sie I, Waters RL. Late complications of the weight-bearing upper extremity in the paraplegic patient. *Clin Orthop.* 1988, 233:132–135.

204. Sie IH, Waters RL, Adkins RH, Gellman H. Upper extremity pain in the postrehabilitation spinal cord injured patient. *Arch Phys Med Rehabil.* 1992, 73(1):44–48.

205. Pentland WE, Twomey LT. Upper limb function in persons with long term paraplegia and implications for independence: part I. *Paraplegia.* 1994, 32(4):211–218.

206. Eide PK. Pathophysiological mechanisms of central neuropathic pain after spinal cord injury. *Spinal Cord.* 1998, 36(9):601–612.

207. Chen D, Nussbaum SB. Gastrointestinal disorders. In: Kirshblum S, Campagnolo DI, DeLisa JA, eds. *Spinal Cord Medicine.* Philadelphia: Lippincott Williams Wilkins, 2002:155–163.

208. Berczeller P, Bezkor M. *Medical Complications of Quadriplegia.* Chicago: Year Book, 1986.

209. Soderstrom CA, Ducker TB. Increased susceptibility of patients with cervical cord lesions to peptic gastrointestinal complications. *J Trauma.* 1985, 25(11):1030–1038.

210. Frost FS. Spinal cord injury: gastrointestinal implications and management. *Top Spinal Cord Inj Rehabil.* 1998, 4(2):56–80.

211. Lu WY, Rhoney DH, Boling WB, et al. A review of stress ulcer prophylaxis in the neurosurgical intensive care unit. *Neurosurgery.* 1997, 41(2):416–425, discussion 425–426.

212. Cardenas DD, Farrell-Roberts L, Sipski ML, Rubner D. Management of gastrointestinal, genitourinary, and sexual function. In: Stover SL, DeLisa JA, Whiteneck GG, eds. *Spinal Cord Injury: Clinical Outcomes from the Model Systems.* Gaithersburg, MD: Aspen, 1995:120–144.

213. Consortium for Spinal Cord Medicine. *Neurogenic Bowel Management in Adults with Spinal Cord Injury.* Washington, DC: Paralyzed Veterans of America, 1998.

214. De Looze D, Van Laere M, De Muynck M, et al. Constipation and other chronic gastrointestinal problems in spinal cord injury patients. *Spinal Cord.* 1998, 36(1):63–66.

215. Hall MK, Hackler RH, Zampieri TA, Zampieri JB. Renal calculi in spinal cord–injured patient: association with reflux, bladder stones, and Foley catheter drainage. *Urology.* 1989, 34(3):126–128.

216. Chen D. Treatment and prevention of thromboembolism after spinal cord injury. *Top Spinal Cord Inj Rehabil.* 2003, 9(1):14–25.

217. Willner D, Shatz O, Cremisi G, et al. Acute spinal cord injury, Part II: major issues in the management of spinal cord injuries. *Contemp Crit Care.* 2006, 3(10):1–55.

218. Consortium for Spinal Cord Medicine. *Prevention of Thromboembolism in Spinal Cord Injury.* 2nd ed. Washington, DC: Paralyzed Veterans of America, 1999.

219. McCagg C. Postoperative management and acute rehabilitation of patients with spinal cord injuries. *Orthop Clin North Am.* 1986, 17(1):171–182.

220. Waring WP, Karunas RS. Acute spinal cord injuries and the incidence of clinically occurring thromboembolic disease. *Paraplegia.* 1991, 29(1):8–16.

221. Ragnarsson KT, Hall KM, Wilmot CB, Carter RE. Management of pulmonary, cardiovascular, and metabolic conditions after spinal cord injury. In: Stover SL, DeLisa JA, Whiteneck GG, eds. *Spinal Cord Injury: Clinical Outcomes from the Model Systems.* Gaithersburg, MD: Aspen, 1995:79–99.

222. Curt A, Nitsche B, Rodic B, et al. Assessment of autonomic dysreflexia in patients with spinal cord injury. *J Neurol Neurosurg Psychiatry.* 1997, 62(5):473–477.

223. Nitsche B, Perschak H, Curt A, Dietz V. Loss of circadian blood pressure variability in complete tetraplegia. *J Hum Hypertens.* 1996, 10(5):311–317.

224. Colachis SC. Autonomic hyperreflexia with spinal cord injury. *Top Spinal Cord Inj Rehabil.* 1997, 3(1):71–81.

225. Johnson RL, Gerhart KA, McCray J, Menconi JC, Whiteneck GG. Secondary conditions following spinal cord injury in a population-based sample. *Spinal Cord.* 1998, 36(1):45–50.

226. Vapnek J. Autonomic dysreflexia. *Top Spinal Cord Inj Rehabil.* 1997, 2(4):54–69.

227. Consortium for Spinal Cord Medicine. *Acute Management of Autonomic Dysreflexia: Adults with Spinal Cord Injury Presenting to Health-Care Facilities.* 2nd ed. Washington, DC: Paralyzed Veterans of America, 2001.

228. Weaver LC, Cassam AK, Krassioukov AV, Llewellyn-Smith IJ. Changes in immunoreactivity for growth associated protein-43 suggest reorganization of synapses on spinal sympathetic neurons after cord transection. *Neuroscience.* 1997, 81(2):535–551.

229. Zhou GC, Yu J, Tang HH, Shi J. The determination of vasoactive substances during autonomic dysreflexia. *Spinal Cord.* 1997, 35(6):390–393.

230. Branco F, Cardenas DD, Svircev JN. Spinal cord injury: a comprehensive review. *Phys Med Rehabil Clin N Am.* 2007, 18(4):651–679, v.

231. McGuire TJ, Kumar VN. Autonomic dysreflexia in the spinal cord-injured. What the physician should know about this medical emergency. *Postgrad Med.* 1986, 80(2):81–84, 89.

232. Cardus D, Ribas-Cardus F, McTaggart WG. Coronary risk in spinal cord injury: assessment following a multivariate approach. *Arch Phys Med Rehabil.* 1992, 73(10):930–933.

233. Imai K, Kadowaki T, Aizawa Y, Fukutomi K. Morbidity rates of complications in persons with spinal cord injury according to the site of injury and with special reference to hypertension. *Paraplegia.* 1994, 32(4):246–252.

234. Bauman WA, Raza M, Spungen AM, Machac J. Cardiac stress testing with thallium-201 imaging reveals silent ischemia in individuals with paraplegia. *Arch Phys Med Rehabil.* 1994, 75(9): 946–950.

235. Bauman WA, Spungen AM, Raza M, et al. Coronary artery disease: metabolic risk factors and latent disease in individuals with paraplegia. *Mt Sinai J Med.* 1992, 59(2):163–168.

236. Yekutiel M, Brooks ME, Ohry A, et al. The prevalence of hypertension, ischaemic heart disease and diabetes in traumatic spinal cord injured patients and amputees. *Paraplegia.* 1989, 27(1):58–62.

237. Ragnarsson KT, Stein AB, Spungen AM, Bauman WA. Medical complications after spinal cord injury: spasticity, pain, and endocrine/metabolic changes. *Top Spinal Cord Inj Rehabil.* 2004, 10(2):86–106.

238. Bauman WA, Adkins RH, Spungen AM, et al. The effect of residual neurological deficit on serum lipoproteins in individuals with chronic spinal cord injury. *Spinal Cord.* 1998, 36(1):13–17.

239. Dearwater SR, LaPorte RE, Robertson RJ, et al. Activity in the spinal cord-injured patient: an epidemiologic analysis of metabolic parameters. *Med Sci Sports Exerc.* 1986, 18(5):541–544.

240. Korres DS, Boscainos PJ, Papagelopoulos PJ, et al. Multiple level noncontiguous fractures of the spine. *Clin Orthop Relat Res.* 2003, 411:95–102.

241. Wittenberg RH, Hargus S, Steffen R, Muhr G, Botel U. Noncontiguous unstable spine fractures. *Spine.* 2002, 27(3):254–257.

242. Jacobs SR, Yeaney NK, Herbison GJ, Ditunno JF Jr. Future ambulation prognosis as predicted by somatosensory evoked potentials in motor complete and incomplete quadriplegia. *Arch Phys Med Rehabil.* 1995, 76(7):635–641.

243. Skold C, Levi R, Seiger A. Spasticity after traumatic spinal cord injury: nature, severity, and location. *Arch Phys Med Rehabil.* 1999, 80(12):1548–1557.

CHAPTER 3

1. Consortium for Spinal Cord Medicine. *Early Acute Management in Adults with Spinal Cord Injury: A Clinical Practice Guideline for Health-Care Providers.* Washington, DC: Paralyzed Veterans of America, 2008.

2. Domeier RM, Frederiksen SM, Welch K. Prospective performance assessment of an out-of-hospital protocol for selective spine immobilization using clinical spine clearance criteria. *Ann Emerg Med.* 2005, 46(2):123–131.

3. Whetstone W. Prehospital management of SCI individuals with extremity fractures. *Top Spinal Cord Inj Rehabil.* 2005, 11(1):11–17.

4. Muhr MD, Seabrook DL, Wittwer LK. Paramedic use of a spinal injury clearance algorithm reduces spinal immobilization in the out-of-hospital setting. *Prehosp Emerg Care.* 1999, 3(1):1–6.

5. Poelstra K, Vaccaro A, Rao S, et al. Emergency transport and radiographic evaluation following spinal cord injury. *Top Spinal Cord Inj Rehabil.* 2006, 12(1):22–37.

6. Marion DW. Head and spinal cord injury. *Neurol Clin.* 1998, 16(2):485–502.

7. Wang D, Teddy PJ, Henderson NJ, et al. Mobilization of patients after spinal surgery for acute spinal cord injury. *Spine.* 2001, 26(20):2278–2282.

8. Aung TS, el Masry WS. Audit of a British Centre for spinal injury. *Spinal Cord.* 1997, 35(3):147–150.

9. Carvell JE, Grundy DJ. Complications of spinal surgery in acute spinal cord injury. *Paraplegia.* 1994, 32(6):389–395.

10. Dalyan M, Sherman A, Cardenas DD. Factors associated with contractures in acute spinal cord injury. *Spinal Cord.* 1998, 36(6):405–408.

11. DeVivo MJ, Kartus PL, Stover SL, Fine PR. Benefits of early admission to an organised spinal cord injury care system. *Paraplegia.* 1990, 28(9):545–555.

12. Waters R, Apple D, Meyer P, et al. Emergency and acute management of spine trauma. In: Stover S, DeLisa J, Whiteneck G, eds. *Spinal Cord Injury: Clinical Outcomes from the Model Systems.* Gaithersburg, MD: Aspen, 1995:56–78.

13. Wells JD, Nicosia S. The effects of multidisciplinary team care for acute spinal cord injury patients. *J Am Paraplegia Soc.* 1993, 16(1):23–29.

14. Barboi C, Peruzzi W. Acute medical management of spinal cord injury. In: Lin V, ed. *Spinal Cord Medicine: Principles and Practice.* New York: Demos, 2003:113–123.

15. Benzel E, Doezema D. Prehospital management of the spinally injured patient. In: Narayan R, Wilberger J, Povlishock J, eds. *Neurotrauma.* New York: McGraw-Hill, 1996:1113–1120.

16. Chesnut R. Emergency management of spinal cord injury. In: Narayan R, Wilberger J, Povlishock J, eds. *Neurotrauma.* New York: McGraw-Hill, 1996:1121–1138.

17. Fehlings MG, Louw D. Initial stabilization and medical management of acute spinal cord injury. *Am Fam Physician.* 1996, 54(1):155–162.

18. Yu D. A crash course in spinal cord injury. *Postgrad Med.* 1998, 104(2):109–110, 113–106, 119–122.

19. McBride DQ, Rodts GE. Intensive care of patients with spinal trauma. *Neurosurg Clin N Am.* 1994, 5(4):755–766.

20. Hurlbert RJ. Strategies of medical intervention in the management of acute spinal cord injury. *Spine.* 2006, 31(Suppl 11): S16–S21, discussion S36.

21. Tator C. Current primary to tertiary prevention of spinal cord injury. *Top Spinal Cord Inj Rehabil.* 2004, 10(1):1–14.

22. Finkelstein J, Anderson P. Surgical management of cervical instability. In: Capen D, Haye W, eds. *Comprehensive Management of Spine Trauma.* St. Louis: Mosby, 1998:144–184.

23. Arnold P, Filardi T, Strang R, McMahon J. Early neurologic assessment of the patient with spinal cord injury. *Top Spinal Cord Inj Rehabil.* 2006, 12(1):38–48.

24. Levi AD, Hurlbert RJ, Anderson P, et al. Neurologic deterioration secondary to unrecognized spinal instability following trauma—a multicenter study. *Spine.* 2006, 31(4):451–458.

25. Graber MA, Kathol M. Cervical spine radiographs in the trauma patient. *Am Fam Physician.* 1999, 59(2):331–342.

26. Stassen NA, Williams VA, Gestring ML, et al. Magnetic resonance imaging in combination with helical computed tomography provides a safe and efficient method of cervical spine clearance in the obtunded trauma patient. *J Trauma.* 2006, 60(1):171–177.

27. McLain RF, Benson DR. Missed cervical dissociation—recognizing and avoiding potential disaster. *J Emerg Med.* 1998, 16(2):179–183.

28. Quencer RM, Nunez D, Green BA. Controversies in imaging acute cervical spine trauma. *AJNR Am J Neuroradiol.* 1997, 18(10):1866–1868.

29. Chen TY, Lee ST, Lui TN, et al. Efficacy of surgical treatment in traumatic central cord syndrome. *Surg Neurol.* 1997, 48(5):435–440, discussion 441.

30. Fehlings MG, Rao SC, Tator CH, et al. The optimal radiologic method for assessing spinal canal compromise and cord compression in patients with cervical spinal cord injury. Part II: results of a multicenter study. *Spine.* 1999, 24(6):605–613.

31. Kulkarni MV, McArdle CB, Kopanicky D, et al. Acute spinal cord injury: MR imaging at 1.5 T. *Radiology.* 1987, 164(3): 837–843.

32. Nesathurai S. Steroids and spinal cord injury: revisiting the NASCIS 2 and NASCIS 3 trials. *J Trauma.* 1998, 45(6): 1088–1093.

33. Poelstra K, Vaccaro A, Rao S, et al. Pharmacologic neuroprotection in patients with spinal cord injury and the efficacy of

early decompressive surgery. *Top Spinal Cord Inj Rehabil.* 2006, 12(2):63–76.

34. Vale FL, Burns J, Jackson AB, Hadley MN. Combined medical and surgical treatment after acute spinal cord injury: results of a prospective pilot study to assess the merits of aggressive medical resuscitation and blood pressure management. *J Neurosurg.* 1997, 87(2):239–246.

35. Frisch R, Antonacci M. Spinal cord injury repair strategies. *Top Spinal Cord Inj Rehabil.* 2005, 10(4):1–31.

36. Kwon BK, Mann C, Sohn HM, et al. Hypothermia for spinal cord injury. *Spine J.* 2008, 8(6):859–874.

37. Cheng H, Cao Y, Olson L. Spinal cord repair in adult paraplegic rats: partial restoration of hind limb function. *Science.* 1996, 273(5274):510–513.

38. Gimenez Y, Ribotta M, Privat A. Biological interventions for spinal cord injury. *Curr Opin Neurol.* 1998, 11(6):647–654.

39. Zompa EA, Cain LD, Everhart AW, et al. Transplant therapy: recovery of function after spinal cord injury. *J Neurotrauma.* 1997, 14(8):479–506.

40. Bregman BS, Kunkel-Bagden E, Schnell L, et al. Recovery from spinal cord injury mediated by antibodies to neurite growth inhibitors. *Nature.* 1995, 378(6556):498–501.

41. Tator CH. Review of treatment trials in human spinal cord injury: issues, difficulties, and recommendations. *Neurosurgery.* 2006, 59(5):957–982, discussion 982–987.

42. Lu J, Waite P. Advances in spinal cord regeneration. *Spine.* 1999, 24(9):926–930.

43. Tator CH. Biology of neurological recovery and functional restoration after spinal cord injury. *Neurosurgery.* 1998, 42(4):696–707, discussion 707–698.

44. Rechtine GR II. Nonoperative management and treatment of spinal injuries. *Spine.* 2006, 31(Suppl 11):S22–S27, discussion S36.

45. Campagnolo D, Heary RF. Acute medical and surgical management of spinal cord injury. In: Kirshblum S, Campagnolo D, DeLisa J, eds. *Spinal Cord Medicine.* Philadelphia: Lippincott Williams & Wilkins, 2002:96–107.

46. Przybylski G, Marion D. Injury to the vertebrae and spinal cord. In: Feliciano D, Moore E, Mattox K, eds. *Trauma.* 3rd ed. Stamford, CT: Appleton & Lange, 1996:307–327.

47. Donovan WH, Kopanicky D, Stolzmann E, Carter R. The neurological and skeletal outcome in patients with closed cervical spinal cord injury. *J Neurosurg.* 1987, 66(5):690–694.

48. Meyer P. *Surgery of Spine Trauma.* New York: Churchill Livingstone, 1989.

49. Wang J, Delamarter R. Lumbar fractures of the spine. In: Capen D, Haye W, eds. *Comprehensive Management of Spine Trauma.* St. Louis: Mosby, 1998:214–234.

50. Castillo RG, Bell J. Cervical spine injury. Stabilization and management. *Postgrad Med.* 1988, 83(7):131–132, 135–138.

51. Dickman C, Zerick W. Cervical, thoracic, and lumbar orthoses. In: Narayan R, Wilberger J, Povlishock J, eds. *Neurotrauma.* New York: McGraw-Hill, 1996:1139–1147.

52. Wimberley D, Goyal N, Goins M, et al. Advances in surgical techniques and instrumentation and their impact on the spinal cord injury rehabilitation process. *Top Spinal Cord Inj Rehabil.* 2004, 10(2):35–48.

53. Zimmerman A, Yoshida G. Prioritization and treatment of patients with thoracolumbar trauma and multiple injuries. *Top Spinal Cord Inj Rehabil.* 2005, 11(1):30–39.

54. Daffner S, Vaccaro A, Katsos M, Grauer J. Advances in operative stabilization for unstable cervical spine injuries: implications for early mobilization and rehabilitation. *Top Spinal Cord Inj Rehabil.* 2003, 9(1):1–13.

55. McKinley W, Meade MA, Kirshblum S, Barnard B. Outcomes of early surgical management versus late or no surgical intervention after acute spinal cord injury. *Arch Phys Med Rehabil.* 2004, 85(11):1818–1825.

56. Farmer J, Vaccaro A, Albert TJ, et al. Neurologic deterioration after cervical spinal cord injury. *J Spinal Disord.* 1998, 11(3):192–196.

57. Mirza SK, Krengel WF III, Chapman JR, et al. Early versus delayed surgery for acute cervical spinal cord injury. *Clin Orthop Relat Res.* 1999, 359:104–114.

58. Savas P, Vaccaro A. Surgical management for thoracolumbar spinal injuries. In: Lin V, ed. *Spinal Cord Medicine: Principles and Practice.* New York: Demos, 2003:143–151.

59. Shaffrey CI, Shaffrey ME, Whitehill R, Nockels RP. Surgical treatment of thoracolumbar fractures. *Neurosurg Clin N Am.* 1997, 8(4):519–540.

60. Bono C, Vives M, Kauffman C. Cervical injuries: indications and options for surgery. In: Lin V, ed. *Spinal Cord Medicine: Principles and Practice.* New York: Demos, 2003:131–141.

61. Cooper P. Use of lateral mass plates for stabilization of the lower cervical spine. In: Fessler R, Haid R, eds. *Current Techniques in Spinal Stabilization.* New York: McGraw-Hill, 1996:129–138.

62. Kalfas I. Cervical spine stabilization: surgical techniques. In: Narayan R, Wilberger J, Povlishock J, eds. *Neurotrauma.* New York: McGraw-Hill, 1996:1179–1192.

63. Vaccaro A, Silveri C, Balderston R. Nonsurgical and surgical management of fractures at the thoracolumbar junction. In: Capen D, Haye W, eds. *Comprehensive Management of Spine Trauma.* St. Louis: Mosby, 1998:199–213.

64. Botel U, Glaser E, Niedeggen A. The surgical treatment of acute spinal paralysed patients. *Spinal Cord.* 1997, 35(7):420–428.

65. Harms J, Tabasso G. *Instrumented Spinal Surgery: Principles and Technique.* New York: Thieme, 1999.

66. Apple D, Perez M. Prospective study of orthotic use after operative stabilization of traumatic thoracic and lumbar fractures. *Top Spinal Cord Inj Rehabil.* 2006, 12(2):77–82.

67. Brown C, Chow G. Orthoses for spinal trauma and postoperative care. In: Goldberg B, Hsu J, eds. *Atlas of Assistive Devices.* 3rd ed. St. Louis: Mosby, 1997:251–258.

68. Nelson R. Nonsurgical management of cervical spine instability. In: Capen D, Haye W, eds. *Comprehensive Management of Spine Trauma.* St Louis: Mosby, 1998:134–133.

69. Richter D, Latta LL, Milne EL, et al. The stabilizing effects of different orthoses in the intact and unstable upper cervical spine: a cadaver study. *J Trauma.* 2001, 50(5):848–854.

70. Johnson RM, Hart DL, Simmons EF, et al. Cervical orthoses. A study comparing their effectiveness in restricting cervical motion in normal subjects. *J Bone Joint Surg Am.* 1977, 59(3):332–339.

71. Vaccaro A, Lavernia C, Bottle M, et al. Spinal orthoses in the management of spinal trauma. In: Levine A, Eismont F, Garfin S, Zigler J, eds. *Spine Trauma.* Philadelphia: Saunders, 1998:171–194.

72. Wang G, Moskal J, Albert T, et al. The effect of halo-vest length on stability of the cervical spine. *J Bone Joint Surg.* 1988, 70-A(3):357–360.

73. Haak M, Bernardoni G. Conservative management of cervical spine injuries. *Top Spinal Cord Inj Rehabil.* 2004, 9(3):33–38.

74. Benzel EC, Hadden TA, Saulsbery CM. A comparison of the Minerva and halo jackets for stabilization of the cervical spine. *J Neurosurg.* 1989, 70(3):411–414.

75. Graziano G, Charles L. Spinal orthoses. In: An H, ed. *Principles and Techniques of Spine Surgery.* Baltimore: Williams & Wilkins, 1998:641–652.

76. Millington PJ, Ellingsen JM, Hauswirth BE, Fabian PJ. Thermoplastic Minerva body jacket—a practical alternative to current methods of cervical spine stabilization. A clinical report. *Phys Ther.* 1987, 67(2):223–225.

77. Nawoczenski D, Rinehart M, Duncanson P, Brown B. Physical management. In: Buchanan L, Nawoczenski D, eds. *Spinal*

Cord Injury: Concepts and Management Approaches. Baltimore: Williams & Wilkins, 1987:123–184.

78. Ayyappa E, Downs K. Spinal orthoses. In: Lin V, ed. *Spinal Cord Medicine: Principles and Practice.* New York: Demos, 2003:655–662.

79. Botte MJ, Byrne TP, Abrams RA, Garfin SR. The halo skeletal fixator: current concepts of application and maintenance. *Orthopedics.* 1995, 18(5):463–471.

80. Bucci MN, Dauser RC, Maynard FA, Hoff JT. Management of post-traumatic cervical spine instability: operative fusion versus halo vest immobilization. Analysis of 49 cases. *J Trauma.* 1988, 28(7):1001–1006.

81. Crum NA. Signs of temporomandibular joint dysfunction in spinal cord injured patients wearing halo braces: a clinical report. *Phys Ther.* 1990, 70(2):132–137.

82. Garfin SR, Botte MJ, Triggs KJ, Nickel VL. Subdural abscess associated with halo-pin traction. *J Bone Joint Surg Am.* 1988, 70(9):1338–1340.

83. Garfin SR, Botte MJ, Waters RL, Nickel VL. Complications in the use of the halo fixation device. *J Bone Joint Surg Am.* 1986, 68(3):320–325.

84. Glaser JA, Whitehill R, Stamp WG, Jane JA. Complications associated with the halo-vest. A review of 245 cases. *J Neurosurg.* 1986, 65(6):762–769.

85. Lee TT, Green BA, Petrin DR. Treatment of stable burst fracture of the atlas (Jefferson fracture) with rigid cervical collar. *Spine.* 1998, 23(18):1963–1967.

86. Whitehill R, Richman J, Glaser JA. Failure of immobilization of the cervical spine by the halo vest. A report of five cases. *J Bone Joint Surg.* 1986, 68-A(3):326–332.

87. Botte MJ, Garfin SR, Byrne TP, et al. The halo skeletal fixator. Principles of application and maintenance. *Clin Orthop Relat Res.* 1989, 239:12–18.

88. New York University. *Spinal Orthotics.* New York: New York University Post-Graduate Medical School, 1983.

89. Askins V, Eismont FJ. Efficacy of five cervical orthoses in restricting cervical motion. A comparison study. *Spine.* 1997, 22(11):1193–1198.

90. Janssen T, Glaser R, Shuster D. Clinical efficacy of electrical stimulation exercise training: effects on health, fitness, and function. *Top Spinal Cord Inj Rehabil.* 1998, 3(3):33–49.

91. Sandler AJ, Dvorak J, Humke T, et al. The effectiveness of various cervical orthoses. An in vivo comparison of the mechanical stability provided by several widely used models. *Spine.* 1996, 21(14):1624–1629.

92. Gavin TM, Carandang G, Havey R, et al. Biomechanical analysis of cervical orthoses in flexion and extension: a comparison of cervical collars and cervical thoracic orthoses. *J Rehabil Res Dev.* 2003, 40(6):527–537.

93. Fishman S, Berger N, Edelstein J, Springer W. Spinal orthoses. In: Bunch W, Keagy R, Kritter L, Kruger L, Letts M, Lonstein J, eds. *Atlas of Orthotics: Biomechanical Principles and Application.* 2nd ed. St Louis: Mosby, 1985:238–256.

94. Ragnarsson K, Stein AB, Kirshblum S. Rehabilitation and comprehensive care of the person with spinal cord injury. In: Capen D, Haye W, eds. *Comprehensive Management of Spine Trauma.* St Louis: Mosby, 1998:365–413.

95. Axelsson P, Johnsson R, Stromqvist B. Lumbar orthosis with unilateral hip immobilization. Effect on intervertebral mobility determined by roentgen stereophotogrammetric analysis. *Spine.* 1993, 18(7):876–879.

96. Glaser JA, Jaworski BA, Cuddy BG, et al. Variation in surgical opinion regarding management of selected cervical spine injuries. A preliminary study. *Spine.* 1998, 23(9):975–982, discussion 983.

97. Tator C, Fehlings M, Thorpe K, Taylor W. Current use and timing of spinal surgery for management of acute spinal cord injury in North America: results of a retrospective multicenter study. *J Neurosurg.* 1999, 91(Suppl 1):12–18.

98. Ashe M, Craven C, Eng J, Krassioukov A. Prevention and treatment of bone loss after a spinal cord injury: a systematic review. *Top Spinal Cord Inj Rehabil.* 2007, 13(1):123–145.

99. Consortium for Spinal Cord Medicine. *Clinical Practice Guideline: Prevention of Thromboembolism in Spinal Cord Injury.* 2nd ed. Washington, DC: Paralyzed Veterans of America, 1999.

100. Consortium for Spinal Cord Medicine. *Clinical Practice Guidelines: Acute Management of Autonomic Dysreflexia: Adults with Spinal Cord Injury Presenting to Health-Care Facilities.* Washington, DC: Paralyzed Veterans of America, 2001.

101. Karch AM. *Lippincott's Nursing Drug Guide.* Philadelphia: Lippincott, 2000.

102. Scelza W, Shatzer M. Pharmacology of spinal cord injury: basic mechanism of action and side effects of commonly used drugs. *J Neurol Phys Ther.* 2003, 27(3):101–108.

103. Shannon MT, Wilson BA, Stang CL. *Health Professional's Drug Guide.* Upper Saddle River, NJ: Prentice Hall, 2003.

104. van Kuijk AA, Geurts AC, van Kuppevelt HJ. Neurogenic heterotopic ossification in spinal cord injury. *Spinal Cord.* 2002, 40(7):313–326.

105. Royster R, Barboi C, Peruzzi W. Critical care in the acute cervical spinal cord injury. *Top Spinal Cord Inj Rehabil.* 2004, 9(3):11–32.

106. Rodts G, Haid R. Intensive care management of spinal cord injury. In: Narayan R, Willberger J, Povlishock J, eds. *Neurotrauma.* New York: McGraw-Hill, 1996:1201–1212.

107. Lu WY, Rhoney DH, Boling WB, et al. A review of stress ulcer prophylaxis in the neurosurgical intensive care unit. *Neurosurgery.* 1997, 41(2):416–425, discussion 425–416.

108. Tryba M, Cook D. Current guidelines on stress ulcer prophylaxis. *Drugs.* 1997, 54(4):581–596.

109. Curry K, Casady L. The relationship between extended periods of immobility and decubitus ulcer formation in the acutely spinal cord–injured individual. *J Neurosci Nurs.* 1992, 24(4):185–189.

110. Linares HA, Mawson AR, Suarez E, Biundo JJ. Association between pressure sores and immobilization in the immediate post-injury period. *Orthopedics.* 1987, 10(4):571–573.

111. Frost FS. Role of rehabilitation after spinal cord injury. *Urol Clin North Am.* 1993, 20(3):549–559.

112. Naso F. Cardiovascular problems in patients with spinal cord injury. *Phys Med Rehabil Clin N Am.* 1992, 3(4):741–749.

113. Sabharwal S. Cardiovascular dysfunction in spinal cord disorders. In: Lin V, ed. *Spinal Cord Medicine: Principles and Practice.* New York: Demos, 2003:179–192.

114. Gittler MS. Acute rehabilitation in Cervical Spinal Cord Injury. *Top Spinal Cord Inj Rehabil.* 2004, 9(3):60–73.

115. Krassioukov AV, Karlsson AK, Wecht JM, et al. Assessment of autonomic dysfunction following spinal cord injury: rationale for additions to International Standards for Neurological Assessment. *J Rehabil Res Dev.* 2007, 44(1):103–112.

116. Phillips WT, Kiratli BJ, Sarkarati M, et al. Effect of spinal cord injury on the heart and cardiovascular fitness. *Curr Probl Cardiol.* 1998, 23(11):641–716.

117. Vapnek J. Autonomic dysreflexia. *Top Spinal Cord Inj Rehabil.* 1997, 2(4):54–69.

118. Bycroft J, Shergill IS, Chung EA, et al. Autonomic dysreflexia: a medical emergency. *Postgrad Med J.* 2005, 81(954):232–235.

119. Blackmer J. Rehabilitation medicine: 1. Autonomic dysreflexia. *CMAJ.* 2003, 169(9):931–935.

120. Yarkony G. Medical and physical complications in spinal cord injury. In: Yarkony G, ed. *Spinal Cord Injury: Medical Management and Rehabilitation.* Gaithersburg, MD: Aspen, 1994: 17–25.

121. Turpie A. Thrombosis prevention and treatment in spinal cord injured patients. In: Bloch R, Basbaum M, eds. *Management of Spinal Cord Injuries.* Baltimore: William & Wilkins, 1986: 212–240.

122. Furlan JC, Fehlings MG. Role of screening tests for deep venous thrombosis in asymptomatic adults with acute spinal cord injury: an evidence-based analysis. *Spine*. 2007, 32(17):1908–1916.

123. Willner D, Shatz O, Cremisi G, et al. Acute spinal cord injury, Part II: major issues in the management of spinal cord injuries. *Contemp Crit Care*. 2006, 3(10):1–55.

124. Bauman WA, Spungen AM, Raza M, et al. Coronary artery disease: metabolic risk factors and latent disease in individuals with paraplegia. *Mt Sinai J Med*. 1992, 59(2):163–168.

125. DeVivo MJ, Black KJ, Stover SL. Causes of death during the first 12 years after spinal cord injury. *Arch Phys Med Rehabil*. 1993, 74(3):248–254.

126. DeVivo MJ. Long-term survival and causes of death. In: Stover SL, DeLisa JA, Whiteneck GG, eds. *Spinal Cord Injury: Clinical Outcomes from the Model Systems*. Gaithersburg, MD: Aspen, 1995:289–316.

127. Stiens S, Johnson M, Lyman P. Cardiac rehabilitation in patients with spinal cord injuries. *Phys Med Rehabil Clin N Am*. 1995, 2(6):263–296.

128. Nash M. Exercise as a health-promoting activity following spinal cord injury. *J Neurol Phys Ther*. 2005, 29(2):87–103.

129. National Spinal Cord Injury Statistical Center. Annual Report for the Model Spinal Cord Injury Care Systems. 2007, http://www.spinalcord.uab.edu. Accessed 12/15/08.

130. Warburton D, Eng JJ, Krassioukov A, Sproule S. Cardiovascular health and exercise rehabilitation in spinal cord injury. *Top Spinal Cord Inj Rehabil*. 2007, 13(1):98–122.

131. Chase T. Physical fitness strategies. In: Lanig I, Chase T, Butt L, et al, eds. *A Practical Guide to Health Promotion after Spinal Cord Injury*. Gaithersburg, MD: Aspen, 1996:243–291.

132. Hooker SP, Wells CL. Effects of low- and moderate-intensity training in spinal cord-injured persons. *Med Sci Sports Exerc*. 1989, 21(1):18–22.

133. Capoor J, Stein AB. Aging with spinal cord injury. *Phys Med Rehabil Clin N Am*. 2005, 16(1):129–161.

134. Jacobs PL, Nash MS. Exercise recommendations for individuals with spinal cord injury. *Sports Med*. 2004, 34(11):727–751.

135. Hicks AL, Martin KA, Ditor DS, et al. Long-term exercise training in persons with spinal cord injury: effects on strength, arm ergometry performance and psychological well-being. *Spinal Cord*. 2003, 41(1):34–43.

136. Jacobs PL, Nash MS, Rusinowski JW. Circuit training provides cardiorespiratory and strength benefits in persons with paraplegia. *Med Sci Sports Exerc*. 2001, 33(5):711–717.

137. Barstow TJ, Scremin AM, Mutton DL, et al. Changes in gas exchange kinetics with training in patients with spinal cord injury. *Med Sci Sports Exerc*. 1996, 28(10):1221–1228.

138. Cowell LL, Squires WG, Raven PB. Benefits of aerobic exercise for the paraplegic: a brief review. *Med Sci Sports Exerc*. 1986, 18(5):501–508.

139. DiCarlo SE. Effect of arm ergometry training on wheelchair propulsion endurance of individuals with quadriplegia. *Phys Ther*. 1988, 68(1):40–44.

140. Glaser RM. Functional neuromuscular stimulation. Exercise conditioning of spinal cord injured patients. *Int J Sports Med*. 1994, 15(3):142–148.

141. Hoffman MD. Cardiorespiratory fitness and training in quadriplegics and paraplegics. *Sports Med*. 1986, 3(5):312–330.

142. Hooker SP, Scremin AM, Mutton DL, et al. Peak and submaximal physiologic responses following electrical stimulation leg cycle ergometer training. *J Rehabil Res Dev*. 1995, 32(4):361–366.

143. Nash M. Exercise reconditioning of the heart and peripheral circulation after spinal cord injury. *Top Spinal Cord Inj Rehabil*. 1998, 3(3):1–15.

144. Yakura JS, Waters RL, Adkins RH. Changes in ambulation parameters in spinal cord injury individuals following rehabilitation. *Paraplegia*. 1990, 28(6):364–370.

145. Kilkens OJ, Dallmeijer AJ, Nene AV, et al. The longitudinal relation between physical capacity and wheelchair skill performance during inpatient rehabilitation of people with spinal cord injury. *Arch Phys Med Rehabil*. 2005, 86(8):1575–1581.

146. Laskin J, James S, Cantwell B. A fitness and wellness program for people with spinal cord injury. *Top Spinal Cord Inj Rehabil*. 1997, 3(1):16–33.

147. Lammerste D. Maintaining health long-term with spinal cord injury. *Top Spinal Cord Inj Rehabil*. 2001, 6(3):1–21.

148. Rimmer JH. Exercise and physical activity in persons aging with a physical disability. *Phys Med Rehabil Clin N Am*. 2005, 16(1):41–56.

149. Washburn RA, Figoni SF. Physical activity and chronic cardiovascular disease prevention in spinal cord injury: a comprehensive literature review. *Top Spinal Cord Inj Rehabil*. 1998, 3(3):16–32.

150. Hart A, Malone T, English T. Shoulder function and rehabilitation implications for the wheelchair racing athlete. *Top Spinal Cord Inj Rehabil*. 1998, 3(3):50–65.

151. Bauman WA, Garland DE, Schwartz E. Calcium metabolism and osteoporosis in individuals with spinal cord injury. *Top Spinal Cord Inj Rehabil*. 1997, 2(4):84–95.

152. BeDell KK, Scremin AM, Perell KL, Kunkel CF. Effects of functional electrical stimulation-induced lower extremity cycling on bone density of spinal cord–injured patients. *Am J Phys Med Rehabil*. 1996, 75(1):29–34.

153. Bloomfield SA, Mysiw WJ, Jackson RD. Bone mass and endocrine adaptations to training in spinal cord injured individuals. *Bone*. 1996, 19(1):61–68.

154. Kunkel CF, Scremin AM, Eisenberg B, et al. Effect of "standing" on spasticity, contracture, and osteoporosis in paralyzed males. *Arch Phys Med Rehabil*. 1993, 74(1):73–78.

155. Leeds EM, Klose KJ, Ganz W, et al. Bone mineral density after bicycle ergometry training. *Arch Phys Med Rehabil*. 1990, 71(3):207–209.

156. Needhan-Shropshire B, Broton J, Klose KJ, et al. Evaluation of a training program for persons with SCI paraplegia using the Parastep 1 ambulation system: part 3. Lack of effect on bone mineral density. *Arch Phys Med Rehabil*. 1997, 78(8):799–803.

157. de Bruin ED, Frey-Rindova P, Herzog RE, et al. Changes of tibia bone properties after spinal cord injury: effects of early intervention. *Arch Phys Med Rehabil*. 1999, 80(2):214–220.

158. Freebourn TM, Barber DB, Able AC. The treatment of immature heterotopic ossification in spinal cord injury with combination surgery, radiation therapy and NSAID. *Spinal Cord*. 1999, 37(1):50–53.

159. Banovac K, Gonzalez F. Evaluation and management of heterotopic ossification in patients with spinal cord injury. *Spinal Cord*. 1997, 35(3):158–162.

160. Meiners T, Abel R, Bohm V, Gerner HJ. Resection of heterotopic ossification of the hip in spinal cord injured patients. *Spinal Cord*. 1997, 35(7):443–445.

161. Finnerup NB, Jensen TS. Spinal cord injury pain—mechanisms and treatment. *Eur J Neurol*. 2004, 11(2):73–82.

162. Siddall P, Middleton J. A proposed algorithm for the management of pain following spinal cord injury. *Spinal Cord*. 2006, 44:67–77.

163. Irwin R, Restrepo J, Sherman A. Musculoskeletal pain in persons with spinal cord injury. *Top Spinal Cord Inj Rehabil*. 2007, 13(2):43–57.

164. Consortium for Spinal Cord Medicine. *Preservation of Upper Limb Function Following Spinal Cord Injury: A Clinical Practice Guideline for Health-Care Professionals*. Washington, DC: Paralyzed Veterans of America, 2005.

165. Nicholson BD. Evaluation and treatment of central pain syndromes. *Neurology*. 2004, 62(5 Suppl 2):S30–36.

166. Wrigley P, Siddall P. Pharmacological interventions for neuropathic pain following spinal cord injury: an update. *Top Spinal Cord Inj Rehabil*. 2007, 13(2):58–71.

167. Ehde D, Jensen M. Psychological treatments for pain management in persons with spinal cord injury: cognitive therapy and self-hypnosis training. *Top Spinal Cord Inj Rehabil.* 2007, 13(2): 72–80.

168. Adams MM, Hicks AL. Spasticity after spinal cord injury. *Spinal Cord.* 2005, 43(10):577–586.

169. Aydin G, Tomruk S, Keles I, et al. Transcutaneous electrical nerve stimulation versus baclofen in spasticity: clinical and electrophysiologic comparison. *Am J Phys Med Rehabil.* 2005, 84(8):584–592.

170. Hsieh J, Wolfe D, Connolly S. Spasticity after spinal cord injury: an evidence-based review of current interventions. *Top Spinal Cord Inj Rehabil.* 2007, 13(1):81–97.

171. Ragnarsson KT, Stein AB, Spungen AM, Bauman WA. Medical complications after spinal cord injury: spasticity, pain, and endocrine/metabolic changes. *Top Spinal Cord Inj Rehabil.* 2004, 10(2):86–106.

172. Stein AB, Pomerantz F, Schechtman J. Evaluation and management of spasticity in spinal cord injury. *Top Spinal Cord Inj Rehabil.* 1997, 2(4):70–83.

173. Gianino J. Intrathecal baclofen for spinal spasticity: implications for nursing practice. *J Neurosci Nurs.* 1993, 25(4):254–264.

174. Gracies JM, Nance P, Elovic E, et al. Traditional pharmacological treatments for spasticity. Part II: general and regional treatments. *Muscle Nerve.* 1997, (Suppl 6):S92–S120.

175. Moore DP. Helping your patients with spasticity reach maximal function. *Postgrad Med.* 1998, 104(2):123–126, 129–131, 135.

176. Azouvi P, Mane M, Thiebaut JB, et al. Intrathecal baclofen administration for control of severe spinal spasticity: functional improvement and long-term follow-up. *Arch Phys Med Rehabil.* 1996, 77(1):35–39.

177. Gracies JM, Elovic E, McGuire J, Simpson DM. Traditional pharmacological treatments for spasticity. Part I: local treatments. *Muscle Nerve.* 1997, (Suppl 6):S61–91.

178. Holicky R. *Roll Models: People Who Live Successfully Following Spinal Cord Injury And How They Do It.* Victoria, BC, Canada: Trafford, 2004.

179. Kwan I, Bunn F, Roberts I. Spinal immobilzation for trauma patients. *Cochrane Database Syst Rev.* 2001, 2(CD002803).

180. Morris CG, McCoy EP, Lavery GG. Spinal immobilisation for unconscious patients with multiple injuries. *BMJ.* 2004, 329(7464):495–499.

181. Bracken MB, Holford TR. Effects of timing of methylprednisolone or naloxone administration on recovery of segmental and long-tract neurological function in NASCIS 2. *J Neurosurg.* 1993, 79(4):500–507.

182. Bracken MB, Shepard MJ, Collins WF, et al. A randomized, controlled trial of methylprednisolone or naloxone in the treatment of acute spinal-cord injury. Results of the Second National Acute Spinal Cord Injury Study. *N Engl J Med.* 1990, 322(20):1405–1411.

183. Bracken MB, Shepard MJ, Holford TR, et al. Administration of methylprednisolone for 24 or 48 hours or tirilazad mesylate for 48 hours in the treatment of acute spinal cord injury. Results of the Third National Acute Spinal Cord Injury Randomized Controlled Trial. National Acute Spinal Cord Injury Study. *JAMA.* 1997, 277(20):1597–1604.

184. Heary RF, Vaccaro AR, Mesa JJ, et al. Steroids and gunshot wounds to the spine. *Neurosurgery.* 1997, 41(3):576–583, discussion 583–584.

185. Prendergast M, Saxe J, Ledgerwood A, et al. Massive steroids do not reduce the zone of injury after penetrating spinal cord injury. *J Trauma.* 1994, 37(4):576–579.

186. Coleman WP, Benzel D, Cahill DW, et al. A critical appraisal of the reporting of the National Acute Spinal Cord Injury Studies (II and III) of methylprednisolone in acute spinal cord injury. *J Spinal Disord.* 2000, 13(3):185–199.

187. McGuire RA, Neville S, Green BA, Watts C. Spinal instability and the log-rolling maneuver. *J Trauma.* 1987, 27(5): 525–531.

188. Rechtine GR, Conrad BP, Bearden BG, Horodyski M. Biomechanical analysis of cervical and thoracolumbar spine motion in intact and partially and completely unstable cadaver spine models with kinetic bed therapy or traditional log roll. *J Trauma.* 2007, 62(2):383–388, discussion 388.

189. Shen WJ, Shen YS. Nonsurgical treatment of three-column thoracolumbar junction burst fractures without neurologic deficit. *Spine.* 1999, 24(4):412–415.

190. Bernardoni GP, Gavin TM. Comparison between custom and noncustom spinal orthoses. *Phys Med Rehabil Clin N Am.* 2006, 17(1):73–89.

191. Fredericks C. Clinical presentations in disorders of motor function. In: Fredericks C, Saladin L, eds. *Pathophysiology of the Motor Systems: Principles and Clinical Presentations.* Philadelphia: F.A. Davis, 1996:257–288.

192. Mayer NH. Clinicophysiologic concepts of spasticity and motor dysfunction in adults with an upper motoneuron lesion. *Muscle Nerve.* 1997, 20(Suppl 6):S1–S13.

193. Priebe MM, Sherwood AM, Thornby JI, et al. Clinical assessment of spasticity in spinal cord injury: a multidimensional problem. *Arch Phys Med Rehabil.* 1996, 77(7):713–716.

CHAPTER 4

1. Hockenberry J. *Moving Violations: War Zones, Wheelchairs, and Declarations of Independence.* New York: Hyperion, 1995.

2. Elliott T, Kurylo M, Rivera P. Positive growth following acquired physical disability. In: Snyder C, Lopez S, eds. *Handbook of Positive Psychology.* New York: Oxford University Press, 2005: 687–699.

3. Anderson D, Dumont S, Azzaria L, et al. Determinants of return to work among spinal cord injury patients: a literature review. *J Vocat Rehabil.* 2007, 27(1):57–68.

4. Boschen KA, Tonack M, Gargaro J. Long-term adjustment and community reintegration following spinal cord injury. *Int J Rehabil Res.* 2003, 26(3):157–164.

5. Franceschini M, Di Clemente B, Rampello A, et al. Longitudinal outcome 6 years after spinal cord injury. *Spinal Cord.* 2003, 41(5):280–285.

6. Dijkers M, Abela M, Gans B, Gordon W. The aftermath of spinal cord injury. In: Stover S, DeLisa J, Whiteneck G, eds. *Spinal Cord Injury: Clinical Outcomes from the Model Systems.* Gaithersburg, MD: Aspen, 1995:185–212.

7. Hall K, Harper B, Whiteneck G. Follow-up study of individuals with high tetraplegia (C1–C4) 10 to 21 years postinjury. *Top Spinal Cord Inj Rehabil.* 1997, 2(3):107–117.

8. Krause JS, Anson CA. Employment after spinal cord injury: relation to selected participant characteristics. *Arch Phys Med Rehabil.* 1996, 77(8):737–743.

9. Ville I, Ravaud JF. Work, non-work and consequent satisfaction after spinal cord injury. *Int J Rehabil Res.* 1996, 19(3):241–252.

10. Holicky R. What consumers tell us. *Top Spinal Cord Inj Rehabil.* 1997, 2(3):118–123.

11. Johnson RL, Gerhart KA, McCray J, et al. Secondary conditions following spinal cord injury in a population-based sample. *Spinal Cord.* 1998, 36(1):45–50.

12. DeSanto-Madeya S. The meaning of living with spinal cord injury 5 to 10 years after the injury. *West J Nurs Res.* 2006, 28(3):265–289, discussion 290–263.

13. McGowan MB, Roth S. Family functioning and functional independence in spinal cord injury adjustment. *Paraplegia.* 1987, 25(4):357–365.

14. Urey J, Henggeler S. Marital adjustment following spinal cord injury. *Arch Phys Med Rehabil.* 1987, 68(2):69–74.

15. Isaksson G, Skar L, Lexell J. Women's perception of changes in the social network after a spinal cord injury. *Disabil Rehabil.* 2005, 27(17):1013–1021.

16. Trieschmann R. *Spinal Cord Injuries: Psychological, Social, and Vocational Rehabilitation.* New York: Demos, 1988.

17. Trieschmann R. The psychosocial adjustment to spinal cord injury. In: Block R, Basbaum M, eds. *Management of Spinal Cord Injuries.* Baltimore: Williams & Wilkins, 1986:302–319.

18. Corbet B, Dobbs J, Bonin B, eds. *Spinal Network: The Total Wheelchair Resource Book.* 3rd ed. Santa Monica, CA: Nine Lives Press, 2002.

19. Krueger D. Psychological rehabilitation of physical trauma and disability. In: Krueger D, ed. *Rehabilitation Psychology: A Comprehensive Textbook.* Rockville, MD: Aspen, 1984:3–13.

20. Schneider J. *Stress, Loss, and Grief: Understanding Their Origins and Growth Potential.* Baltimore: University Park Press, 1984.

21. Maddox S. *Spinal Network.* Boulder, CO: Spinal Network, 1987.

22. English R. Combating stigma towards physically disabled persons. In: Marinelli R, Orto AD, eds. *The Psychological and Social Impact of Physical Disability.* New York: Springer, 1977:183–193.

23. Gilliland B, James R. *Crisis Intervention Strategies.* Pacific Grove, CA: Brooks/Cole, 1988.

24. Stubbins J. The politics of disability. In: Yuker H, ed. *Attitudes toward Persons with Disabilities.* New York: Springer, 1988:22–32.

25. Tunks E, Bahry N, Basbaum M. The resocialization process after spinal cord injury. In: Bloch R, Basbaum M, eds. *Management of Spinal Cord Injuries.* Baltimore: Williams & Wilkins, 1986:387–409.

26. Chesler M, Chesney B. Self-help groups: empowerment attitudes and behaviors of disabled or chronically ill persons. In: Yuker H, ed. *Attitudes toward Persons with Disabilities.* New York: Springer, 1988:230–245.

27. McCarthy H. Attitudes that affect employment opportunities for persons with disabilities. In: Yuker H, ed. *Attitudes toward Persons with Disabilities.* New York: Springer, 1988:246–261.

28. DeJong G, Branch LG, Corcoran PJ. Independent living outcomes in spinal cord injury: multivariate analyses. *Arch Phys Med Rehabil.* 1984, 65(2):66–73.

29. Wolfensberger W, Tullman S. A brief outline of the principle of normalization. *Rehabil Psychol.* 1982, 27:131–145.

30. Fichten C. Students with physical disabilities in higher education: attitudes and beliefs that affect integration. In: Yuker H, ed. *Attitudes toward Persons with Disabilities.* New York: Springer, 1988:171–186.

31. Lindemann J. *Psychological and Behavioral Aspects of Physical Disability: A Manual for Health Practitioners.* New York: Plenum Press, 1981.

32. Weinberg N. Another perspective: attitudes of persons with disabilities. In: Yuker H, ed. *Attitudes toward Persons with Disabilities.* New York: Springer, 1988:141–153.

33. Karp G, Klein SD, eds. *From There to Here.* Horsham, PA: No Limits Communications, 2004.

34. Haney M, Rabin B. Modifying attitudes toward disabled persons while resocializing spinal cord injured patients. *Arch Phys Med Rehabil.* 1984, 65(8):431–436.

35. Hammell KR. Psychosocial outcome following spinal cord injury. *Paraplegia.* 1994, 32(11):771–779.

36. Berlowitz DJ, Brown DJ, Campbell DA, Pierce RJ. A longitudinal evaluation of sleep and breathing in the first year after cervical spinal cord injury. *Arch Phys Med Rehabil.* 2005, 86(6):1193–1199.

37. North NT. The psychological effects of spinal cord injury: a review. *Spinal Cord.* 1999, 37(10):671–679.

38. Crossman MW. Sensory deprivation in spinal cord injury—an essay. *Spinal Cord.* 1996, 34(10):573–577.

39. Richards JS, Seitz MR, Eisele WA. Auditory processing in spinal cord injury: a preliminary investigation from a sensory

deprivation perspective. *Arch Phys Med Rehabil.* 1986, 67(2): 115–117.

40. Sand A, Karlberg I, Kreuter M. Spinal cord injured persons' conceptions of hospital care, rehabilitation, and a new life situation. *Scand J Occup Ther.* 2006, 13(3):183–192.

41. Siosteen A, Kreuter M, Lampic C, Persson LO. Patient-staff agreement in the perception of spinal cord lesioned patients' problems, emotional well-being, and coping pattern. *Spinal Cord.* 2005, 43(3):179–186.

42. Gerhart K. Quality of life: the danger of differing perceptions. *Top Spinal Cord Inj Rehabil.* 1997, 2(3):78–84.

43. Howell T, Fullerton DT, Harvey RF, Klein M. Depression in spinal cord injured patients. *Paraplegia.* 1981, 19(5):284–288.

44. Lawson NC. Significant events in the rehabilitation process: the spinal cord patient's point of view. *Arch Phys Med Rehabil.* 1978, 59(12):573–579.

45. Corbet B. *Options: Spinal Cord Injury and the Future.* Denver: Hirschfeld Press, 1980.

46. Krause JS. Longitudinal changes in adjustment after spinal cord injury: a 15-year study. *Arch Phys Med Rehabil.* 1992, 73(6):564–568.

47. Bach JR, Tilton MC. Life satisfaction and well-being measures in ventilator assisted individuals with traumatic tetraplegia. *Arch Phys Med Rehabil.* 1994, 75(6):626–632.

48. Westgren N, Levi R. Quality of life and traumatic spinal cord injury. *Arch Phys Med Rehabil.* 1998, 79(11):1433–1439.

49. Kemp BJ, Krause JS. Depression and life satisfaction among people ageing with post-polio and spinal cord injury. *Disabil Rehabil.* 1999, 21(5–6):241–249.

50. Dijkers MP. Correlates of life satisfaction among persons with spinal cord injury. *Arch Phys Med Rehabil.* 1999, 80(8):867–876.

51. DeSantis N, Becker B. Building a durable relationship: avoiding catastrophe between the therapeutic team and the patient with a new spinal cord injury. *Top Spinal Cord Inj Rehabil.* 1999, 4(3):29–35.

52. Elliott TR, Frank RG. Depression following spinal cord injury. *Arch Phys Med Rehabil.* 1996, 77(8):816–823.

53. Moverman R. Psychosocial factors in spinal cord injury. In: Lin V, ed. *Spinal Cord Medicine: Principles and Practice.* New York: Demos, 2003:931–939.

54. Elfstrom ML, Kreuter M, Ryden A, et al. Effects of coping on psychological outcome when controlling for background variables: a study of traumatically spinal cord lesioned persons. *Spinal Cord.* 2002, 40(8):408–415.

55. Frank RG, Elliott TR, Buckelew SP, Haut AE. Age as a factor in response to spinal cord injury. *Am J Phys Med Rehabil.* 1988, 67(3):128–131.

56. Galvin LR, Godfrey HP. The impact of coping on emotional adjustment to spinal cord injury (SCI): review of the literature and application of a stress appraisal and coping formulation. *Spinal Cord.* 2001, 39(12):615–627.

57. Martz E. Associations and predictors of posttraumatic stress levels according to person-related, disability-related, and trauma-related variables among individuals with spinal cord injuries. *Rehabil Psychol.* 2005, 50(2):149–157.

58. Schmitt M, Elliott T. Verbal learning ability and adjustment to recent-onset spinal cord injury. *Rehabil Psychol.* 2004, 49(4): 288–294.

59. Glass CA, Jackson HF, Dutton J, et al. Estimating social adjustment following spinal trauma—II: population trends and effects of compensation on adjustment. *Spinal Cord.* 1997, 35(6):349–357.

60. Green BC, Pratt CC, Grigsby TE. Self-concept among persons with long-term spinal cord injury. *Arch Phys Med Rehabil.* 1984, 65(12):751–754.

61. Krause JS. Aging and life adjustment after spinal cord injury. *Spinal Cord.* 1998, 36(5):320–328.

62. Kreuter M, Sullivan M, Dahllof AG, Siosteen A. Partner relationships, functioning, mood and global quality of life in

persons with spinal cord injury and traumatic brain injury. *Spinal Cord.* 1998, 36(4):252–261.

63. Sammallahti P, Kannisto M, Aalberg V. Psychological defenses and psychiatric symptoms in adults with pediatric spinal cord injuries. *Spinal Cord.* 1996, 34(11):669–672.

64. Servoss A, Krueger D. Normal vs. pathological grief and mourning: some precursors. In: Krueger D, ed. *Emotional Rehabilitation of Physical Trauma and Disability.* New York: SP Medical & Scientific Books, 1984:45–49.

65. McColl MA, Skinner H. Assessing inter- and intrapersonal resources: social support and coping among adults with a disability. *Disabil Rehabil.* 1995, 17(1):24–34.

66. Larsson M, Nordlund A, Nygard L, et al. Perceptions of participation and predictors of perceived problems with participation in persons with spinal cord injury. *J Rehabil Med.* 2005, 37(1):3–8.

67. Nielsen M. Prevalence of posttraumatic stress disorder in persons with spinal cord injuries: the mediating effect of social support. *Rehabil Psychol.* 2003, 48(4):289–295.

68. Kennedy P, Lude P, Taylor N. Quality of life, social participation, appraisals and coping post spinal cord injury: a review of four community samples. *Spinal Cord.* 2006, 44(2):95–105.

69. Saravanan B, Manigandan C, Macaden A, et al. Re-examining the psychology of spinal cord injury: a meaning centered approach from a cultural perspective. *Spinal Cord.* 2001, 39(6):323–326.

70. Bombardier CH, Richards JS, Krause JS, et al. Symptoms of major depression in people with spinal cord injury: implications for screening. *Arch Phys Med Rehabil.* 2004, 85(11):1749–1756.

71. Kalpakjian CZ, Albright KJ. An examination of depression through the lens of spinal cord injury: comparative prevalence rates and severity in women and men. *Womens Health Issues.* 2006, 16(6):380–388.

72. Cushman LA, Hassett J. Spinal cord injury: 10 and 15 years after. *Paraplegia.* 1992, 30(10):690–696.

73. Daverat P, Petit H, Kemoun G, et al. The long term outcome in 149 patients with spinal cord injury. *Paraplegia.* 1995, 33(11):665–668.

74. Fuhrer MJ, Rintala DH, Hart KA, et al. Relationship of life satisfaction to impairment, disability, and handicap among persons with spinal cord injury living in the community. *Arch Phys Med Rehabil.* 1992, 73(6):552–557.

75. Gerhart KA, Weitzenkamp DA, Kennedy P, et al. Correlates of stress in long-term spinal cord injury. *Spinal Cord.* 1999, 37(3):183–190.

76. Goldberg RT, Freed MM. Vocational development of spinal cord injury patients: an 8-year follow-up. *Arch Phys Med Rehabil.* 1982, 63(5):207–210.

77. Gorman C, Kennedy P, Hamilton LR. Alterations in self-perceptions following childhood onset of spinal cord injury. *Spinal Cord.* 1998, 36(3):181–185.

78. Macleod L, Macleod G. Control cognitions and psychological disturbance in people with contrasting physically disabling conditions. *Disabil Rehabil.* 1998, 20(12):448–456.

79. Malec J, Neimeyer R. Psychologic prediction of duration of inpatient spinal cord injury rehabilitation and performance of self-care. *Arch Phys Med Rehabil.* 1983, 64(8):359–363.

80. Post MW, de Witte LP, van Asbeck FW, et al. Predictors of health status and life satisfaction in spinal cord injury. *Arch Phys Med Rehabil.* 1998, 79(4):395–401.

81. Scivoletto G, Petrelli A, Di Lucente L, Castellano V. Psychological investigation of spinal cord injury patients. *Spinal Cord.* 1997, 35(8):516–520.

82. Hartkopp A, Bronnum-Hansen H, Seidenschnur AM, Biering-Sorensen F. Suicide in a spinal cord injured population: its relation to functional status. *Arch Phys Med Rehabil.* 1998, 79(11):1356–1361.

83. Gerhart KA, Johnson RL, Whiteneck GG. Health and psychosocial issues of individuals with incomplete and resolving spinal cord injuries. *Paraplegia.* 1992, 30(4):282–287.

84. Ducharme S, Ducharme J. Psychological adjustment to spinal cord injury. In: Krueger D, ed. *Emotional Rehabilitation of Physical Trauma and Disability.* New York: SP Medical & Scientific Books, 1984:149–156.

85. Brown R, Hughston E. *Behavioral and Social Rehabilitation and Training.* New York: Wiley, 1987.

86. Lustig D. The adjustment process for individuals with spinal cord injury: the effect of perceived premorbid sense of coherence. *Rehabil Couns Bull.* 2005, 48(3):146–156.

87. Fichtenbaum J, Kirshblum S. Psychologic adaptation to spinal cord injury. In: Kirshblum S, Campagnolo DI, DeLisa JA, eds. *Spinal Cord Medicine.* Philadelphia: Lippincott Williams & Wilkins, 2002:299–311.

88. Jackson S, Hough S. Adjustment to the process of grief following spinal cord injury/dysfunction. *SCI Psychosoc Process.* 2004, 17(3):145, 150–155.

89. Bracken MB, Shepard MJ, Webb SB Jr. Psychological response to acute spinal cord injury: an epidemiological study. *Paraplegia.* 1981, 19(5):271–283.

90. Macleod AD. Self-neglect of spinal injured patients. *Paraplegia.* 1988, 26(5):340–349.

91. Pinkerton AC, Griffin ML. Rehabilitation outcomes in females with spinal cord injury: a follow-up study. *Paraplegia.* 1983, 21(3):166–175.

92. Carlson CE. Conceptual style and life satisfaction following spinal cord injury. *Arch Phys Med Rehabil.* 1979, 60(8):346–352.

93. Richards JS. Psychologic adjustment to spinal cord injury during first postdischarge year. *Arch Phys Med Rehabil.* 1986, 67(6):362–365.

94. Whiteneck G, Forcheimer M, Krause J. Quality of life and health in the last years after spinal cord injury. *Top Spinal Cord Inj Rehabil.* 2007, 12(3):77–90.

95. Noyes R. The existential crisis of serious illness. In: Krueger D, ed. *Emotional Rehabilitation of Physical Trauma and Disability.* New York: SP Medical & Scientific Books, 1984:51–61.

96. Crewe N. Gains and losses due to spinal cord injury: views across 20 years. *Top Spinal Cord Inj Rehabil.* 1996, 2(2):46–57.

97. Holicky R. *Roll Models: People Who Live Successfully Following Spinal Cord Injury And How They Do It.* Victoria, BC, Canada: Trafford, 2004.

98. Kishi Y, Robinson RG, Forrester AW. Comparison between acute and delayed onset major depression after spinal cord injury. *J Nerv Ment Dis.* 1995, 183(5):286–292.

99. MacDonald MR, Nielson WR, Cameron MG. Depression and activity patterns of spinal cord injured persons living in the community. *Arch Phys Med Rehabil.* 1987, 68(6):339–343.

100. Elliott T, Kennedy P. Treatment of depression following spinal cord injury: an evidence-based review. *Rehabil Psychol.* 2004, 49:134–139.

101. Chung MC, Preveza E, Papandreou K, Prevezas N. Spinal cord injury, posttraumatic stress, and locus of control among the elderly: a comparison with young and middle-aged patients. *Psychiatry.* 2006, 69(1):69–80.

102. Craig A, Hancock K, Dickson H. Improving the long-term adjustment of spinal cord injured persons. *Spinal Cord.* 1999, 37(5):345–350.

103. Dijkers M. Community integration: conceptual issues and measurement approaches in rehabilitation research. *Top Spinal Cord Inj Rehabil.* 1998, 4(1):1–15.

104. Hansen N, Forchheimer M, Tate D, Luera G. Relationships among community reintegration, coping strategies, and life satisfaction in a sample of persons with spinal cord injury. *Top Spinal Cord Inj Rehabil.* 1998, 4(1):56–72.

105. Roush SE. Health professionals as contributors to attitudes toward persons with disabilities. A special communication. *Phys Ther*. 1986, 66(10):1551–1554.

106. Wright B. Attitudes and the fundamental negative bias: conditions and corrections. In: Yuker H, ed. *Attitudes toward Persons with Disabilities*. New York: Springer, 1988:3–21.

107. DeJong G. Independent living: from social movement to analytic paradigm. *Arch Phys Med Rehabil*. 1979, 60(10):435–446.

108. Nosek MA, Parker RM, Larsen S. Psychosocial independence and functional abilities: their relationship in adults with severe musculoskeletal impairments. *Arch Phys Med Rehabil*. 1987, 68(12):840–845.

109. Halstead LS, Rintala DH, Kanellos M, et al. The innovative rehabilitation team: an experiment in team building. *Arch Phys Med Rehabil*. 1986, 67(6):357–361.

110. Reeve C. *Nothing is Impossible: Reflections on a New Life*. New York: Ballantine Books, 2002.

111. Park L. Barriers to normality for the handicapped adult in the United States. In: Marinelli R, Orto AD, eds. *The Psychological and Social Impact of Physical Disability*. New York: Springer, 1977:25–33.

112. Lys K, Pernice R. Perceptions of positive attitudes toward people with spinal cord injury. *Int J Rehabil Res*. 1995, 18(1):35–43.

113. Osterweis M, Solomon F, Green M. *Bereavement: Reactions, Consequences, and Care*. Washington, DC: National Academy Press, 1984.

114. Hoff L. *People in Crisis: Understanding and Helping*. Redwood City, CA: Addison-Wesley, 1989.

115. Brockopp DY, Hayko D, Davenport W, Winscott C. Personal control and the needs for hope and information among adults diagnosed with cancer. *Cancer Nurs*. 1989, 12(2):112–116.

116. Northouse P, Northouse L. *Health Communication: A Handbook for Health Professionals*. Englewood Cliffs, NJ: Prentice Hall, 1985.

117. Decker N. Brief psychotherapy of chronic illness. In: Krueger D, ed. *Emotional Rehabilitation of Physical Trauma and Disability*. New York: SP Medical & Scientific Books, 1984:195–218.

118. Judd FK, Brown DJ. Psychiatry in the spinal injuries unit. *Paraplegia*. 1987, 25(3):254–257.

119. Judd FK, Brown DJ. The psychosocial approach to rehabilitation of the spinal cord injured patient. *Paraplegia*. 1988, 26(6):419–424.

120. Consortium for Spinal Cord Medicine. *Depression Following Spinal Cord Injury: A Clinical Practice Guideline for Primary Care Physicians*. Washington, DC: Paralyzed Veterans of America, 1998.

121. Elliott T, Jackson W. Psychologic assessment in spinal cord injury rehabilitation: benefiting patient, treatment team, and health care delivery system. *Top Spinal Cord Inj Rehabil*. 1996, 2(2):34–45.

122. Heinemann AW, Keen M, Donohue R, Schnoll S. Alcohol use by persons with recent spinal cord injury. *Arch Phys Med Rehabil*. 1988, 69(8):619–624.

123. Young ME, Rintala DH, Rossi CD, et al. Alcohol and marijuana use in a community-based sample of persons with spinal cord injury. *Arch Phys Med Rehabil*. 1995, 76(6):525–532.

124. Rohrer K, Adelman B, Puckett J, et al. Rehabilitation in spinal cord injury: use of a patient-family group. *Arch Phys Med Rehabil*. 1980, 61(5):225–229.

125. Lasky R, Orto AD, Marinelli R. Structured experimental therapy: a group approach to rehabilitation. In: Marinelli R, Orto AD, eds. *The Psychological and Social Impact of Physical Disability*. New York: Springer, 1977:319–333.

126. Moeller T, Hartman D. The group psychotherapy process in rehabilitation settings. In: Krueger D, ed. *Emotional Rehabilitation of Physical Trauma and Disability*. New York: SP Medical & Scientific Books, 1984:219–233.

127. Patterson R, Bushnik T, Burdsall D, Wright J. Considerations of peer support for persons with high tetraplegia. *Top Spinal Cord Inj Rehabil*. 2005, 10(3):30–37.

128. Veith E, Sherman J, Pellino T, Yasui N. Qualitative analysis of the peer-mentoring relationship among individuals with spinal cord injury. *Rehabil Psychol*. 2006, 51(4):289–298.

129. Cogswell B. Self-socialization: readjustment of paraplegics in the community. In: Marinelli R, Orto AD, eds. *The Psychological and Social Impact of Physical Disability*. New York: Springer, 1977:151–159.

130. Yuker H. The effects of contact on attitudes toward disabled persons: some empirical generalizations. In: Yuker H, ed. *Attitudes toward Persons with Disabilities*. New York: Springer, 1988:262–274.

131. Horne M. Modifying peer attitudes toward the handicapped: procedures and research issues. In: Yuker H, ed. *Attitudes toward Persons with Disabilities*. New York: Springer, 1988:203–222.

132. Craig AR, Hancock K, Dickson H, Chang E. Long-term psychological outcomes in spinal cord injured persons: results of a controlled trial using cognitive behavior therapy. *Arch Phys Med Rehabil*. 1997, 78(1):33–38.

133. Kennedy P, Duff J, Evans M, Beedie A. Coping effectiveness training reduces depression and anxiety following traumatic spinal cord injuries. *Br J Clin Psychol*. 2003, 42(Pt 1):41–52.

134. Craig AR, Hancock K, Chang E, Dickson H. Immunizing against depression and anxiety after spinal cord injury. *Arch Phys Med Rehabil*. 1998, 79(4):375–377.

135. Quigley MC. Impact of spinal cord injury on the life roles of women. *Am J Occup Ther*. 1995, 49(8):780–786.

136. Post M, Noreau L. Quality of life after spinal cord injury. *J Neurol Phys Ther*. 2005, 29(3):139–146.

137. Nichols S, Brasile F. The role of recreational therapy in physical medicine. *Top Spinal Cord Inj Rehabil*. 1998, 3(3):89–98.

138. Morgan D. Not all sadness can be treated with antidepressants. *W V Med J*. 1980, 76(6):136–137.

139. Sherman J, DeVinney D. Social support and adjustment after spinal cord injury: influence of past peer-mentoring experiences and current live-in partner. *Rehabil Psychol*. 2004, 49(2):140–149.

140. Jaques M, Patterson K. The self-help group model: a review. In: Marinelli R, Orto AD, eds. *The Psychological and Social Impact of Physical Disability*. New York: Springer, 1977:270–281.

141. Stewart R, Bhagwanjee A. Promoting group empowerment and self-reliance through participatory research: a case study of people with physical disability. *Disabil Rehabil*. 1999, 21(7):338–345.

142. Fuhrer MJ, Rossi LD, Gerken L, et al. Relationships between independent living centers and medical rehabilitation programs. *Arch Phys Med Rehabil*. 1990, 71(7):519–522.

143. Forcheimer M, Tate D. Enhancing community re-integration following spinal cord injury. *NeuroRehabilitation*. 2004, 19(2):103–113.

144. Robinson K. A primer on independent living centers. In: Corbet B, Dobbs J, Bonin B, eds. *Spinal Network: The Total Wheelchair Resource Book*. Santa Monica, CA: Nine Lives Press, 2002:387–388.

145. Tate D, Forchheimer M. Enhancing community reintegration after impatient rehabilitation for persons with spinal cord injury. *Top Spinal Cord Inj Rehabil*. 1998, 4(1):42–55.

146. Krause JS. Employment after spinal cord injury. *Arch Phys Med Rehabil*. 1992, 73(2):163–169.

147. Dijkers M. Quality of life after spinal cord injury: a meta analysis of the effects of disablement components. *Spinal Cord*. 1997, 35(12):829–840.

148. Hess D, Meade M, Forchheimer M, Tate D. Psychological well-being and intensity of employment in individuals with a spinal cord injury. *Top Spinal Cord Inj Rehabil*. 2004, 9(4):1–10.

149. Krause JS. Years to employment after spinal cord injury. *Arch Phys Med Rehabil*. 2003, 84(9):1282–1289.

150. Hills L, Cullen E. A study into the employment trends of individuals treated at a spinal cord injury centre. *Int J Ther Rehabil*. 2007, 14(8):350–355.

151. Dorsett P, Geraghty T. Depression and adjustment after spinal cord injury: a three year longitudinal study. *Top Spinal Cord Inj Rehabil*. 2004, 9(4):43–56.

152. Brown M, Gordon WA, Ragnarsson K. Unhandicapping the disabled: what is possible? *Arch Phys Med Rehabil*. 1987, 68(4): 206–209.

153. World Health Organization. Towards a Common Language for Functioning, Disability and Health: ICF. 2002, http://www.who.int/classifications/icf/training/icfbeginnersguide.pdf. Accessed 9/9/08.

154. Krause J. Aging and self-reported barriers to employment after spinal cord injury. *Top Spinal Cord Inj Rehabil*. 2001, 6(3): 102–115.

155. Atwell S, Hudson L. Social security legislation creates Ticket to Work and Work Incentives Improvement Act. *Top Spinal Cord Inj Rehabil*. 2004, 9(4):26–32.

156. American Psychiatric Association. *Diagnostic and Statistical Manual of Mental Disorders: DSM-IV-TR*. 4th ed. Washington, DC: American Psychiatric Association, 2000.

CHAPTER 5

1. Cardenas DD, Hoffman JM, Kirshblum S, McKinley W. Etiology and incidence of rehospitalization after traumatic spinal cord injury: a multicenter analysis. *Arch Phys Med Rehabil*. 2004, 85(11):1757–1763.

2. Richards J, Waites K, Chen Y, et al. The epidemiology of secondary conditions following spinal cord injury. *Top Spinal Cord Inj Rehabil*. 2004, 10(1):15–29.

3. da Paz AC, Beraldo PS, Almeida MC, et al. Traumatic injury to the spinal cord. Prevalence in Brazilian hospitals. *Paraplegia*. 1992, 30(9):636–640.

4. Walter JS, Sacks J, Othman R, et al. A database of self-reported secondary medical problems among VA spinal cord injury patients: its role in clinical care and management. *J Rehabil Res Dev*. 2002, 39(1):53–61.

5. Knutsdottir S. Spinal cord injuries in Iceland 1973–1989. A follow up study. *Paraplegia*. 1993, 31(1):68–72.

6. Nakajima A, Honda S, Yoshimura S, et al. The disease pattern and causes of death of spinal cord injured patients in Japan. *Paraplegia*. 1989, 27(3):163–171.

7. Yarkony G, Heinemann AW. Pressure ulcers. In: Stover SL, DeLisa JA, Whiteneck GG, eds. *Spinal Cord Injury: Clinical Outcomes from the Model Systems*. Gaithersburg, MD: Aspen, 1995:100–119.

8. Jan J, Brienza D. Technology for pressure ulcer prevention. *Top Spinal Cord Inj Rehabil*. 2006, 11(4):30–41.

9. Niazi ZB, Salzberg CA, Byrne DW, Viehbeck M. Recurrence of initial pressure ulcer in persons with spinal cord injuries. *Adv Wound Care*. 1997, 10(3):38–42.

10. Byrne DW, Salzberg CA. Major risk factors for pressure ulcers in the spinal cord disabled: a literature review. *Spinal Cord*. 1996, 34(5):255–263.

11. Krause JS. Skin sores after spinal cord injury: relationship to life adjustment. *Spinal Cord*. 1998, 36(1):51–56.

12. Vidal J, Sarrias M. An analysis of the diverse factors concerned with the development of pressure sores in spinal cord injured patients. *Paraplegia*. 1991, 29(4):261–267.

13. Anson CA, Shepherd C. Incidence of secondary complications in spinal cord injury. *Int J Rehabil Res*. 1996, 19(1):55–66.

14. Fuhrer MJ, Garber SL, Rintala DH, et al. Pressure ulcers in community-resident persons with spinal cord injury: prevalence and risk factors. *Arch Phys Med Rehabil*. 1993, 74(11):1172–1177.

15. Salzberg CA, Byrne DW, Cayten CG, et al. A new pressure ulcer risk assessment scale for individuals with spinal cord injury. *Am J Phys Med Rehabil*. 1996, 75(2):96–104.

16. Consortium for Spinal Cord Medicine. *Pressure Ulcer Prevention and Treatment Following Spinal Cord Injury: A Clinical Practice Guideline for Health-Care Professionals*. Washington, DC: Paralyzed Veterans of America, 2000.

17. Elliott R, Bush B, Chen Y. Social problem-solving abilities predict pressure sore occurrence in the first 3 years of spinal cord injury. *Rehabil Psychol*. 2006, 51(1):69–77.

18. Krause JS, Broderick L. Patterns of recurrent pressure ulcers after spinal cord injury: identification of risk and protective factors 5 or more years after onset. *Arch Phys Med Rehabil*. 2004, 85(8):1257–1264.

19. Krause JS, Vines CL, Farley TL, et al. An exploratory study of pressure ulcers after spinal cord injury: relationship to protective behaviors and risk factors. *Arch Phys Med Rehabil*. 2001, 82(1):107–113.

20. Burr RG, Clift-Peace L, Nuseibeh I. Haemoglobin and albumin as predictors of length of stay of spinal injured patients in a rehabilitation centre. *Paraplegia*. 1993, 31(7):473–478.

21. Johnson RL, Gerhart KA, McCray J, et al. Secondary conditions following spinal cord injury in a population-based sample. *Spinal Cord*. 1998, 36(1):45–50.

22. Lehman CA. Risk factors for pressure ulcers in the spinal cord injured in the community. *SCI Nurs*. 1995, 12(4):110–114.

23. Linares HA, Mawson AR, Suarez E, Biundo JJ. Association between pressure sores and immobilization in the immediate post-injury period. *Orthopedics*. 1987, 10(4):571–573.

24. McGlinchey-Berroth R, Morrow L, Ahlquist M, et al. Late-life spinal cord injury and aging with a long term injury: characteristics of two emerging populations. *J Spinal Cord Med*. 1995, 18(3):183–193.

25. Menter R, Hudson L. Effects of age at injury and the aging process. In: Stover S, DeLisa J, Whiteneck J, eds. *Spinal Cord Injury: Clinical Outcomes from the Model Systems*. Gaithersburg, MD: Aspen, 1995:272–288.

26. Rochon PA, Beaudet MP, McGlinchey-Berroth R, et al. Risk assessment for pressure ulcers: an adaptation of the National Pressure Ulcer Advisory Panel risk factors to spinal cord injured patients. *J Am Paraplegia Soc*. 1993, 16(3): 169–177.

27. Salzberg CA, Byrne DW, Cayten CG, et al. Predicting and preventing pressure ulcers in adults with paralysis. *Adv Wound Care*. 1998, 11(5):237–246.

28. Sumiya T, Kawamura K, Tokuhiro A, et al. A survey of wheelchair use by paraplegic individuals in Japan. Part 2: prevalence of pressure sores. *Spinal Cord*. 1997, 35(9):595–598.

29. Uveges J. Psychosocial correlates of pressure ulcers. *Top Spinal Cord Inj Rehabil*. 1996, 2(1):51–56.

30. Garber SL, Rintala DH. Pressure ulcers in veterans with spinal cord injury: a retrospective study. *J Rehabil Res Dev*. 2003, 40(5):433–441.

31. Gunnewicht BR. Pressure sores in patients with acute spinal cord injury. *J Wound Care*. 1995, 4(10):452–454.

32. Rodriguez GP, Claus-Walker J, Kent MC, Garza HM. Collagen metabolite excretion as a predictor of bone- and skin-related complications in spinal cord injury. *Arch Phys Med Rehabil*. 1989, 70(6):442–444.

33. Mawson AR, Siddiqui FH, Biundo JJ Jr. Enhancing host resistance to pressure ulcers: a new approach to prevention. *Prev Med*. 1993, 22(3):433–450.

34. Brienza DM, Karg PE. Seat cushion optimization: a comparison of interface pressure and tissue stiffness characteristics for spinal cord injured and elderly patients. *Arch Phys Med Rehabil*. 1998, 79(4):388–394.

35. Hobson DA. Comparative effects of posture on pressure and shear at the body-seat interface. *J Rehabil Res Dev*. 1992, 29(4):21–31.

36. Gildsorf P, Patterson R, Fisher S. Thirty-minute continuous sitting force measurements with different support surfaces in

the spinal cord injured and able-bodied. *J Rehabil Res Dev.* 1991, 28(4):33–38.

37. Ditunno JF Jr, Formal CS. Chronic spinal cord injury. *N Engl J Med.* 1994, 330(8):550–556.

38. Vohra RK, McCollum CN. Pressure sores. *BMJ.* 1994, 309(6958):853–857.

39. Yarkony GM. Pressure ulcers: a review. *Arch Phys Med Rehabil.* 1994, 75(8):908–917.

40. Maklebust J. Choosing the right support surface. *Adv Skin Wound Care.* 2005, 18(3):158–161.

41. Bergstrom N, Allman R, Carlson C, et al. *Pressure Ulcers in Adults: Prediction and Prevention. Clinical Practice Guideline, Number 3.* AHCR Publication No. 92-0047. Rockville, MD: U.S. Department of Health and Human Services. Public Health Service, Agency for Health Care Policy and Research, 1992.

42. Patterson RP, Fisher SV. Sitting pressure-time patterns in patients with quadriplegia. *Arch Phys Med Rehabil.* 1986, 67(11):812–814.

43. DeVivo MJ, Kartus PL, Stover SL, et al. Cause of death for patients with spinal cord injuries. *Arch Intern Med.* 1989, 149(8):1761–1766.

44. Dumurgier C, Pujol G, Chevalley J, et al. Pressure sore carcinoma: a late but fulminant complication of pressure sores in spinal cord injury patients: case reports. *Paraplegia.* 1991, 29(6):390–395.

45. National Spinal Cord Injury Statistical Center. Annual Report for the Model Spinal Cord Injury Care Systems. 2007, http://www.spinalcord.uab.edu. Accessed 12/15/08.

46. Aung TS, el Masry WS. Audit of a British Centre for spinal injury. *Spinal Cord.* 1997, 35(3):147–150.

47. Sapountzi-Krepia D, Soumilas A, Papadakis N, et al. Post traumatic paraplegics living in Athens: the impact of pressure sores and UTIs on everyday life activities. *Spinal Cord.* 1998, 36(6):432–437.

48. McBride DQ, Rodts GE. Intensive care of patients with spinal trauma. *Neurosurg Clin N Am.* 1994, 5(4):755–766.

49. Wound Ostomy and Continence Nurses Society. *Guideline for the Prevention and Management of Pressure Ulcers.* Glenview, IL: Wound, Ostomy, and Continence Nurses Society, 2003.

50. Royster R, Barboi C, Peruzzi W. Critical care in the acute cervical spinal cord injury. *Top Spinal Cord Inj Rehabil.* 2004, 9(3):11–32.

51. Shenaq SM, Dinh TA. Decubitus ulcers. How to prevent them—and intervene should prevention fail. *Postgrad Med.* 1990, 87(4):91–95.

52. Frost FS. Role of rehabilitation after spinal cord injury. *Urol Clin North Am.* 1993, 20(3):549–559.

53. Macklebust J. Pressure ulcers: etiology and prevention. *Nurs Clin North Am.* 1987, 22(2):359–377.

54. Gittler M. Acute rehabilitation in cervical spinal cord injury. *Top Spinal Cord Inj Rehabil.* 2004, 9(3):60–73.

55. Willey T. High-tech beds and mattress overlays. A decision guide. *Am J Nurs.* 1989, 89(9):1142–1145.

56. Kennedy E, Stover S, Fine P, eds. *Spinal Cord Injury: The Facts and Figures.* Birmingham, AL: The University of Alabama Spinal Cord Injury Statistical Center, 1986.

57. Nawoczenski D. Pressure sores: prevention and management. In: Buchanan J, Nawoczenski D, eds. *Spinal Cord Injury: Concepts and Management Approaches.* Baltimore: Williams & Wilkins, 1987:99–121.

58. Bergstrom N, Allman R, Carlson C, et al. *Treatment of Pressure Ulcers. Clinical Practice Guideline, Number 15.* AHCPR Publication No. 95-0652. Rockville, MD: Department of Health and Human Services. Public Health Service, Agency for Health Care Policy and Research, 1994.

59. Bates-Jensen B. Pressure ulcers: pathophysiology and prevention. In: Sussman C, Bates-Jensen B, eds. *Wound Care: A Collaborative Practice Manual for Physical Therapists and Nurses.* Gaithersburg, MD: Aspen, 2001:325–360.

60. Seiler WO, Allen S, Stahelin HB. Influence of the 30 degrees laterally inclined position and the "super-soft" 3-piece mattress on skin oxygen tension on areas of maximum pressure—implications for pressure sore prevention. *Gerontology.* 1986, 32(3):158–166.

61. Kirk P. Pressure ulcer management following spinal cord injury. *Top Spinal Cord Inj Rehabil.* 1996, 2(1):9–20.

62. Stewart P, Wharton GW. Bridging: an effective and practical method of preventive skin care for the immobilized person. *South Med J.* 1976, 69(11):1469–1473.

63. National Collaborating Centre for Nursing and Supportive Care. *The Use of Pressure-Relieving Devices (Beds, Mattresses and Overlays) for the Prevention of Pressure Ulcers in Primary and Secondary Care.* London: National Institute for Clinical Excellence, 2003.

64. National Pressure Ulcer Advisory Panel. *Terms and Definitions Related to Support Surfaces.* 2007, http://www.npuap.org. Accessed 02/6/09.

65. Brienza DM, Geyer MJ. Using support surfaces to manage tissue integrity. *Adv Skin Wound Care.* 2005, 18(3):151–157.

66. Fletcher J. Types of pressure-relieving equipment available: 1. *Br J Nurs.* 1996, 5(11):694, 696, 698 passim.

67. Thompson P, Anderson J, Langemo D, et al. Support surfaces: definitions and utilization for patient care. *Adv Skin Wound Care.* 2008, 21(6):264–266.

68. Petrie LA, Hummel RS III. A study of interface pressure for pressure reduction and relief mattresses. *J Enterostom Ther.* 1990, 17(5):212–216.

69. Economides NG, Skoutakis VA, Carter CA, Smith VH. Evaluation of the effectiveness of two support surfaces following myocutaneous flap surgery. *Adv Wound Care.* 1995, 8(1):49–53.

70. Cooper PJ, Gray DG, Mollison J. A randomised controlled trial of two pressure-reducing surfaces. *J Wound Care.* 1998, 7(8):374–376.

71. Catz A, Zifroni A, Philo O. Economic assessment of pressure sore prevention using a computerized mattress system in patients with spinal cord injury. *Disabil Rehabil.* 2005, 27(21):1315–1319.

72. McLeod AG. Principles of alternating pressure surfaces. *Adv Wound Care.* 1997, 10(7):30–36.

73. Gunnewicht BR. Management of pressure sores in a spinal injuries unit. *J Wound Care.* 1996, 5(1):36–39.

74. Mayall J, Desharnais G. *Positioning in a Wheelchair: A Guide for Professional Caregivers of the Disabled Adult.* 2nd ed. Thorofare, NJ: Slack, 1995.

75. Peterson MJ, Adkins HV. Measurement and redistribution of excessive pressures during wheelchair sitting. *Phys Ther.* 1982, 62(7):990–994.

76. Koo TK, Mak AF, Lee YL. Posture effect on seating interface biomechanics: comparison between two seating cushions. *Arch Phys Med Rehabil.* 1996, 77(1):40–47.

77. Cooper R. *Wheelchair Selection and Configuration.* New York: Demos, 1998.

78. Gilsdorf P, Patterson R, Fisher S. Thirty-minute continuous sitting force measurements with different support surfaces in the spinal cord injured and able-bodied. *J Rehabil Res Dev.* 1991, 28(4):33–38.

79. Karp G. *Choosing a Wheelchair: A Guide for Optimal Independence.* Sebastopol, CA: O'Reilly & Associates, 1998.

80. Ragnarsson KT. Prescription considerations and a comparison of conventional and lightweight wheelchairs. *J Rehabil Res Dev Clin Suppl.* 1990, (2):8–16.

81. Wilson A. *How to Select and Use Manual Wheelchairs.* Topping, VA: Rehabilitation Press, 1992.

82. Brubaker C. Ergonomic considerations. *J Rehabil Res Dev Clin Suppl.* 1990, (2):37–48.

83. Maklebust J. Pressure ulcers: etiology and prevention. *Nurs Clin North Am.* 1987, 22(2):359–377.

84. Krey CH, Calhoun CL. Utilizing research in wheelchair and seating selection and configuration for children with injury/dysfunction of the spinal cord. *J Spinal Cord Med*. 2004, 27(Suppl 1):S29–S37.

85. Burns SP, Betz KL. Seating pressures with conventional and dynamic wheelchair cushions in tetraplegia. *Arch Phys Med Rehabil*. 1999, 80(5):566–571.

86. Dabnichki P, Taktak D. Pressure variation under the ischial tuberosity during a push cycle. *Med Eng Phys*. 1998, 20(4):242–256.

87. Kernozek TW, Lewin JE. Seat interface pressures of individuals with paraplegia: influence of dynamic wheelchair locomotion compared with static seated measurements. *Arch Phys Med Rehabil*. 1998, 79(3):313–316.

88. Consortium for Spinal Cord Medicine. *Preservation of Upper Limb Function Following Spinal Cord Injury: A Clinical Practice Guideline for Health-Care Professionals*. Washington, DC: Paralyzed Veterans of America, 2005.

89. Ferguson-Pell MW. Seat cushion selection. *J Rehabil Res Dev Clin Suppl*. 1990, (2):49–73.

90. Sprigle S, Chung KC, Brubaker CE. Reduction of sitting pressures with custom contoured cushions. *J Rehabil Res Dev*. 1990, 27(2):135–140.

91. Seymour RJ, Lacefield WE. Wheelchair cushion effect on pressure and skin temperature. *Arch Phys Med Rehabil*. 1985, 66(2):103–108.

92. Takechi H, Tokuhiro A. Evaluation of wheelchair cushions by means of pressure distribution mapping. *Acta Med Okayama*. 1998, 52(5):245–254.

93. Nixon V. *Spinal Cord Injury: A Guide to Functional Outcomes in Physical Therapy Management*. Rockville, MD: Aspen, 1985.

94. Williams C. RoHo Dry Floatation system: an alternative means of pressure relief. *Br J Nurs*. 1998–1999, 7(22):1400, 1402–1404.

95. Krouskop TA, Williams R, Noble P, Brown J. Inflation pressure effect on performance of air-filled wheelchair cushions. *Arch Phys Med Rehabil*. 1986, 67(2):126–128.

96. Cochran GV, Palmieri V. Development of test methods for evaluation of wheelchair cushions. *Bull Prosthet Res*. 1980, 10(33):9–30.

97. Henderson JL, Price SH, Brandstater ME, Mandac BR. Efficacy of three measures to relieve pressure in seated persons with spinal cord injury. *Arch Phys Med Rehabil*. 1994, 75(5):535–539.

98. Wagner D, Fox M, Ellis E. Developing a successful interdisciplinary seating program. *Ostomy Wound Manage*. 1994, 40(1):32–34, 36–38, 40–31.

99. Pires M, Adkins R. Pressure ulcers and spinal cord injury: scope of the problem. *Top Spinal Cord Inj Rehabil*. 1996, 2(1):1–8.

100. Basta SM. Pressure sore prevention education with the spinal cord injured. *Rehabil Nurs*. 1991, 16(1):6–8.

101. Rodriguez GP, Garber SL. Prospective study of pressure ulcer risk in spinal cord injury patients. *Paraplegia*. 1994, 32(3):150–158.

102. Fine C. Utilizing a day hospital program as part of a pressure ulcer management program continuum. *Top Spinal Cord Inj Rehabil*. 1996, 2(1):42–50.

103. Garber SL, Rintala DH, Holmes SA, Rodriguez GP, Friedman J. A structured educational model to improve pressure ulcer prevention knowledge in veterans with spinal cord dysfunction. *J Rehabil Res Dev*. 2002, 39(5):575–588.

104. Dover H, Pickard W, Swain I, Grundy D. The effectiveness of a pressure clinic in preventing pressure sores. *Paraplegia*. 1992, 30(4):267–272.

105. King T, Temkin A, Vesmarovich S. Taking charge: a proactive nursing approach to skin management. *Top Spinal Cord Inj Rehabil*. 1996, 2(1):21–25.

106. Wolfe D, Potter P, Sequeira K. Overcoming challenges: the role of rehabilitation in educating individuals with SCI to reduce secondary conditions. *Top Spinal Cord Inj Rehabil*. 2004, 10(1):41–50.

107. Registered Nurses' Association of Ontario. *Assessment and Management of Stage I to IV Pressure Ulcers*. Toronto: Registered Nurses' Association of Ontario, 2007.

108. Bates-Jensen BM. The Pressure Sore Status Tool a few thousand assessments later. *Adv Wound Care*. 1997, 10(5):65–73.

109. Ferrell BA. The Sessing Scale for measurement of pressure ulcer healing. *Adv Wound Care*. 1997, 10(5):78–80.

110. Krasner D. Wound Healing Scale, version 1.0: a proposal. *Adv Wound Care*. 1997, 10(5):82–85.

111. Sussman C, Swanson G. Utility of the Sussman Wound Healing Tool in predicting wound healing outcomes in physical therapy. *Adv Wound Care*. 1997, 10(5):74–77.

112. Thomas DR. Existing tools: are they meeting the challenges of pressure ulcer healing? *Adv Wound Care*. 1997, 10(5):86–90.

113. Xakellis GC Jr, Frantz RA. Pressure ulcer healing: what is it? What influences it? How is it measured? *Adv Wound Care*. 1997, 10(5):20–26.

114. Thomas DR, Rodeheaver GT, Bartolucci AA, et al. Pressure ulcer scale for healing: derivation and validation of the PUSH tool. The PUSH Task Force. *Adv Wound Care*. 1997, 10(5):96–101.

115. National Pressure Ulcer Advisory Panel. Pressure ulcers prevalence, cost and risk assessment: consensus development conference statement. *Decubitus*. 1989, 2(2):24–28.

116. Black J, Baharestani MM, Cuddigan J, et al. National Pressure Ulcer Advisory Panel's updated pressure ulcer staging system. *Adv Skin Wound Care*. 2007, 20(5):269–274.

117. National Pressure Ulcer Advisory Panel. Updated Staging System. 2007, http://www.npuap.org. Accessed 2/6/09.

118. Bergstrom N, Allman R, Alvarez O, et al. Pressure ulcer treatment: quick reference guide for clinicians. *Adv Wound Care*. 1995, 8(2):22–44.

119. Knight AL. Medical management of pressure sores. *J Fam Pract*. 1988, 27(1):95–100.

120. Harrow JJ, Malassigne P, Nelson AL, et al. Design and evaluation of a stand-up motorized prone cart. *J Spinal Cord Med*. 2007, 30(1):50–61.

121. Nelson A, Malassigne P, Cors M, et al. Patient evaluation of prone carts used in spinal cord injury. *SCI Nurs*. 1996, 13(2):39–44.

122. Bristow JV, Goldfarb EH, Green M. Clinitron therapy: is it effective? *Geriatr Nurs*. 1987, 8(3):120–124.

123. Goode PS, Allman RM. The prevention and management of pressure ulcers. *Med Clin North Am*. 1989, 73(6):1511–1524.

124. Bates-Jensen B. Management of exudate and infection. In: Sussman C, Bates-Jensen B, eds. *Wound Care: A Collaborative Practice Manual for Physical Therapists and Nurses*. Gaithersburg, MD: Aspen, 2001:216–234.

125. Abramowicz M. Treatment of pressure ulcers. *Med Lett Drugs Ther*. 1990, 32(812):17–18.

126. Feedar J. Clinical management of chronic wounds. In: McCulloch J, Kloth LC, Feedar J, eds. *Wound Healing: Alternatives in Management*. 2nd ed. Philadelphia: F.A. Davis, 1995:137–176.

127. Rodeheaver G, Baharestani MM, Brabec ME, et al. Wound healing and wound management: focus on debridement. An interdisciplinary round table, September 18, 1992, Jackson Hole, WY. *Adv Wound Care*. 1994, 7(1):22–24, 26–29, 32–26, quiz 37–29.

128. Whittle H, Fletcher C, Hoskin A, Campbell K. Nursing management of pressure ulcers using a hydrogel dressing protocol: four case studies. *Rehabil Nurs*. 1996, 21(5):239–242.

129. Akers TK, Gabrielson AL. The effect of high voltage galvanic stimulation on the rate of healing of decubitus ulcers. *Biomed Sci Instrum*. 1984, 20:99–100.

130. Griffin JW, Tooms RE, Mendius RA, et al. Efficacy of high voltage pulsed current for healing of pressure ulcers in patients

with spinal cord injury. *Phys Ther.* 1991, 71(6):433–442, discussion 442–444.

131. Kloth LC, Feedar JA. Acceleration of wound healing with high voltage, monophasic, pulsed current. *Phys Ther.* 1988, 68(4):503–508.

132. Carley PJ, Wainapel SF. Electrotherapy for acceleration of wound healing: low intensity direct current. *Arch Phys Med Rehabil.* 1985, 66(7):443–446.

133. Gault W, Gatens P. Use of low intensity direct current in management of ischemic skin ulcers. *Phys Ther.* 1976, 56(3):265–269.

134. Salzberg CA, Cooper-Vastola SA, et al. The effects of non-thermal pulsed electromagnetic energy on wound healing of pressure ulcers in spinal cord-injured patients: a randomized, double-blind study. *Ostomy Wound Manage.* 1995, 41(3):42–44, 46, 48 passim.

135. Hess C. *Wound Care: Nurse's Clinical Guide.* Springhouse, PA: Springhouse, 1995.

136. Nussbaum EL, Biemann I, Mustard B. Comparison of ultrasound/ultraviolet-C and laser for treatment of pressure ulcers in patients with spinal cord injury. *Phys Ther.* 1994, 74(9):812–823, discussion 824–825.

137. Gogia P. Low-energy laser in wound management. In: Gogia P, ed. *Clinical Wound Management.* Thorofare, NJ: Slack, 1995:165–172.

138. Baynham SA, Kohlman P, Katner HP. Treating stage IV pressure ulcers with negative pressure therapy: a case report. *Ostomy Wound Manage.* 1999, 45(4):28–32, 34–25.

139. Morykwas MJ, Argenta LC, Shelton-Brown EI, McGuirt W. Vacuum-assisted closure: a new method for wound control and treatment: animal studies and basic foundation. *Ann Plast Surg.* 1997, 38(6):553–562.

140. Cuddigan J, Frantz RA. Pressure ulcer research: pressure ulcer treatment. A monograph from the National Pressure Ulcer Advisory Panel. *Adv Wound Care.* 1998, 11(6):294–300, quiz 302.

141. Montgomerie JZ. Infections in patients with spinal cord injuries. *Clin Infect Dis.* 1997, 25(6):1285–1290, quiz 1291–1292.

142. Kierney PC, Cardenas DD, Engrav LH, et al. Limb-salvage in reconstruction of recalcitrant pressure sores using the inferiorly based rectus abdominis myocutaneous flap. *Plast Reconstr Surg.* 1998, 102(1):111–116.

143. Pena MM, Drew GS, Smith SJ, Given KS. The inferiorly based rectus abdominis myocutaneous flap for reconstruction of recurrent pressure sores. *Plast Reconstr Surg.* 1992, 89(1):90–95.

144. Peters JW, Johnson GE. Proximal femurectomy for decubitus ulceration in the spinal cord injury patient. *Paraplegia.* 1990, 28(1):55–61.

145. Disa JJ, Carlton JM, Goldberg NH. Efficacy of operative cure in pressure sore patients. *Plast Reconstr Surg.* 1992, 89(2):272–278.

146. Salzberg CA, Gray BC, Petro JA, Salisbury RE. The perioperative antimicrobial management of pressure ulcers. *Decubitus.* 1990, 3(2):24–26.

147. Garg M, Rubayi S, Montgomerie JZ. Postoperative wound infections following myocutaneous flap surgery in spinal injury patients. *Paraplegia.* 1992, 30(10):734–739.

148. Black JM, Black SB. Surgical management of pressure ulcers. *Nurs Clin North Am.* 1987, 22(2):429–438.

149. Goldstein B, Sanders JE, Benson B. Pressure ulcers in SCI: does tension stimulate wound healing? *Am J Phys Med Rehabil.* 1996, 75(2):130–133.

150. Rubayi S. Reconstructive surgery of pressure ulcers around the pelvic region. *Top Spinal Cord Inj Rehabil.* 2003, 9(2):20–23.

151. Bobel LM. Nutritional implications in the patient with pressure sores. *Nurs Clin North Am.* 1987, 22(2):379–390.

152. Brylinsky CM. Nutrition and wound healing: an overview. *Ostomy Wound Manage.* 1995, 41(10):14–16, 18, 20–12 passim, quiz 25–26.

153. Ahrens T, Kollef M, Stewart J, Shannon W. Effect of kinetic therapy on pulmonary complications. *Am J Crit Care.* 2004, 13(5):376–383.

154. McGuire RA, Green BA, Eismont FJ, Watts C. Comparison of stability provided to the unstable spine by the kinetic therapy table and the Stryker frame. *Neurosurgery.* 1988, 22(5):842–845.

CHAPTER 6

1. DeVivo MJ, Krause JS, Lammertse DP. Recent trends in mortality and causes of death among persons with spinal cord injury. *Arch Phys Med Rehabil.* 1999, 80(11):1411–1419.

2. National Spinal Cord Injury Statistical Center. Annual Report for the Model Spinal Cord Injury Care Systems. 2007, http://www.spinalcord.uab.edu. Accessed 12/15/08.

3. Martini F. *Fundamentals of Anatomy and Physiology.* 4th ed. Upper Saddle River, NJ: Prentice Hall, 1998.

4. Rosse C, Gaddum-Rosse P. *Hollinshead's Textbook of Anatomy.* 5th ed. Philadelphia: Lippincott-Raven, 1997.

5. Snell R. *Clinical Anatomy for Medical Students.* 5th ed. Boston: Little, Brown, 1995.

6. Brannon F, Foley M, Starr J, Saul L. *Cardiopulmonary Rehabilitation: Basic Theory and Application.* 3rd ed. Philadelphia: F.A. Davis, 1998.

7. Neumann D. *Kinesiology of the Musculoskeletal System.* St. Louis: Mosby, 2002.

8. Dean E. Cardiopulmonary anatomy. In: Frownfelter D, Dean E, eds. *Cardiovascular and Pulmonary Physical Therapy: Evidence and Practice.* 4th ed. St. Louis: Mosby Elsevier, 2006:53–72.

9. Bach JR, Saporito LR. Criteria for extubation and tracheostomy tube removal for patients with ventilatory failure. A different approach to weaning. *Chest.* 1996, 110(6):1566–1571.

10. Madama V. *Pulmonary Function Testing and Cardiopulmonary Stress Testing.* Albany, NY: Delmar, 1993.

11. Wang AY, Jaeger RJ, Yarkony GM, Turba RM. Cough in spinal cord injured patients: the relationship between motor level and peak expiratory flow. *Spinal Cord.* 1997, 35(5):299–302.

12. Guyton A, Hall J. *Textbook of Medical Physiology.* 11th ed. Philadelphia: Elsevier Saunders, 2006.

13. McArdle W, Katch F, Katch V. *Essentials in Exercise Physiology.* 2nd ed. Philadelphia: Lippincott Williams & Wilkins, 2000.

14. Vander A, Sherman J, Luciano D. *Human Physiology: The Mechanisms of Body Function.* 7th ed. New York: McGraw-Hill, 1998.

15. Mansel JK, Norman JR. Respiratory complications and management of spinal cord injuries. *Chest.* 1990, 97(6):1446–1452.

16. Kendall F, McCreary E, Provance P. *Muscles: Testing and Function.* 4th ed. Baltimore: Williams & Wilkins, 1993.

17. Lanig IS, Lammerste DP. The respiratory system in spinal cord injury. *Phys Med Rehabil Clin N Am.* 1992, 3(4):725–740.

18. Moore K. *Clinically Oriented Anatomy.* Baltimore: Williams & Wilkins, 1992.

19. McMinn R. *Last's Anatomy: Regional and Applied.* 9th ed. New York: Churchill Livingstone, 1994.

20. Derenne JP, Macklem PT, Roussos C. The respiratory muscles: mechanics, control, and pathophysiology, Part II. *Am Rev Respir Dis.* 1978, 118(2):373–390.

21. Brown R, DiMarco AF, Hoit JD, Garshick E. Respiratory dysfunction and management in spinal cord injury. *Respir Care.* 2006, 51(8):853–868, discussion 869–870.

22. Winslow C, Rozovsky J. Effect of spinal cord injury on the respiratory system. *Am J Phys Med Rehabil.* 2003, 82(10):803–814.

23. Derenne JP, Macklem PT, Roussos C. The respiratory muscles: mechanics, control, and pathophysiology, Part I. *Am Rev Respir Dis.* 1978, 118(1):119–133.

24. Frownfelter D, Massery M. Body mechanics—the art of positioning and moving patients. In: Frownfelter D, Dean E, eds.

Cardiovascular and Pulmonary Physical Therapy: Evidence and Practice. 4th ed. St. Louis: Mosby Elsevier, 2006:749–758.

25. Landers M, Barker G, Wallentine S, et al. A comparison of tidal volume, breathing frequency, and minute ventilation between two sitting postures in healthy adults. *Physiother Theory Pract.* 2003, 19(2):109–119.

26. Frownfelter D, Massery M. Facilitating airway clearance with coughing techniques. In: Frownfelter D, Dean E, eds. *Cardiovascular and Pulmonary Physical Therapy: Evidence and Practice.* 4th ed. St. Louis: Mosby Elsevier, 2006:363–376.

27. Bach JR, Smith WH, Michaels J, et al. Airway secretion clearance by mechanical exsufflation for post-poliomyelitis ventilator-assisted individuals. *Arch Phys Med Rehabil.* 1993, 74(2):170–177.

28. Linder SH. Functional electrical stimulation to enhance cough in quadriplegia. *Chest.* 1993, 103(1):166–169.

29. Yarkony G, Jaeger R, Gittler M. Cough in tetraplegia. *Top Spinal Cord Inj Rehabil.* 1997, 3(1):67–70.

30. Roth EJ, Lu A, Primack S, et al. Ventilatory function in cervical and high thoracic spinal cord injury. Relationship to level of injury and tone. *Am J Phys Med Rehabil.* 1997, 76(4):262–267.

31. Peterson W, Kirshblum S. Pulmonary management of spinal cord injury. In: Kirshblum S, Campagnolo D, De Lisa J, eds. *Spinal Cord Medicine.* Philadelphia: Lippincott Williams & Wilkins, 2002:135–154.

32. Keen M. Management of the ventilator-dependent patient with quadriplegia. In: Yarkony G, ed. *Spinal Cord Injury: Medical Management and Rehabilitation.* Gaithersburg, MD: Aspen, 1994:129–135.

33. Peterson W, Charlifue W, Gerhart A, Whiteneck G. Two methods of weaning persons with quadriplegia from mechanical ventilators. *Paraplegia.* 1994, 32(2):98–103.

34. Consortium for Spinal Cord Medicine. *Respiratory Management Following Spinal Cord Injury: A Clinical Practice Guideline for Health-Care Professionals.* Washington, DC: Paralyzed Veterans of America, 2005.

35. Wallbom A, Naran B, Thomas E. Acute ventilator management and weaning in individuals with high tetraplegia. *Top Spinal Cord Inj Rehabil.* 2005, 10(3):1–7.

36. Ledsome JR, Sharp JM. Pulmonary function in acute cervical cord injury. *Am Rev Respir Dis.* 1981, 124(1):41–44.

37. Jackson AB, Groomes TE. Incidence of respiratory complications following spinal cord injury. *Arch Phys Med Rehabil.* 1994, 75(3):270–275.

38. Estenne M, Knoop C, Vanvaerenbergh J, et al. The effect of pectoralis muscle training in tetraplegic subjects. *Am Rev Respir Dis.* 1989, 139(5):1218–1222.

39. Linn WS, Adkins RH, Gong H Jr, Waters RL. Pulmonary function in chronic spinal cord injury: a cross-sectional survey of 222 southern California adult outpatients. *Arch Phys Med Rehabil.* 2000, 81(6):757–763.

40. Mateus SR, Beraldo PS, Horan TA. Cholinergic bronchomotor tone and airway caliber in tetraplegic patients. *Spinal Cord.* 2006, 44(5):269–274.

41. Schilero GJ, Grimm DR, Bauman WA, et al. Assessment of airway caliber and bronchodilator responsiveness in subjects with spinal cord injury. *Chest.* 2005, 127(1):149–155.

42. Alvarez SE, Peterson M, Lunsford BR. Respiratory treatment of the adult patient with spinal cord injury. *Phys Ther.* 1981, 61(12):1737–1745.

43. Chen CF, Lien IN, Wu MC. Respiratory function in patients with spinal cord injuries: effects of posture. *Paraplegia.* 1990, 28(2):81–86.

44. Estenne M, De Troyer A. Mechanism of the postural dependence of vital capacity in tetraplegic subjects. *Am Rev Respir Dis.* 1987, 135(2):367–371.

45. Baydur A, Adkins RH, Milic-Emili J. Lung mechanics in individuals with spinal cord injury: effects of injury level and posture. *J Appl Physiol.* 2001, 90(2):405–411.

46. Haas F, Axen K, Pineda H, et al. Temporal pulmonary function changes in cervical cord injury. *Arch Phys Med Rehabil.* 1985, 66(3):139–144.

47. Como JJ, Sutton ER, McCunn M, et al. Characterizing the need for mechanical ventilation following cervical spinal cord injury with neurologic deficit. *J Trauma.* 2005, 59(4):912–916, discussion 916.

48. Bach JR, Hunt D, Horton JA III. Traumatic tetraplegia: noninvasive respiratory management in the acute setting. *Am J Phys Med Rehabil.* 2002, 81(10):792–797.

49. Bach JR, Wang TG. Pulmonary function and sleep disordered breathing in patients with traumatic tetraplegia: a longitudinal study. *Arch Phys Med Rehabil.* 1994, 75(3):279–284.

50. Scanlon PD, Loring SH, Pichurko BM, et al. Respiratory mechanics in acute quadriplegia. Lung and chest wall compliance and dimensional changes during respiratory maneuvers. *Am Rev Respir Dis.* 1989, 139(3):615–620.

51. Linn WS, Spungen AM, Gong H Jr, et al. Forced vital capacity in two large outpatient populations with chronic spinal cord injury. *Spinal Cord.* 2001, 39(5):263–268.

52. Tow AM, Graves DE, Carter RE. Vital capacity in tetraplegics twenty years and beyond. *Spinal Cord.* 2001, 39(3):139–144.

53. Ahmed QA. Metabolic complications of obstructive sleep apnea syndrome. *Am J Med Sci.* 2008, 335(1):60–64.

54. Benjamin JA, Lewis KE. Sleep-disordered breathing and cardiovascular disease. *Postgrad Med J.* 2008, 84(987):15–22.

55. Olson EJ, Park JG, Morgenthaler TI. Obstructive sleep apnea-hypopnea syndrome. *Prim Care.* 2005, 32(2):329–359.

56. Punjabi NM. The epidemiology of adult obstructive sleep apnea. *Proc Am Thorac Soc.* 2008, 5(2):136–143.

57. Berlowitz DJ, Brown DJ, Campbell DA, Pierce RJ. A longitudinal evaluation of sleep and breathing in the first year after cervical spinal cord injury. *Arch Phys Med Rehabil.* 2005, 86(6):1193–1199.

58. Burns SP, Kapur V, Yin KS, Buhrer R. Factors associated with sleep apnea in men with spinal cord injury: a population-based case-control study. *Spinal Cord.* 2001, 39(1):15–22.

59. Leduc BE, Dagher JH, Mayer P, et al. Estimated prevalence of obstructive sleep apnea-hypopnea syndrome after cervical cord injury. *Arch Phys Med Rehabil.* 2007, 88(3):333–337.

60. Stockhammer E, Tobon A, Michel F, et al. Characteristics of sleep apnea syndrome in tetraplegic patients. *Spinal Cord.* 2002, 40(6):286–294.

61. Frownfelter D, Massery M. Facilitating ventilation patterns and breathing strategies. In: Frownfelter D, Dean E, eds. *Cardiovascular and Pulmonary Physical Therapy: Evidence and Practice.* 4th ed. St. Louis: Mosby Elsevier, 2006:377–403.

62. Berly M, Shem K. Respiratory management during the first five days after spinal cord injury. *J Spinal Cord Med.* 2007, 30(4):309–318.

63. Marshall S, Marshall L, Vos H, Chesnut R. *Neuroscience Critical Care: Pathophysiology and Patient Management.* Philadelphia: Saunders, 1990.

64. Ragnarsson K, Hall K, Wilmot C, Carter E. Management of pulmonary, cardiovascular, and metabolic conditions after spinal cord injury. In: Stover S, De Lisa J, Whiteneck G, eds. *Spinal Cord Injury: Clinical Outcomes from the Model Systems.* Gaithersburg, MD: Aspen, 1995:79–90.

65. McDonagh D, Borel C. Ventilatory management in the neurosciences critical care unit. In: Suarez J, ed. *Critical Care Neurology and Neurosurgery.* Totowa, NJ: Humana, 2004: 151–166.

66. Brady S, Miserendino R, Statkus D, et al. Predictors to dysphagia and recovery after cervical spinal cord injury during acute rehabilitation. *J Appl Res.* 2004, 4(1):1–11.

67. Shem K, Castillo K, Naran B. Factors associated with dysphagia in individuals with high tetraplegia. *Top Spinal Cord Inj Rehabil.* 2005, 10(3):8–18.

68. Wolf C, Meiners TH. Dysphagia in patients with acute cervical spinal cord injury. *Spinal Cord.* 2003, 41(6):347–353.

69. Kirshblum S, Johnston MV, Brown J, et al. Predictors of dysphagia after spinal cord injury. *Arch Phys Med Rehabil.* 1999, 80(9):1101–1105.

70. Lemons VR, Wagner FC Jr. Respiratory complications after cervical spinal cord injury. *Spine.* 1994, 19(20):2315–2320.

71. Richards J, Waites K, Chen Y, et al. The epidemiology of secondary conditions following spinal cord injury. *Top Spinal Cord Inj Rehabil.* 2004, 10(1):15–29.

72. DeVivo MJ, Ivie CS III. Life expectancy of ventilator-dependent persons with spinal cord injuries. *Chest.* 1995, 108(1):226–232.

73. DeVivo MJ, Stover SL, Black KJ. Prognostic factors for 12-year survival after spinal cord injury. *Arch Phys Med Rehabil.* 1992, 73(2):156–162.

74. Derenne JP, Macklem PT, Roussos C. The respiratory muscles: mechanics, control, and pathophysiology. Part III. *Am Rev Respir Dis.* 1978, 118(3):581–601.

75. Wetzel J, Lunsford B, Peterson M, Alavarez S. Respiratory rehabilitation of the patient with a spinal cord injury. In: Irwin S, Tecklin J, eds. *Cardiopulmonary Physical Therapy.* 3rd ed. St. Louis: Mosby, 1995:579–603.

76. Rinehart M, Nawoczenski D. Respiratory care. In: Buchanan L, Nawoczenski D, eds. *Spinal Cord Injury: Concepts and Management Approaches.* Baltimore: Williams & Wilkins, 1987:61–79.

77. Roth EJ, Nussbaum SB, Berkowitz M, et al. Pulmonary function testing in spinal cord injury: correlation with vital capacity. *Paraplegia.* 1995, 33(8):454–457.

78. Johnson K, Grant T, Peterson P. Ventilator weaning for the patient with high-level tetraplegia. *Top Spinal Cord Inj Rehabil.* 1997, 2(3):11–20.

79. Kang S, Shin J, Park C, et al. Relationship between inspiratory muscle strength and cough capacity in cervical spinal cord injured patients. *Spinal Cord.* 2006, 44(4):242–248.

80. Mengelkoch LJ, Martin D, Lawler J. A review of the principles of pulse oximetry and accuracy of pulse oximeter estimates during exercise. *Phys Ther.* 1994, 74(1):40–49.

81. McBride DQ, Rodts GE. Intensive care of patients with spinal trauma. *Neurosurg Clin N Am.* 1994, 5(4):755–766.

82. Wicks AB, Menter RR. Long-term outlook in quadriplegic patients with initial ventilator dependency. *Chest.* 1986, 90(3):406–410.

83. Bach JR. Inappropriate weaning and late onset ventilatory failure of individuals with traumatic spinal cord injury. *Paraplegia.* 1993, 31(7):430–438.

84. Gerold K, Nussbaum E. Understanding mechanical ventilation. *Phys Ther Pract.* 1994, 3(2):81–91.

85. Peterson WP, Barbalata L, Brooks CA, et al. The effect of tidal volume on the time to wean persons with high tetraplegia from ventilators. *Spinal Cord.* 1999, 37(4):284–288.

86. Peterson P, Brooks C, Mellick D, Whiteneck G. Protocol for ventilator management in high tetraplegia. *Top Spinal Cord Inj Rehabil.* 1997, 2(3):101–106.

87. Bach J. Noninvasive alternatives for tracheostomy for managing respiratory muscle dysfunction in spinal cord injury. *Top Spinal Cord Inj Rehabil.* 1997, 2(3):49–58.

88. Bach JR, Alba AS. Intermittent abdominal pressure ventilator in a regimen of noninvasive ventilatory support. *Chest.* 1991, 99(3):630–636.

89. Bach JR, Alba AS, Saporito LR. Intermittent positive pressure ventilation via the mouth as an alternative to tracheostomy for 257 ventilator users. *Chest.* 1993, 103(1):174–182.

90. Hess DR. Noninvasive ventilation in neuromuscular disease: equipment and application. *Respir Care.* 2006, 51(8):896–911, discussion 911–912.

91. Bach JR. A comparison of long-term ventilatory support alternatives from the perspective of the patient and care giver. *Chest.* 1993, 104(6):1702–1706.

92. Bach JR. Update and perspectives on noninvasive respiratory muscle aids. Part 1: the inspiratory aids. *Chest.* 1994, 105(4):1230–1240.

93. Miller HJ, Thomas E, Wilmot CB. Pneumobelt use among high quadriplegic population. *Arch Phys Med Rehabil.* 1988, 69(5):369–372.

94. Linton DM. Cuirass ventilation: a review and update. *Crit Care Resusc.* 2005, 7(1):22–28.

95. DiMarco AF, Onders RP, Ignagni A, Kowalski KE. Inspiratory muscle pacing in spinal cord injury: case report and clinical commentary. *J Spinal Cord Med.* 2006, 29(2):95–108.

96. Zimmer MB, Nantwi K, Goshgarian HG. Effect of spinal cord injury on the respiratory system: basic research and current clinical treatment options. *J Spinal Cord Med.* 2007, 30(4):319–330.

97. Esclarin A, Bravo P, Arroyo O, et al. Tracheostomy ventilation versus diaphragmatic pacemaker ventilation in high spinal cord injury. *Paraplegia.* 1994, 32(10):687–693.

98. Vincken W, Corne L. Improved arterial oxygenation by diaphragmatic pacing in quadriplegia. *Crit Care Med.* 1987, 15(9):872–873.

99. Yarkony G, Jaeger R. Phrenic nerve pacemakers for tetraplegia. *Top Spinal Cord Inj Rehabil.* 1995, 1(1):77–82.

100. Cruzado D, Jones M, Segebart S, McDonagh J. Resistive inspiratory muscle training improves inspiratory muscle strength in subjects with cervical spinal cord injury. *Neurol Rep.* 2002, 26(1):3–7.

101. Liaw MY, Lin MC, Cheng PT, et al. Resistive inspiratory muscle training: its effectiveness in patients with acute complete cervical cord injury. *Arch Phys Med Rehabil.* 2000, 81(6):752–756.

102. Derrickson J, Ciesla N, Simpson N, Imle PC. A comparison of two breathing exercise programs for patients with quadriplegia. *Phys Ther.* 1992, 72(11):763–769.

103. Gross D, Ladd HW, Riley EJ, et al. The effect of training on strength and endurance of the diaphragm in quadriplegia. *Am J Med.* 1980, 68(1):27–35.

104. Rutchik A, Weissman AR, Almenoff PL, et al. Resistive inspiratory muscle training in subjects with chronic cervical spinal cord injury. *Arch Phys Med Rehabil.* 1998, 79(3):293–297.

105. Lin KH, Chuang CC, Wu HD, et al. Abdominal weight and inspiratory resistance: their immediate effects on inspiratory muscle functions during maximal voluntary breathing in chronic tetraplegic patients. *Arch Phys Med Rehabil.* 1999, 80(7):741–745.

106. Wetzel J. Respiratory evaluation and treatment. In: Adkins H, ed. *Spinal Cord Injury.* New York: Churchill Livingstone, 1985:75–98.

107. Loveridge B, Badour M, Dubo H. Ventilatory muscle endurance training in quadriplegia: effects on breathing pattern. *Paraplegia.* 1989, 27(5):329–339.

108. Silva AC, Neder JA, Chiurciu MV, et al. Effect of aerobic training on ventilatory muscle endurance of spinal cord injured men. *Spinal Cord.* 1998, 36(4):240–245.

109. Bianchi C, Grandi M, Felisari G. Efficacy of glossopharyngeal breathing for a ventilator-dependent, high-level tetraplegic patient after cervical cord tumor resection and tracheotomy. *Am J Phys Med Rehabil.* 2004, 83(3):216–219.

110. Bach JR, Alba AS. Noninvasive options for ventilatory support of the traumatic high level quadriplegic patient. *Chest.* 1990, 98(3):613–619.

111. Warren VC. Glossopharyngeal and neck accessory muscle breathing in a young adult with C2 complete tetraplegia resulting in ventilator dependency. *Phys Ther.* 2002, 82(6):590–600.

112. Clough P, Lindenauer D, Hayes M, Zekany B. Guidelines for routine respiratory care of patients with spinal cord injury. A clinical report. *Phys Ther.* 1986, 66(9):1395–1402.

113. Massery M. What's positioning got to do with it? *Neurol Rep.* 1994, 18(3):11–14.

114. Boaventura C, Gastaldi A, Silveira J, et al. Effect of an abdominal binder on the efficacy of respiratory muscles in seated and supine tetraplegic subjects. *Physiotherapy*. 2003, 89(5):290–295.

115. McCool FD, Pichurko BM, Slutsky AS, et al. Changes in lung volume and rib cage configuration with abdominal binding in quadriplegia. *J Appl Physiol*. 1986, 60(4):1198–1202.

116. Esteban A, Frutos F, Tobin MJ, et al. A comparison of four methods of weaning patients from mechanical ventilation. Spanish Lung Failure Collaborative Group. *N Engl J Med*. 1995, 332(6):345–350.

117. Bach JR. New approaches in the rehabilitation of the traumatic high level quadriplegic. *Am J Phys Med Rehabil*. 1991, 70(1):13–19.

118. Gutierrez C, Harrow J, Haines F. Using an evidence-based protocol to guide rehabilitation and weaning of ventilator-dependent cervical spinal cord injury patients. *J Rehabil Res Dev*. 2003, 40(5):99–110.

119. Bach J. Mechanical insufflation-exsufflation: comparison of peak expiratory flows with manually assisted and unassisted coughing techniques. *Chest*. 1993, 104(5):1553–1562.

120. Jaeger RJ, Turba RM, Yarkony GM, Roth EJ. Cough in spinal cord injured patients: comparison of three methods to produce cough. *Arch Phys Med Rehabil*. 1993, 74(12):1358–1361.

121. Zupan A, Savrin R, Erjavec T, et al. Effects of respiratory muscle training and electrical stimulation of abdominal muscles on respiratory capabilities in tetraplegic patients. *Spinal Cord*. 1997, 35(8):540–545.

122. Massery M. Manual breathing and coughing aids. *Phys Med Rehabil Clin N Am*. 1996, 7(2):407–422.

123. Liszner K, Feinberg M. Cough assist strategy for pulmonary toileting in ventilator-dependent spinal cord injured patients. *Rehabil Nurs*. 2006, 31(5):218–221.

124. Schmitt J, Stiens S, Trincher R, et al. Survey of use of the insufflator-exsufflator in patients with spinal cord injury. *J Spinal Cord Med*. 2007, 30(2):127–130.

125. Bach JR. Respiratory muscle aids for the prevention of pulmonary morbidity and mortality. *Semin Neurol*. 1995, 15(1):72–83.

126. Garstang SV, Kirshblum SC, Wood KE. Patient preference for in-exsufflation for secretion management with spinal cord injury. *J Spinal Cord Med*. 2000, 23(2):80–85.

127. Morgan M, Silver J, Williams S. The respiratory system of the spinal cord patient. In: Bloch R, Basbaum M, eds. *Management of Spinal Cord Injuries*. Baltimore: Williams & Wilkins, 1986:78–116.

128. Brownlee S, Williams S. Physiotherapy in the respiratory care of patients with high spinal injury. *Physiotherapy*. 1987, 73(3):148–152.

129. Burns SP, Rad MY, Bryant S, Kapur V. Long-term treatment of sleep apnea in persons with spinal cord injury. *Am J Phys Med Rehabil*. 2005, 84(8):620–626.

130. Hall K, Harper B, Whiteneck G. Follow-up study of individuals with high tetraplegia (C1–C4) 10 to 21 years postinjury. *Top Spinal Cord Inj Rehabil*. 1997, 2(3):107–117.

131. Capoor J, Stein AB. Aging with spinal cord injury. *Phys Med Rehabil Clin N Am*. 2005, 16(1):129–161.

132. Garshick E, Kelley A, Cohen SA, et al. A prospective assessment of mortality in chronic spinal cord injury. *Spinal Cord*. 2005, 43(7):408–416.

133. Gilgoff IS, Barras DM, Jones MS, Adkins HV. Neck breathing: a form of voluntary respiration for the spine-injured ventilator-dependent quadriplegic child. *Pediatrics*. 1988, 82(5):741–745.

134. Bluechardt MH, Wiens M, Thomas SG, Plyley MJ. Repeated measurements of pulmonary function following spinal cord injury. *Paraplegia*. 1992, 30(11):768–774.

135. Brooks D, O'Brien K. Is inspiratory muscle training effective for individuals with cervical spinal cord injury? A qualitative systematic review. *Clin Rehabil*. 2005, 19(3):237–246.

136. Van Houtte S, Vanlandewijck Y, Gosselink R. Respiratory muscle training in persons with spinal cord injury: a systematic review. *Respir Med*. 2006, 100(11):1886–1895.

137. Taylor PN, Tromans AM, Harris KR, Swain ID. Electrical stimulation of abdominal muscles for control of blood pressure and augmentation of cough in a C3/4 level tetraplegic. *Spinal Cord*. 2002, 40(1):34–36.

138. Lin VW, Singh H, Chitkara RK, Perkash I. Functional magnetic stimulation for restoring cough in patients with tetraplegia. *Arch Phys Med Rehabil*. 1998, 79(5):517–522.

139. DiMarco AF, Kowalski KE, Geertman RT, Hromyak DR. Spinal cord stimulation: a new method to produce an effective cough in patients with spinal cord injury. *Am J Respir Crit Care Med*. 2006, 173(12):1386–1389.

CHAPTER 7

1. American Spinal Injury Association. *International Standards for Neurological Classification of Spinal Cord Injury*. Atlanta: American Spinal Injury Association, 2000, reprinted 2008.

2. Ditunno JF Jr, Graziani V, Tessler A. Neurological assessment in spinal cord injury. *Adv Neurol*. 1997, 72:325–333.

3. Graziani V, Crozier K, Selby-Silverstein L. Lower extremity function following spinal cord injury. *Top Spinal Cord Inj Rehabil*. 1996, 1(4):46–55.

4. Mange KC, Ditunno JF Jr, Herbison GJ, Jaweed MM. Recovery of strength at the zone of injury in motor complete and motor incomplete cervical spinal cord injured patients. *Arch Phys Med Rehabil*. 1990, 71(8):562–565.

5. Waters RL, Adkins RH, Yakura JS, Sie I. Motor and sensory recovery following incomplete paraplegia. *Arch Phys Med Rehabil*. 1994, 75(1):67–72.

6. Waters RL, Adkins RH, Yakura JS, Sie I. Motor and sensory recovery following complete tetraplegia. *Arch Phys Med Rehabil*. 1993, 74(3):242–247.

7. Waters RL, Adkins RH, Yakura JS, Sie I. Motor and sensory recovery following incomplete tetraplegia. *Arch Phys Med Rehabil*. 1994, 75(3):306–311.

8. Waters RL. Functional prognosis of spinal cord injuries. *J Spinal Cord Med*. 1996, 19(2):89–92.

9. Maynard F, Karunas R, Adkins R, et al. Management of the neuromusculoskeletal systems. In: Stover S, DeLisa J, Whiteneck G, eds. *Spinal Cord Injury: Clinical Outcomes from the Model Systems*. Gaithersburg, MD: Aspen, 1995:145–169.

10. Parke B, Penn RD, Savoy SM, Corcos D. Functional outcome after delivery of intrathecal baclofen. *Arch Phys Med Rehabil*. 1989, 70(1):30–32.

11. Cook KF, Teal CR, Engebretson JC, et al. Development and validation of Patient Reported Impact of Spasticity Measure (PRISM). *J Rehabil Res Dev*. 2007, 44(3):363–372.

12. Fredericks C. Clinical presentations in disorders of motor function. In: Fredericks C, Saladin L, eds. *Pathophysiology of the Motor Systems: Principles and Clinical Presentations*. Philadelphia: F.A. Davis, 1996:257–288.

13. Rymer Z. Spasticity: pathophysiology and implications for measurement. *Neurol Rep*. 1997, 21(3):73–75.

14. Bohannon R, Smith M. Interrater reliability of a modified Ashworth scale of muscle spasticity. *Phys Ther*. 1987, 67(2):206–207.

15. Priebe MM, Sherwood AM, Thornby JI, et al. Clinical assessment of spasticity in spinal cord injury: a multidimensional problem. *Arch Phys Med Rehabil*. 1996, 77(7):713–716.

16. Finkbeiner K, Russo S. *Physical Therapy Management of Spinal cord Injury: Accent on Independence*. Fisherville, VA: Woodrow Wilson Rehabilitation Center, 1990.

17. Deutsch A, Braun S, Granger C. The Functional Independence Measure (FIM Instrument). *J Rehabil Outcome Meas*. 1997, 1(2):67–71.

18. Harvey LA, Batty J, Fahey A. Reliability of a tool for assessing mobility in wheelchair-dependent paraplegics. *Spinal Cord.* 1998, 36(6):427–431.

19. Kilkens OJ, Post MW, Dallmeijer AJ, et al. Wheelchair skills tests: a systematic review. *Clin Rehabil.* 2003, 17(4):418–430.

20. Kilkens OJ, Dallmeijer AJ, De Witte LP, et al. The wheelchair circuit: construct validity and responsiveness of a test to assess manual wheelchair mobility in persons with spinal cord injury. *Arch Phys Med Rehabil.* 2004, 85(3):424–431.

21. Kirby RL, Swuste J, Dupuis DJ, et al. The wheelchair skills test: a pilot study of a new outcome measure. *Arch Phys Med Rehabil.* 2002, 83(1):10–18.

22. Routhier F, Desrosiers J, Vincent C, Nadeau S. Reliability and construct validity studies of an obstacle course assessment of wheelchair user performance. *Int J Rehabil Res.* 2005, 28(1):49–56.

23. Kirby RL, Dupuis DJ, Macphee AH, et al. The wheelchair skills test (version 2.4): measurement properties. *Arch Phys Med Rehabil.* 2004, 85(5):794–804.

24. van Hedel HJ, Wirz M, Dietz V. Assessing walking ability in subjects with spinal cord injury: validity and reliability of 3 walking tests. *Arch Phys Med Rehabil.* 2005, 86(2):190–196.

25. van Hedel HJ, Wirz M, Curt A. Improving walking assessment in subjects with an incomplete spinal cord injury: responsiveness. *Spinal Cord.* 2006, 44(6):352–356.

26. Ditunno JF Jr, Burns AS, Marino RJ. Neurological and functional capacity outcome measures: essential to spinal cord injury clinical trials. *J Rehabil Res Dev.* 2005, 42(3 Suppl 1):35–41.

27. Dittuno PL, Ditunno JF Jr. Walking index for spinal cord injury (WISCI II): scale revision. *Spinal Cord.* 2001, 39(12):654–656.

28. Field-Fote EC, Fluet GG, Schafer SD, et al. The Spinal Cord Injury Functional Ambulation Inventory (SCI-FAI). *J Rehabil Med.* 2001, 3(4):177–181.

29. Dittmar S. Overview: a functional approach to measurement of rehabilitation outcomes. In: Dittmar S, Gresham G, eds. *Functional Assessment and Outcome Measures for the Rehabilitation Health Professional.* Gaithersburg, MD: Aspen, 1997:1–15.

30. Marino R, Stineman M. Functional assessment in spinal cord injury. *Top Spinal Cord Inj Rehabil.* 1996, 1(4):32–45.

31. Bryden A, Sinnott A, Mulcahey M. Innovative strategies for improving upper extremity function in tetraplegia and considerations for measuring functional outcomes. *Top Spinal Cord Inj Rehabil.* 2005, 10(4):75–93.

32. Marino R. Neurological and functional outcomes in spinal cord injury: review and recommendations. *Top Spinal Cord Inj Rehabil.* 2005, 10(4):51–64.

33. Anderson K, Aito S, Atkins M, et al. Functional recovery measures for spinal cord injury: an evidence-based review for clinical practice and research. *J Spinal Cord Med.* 2008, 31(2):133–144.

34. Catz A, Itzkovich M. Spinal cord independence measure: comprehensive ability rating scale for the spinal cord lesion patient. *J Rehabil Res Dev.* 2007, 44(1):65–68.

35. Catz A, Itzkovich M, Agranov E, et al. SCIM—spinal cord independence measure: a new disability scale for patients with spinal cord lesions. *Spinal Cord.* 1997, 35(12):850–856.

36. Catz A, Itzkovich M, Agranov E, et al. The spinal cord independence measure (SCIM): sensitivity to functional changes in subgroups of spinal cord lesion patients. *Spinal Cord.* 2001, 39(2):97–100.

37. Itzkovich M, Tripolski M, Zeilig G, et al. Rasch analysis of the Catz-Itzkovich spinal cord independence measure. *Spinal Cord.* 2002, 40(8):396–407.

38. Itzkovich M, Gelernter I, Biering-Sorensen F, et al. The Spinal Cord Independence Measure (SCIM) version III: reliability and validity in a multi-center international study. *Disabil Rehabil.* 2007, 29(24):1926–1933.

39. Dittmar S, Gresham G, eds. *Functional Assessment and Outcome Measures for the Rehabilitation Health Professional.* Gaithersburg, MD: Aspen, 1997.

40. Yavuz N, Tezyurek M, Akyuz M. A comparison of two functional tests in quadriplegia: the quadriplegia index of function and the functional independence measure. *Spinal Cord.* 1998, 36(12):832–837.

41. Gresham GE, Labi ML, Dittmar SS, et al. The Quadriplegia Index of Function (QIF): sensitivity and reliability demonstrated in a study of thirty quadriplegic patients. *Paraplegia.* 1986, 24(1):38–44.

42. Basmajian J, ed. *Physical Rehabilitation Outcome Measures.* Toronto, Ontario: Canadian Physiotherapy Association, 1994.

43. Shah S, Vanclay F, Cooper B. Improving the sensitivity of the Barthel Index for stroke rehabilitation. *J Clin Epidemiol.* 1989, 42(8):703–709.

44. Hocking C, Williams M, Broad J, Baskett J. Sensitivity of Shah, Vanclay and Cooper's modified Barthel Index. *Clin Rehabil.* 1999, 13(2):141–147.

45. Noreau L, Fougeyrollas P, Post M, Asano M. Participation after spinal cord injury: the evolution of conceptualization and measurement. *J Neurol Phys Ther.* 2005, 29(3):147–156.

46. Siddall PJ, Loeser JD. Pain following spinal cord injury. *Spinal Cord.* 2001, 39(2):63–73.

47. Siddall PJ, Middleton JW. A proposed algorithm for the management of pain following spinal cord injury. *Spinal Cord.* 2006, 44(2):67–77.

48. American Physical Therapy Association. *Guide to Physical Therapist Practice.* Revised 2nd ed. Alexandria, VA: American Physical Therapy Association, 2003.

49. Consortium for Spinal Cord Medicine. *Outcomes Following Traumatic Spinal Cord Injury: Clinical Practice Guidelines for Health-Care Professionals.* Washington, DC: Paralyzed Veterans of America, 1999.

50. Zampa A, Zacquini S, Rosin C, et al. Relationship between neurological level and functional recovery in spinal cord injury patients after rehabilitation. *Eur Medicophys.* 2003, 39(2):69–78.

51. Daverat P, Petit H, Kemoun G, et al. The long term outcome in 149 patients with spinal cord injury. *Paraplegia.* 1995, 33(11):665–668.

52. Lazar RB, Yarkony GM, Ortolano D, et al. Prediction of functional outcome by motor capability after spinal cord injury. *Arch Phys Med Rehabil.* 1989, 70(12):819–822.

53. Ota T, Akaboshi K, Nagata M, et al. Functional assessment of patients with spinal cord injury: measured by the motor score and the Functional Independence Measure. *Spinal Cord.* 1996, 34(9):531–535.

54. Saboe LA, Darrah JM, Pain KS, Guthrie J. Early predictors of functional independence 2 years after spinal cord injury. *Arch Phys Med Rehabil.* 1997, 78(6):644–650.

55. Waters RL, Yakura JS, Adkins R, Barnes G. Determinants of gait performance following spinal cord injury. *Arch Phys Med Rehabil.* 1989, 70(12):811–818.

56. Welch RD, Lobley SJ, O'Sullivan SB, Freed MM. Functional independence in quadriplegia: critical levels. *Arch Phys Med Rehabil.* 1986, 67(4):235–240.

57. Stevenson VL, Playford ED, Langdon DW, Thompson AJ. Rehabilitation of incomplete spinal cord pathology: factors affecting prognosis and outcome. *J Neurol.* 1996, 243(9):644–647.

58. Ditunno JF, Cohen ME, Formal C, Whiteneck GG. Functional outcomes. In: Stover SL, DeLisa JA, Whiteneck GG, eds. *Spinal Cord Injury: Clinical Outcomes from the Model Systems.* Gaithersburg, MD: Aspen, 1995:170–184.

59. Grover J, Gellman H, Waters RL. The effect of a flexion contracture of the elbow on the ability to transfer in patients who have quadriplegia at the sixth cervical level. *J Bone Joint Surg Am.* 1996, 78(9):1397–1400.

60. Penrod LE, Hegde SK, Ditunno JF Jr. Age effect on prognosis for functional recovery in acute, traumatic central cord syndrome. *Arch Phys Med Rehabil.* 1990, 71(12):963–968.

61. Roth EJ, Lawler MH, Yarkony GM. Traumatic central cord syndrome: clinical features and functional outcomes. *Arch Phys Med Rehabil*. 1990, 71(1):18–23.

62. Yarkony G, Heinemann A. Pressure ulcers. In: Stover S, DeLisa J, Whiteneck G, eds. *Spinal Cord Injury: Clinical Outcomes from the Model Systems*. Gaithersburg, MD: Aspen, 1995:100–119.

63. Macciocchi SN, Bowman B, Coker J, et al. Effect of co-morbid traumatic brain injury on functional outcome of persons with spinal cord injuries. *Am J Phys Med Rehabil*. 2004, 83(1):22–26.

64. Scivoletto G, Morganti B, Ditunno P, et al. Effects on age on spinal cord lesion patients' rehabilitation. *Spinal Cord*. 2003, 41(8):457–464.

65. Atrice MB, Morrison SA, McDowell SL, et al. Traumatic spinal cord injury. In: Umphred DA, ed. *Neurological Rehabilitation*. 5th ed. St. Louis: Mosby Elsevier, 2007:605–657.

66. Ford J, Duckworth B. *Physical Management for the Quadriplegic Patient*. 2nd ed. Philadelphia: F.A. Davis, 1987.

67. Nixon V. *Spinal Cord Injury: A Guide to Functional Outcomes in Physical Therapy Management*. Rockville, MD: Aspen, 1985.

68. Little JW, Micklesen P, Umlauf R, Britell C. Lower extremity manifestations of spasticity in chronic spinal cord injury. *Am J Phys Med Rehabil*. 1989, 68(1):32–36.

69. Robinson CJ, Kett NA, Bolam JM. Spasticity in spinal cord injured patients: 2. Initial measures and long-term effects of surface electrical stimulation. *Arch Phys Med Rehabil*. 1988, 69(10):862–868.

70. Boss BJ, Pecanty L, McFarland SM, Sasser L. Self-care competence among persons with spinal cord injury. *SCI Nurs*. 1995, 12(2):48–53.

71. Yarkony GM, Roth EJ, Heinemann AW, et al. Functional skills after spinal cord injury rehabilitation: three-year longitudinal follow-up. *Arch Phys Med Rehabil*. 1988, 69(2):111–114.

72. Akmal M, Trivedi R, Sutcliffe J. Functional outcome in trauma patients with spinal injury. *Spine*. 2003, 28(2):180–185.

73. Ditunno JF Jr, Sipski ML, Posuniak EA, et al. Wrist extensor recovery in traumatic quadriplegia. *Arch Phys Med Rehabil*. 1987, 68(5 Pt 1):287–290.

74. Kirshblum S, Millis S, McKinley W, Tulsky D. Late neurologic recovery after traumatic spinal cord injury. *Arch Phys Med Rehabil*. 2004, 85(11):1811–1817.

75. Kirshblum SC, O'Connor KC. Predicting neurologic recovery in traumatic cervical spinal cord injury. *Arch Phys Med Rehabil*. 1998, 79(11):1456–1466.

76. Pollard ME, Apple DF. Factors associated with improved neurologic outcomes in patients with incomplete tetraplegia. *Spine*. 2003, 28(1):33–39.

77. Waters RL, Yakura JS, Adkins RH, Sie I. Recovery following complete paraplegia. *Arch Phys Med Rehabil*. 1992, 73(9):784–789.

78. Randall KE, McEwen IR. Writing patient-centered functional goals. *Phys Ther*. 2000, 80(12):1197–1203.

79. Corbet B. *Options: Spinal Cord Injury and the Future*. Denver: Hirschfeld, 1980.

80. DeJong C, Sutton J. Managed care and catastrophic injury: the case of spinal cord injury. *Top Spinal Cord Inj Rehabil*. 1998, 3(4):1–16.

81. Parsons K. Impact of managed care on spinal cord injury physicians and their patients. *Top Spinal Cord Inj Rehabil*. 1998, 3(4):28–35.

82. Burgess C. Managed care and its effects on how we deliver services. *Top Spinal Cord Inj Rehabil*. 1998, 3(4):17–27.

83. Noreau L, Vachon J. Comparison of three methods to assess muscular strength in individuals with spinal cord injury. *Spinal Cord*. 1998, 36(10):716–723.

84. Sisto SA, Dyson-Hudson T. Dynamometry testing in spinal cord injury. *J Rehabil Res Dev*. 2007, 44(1):123–136.

Chapter 8

1. Hislop H, Montgomery J. *Daniels and Worthingham's Muscle Testing: Techniques of Manual Examination*. Philadelphia: Saunders, 1995.

2. Kendall FP, McCreary EK, Provance P, et al. *Muscles: Testing and Function, with Posture and Pain*. 5th ed. Philadelphia: Lippincott, Williams & Wilkins, 2005.

3. Harvey L. Principles of conservative management for a non-orthotic tenodesis grip in tetraplegics. *J Hand Ther*. 1996, 9(3):238–242.

4. Marciello MA, Herbison GJ, Cohen ME, Schmidt R. Elbow extension using anterior deltoids and upper pectorals in spinal cord-injured subjects. *Arch Phys Med Rehabil*. 1995, 76(5):426–432.

5. Harvey LA, Crosbie J. Weight bearing through flexed upper limbs in quadriplegics with paralyzed triceps brachii muscles. *Spinal Cord*. 1999, 37(11):780–785.

6. Harvey LA, Crosbie J. Biomechanical analysis of a weight-relief maneuver in C5 and C6 quadriplegia. *Arch Phys Med Rehabil*. 2000, 81(4):500–505.

7. Beninato M, O'Kane KS, Sullivan PE. Relationship between motor FIM and muscle strength in lower cervical-level spinal cord injuries. *Spinal Cord*. 2004, 42(9):533–540.

8. Duran FS, Lugo L, Ramirez L, Eusse E. Effects of an exercise program on the rehabilitation of patients with spinal cord injury. *Arch Phys Med Rehabil*. 2001, 82(10):1349–1354.

9. Fujiwara T, Hara Y, Akaboshi K, Chino N. Relationship between shoulder muscle strength and functional independence measure (FIM) score among C6 tetraplegics. *Spinal Cord*. 1999, 37(1):58–61.

10. Kilkens OJ, Dallmeijer AJ, Nene AV, et al. The longitudinal relation between physical capacity and wheelchair skill performance during inpatient rehabilitation of people with spinal cord injury. *Arch Phys Med Rehabil*. 2005, 86(8):1575–1581.

11. Fredericks C. Skeletal muscle: the somatic effector. In: Fredericks C, Saladin L, eds. *Pathophysiology of the Motor Systems: Principles and Clinical Presentations*. Philadelphia: F.A. Davis, 1996:30–61.

12. Jacobs PL, Nash MS. Exercise recommendations for individuals with spinal cord injury. *Sports Med*. 2004, 34(11):727–751.

13. Delitto A, Snyder-Mackler L, Robinson A. Electrical stimulation of muscle: techniques and applications. In: Robinson J, Snyder-Mackler L, eds. *Clinical Electrophysiology: Electrotherapy and Electrophysiological Testing*. 2nd ed. Baltimore: Williams & Wilkins, 1995:121–153.

14. Hooker DN. Electrical stimulating currents. In: Prentice WE, ed. *Therapeutic Modalities for Physical Therapists*. 2nd ed. New York: McGraw-Hill, 2002:72–132.

15. O'Sullivan SB. Strategies to improve motor function. In: O'Sullivan SB, Schmitz TJ, eds. *Physical Rehabilitation*. 5th ed. Philadelphia: F.A. Davis, 2007:471–522.

16. Wolfe G, Adams JM. Electromyography and electrical stimulation. In: Umphred DA, ed. *Neurological Rehabilitation*. 5th ed. St. Louis: Mosby Elsevier, 2007:1005–1035.

17. Bohannon R. Orthopaedic problems in the neurologic patient. In: Donatelli R, Wooden M, eds. *Orthopaedic Physical Therapy*. 2nd ed. New York: Churchill Livingstone, 1994:675–695.

18. Schmidt R. Motor learning principles for physical therapy. In: Lister M, ed. *Contemporary Management of Motor control Problems: Proceedings of the II STEP Conference*. Fredericksburg, VA: Foundation for Physical Therapy, 1991:49–63.

19. Fell D. Progressing therapeutic intervention in patients with neuromuscular disorders: a framework to assist clinical decision making. *J Neurol Phys Ther*. 2004, 28(1):35–46.

20. Schmidt R, Lee T. *Motor Control and Learning: A Behavioral Emphasis*. 2nd ed. Champaign, IL: Human Kinetics, 1999.

21. Marley T, Ezekiel H, Lehto N, et al. Application of motor learning principles: the physiotherapy client as a problem-solver. II. Scheduling practice. *Physiother Can*. 2000, 52(4):315–320.

22. Shumway-Cook A, Woollacott M. *Motor Control: Translating Research into Clinical Practice*. 3rd ed. Philadelphia: Lippincott Williams & Wilkins, 2007.

23. Nicholson D. Motor learning. In: Fredericks C, Saladin L, eds. *Pathophysiology of the Motor Systems: Principles and Clinical Presentations*. Philadelphia: F.A. Davis, 1996:238–254.

24. Allison LK, Fuller K. Balance and vestibular disorders. In: Umphred DA, ed. *Neurological Rehabilitation*. 5th ed. St. Louis: Mosby Elsevier, 2007:732–774.

25. Sullivan P, Markos P, Minor M. *An Integrated Approach to Therapeutic Exercises: Theory and Clinical Application*. Reston, VA: Reston, 1982.

26. Umphred DA, Byl NN, Lazaro RT, Roller ML. Interventions for clients with movement limitations. In: Umphred DA, ed. *Neurological Rehabilitation*. 5th ed. St. Louis: Mosby Elsevier, 2007:187–281.

27. Winstein C. Designing practice for motor learning: clinical implications. In: Lister M, ed. *Contemporary Management of Motor Control Problems: Proceedings of the II STEP Conference*. Fredericksburg, VA: Foundation for Physical Therapy, 1991:65–76.

28. Finkbeiner K, Russo S. *Physical Therapy Management of Spinal Cord Injury: Accent on Independence*. Fisherville, VA: Woodrow Wilson Rehabilitation Center, 1990.

29. Maynard F, Karunas R, Adkins R, et al. Management of the neuromusculoskeletal systems. In: Stover S, DeLisa J, Whiteneck G, eds. *Spinal Cord Injury: Clinical Outcomes from the Model Systems*. Gaithersburg, MD: Aspen, 1995:145–169.

30. Mulroy SJ, Farrokhi S, Newsam CJ, Perry J. Effects of spinal cord injury level on the activity of shoulder muscles during wheelchair propulsion: an electromyographic study. *Arch Phys Med Rehabil*. 2004, 85(6):925–934.

31. van Drongelen S, de Groot S, Veeger HE, et al. Upper extremity musculoskeletal pain during and after rehabilitation in wheelchair-using persons with a spinal cord injury. *Spinal Cord*. 2006, 44(3):152–159.

32. Boninger ML, Cooper RA, Robertson RN, Shimada SD. Three-dimensional pushrim forces during two speeds of wheelchair propulsion. *Am J Phys Med Rehabil*. 1997, 76(5):420–426.

33. Gellman H, Sie I, Waters RL. Late complications of the weight-bearing upper extremity in the paraplegic patient. *Clin Orthop Relat Res*. 1988, 233:132–135.

34. Boninger ML, Dicianno BE, Cooper RA, et al. Shoulder magnetic resonance imaging abnormalities, wheelchair propulsion, and gender. *Arch Phys Med Rehabil*. 2003, 84(11):1615–1620.

35. Consortium for Spinal Cord Medicine. *Preservation of Upper Limb Function Following Spinal Cord Injury: A Clinical Practice Guideline for Health-Care Professionals*. Washington, DC: Paralyzed Veterans of America, 2005.

36. Nawoczenski DA, Ritter-Soronen JM, Wilson CM, et al. Clinical trial of exercise for shoulder pain in chronic spinal injury. *Phys Ther*. 2006, 86(12):1604–1618.

37. Ditunno JF, Cohen ME, Formal C, Whiteneck GG. Functional outcomes. In: Stover SL, DeLisa JA, Whiteneck GG, eds. *Spinal Cord Injury: Clinical Outcomes from the Model Systems*. Gaithersburg, MD: Aspen, 1995:170–184.

38. Ditunno JF Jr, Stover SL, Freed MM, Ahn JH. Motor recovery of the upper extremities in traumatic quadriplegia: a multicenter study. *Arch Phys Med Rehabil*. 1992, 73(5):431–436.

39. Mange KC, Marino RJ, Gregory PC, et al. Course of motor recovery in the zone of partial preservation in spinal cord injury. *Arch Phys Med Rehabil*. 1992, 73(5):437–441.

40. Mange KC, Ditunno JF Jr, Herbison GJ, Jaweed MM. Recovery of strength at the zone of injury in motor complete and motor incomplete cervical spinal cord injured patients. *Arch Phys Med Rehabil*. 1990, 71(8):562–565.

41. Ditunno JF Jr, Sipski ML, Posuniak EA, et al. Wrist extensor recovery in traumatic quadriplegia. *Arch Phys Med Rehabil*. 1987, 68(5 Pt 1):287–290.

42. Harvey LA, Byak AJ, Ostrovskaya M, et al. Randomised trial of the effects of four weeks of daily stretch on extensibility of hamstring muscles in people with spinal cord injuries. *Aust J Physiother*. 2003, 49(3):176–181.

43. Ben M, Harvey L, Denis S, et al. Does 12 weeks of regular standing prevent loss of ankle mobility and bone mineral density in people with recent spinal cord injuries? *Aust J Physiother*. 2005, 51(4):251–256.

44. Harvey LA, Herbert RD, Glinsky J, et al. Effects of 6 months of regular passive movements on ankle joint mobility in people with spinal cord injury: a randomized controlled trial. *Spinal Cord*. 2009, 47(1):62–66.

45. Harvey LA, Batty J, Crosbie J, et al. A randomized trial assessing the effects of 4 weeks of daily stretching on ankle mobility in patients with spinal cord injuries. *Arch Phys Med Rehabil*. 2000, 81(10):1340–1347.

CHAPTER 9

1. Consortium for Spinal Cord Medicine. *Preservation of Upper Limb Function Following Spinal Cord Injury: A Clinical Practice Guideline for Health-Care Professionals*. Washington, DC: Paralyzed Veterans of America, 2005.

2. Kendall F, McCreary E, Provance P. *Muscles: Testing and Function*. 4th ed. Baltimore: Williams & Wilkins, 1993.

3. Martini F. *Fundamentals of Anatomy and Physiology*. 4th ed. Upper Saddle River, NJ: Prentice Hall, 1998.

4. McMinn R. *Last's Anatomy: Regional and Applied*. 9th ed. New York: Churchill Livingstone, 1994.

5. Moore K. *Clinically Oriented Anatomy*. Baltimore: Williams & Wilkins, 1992.

6. Rosse C, Gaddum-Rosse P. *Hollinshead's Textbook of Anatomy*. 5th ed. Philadelphia: Lippincott-Raven, 1997.

7. Little JW, Micklesen P, Umlauf R, Britell C. Lower extremity manifestations of spasticity in chronic spinal cord injury. *Am J Phys Med Rehabil*. 1989, 68(1):32–36.

8. Maynard F, Karunas R, Adkins R, et al. Management of the neuromusculoskeletal systems. In: Stover S, DeLisa J, Whiteneck G, eds. *Spinal Cord Injury: Clinical Outcomes from the Model Systems*. Gaithersburg, MD: Aspen, 1995: 145–169.

9. Robinson CJ, Kett NA, Bolam JM. Spasticity in spinal cord injured patients: 2. Initial measures and long-term effects of surface electrical stimulation. *Arch Phys Med Rehabil*. 1988, 69(10):862–868.

10. Richter RR, VanSant AF, Newton RA. Description of adult rolling movements and hypothesis of developmental sequences. *Phys Ther*. 1989, 69(1):63–71.

11. O'Sullivan S, Schmitz T. *Physical Laboratory Manual: Focus on Functional Training*. Philadelphia: F.A. Davis, 1998.

12. McCoy JO, VanSant AF. Movement patterns of adolescents rising from a bed. *Phys Ther*. 1993, 73(3):182–193.

13. Shumway-Cook A, Woollacott M. *Motor Control: Translating Research into Clinical Practice*. 3rd ed. Philadelphia: Lippincott Williams & Wilkins, 2007.

CHAPTER 10

1. Nyland J, Quigley P, Huang C, et al. Preserving transfer independence among individuals with spinal cord injury. *Spinal Cord*. 2000, 38(11):649–657.

2. Forslund EB, Granstrom A, Levi R, et al. Transfer from table to wheelchair in men and women with spinal cord

injury: coordination of body movement and arm forces. *Spinal Cord*. 2007, 45(1):41–48.

3. Gagnon D, Nadeau S, Gravel D, et al. Biomechanical analysis of a posterior transfer maneuver on a level surface in individuals with high and low-level spinal cord injuries. *Clin Biomech (Bristol, Avon)*. 2003, 18(4):319–331.

4. Lee TQ, McMahon PJ. Shoulder biomechanics and muscle plasticity: implications in spinal cord injury. *Clin Orthop Relat Res*. 2002, (Suppl 403):S26–S36.

5. Consortium for Spinal Cord Medicine. *Preservation of Upper Limb Function Following Spinal Cord Injury: A Clinical Practice Guideline for Health-Care Professionals*. Washington, DC: Paralyzed Veterans of America, 2005.

6. Kendall F, McCreary E, Provance P. *Muscles: Testing and Function*. 4th ed. Baltimore: Williams & Wilkins, 1993.

7. Martini F. *Fundamentals of Anatomy and Physiology*. 4th ed. Upper Saddle River, NJ: Prentice Hall, 1998.

8. McMinn R. *Last's Anatomy: Regional and Applied*. 9th ed. New York: Churchill Livingstone, 1994.

9. Moore K. *Clinically Oriented Anatomy*. Baltimore: Williams & Wilkins, 1992.

10. Rosse C, Gaddum-Rosse P. *Hollinshead's Textbook of Anatomy*. 5th ed. Philadelphia: Lippincott-Raven, 1997.

11. Burgess C. Managed care and its effects on how we deliver services. *Top Spinal Cord Inj Rehabil*. 1998, 3(4):17–27.

12. Gefen JY, Gelmann AS, Herbison GJ, et al. Use of shoulder flexors to achieve isometric elbow extension in C6 tetraplegic patients during weight shift. *Spinal Cord*. 1997, 35(5):308–313.

13. Marciello MA, Herbison GJ, Cohen ME, Schmidt R. Elbow extension using anterior deltoids and upper pectorals in spinal cord-injured subjects. *Arch Phys Med Rehabil*. 1995, 76(5):426–432.

14. Perry J, Gronley JK, Newsam CJ, et al. Electromyographic analysis of the shoulder muscles during depression transfers in subjects with low-level paraplegia. *Arch Phys Med Rehabil*. 1996, 77(4):350–355.

15. Little JW, Micklesen P, Umlauf R, Britell C. Lower extremity manifestations of spasticity in chronic spinal cord injury. *Am J Phys Med Rehabil*. 1989, 68(1):32–36.

16. Maynard F, Karunas R, Adkins R, et al. Management of the neuromusculoskeletal systems. In: Stover S, DeLisa J, Whiteneck G, eds. *Spinal Cord Injury: Clinical Outcomes from the Model Systems*. Gaithersburg, MD: Aspen, 1995:145–169.

17. Robinson CJ, Kett NA, Bolam JM. Spasticity in spinal cord injured patients: 2. Initial measures and long-term effects of surface electrical stimulation. *Arch Phys Med Rehabil*. 1988, 69(10):862–868.

18. Ditunno J, Cohen M, Formal C, Whiteneck G. Functional outcomes. In: Stover S, DeLisa J, Whiteneck G, eds. *Spinal Cord Injury: Clinical Outcomes from the Model Systems*. Gaithersburg, MD: Aspen, 1995:170–184.

19. Graziani V, Crozier K, Selby-Silverstein L. Lower extremity function following spinal cord injury. *Top Spinal Cord Inj Rehabil*. 1996, 1(4):46–55.

20. Behrman A, Sawyer K, Tomlinson S. "I want to walk": an approach to physical therapy management of the individual with an incomplete spinal cord injury. *Neurol Rep*. 1993, 17(2):7–12.

21. Shumway-Cook A, Woollacott M. *Motor Control: Translating Research into Clinical Practice*. 3rd ed. Philadelphia: Lippincott Williams & Wilkins, 2007.

22. O'Sullivan S, Schmitz T. *Physical Rehabilitation Laboratory Manual: Focus on Functional Training*. Philadelphia: F.A. Davis, 1999.

23. Schmitz TJ. Locomotor training. In: O'Sullivan SB, Schimtz TJ, eds. *Physical Rehabilitation*. 5th ed. Philadelphia: Davis, 2007:523–560.

CHAPTER 11

1. Heinemann AW, Magiera-Planey R, Schiro-Geist C, Gimines G. Mobility for persons with spinal cord injury: an evaluation of two systems. *Arch Phys Med Rehabil*. 1987, 68(2):90–93.

2. Waters R, Lunsford B. Energy costs of paraplegic locomotion. *J Bone Joint Surg Am*. 1985, 67(8):1245–1250.

3. Waters R, Miller L. A physiologic rationale for orthotic prescription in paraplegia. *Clin Prosthet Orthot*. 1987, 11(2):66–73.

4. Hansen R, Tresse S, Gunnarsson RK. Fewer accidents and better maintenance with active wheelchair check-ups: a randomized controlled clinical trial. *Clin Rehabil*. 2004, 18(6):631–639.

5. Consortium for Spinal Cord Medicine. *Preservation of Upper Limb Function Following Spinal Cord Injury: A Clinical Practice Guideline for Health-Care Professionals*. Washington, DC: Paralyzed Veterans of America, 2005.

6. Gaal RP, Rebholtz N, Hotchkiss RD, Pfaelzer PF. Wheelchair rider injuries: causes and consequences for wheelchair design and selection. *J Rehabil Res Dev*. 1997, 34(1):58–71.

7. Kirby RL, Ackroyd-Stolarz SA, Brown MG, et al. Wheelchair-related accidents caused by tips and falls among noninstitutionalized users of manually propelled wheelchairs in Nova Scotia. *Am J Phys Med Rehabil*. 1994, 73(5):319–330.

8. Kirby RL, Sampson MT, Thoren FA, MacLeod DA. Wheelchair stability: effect of body position. *J Rehabil Res Dev*. 1995, 32(4):367–372.

9. Koo TK, Mak AF, Lee YL. Posture effect on seating interface biomechanics: comparison between two seating cushions. *Arch Phys Med Rehabil*. 1996, 77(1):40–47.

10. Peterson MJ, Adkins HV. Measurement and redistribution of excessive pressures during wheelchair sitting. *Phys Ther*. 1982, 62(7):990–994.

11. van Drongelen S, de Groot S, Veeger HE, et al. Upper extremity musculoskeletal pain during and after rehabilitation in wheelchair-using persons with a spinal cord injury. *Spinal Cord*. 2006, 44(3):152–159.

12. Boninger ML, Dicianno BE, Cooper RA, et al. Shoulder magnetic resonance imaging abnormalities, wheelchair propulsion, and gender. *Arch Phys Med Rehabil*. 2003, 84(11):1615–1620.

13. Hastings J, Goldstein B. Paraplegia and the shoulder. *Phys Med Rehabil Clin N Am*. 2004, 15(3):vii, 699–718.

14. Boninger ML, Cooper RA, Robertson RN, Shimada SD. Three-dimensional pushrim forces during two speeds of wheelchair propulsion. *Am J Phys Med Rehabil*. 1997, 76(5):420–426.

15. Gellman H, Sie I, Waters RL. Late complications of the weight-bearing upper extremity in the paraplegic patient. *Clin Orthop Relat Res*. 1988, 233:132–135.

16. Kirshblum S, Druin E, Planten K. Musculoskeletal conditions in chronic spinal cord injury. *Top Spinal Cord Inj Rehabil*. 1997, 2(4):23–35.

17. Kulig K, Rao SS, Mulroy SJ, et al. Shoulder joint kinetics during the push phase of wheelchair propulsion. *Clin Orthop Relat Res*. 1998, 354:132–143.

18. Pentland WE, Twomey LT. Upper limb function in persons with long term paraplegia and implications for independence: part I. *Paraplegia*. 1994, 32(4):211–218.

19. Rodgers MM, Gayle GW, Figoni SF, et al. Biomechanics of wheelchair propulsion during fatigue. *Arch Phys Med Rehabil*. 1994, 75(1):85–93.

20. Sie IH, Waters RL, Adkins RH, Gellman H. Upper extremity pain in the postrehabilitation spinal cord injured patient. *Arch Phys Med Rehabil*. 1992, 73(1):44–48.

21. Boninger ML, Koontz AM, Sisto SA, et al. Pushrim biomechanics and injury prevention in spinal cord injury: recommendations based on CULP-SCI investigations. *J Rehabil Res Dev*. 2005, 42(3 Suppl 1):9–19.

22. Gerhart KA, Bergstrom E, Charlifue SW, et al. Long-term spinal cord injury: functional changes over time. *Arch Phys Med Rehabil*. 1993, 74(10):1030–1034.
23. Curtis KA, Drysdale GA, Lanza RD, et al. Shoulder pain in wheelchair users with tetraplegia and paraplegia. *Arch Phys Med Rehabil*. 1999, 80(4):453–457.
24. Noreau L, Proulx P, Gagnon L, et al. Secondary impairments after spinal cord injury: a population-based study. *Am J Phys Med Rehabil*. 2000, 79(6):526–535.
25. Nyland J, Quigley P, Huang C, et al. Preserving transfer independence among individuals with spinal cord injury. *Spinal Cord*. 2000, 38(11):649–657.
26. Ballinger DA, Rintala DH, Hart KA. The relation of shoulder pain and range-of-motion problems to functional limitations, disability, and perceived health of men with spinal cord injury: a multifaceted longitudinal study. *Arch Phys Med Rehabil*. 2000, 81(12):1575–1581.
27. Krause J. Changes in wheelchair technology: a consumer commentary. *Top Spinal Cord Inj Rehabil*. 1995, 1(1):66–70.
28. Scherer MJ. Outcomes of assistive technology use on quality of life. *Disabil Rehabil*. 1996, 18(9):439–448.
29. Consortium for Spinal Cord Medicine. *Preservation of Upper Limb Function Following Spinal Cord Injury: A Clinical Practice Guideline for Health-Care Professionals*. Washington, DC: Paralyzed Veterans of America, 2005.
30. Axelson P, Minkel J, Chesney D. *A Guide to Wheelchair Selection: How to Use the ANSI/RESNA Wheelchair Standards to Buy a Wheelchair*. Washington, DC: Paralyzed Veteran of America, 1994.
31. Cooper R. *Wheelchair Selection and Configuration*. New York: Demos, 1998.
32. Karp G. *Choosing a Wheelchair: A Guide for Optimal Independence*. Sebastopol, CA: O'Reilly & Associates, 1998.
33. Leonard R. To tilt or recline? *Top Spinal Cord Inj Rehabil*. 1995, 1(1):17–22.
34. Taylor S. Powered mobility evaluation and technology. *Top Spinal Cord Inj Rehabil*. 1995, 1(1):23–36.
35. Chase T. Physical fitness strategies. In: Lanig I, Chase T, Butt L, Hulse K, Johnson K, eds. *A Practical Guide to Health Promotion after Spinal Cord Injury*. Gaithersburg, MD: Aspen, 1996:243–291.
36. Tahamont M, Knowlton RG, Sawka MN, Miles DS. Metabolic responses of women to exercise attributable to long term use of a manual wheelchair. *Paraplegia*. 1986, 24(5):311–317.
37. Hilbers PA, White TP. Effects of wheelchair design on metabolic and heart rate responses during propulsion by persons with paraplegia. *Phys Ther*. 1987, 67(9):1355–1358.
38. Beekman CE, Miller-Porter L, Schoneberger M. Energy cost of propulsion in standard and ultralight wheelchairs in people with spinal cord injuries. *Phys Ther*. 1999, 79(2):146–158.
39. Kreutz D. Manual wheelchairs: prescribing for function. *Top Spinal Cord Inj Rehabil*. 1995, 1(1):1–16.
40. Parziale JR. Standard v lightweight wheelchair propulsion in spinal cord injured patients. *Am J Phys Med Rehabil*. 1991, 70(2):76–80.
41. Gilsdorf P, Patterson R, Fisher S. Thirty-minute continuous sitting force measurements with different support surfaces in the spinal cord injured and able-bodied. *J Rehabil Res Dev*. 1991, 28(4):33–38.
42. Hughes CJ, Weimar WH, Sheth PN, Brubaker CE. Biomechanics of wheelchair propulsion as a function of seat position and user-to-chair interface. *Arch Phys Med Rehabil*. 1992, 73(3):263–269.
43. Kirby RL, McLean AD, Eastwood BJ. Influence of caster diameter on the static and dynamic forward stability of occupied wheelchairs. *Arch Phys Med Rehabil*. 1992, 73(1):73–77.
44. Mayall J, Desharnais G. *Positioning in a Wheelchair: A Guide for Professional Caregivers of the Disabled Adult*. 2nd ed. Thorofare, NJ: Slack, 1995.
45. Veeger D, van der Woude LH, Rozendal RH. The effect of rear wheel camber in manual wheelchair propulsion. *J Rehabil Res Dev*. 1989, 26(2):37–46.
46. Wilson A. *Wheelchairs: A Prescription Guide*. Charlottesville, VA: Rehabilitation Press, 1986.
47. Wilson A. *How to Select and Use Manual Wheelchairs*. Topping, VA: Rehabilitation Press, 1992.
48. DiGiovine C, Koontz A, Boninger M. Advances in manual wheelchair technology. *Top Spinal Cord Inj Rehabil*. 2006, 11(4):1–14.
49. Sawatzky BJ, Kim WO, Denison I. The ergonomics of different tyres and tyre pressure during wheelchair propulsion. *Ergonomics*. 2004, 47(14):1475–1483.
50. Algood SD, Cooper RA, Fitzgerald SG, et al. Impact of a pushrim-activated power-assisted wheelchair on the metabolic demands, stroke frequency, and range of motion among subjects with tetraplegia. *Arch Phys Med Rehabil*. 2004, 85(11):1865–1871.
51. Arva J, Fitzgerald SG, Cooper RA, Boninger ML. Mechanical efficiency and user power requirement with a pushrim activated power assisted wheelchair. *Med Eng Phys*. 2001, 23(10):699–705.
52. Cooper RA, Fitzgerald SG, Boninger ML, et al. Evaluation of a pushrim-activated, power-assisted wheelchair. *Arch Phys Med Rehabil*. 2001, 82(5):702–708.
53. Algood SD, Cooper RA, Fitzgerald SG, et al. Effect of a pushrim-activated power-assist wheelchair on the functional capabilities of persons with tetraplegia. *Arch Phys Med Rehabil*. 2005, 86(3):380–386.
54. Haubert L, Requejo P, Newsam C, Mulroy S. Comparison of energy expenditure and propulsion characteristics in a standard and three pushrim-activated power-assisted wheelchairs. *Top Spinal Cord Inj Rehabil*. 2005, 11(2):64–73.
55. Somers M, Wlodarczyk S. Use of a pushrim-activated, power-assisted wheelchair enhanced mobility for an individual with cervical C5/6 tetraplegia. *Neurol Rep*. 2003, 27(1):22–28.
56. Taylor SJ. Evaluating the client with physical disabilities for wheelchair seating. *Am J Occup Ther*. 1987, 41(11):711–716.
57. Ragone D. Is it worth it? A personal perspective. In: Buchanan L, Nawoczenski D, eds. *Spinal Cord Injury: Concepts and Management Approaches*. Baltimore: Williams & Wilkins, 1987:249–265.
58. Tomlinson J. Maximizing manual wheelchair propulsion for the marginal user. *Neurol Rep*. 1990, 14(3):14–18.
59. Cooper R. *Wheelchair Selection and Configuration*. New York: Demos, 1998.
60. Brubaker C. Ergonomic considerations. *J Rehabil Res Dev Clin Suppl*. 1990, (2):37–48.
61. Alm M, Gutierrez E, Hultling C, Saraste H. Clinical evaluation of seating in persons with complete thoracic spinal cord injury. *Spinal Cord*. 2003, 41(10):563–571.
62. Hastings JD, Fanucchi ER, Burns SP. Wheelchair configuration and postural alignment in persons with spinal cord injury. *Arch Phys Med Rehabil*. 2003, 84(4):528–534.
63. Maurer CL, Sprigle S. Effect of seat inclination on seated pressures of individuals with spinal cord injury. *Phys Ther*. 2004, 84(3):255–261.
64. O'Neil L, Seelye R. Power wheelchair training for patients with marginal upper extremity function. *Neurol Rep*. 1990, 14(3):19–20.
65. Kendall F, McCreary E, Provance P. *Muscles: Testing and Function*. 4th ed. Baltimore: Williams & Wilkins, 1993.
66. Martini F. *Fundamentals of Anatomy and Physiology*. 4th ed. Upper Saddle River, NJ: Prentice Hall, 1998.
67. McMinn R. *Last's Anatomy: Regional and Applied*. 9th ed. New York: Churchill Livingstone, 1994.
68. Moore K. *Clinically Oriented Anatomy*. Baltimore: Williams & Wilkins, 1992.
69. Rosse C, Gaddum-Rosse P. *Hollinshead's Textbook of Anatomy*. 5th ed. Philadelphia: Lippincott-Raven, 1997.

70. Burgess C. Managed care and its effects on how we deliver services. *Top Spinal Cord Inj Rehabil*. 1998, 3(4):17–27.

71. Nobunaga AI. Orthostatic hypotension in spinal cord injury. *Top Spinal Cord Inj Rehabil*. 1997, 4(1):73–80.

72. Naso F. Cardiovascular problems in patients with spinal cord injury. *Phys Med Rehabil Clin N Am*. 1992, 3(4):741–749.

73. Lehmann KG, Lane JG, Piepmeier JM, Batsford WP. Cardiovascular abnormalities accompanying acute spinal cord injury in humans: incidence, time course and severity. *J Am Coll Cardiol*. 1987, 10(1):46–52.

74. Minkel JL. Seating and mobility considerations for people with spinal cord injury. *Phys Ther*. 2000, 80(7):701–709.

75. Henderson JL, Price SH, Brandstater ME, Mandac BR. Efficacy of three measures to relieve pressure in seated persons with spinal cord injury. *Arch Phys Med Rehabil*. 1994, 75(5):535–539.

76. Capoor J, Stein AB. Aging with spinal cord injury. *Phys Med Rehabil Clin N Am*. 2005, 16(1):129–161.

77. McClay I. Electric wheelchair propulsion using a hand control in C4 quadriplegia. A case report. *Phys Ther*. 1983, 63(2):221–223.

78. Robertson RN, Boninger ML, Cooper RA, Shimada SD. Pushrim forces and joint kinetics during wheelchair propulsion. *Arch Phys Med Rehabil*. 1996, 77(9):856–864.

79. Boninger ML, Impink BG, Cooper RA, Koontz AM. Relation between median and ulnar nerve function and wrist kinematics during wheelchair propulsion. *Arch Phys Med Rehabil*. 2004, 85(7):1141–1145.

80. Newsam CJ, Mulroy SJ, Gronley JK, et al. Temporal-spatial characteristics of wheelchair propulsion. Effects of level of spinal cord injury, terrain, and propulsion rate. *Am J Phys Med Rehabil*. 1996, 75(4):292–299.

81. Wolfe GA, Waters R, Hislop HJ. Influence of floor surface on the energy cost of wheelchair propulsion. *Phys Ther*. 1977, 57(9):1022–1027.

82. DiCarlo SE. Effect of arm ergometry training on wheelchair propulsion endurance of individuals with quadriplegia. *Phys Ther*. 1988, 68(1):40–44.

83. Cappozzo A, Felici F, Figura F, et al. Prediction of ramp traversability for wheelchair dependent individuals. *Paraplegia*. 1991, 29(7):470–478.

84. Cooper R, Cooper R, Tolerico M, et al. Advances in electric-powered wheelchairs. *Top Spinal Cord Inj Rehabil*. 2006, 11(4):15–29.

85. Little JW, Micklesen P, Umlauf R, Britell C. Lower extremity manifestations of spasticity in chronic spinal cord injury. *Am J Phys Med Rehabil*. 1989, 68(1):32–36.

86. Maynard F, Karunas R, Adkins R, et al. Management of the neuromusculoskeletal systems. In: Stover S, DeLisa J, Whiteneck G, eds. *Spinal Cord Injury: Clinical Outcomes from the Model Systems*. Gaithersburg, MD: Aspen, 1995:145–169.

87. Robinson CJ, Kett NA, Bolam JM. Spasticity in spinal cord injured patients: 2. Initial measures and long-term effects of surface electrical stimulation. *Arch Phys Med Rehabil*. 1988, 69(10):862–868.

88. Dallmeijer AJ, van der Woude LH, Veeger HE, Hollander AP. Effectiveness of force application in manual wheelchair propulsion in persons with spinal cord injuries. *Am J Phys Med Rehabil*. 1998, 77(3):213–221.

89. Dallmeijer AJ, Kappe YJ, Veeger DH, et al. Anaerobic power output and propulsion technique in spinal cord injured subjects during wheelchair ergometry. *J Rehabil Res Dev*. 1994, 31(2):120–128.

CHAPTER 12

1. Atrice M. Lower extremity orthotic management for the spinal-cord-injured client. *Top Spinal Cord Inj Rehabil*. 2000, 5(4):1–10.

2. Merkel KD, Miller NE, Merritt JL. Energy expenditure in patients with low-, mid-, or high-thoracic paraplegia using Scott-Craig knee-ankle-foot orthoses. *Mayo Clin Proc*. 1985, 60(3):165–168.

3. Noreau L, Richards CL, Comeau F, Tardif D. Biomechanical analysis of swing-through gait in paraplegic and non-disabled individuals. *J Biomech*. 1995, 28(6):689–700.

4. Noreau L, Shephard RJ. Spinal cord injury, exercise and quality of life. *Sports Med*. 1995, 20(4):226–250.

5. Waters RL, Adkins RH, Yakura JS, Sie I. Motor and sensory recovery following incomplete paraplegia. *Arch Phys Med Rehabil*. 1994, 75(1):67–72.

6. Waters RL, Yakura JS, Adkins RH. Gait performance after spinal cord injury. *Clin Orthop Relat Res*. 1993, 288:87–96.

7. Waters RL, Yakura JS, Adkins R, Barnes G. Determinants of gait performance following spinal cord injury. *Arch Phys Med Rehabil*. 1989, 70(12):811–818.

8. Fatone S. A review of the literature pertaining to KAFOs and HKAFOs for ambulation. *J Prosthet Orthot*. 2006, 18(7):137–168.

9. Cerny D, Waters R, Hislop H, Perry J. Walking and wheelchair energetics in persons with paraplegia. *Phys Ther*. 1980, 60(9):1133–1139.

10. Ulkar B, Yavuzer G, Guner R, Ergin S. Energy expenditure of the paraplegic gait: comparison between different walking aids and normal subjects. *Int J Rehabil Res*. 2003, 26(3):213–217.

11. Franceschini M, Baratta S, Zampolini M, et al. Reciprocating gait orthoses: a multicenter study of their use by spinal cord injured patients. *Arch Phys Med Rehabil*. 1997, 78(6):582–586.

12. Hawran S, Biering-Sorensen F. The use of long leg calipers for paraplegic patients: a follow-up study of patients discharged 1973–82. *Spinal Cord*. 1996, 34(11):666–668.

13. Sykes L, Ross ER, Powell ES, Edwards J. Objective measurement of use of the reciprocating gait orthosis (RGO) and the electrically augmented RGO in adult patients with spinal cord lesions. *Prosthet Orthot Int*. 1996, 20(3):182–190.

14. Waters R, Lunsford B. Energy costs of paraplegic locomotion. *J Bone Joint Surg Am*. 1985, 67(8):1245–1250.

15. Chafetz R, Johnston T, Calhoun C. Outcomes in upright mobility in individuals with a spinal cord injury. *Top Spinal Cord Inj Rehabil*. 2005, 10(4):94–108.

16. Heinemann AW, Magiera-Planey R, Schiro-Geist C, Gimines G. Mobility for persons with spinal cord injury: an evaluation of two systems. *Arch Phys Med Rehabil*. 1987, 68(2):90–93.

17. Yarkony GM, Roth EJ, Heinemann AW, et al. Functional skills after spinal cord injury rehabilitation: three-year longitudinal follow-up. *Arch Phys Med Rehabil*. 1988, 69(2):111–114.

18. Behrman AL, Harkema SJ. Locomotor training after human spinal cord injury: a series of case studies. *Phys Ther*. 2000, 80(7):688–700.

19. Behrman AL, Lawless-Dixon AR, Davis SB, et al. Locomotor training progression and outcomes after incomplete spinal cord injury. *Phys Ther*. 2005, 85(12):1356–1371.

20. Wirz M, Zemon DH, Rupp R, et al. Effectiveness of automated locomotor training in patients with chronic incomplete spinal cord injury: a multicenter trial. *Arch Phys Med Rehabil*. 2005, 86(4):672–680.

21. Dobkin B, Apple D, Barbeau H, et al. Weight-supported treadmill vs over-ground training for walking after acute incomplete SCI. *Neurology*. 2006, 66(4):484–493.

22. Dobkin B, Barbeau H, Deforge D, et al. The evolution of walking-related outcomes over the first 12 weeks of rehabilitation for incomplete traumatic spinal cord injury: the multicenter randomized spinal cord injury locomotor trial. *Neurorehabil Neural Repair*. 2007, 21(1):25–35.

23. Lam T, Eng J, Wolfe D, et al. A systematic review of the efficacy of gait rehabilitation strategies for spinal cord injury. *Top Spinal Cord Inj Rehabil*. 2007, 13(1):32–57.

24. Behrman AL, Bowden MG, Nair PM. Neuroplasticity after spinal cord injury and training: an emerging paradigm shift in rehabilitation and walking recovery. *Phys Ther*. 2006, 86(10): 1406–1425.

25. Hicks AL, Adams MM, Martin Ginis K, et al. Long-term body-weight-supported treadmill training and subsequent follow-up in persons with chronic SCI: effects on functional walking ability and measures of subjective well-being. *Spinal Cord*. 2005, 43(5):291–298.

26. Lunsford T, Wallace J. The orthotic prescription. In: Goldberg B, Hsu J, eds. *Atlas of Orthoses and Assistive Devices*. 3rd ed. St. Louis: Mosby, 1997:3–14.

27. Barnett SL, Bagley AM, Skinner HB. Ankle weight effect on gait: orthotic implications. *Orthopedics*. 1993, 16(10):1127–1131.

28. Yang L, Condie DN, Granat MH, et al. Effects of joint motion constraints on the gait of normal subjects and their implications on the further development of hybrid FES orthosis for paraplegic persons. *J Biomech*. 1996, 29(2):217–226.

29. Beekman C, Perry J, Boyd LA, et al. The effects of a dorsiflexion-stopped ankle-foot orthosis on walking in individuals with incomplete spinal cord injury. *Top Spinal Cord Inj Rehabil*. 2000, 5(4):54–62.

30. Peterson M. Ambulation and orthotic management. In: Adkins H, ed. *Spinal Cord Injury*. New York: Churchill Livingstone, 1985:199–217.

31. Michael J. Lower limb orthoses. In: Goldberg B, Hsu J, eds. *Atlas of Orthoses and Assistive Devices*. 3rd ed. St. Louis: Mosby, 1997:209–224.

32. O'Daniel B, Krapfl B. Spinal cord injury. In: Payton O, ed. *Manual of Physical Therapy*. New York: Churchill Livingstone, 1989:69–172.

33. Seleski S. Orthotic prescription principles. *J Spinal Cord Med*. 1996, 19(2):97–98.

34. Zablotny C. Use of orthoses for the adult with neurological involvement. In: Nawoczenski D, Epler M, eds. *Orthotics in Functional Rehabilitation of the Lower Limb*. Philadelphia: Saunders, 1997:205–243.

35. Lehmann J. Lower limb orthotics. In: Redford J, ed. *Orthotics Etcetera*. 3rd ed. Baltimore: Williams & Wilkins, 1986:278–351.

36. New York University. *Lower Limb Orthotics*. New York: New York University Post-Graduate Medical School, 1986.

37. Hurley EA. Use of KAFOs for patients with cerebral vascular accident, traumatic brain injury, and spinal cord injury. *J Prosthet Orthot*. 2006, 18(Proceedings 7):P199–P201.

38. Kaufman KR, Irby SE. Ambulatory KAFOs: A biomechanical engineering perspective. *J Prosthet Orthot*. 2006, 18(Proceedings 7):P175–P182.

39. Yakimovich T, Lemaire ED, Kofman J. Preliminary kinematic evaluation of a new stance-control knee-ankle-foot orthosis. *Clin Biomech (Bristol, Avon)*. 2006, 21(10):1081–1089.

40. Hebert JS, Liggins AB. Gait evaluation of an automatic stance-control knee orthosis in a patient with postpoliomyelitis. *Arch Phys Med Rehabil*. 2005, 86(8):1676–1680.

41. Nene AV, Hermens HJ, Zilvold G. Paraplegic locomotion: a review. *Spinal Cord*. 1996, 34(9):507–524.

42. Kohlmeyer K, Yarkony G. Functional outcome after spinal cord injury rehabilitation. In: Yarkony G, ed. *Spinal Cord Injury: Medical Management and Rehabilitation*. Rockville, MD: Aspen, 1994:9–14.

43. Campbell J, Moore T. Lower extremity orthoses for spinal cord injury. In: Goldberg B, Hsu J, eds. *Atlas of Orthoses and Assistive Devices*. 3rd ed. St. Louis: Mosby, 1997:391–400.

44. Hirokawa S, Solomonow M, Baratta R, D'Ambrosia R. Energy expenditure and fatiguability in paraplegic ambulation using reciprocating gait orthosis and electric stimulation. *Disabil Rehabil*. 1996, 18(3):115–122.

45. Knutson J, Audu M, Triolo R. Interventions for mobility and manipulation after spinal cord injury: a review of orthotic and neuroprosthetic options. *Top Spinal Cord Inj Rehabil*. 2006, 11(4):61–81.

46. Bernardi M, Canale I, Castellano V, et al. The efficiency of walking of paraplegic patients using a reciprocating gait orthosis. *Paraplegia*. 1995, 33(7):409–415.

47. Solomonow M, Baratta R, D'Ambrosia R. Standing and walking after spinal cord injury: experience with the reciprocating gait orthosis powered by electrical muscle stimulation. *Top Spinal Cord Inj Rehabil*. 2000, 5(4):29–53.

48. Miller PC. Orthoses for the pelvic and hip region. In: Nawoczenski D, Epler M, eds. *Orthotics in Functional Rehabilitation of the Lower Limb*. Philadelphia: Saunders, 1997:15–29.

49. Winchester PK, Carollo JJ, Parekh RN, et al. A comparison of paraplegic gait performance using two types of reciprocating gait orthoses. *Prosthet Orthot Int*. 1993, 17(2):101–106.

50. Baardman G, Uzerman MJ, Hermens HJ, et al. The influence of the reciprocal hip joint link in the Advanced Reciprocating Gait Orthosis on standing performance in paraplegia. *Prosthet Orthot Int*. 1997, 21(3):210–221.

51. Dall P, Granat M. The function of the reciprocal link in paraplegic orthotic gait. *J Prosthet Orthot*. 2001, 13(1):10–13.

52. Vogel L, Lubicky J. Pediatric spinal cord injury issues: ambulation. *Top Spinal Cord Inj Rehabil*. 1997, 3(2):37–47.

53. Waters RL, Adkins R, Yakura J, Vigil D. Prediction of ambulatory performance based on motor scores derived from standards of the American Spinal Injury Association. *Arch Phys Med Rehabil*. 1994, 75(7):756–760.

54. Yakura JS, Waters RL, Adkins RH. Changes in ambulation parameters in spinal cord injury individuals following rehabilitation. *Paraplegia*. 1990, 28(6):364–370.

55. Consortium for Spinal Cord Medicine. *Outcomes Following Traumatic Spinal Cord Injury: Clinical Practice Guidelines for Health-Care Professionals*. Washington, DC: Paralyzed Veterans of America, 1999.

56. Kendall F, McCreary E, Provance P. *Muscles: Testing and Function*. 4th ed. Baltimore: Williams & Wilkins, 1993.

57. Martini F. *Fundamentals of Anatomy and Physiology*. 4th ed. Upper Saddle River, NJ: Prentice Hall, 1998.

58. McMinn R. *Last's Anatomy: Regional and Applied*. 9th ed. New York: Churchill Livingstone, 1994.

59. Moore K. *Clinically Oriented Anatomy*. Baltimore: Williams & Wilkins, 1992.

60. Rosse C, Gaddum-Rosse P. *Hollinshead's Textbook of Anatomy*. 5th ed. Philadelphia: Lippincott-Raven, 1997.

61. Waters RL, Miller L. A physiologic rationale for orthotic prescription in paraplegia. *Clin Prosthet Orthot*. 1987, 11(2):66–73.

62. Waters RL, Sie IH, Adkins RH. Rehabilitation of the patient with a spinal cord injury. *Orthop Clin North Am*. 1995, 26(1):117–122.

63. Krawetz P, Nance P. Gait analysis of spinal cord injured subjects: effects of injury level and spasticity. *Arch Phys Med Rehabil*. 1996, 77(7):635–638.

64. Penrod LE, Hegde SK, Ditunno JF Jr. Age effect on prognosis for functional recovery in acute, traumatic central cord syndrome. *Arch Phys Med Rehabil*. 1990, 71(12):963–968.

65. Roth EJ, Lawler MH, Yarkony GM. Traumatic central cord syndrome: clinical features and functional outcomes. *Arch Phys Med Rehabil*. 1990, 71(1):18–23.

66. Vogel LC, Lubicky JP. Ambulation in children and adolescents with spinal cord injuries. *J Pediatr Orthop*. 1995, 15(4):510–516.

67. Tow AM, Kong KH. Central cord syndrome: functional outcome after rehabilitation. *Spinal Cord*. 1998, 36(3):156–160.

68. Kobetic R, Marsolias E, Samame P, Borges G. The next step: artificial walking. In: Rose J, Gamble J, eds. *Human Walking*. 2nd ed. Baltimore: Lippincott Williams & Wilkins, 1994:225–252.

69. Marsolias EB, Kobetic R. Functional electrical stimulation for walking in paraplegia. *J Bone Joint Surg Am*. 1987, 69(5):728–733.

70. Peckham PH. Functional electrical stimulation: current status and future prospects of applications to the neuromuscular system in spinal cord injury. *Paraplegia.* 1987, 25(3):279–288.

71. Thoma H, Frey M, Holle J, et al. State of the art of implanted multichannel devices to mobilize paraplegics. *Int J Rehabil Res.* 1987, 10(4 Suppl 5):86–90.

72. Kralj A, Jaeger R. Functional electrical stimulation for spinal cord injury. In: Yarkony G, ed. *Spinal Cord Injury: Medical Management and Rehabilitation.* Rockville, MD: Aspen, 1994: 175–182.

73. McClelland M, Andrews BJ, Patrick JH, et al. Augmentation of the Oswestry Parawalker orthosis by means of surface electrical stimulation: gait analysis of three patients. *Paraplegia.* 1987, 25(1):32–38.

74. Stallard J, Major RE. The influence of orthosis stiffness on paraplegic ambulation and its implications for functional electrical stimulation (FES) walking systems. *Prosthet Orthot Int.* 1995, 19(2):108–114.

75. Watkins E, Edwards D, Patrick J. ParaWalker paraplegic walking. *Physiotherapy.* 1987, 73(2):99–100.

76. Graupe D, Kohn KH. Transcutaneous functional neuromuscular stimulation of certain traumatic complete thoracic paraplegics for independent short-distance ambulation. *Neurol Res.* 1997, 19(3):323–333.

77. Jaeger RJ. Principles underlying functional electrical stimulation techniques. *J Spinal Cord Med.* 1996, 19(2):93–96.

78. Kobetic R, Triolo RJ, Marsolais EB. Muscle selection and walking performance of multichannel FES systems for ambulation in paraplegia. *IEEE Trans Rehabil Eng.* 1997, 5(1):23–29.

79. Marsolias EB, Kobetic R. Development of a practical electrical stimulation system for restoring gait in the paralyzed patient. *Clin Orthop Relat Res.* 1988, 233:64–74.

80. Smith B. Functional electrical stimulation. *Top Spinal Cord Inj Rehabil.* 1997, 3(2):56–69.

81. Gorman PH. Functional electrical stimulation. In: Lin VW, ed. *Spinal Cord Medicine.* New York: Demos, 2003:733–745.

82. Burns AS, Ditunno JF. Establishing prognosis and maximizing functional outcomes after spinal cord injury: a review of current and future directions in rehabilitation management. *Spine.* 2001, 26(Suppl 24):S137–S145.

83. Spadone R, Merati G, Bertocchi E, et al. Energy consumption of locomotion with orthosis versus Parastep-assisted gait: a single case study. *Spinal Cord.* 2003, 41(2):97–104.

84. Chaplin E. Functional neuromuscular stimulation for mobility in people with spinal cord injuries. The Parastep I system. *J Spinal Cord Med.* 1996, 19(2):99–105.

85. Gallien P, Brissot R, Eyssette M, et al. Restoration of gait by functional electrical stimulation for spinal cord injured patients. *Paraplegia.* 1995, 33(11):660–664.

86. Graupe D, Kohn KH. Functional neuromuscular stimulator for short-distance ambulation by certain thoracic-level spinal-cord-injured paraplegics. *Surg Neurol.* 1998, 50(3):202–207.

87. Peckham P, Gorman P. Functional electrical stimulation in the 21st century. *Top Spinal Cord Inj Rehabil.* 2004, 10(2):126–150.

88. Crozier KS, Cheng LL, Graziani V, et al. Spinal cord injury: prognosis for ambulation based on quadriceps recovery. *Paraplegia.* 1992, 30(11):762–767.

89. Hornby T, Campbell D, Zemon D, Khan J. Clinical and quantitative evaluation of robotic-assisted treadmill walking to retrain ambulation after spinal cord injury. *Top Spinal Cord Inj Rehabil.* 2005, 11(3):1–17.

90. Kim CM, Eng JJ, Whittaker MW. Level walking and ambulatory capacity in persons with incomplete spinal cord injury: relationship with muscle strength. *Spinal Cord.* 2004, 42(3): 156–162.

91. Alander DH, Parker J, Stauffer ES. Intermediate-term outcome of cervical spinal cord-injured patients older than 50 years of age. *Spine.* 1997, 22(11):1189–1192.

92. Burns SP, Golding DG, Rolle WA Jr, et al. Recovery of ambulation in motor-incomplete tetraplegia. *Arch Phys Med Rehabil.* 1997, 78(11):1169–1172.

93. Graziani V, Crozier K, Selby-Silverstein L. Lower extremity function following spinal cord injury. *Top Spinal Cord Inj Rehabil.* 1996, 1(4):46–55.

94. Waters RL. Functional prognosis of spinal cord injuries. *J Spinal Cord Med.* 1996, 19(2):89–92.

95. Newey ML, Sen PK, Fraser RD. The long-term outcome after central cord syndrome: a study of the natural history. *J Bone Joint Surg Br.* 2000, 82(6):851–855.

96. Scivoletto G, Morganti B, Ditunno P, et al. Effects on age on spinal cord lesion patients' rehabilitation. *Spinal Cord.* 2003, 41(8):457–464.

97. Roth EJ, Park T, Pang T, et al. Traumatic cervical Brown-Sequard and Brown-Sequard–plus syndromes: the spectrum of presentations and outcomes. *Paraplegia.* 1991, 29(9):582–589.

98. Crozier KS, Graziani V, Ditunno JF Jr, Herbison GJ. Spinal cord injury: prognosis for ambulation based on sensory examination in patients who are initially motor complete. *Arch Phys Med Rehabil.* 1991, 72(2):119–121.

99. Oleson CV, Burns AS, Ditunno JF, et al. Prognostic value of pinprick preservation in motor complete, sensory incomplete spinal cord injury. *Arch Phys Med Rehabil.* 2005, 86(5):988–992.

100. Behrman AL, Sawyer KL, Tomlinson SS. "I want to walk": an approach to physical therapy management of the individual with an incomplete spinal cord injury. *Neurol Rep.* 1993, 17(2):7–12.

101. Bennett S, Karnes J. *Neurological Disabilities: Assessment and Treatment.* Philadelphia: Lippincott, 1998.

102. Schmitz TJ. Locomotor training. In: O'Sullivan SB, Schimtz TJ, eds. *Physical Rehabilitation.* 5th ed. Philadelphia: F.A. Davis, 2007:523–560.

103. Shumway-Cook A, Woollacott M. *Motor Control: Translating Research into Clinical Practice.* 3rd ed. Philadelphia: Lippincott Williams & Wilkins, 2007.

104. O'Sullivan S, Schmitz T. *Physical Rehabilitation Laboratory Manual: Focus on Functional Training.* Philadelphia: F.A. Davis, 1999.

105. Barbeau H, Ladouceur M, Norman KE, et al. Walking after spinal cord injury: evaluation, treatment, and functional recovery. *Arch Phys Med Rehabil.* 1999, 80(2):225–235.

106. Barbeau H, Rossignol S. Enhancement of locomotor recovery following spinal cord injury. *Curr Opin Neurol.* 1994, 7(6): 517–524.

107. Dietz V, Colombo G, Jensen L. Locomotor activity in spinal man. *Lancet.* 1994, 344(8932):1260–1263.

108. Dietz V, Colombo G, Jensen L, Baumgartner L. Locomotor capacity of spinal cord in paraplegic patients. *Ann Neurol.* 1995, 37(5):574–582.

109. Dietz V, Wirz M, Jensen L. Locomotion in patients with spinal cord injuries. *Phys Ther.* 1997, 77(5):508–516.

110. Gardner MB, Holden MK, Leikauskas JM, Richard RL. Partial body weight support with treadmill locomotion to improve gait after incomplete spinal cord injury: a single-subject experimental design. *Phys Ther.* 1998, 78(4):361–374.

111. Wickelgren I. Teaching the spinal cord to walk. *Science.* 1998, 279(5349):319–321.

112. Field-Fote EC, Lindley SD, Sherman AL. Locomotor training approaches for individuals with spinal cord injury: a preliminary report of walking-related outcomes. *J Neurol Phys Ther.* 2005, 29(3):127–137.

113. Wernig A, Nanassy A, Muller S. Maintenance of locomotor abilities following Laufband (treadmill) therapy in para- and tetraplegic persons: follow-up studies. *Spinal Cord.* 1998, 36(11):744–749.

114. Dobkin BH, Apple D, Barbeau H, et al. Methods for a randomized trial of weight-supported treadmill training versus conventional training for walking during inpatient rehabilitation after

incomplete traumatic spinal cord injury. *Neurorehabil Neural Repair*. 2003, 17(3):153–167.

115. Dobkin BH, Havton LA. Basic advances and new avenues in therapy of spinal cord injury. *Annu Rev Med*. 2004, 55:255–282.

116. Barbeau H. Locomotor training in neurorehabilitation: emerging rehabilitation concepts. *Neurorehabil Neural Repair*. 2003, 17(1):3–11.

117. Galvez JA, Reinkensmeyer DJ. Robotics for gait training after spinal cord injury. *Top Spinal Cord Inj Rehabil*. 2005, 11(2):18–33.

118. Hornby TG, Zemon DH, Campbell D. Robotic-assisted, body-weight-supported treadmill training in individuals following motor incomplete spinal cord injury. *Phys Ther*. 2005, 85(1):52–66.

119. Ferris DP, Sawicki GS, Domingo A. Powered lower limb orthoses for gait rehabilitation. *Top Spinal Cord Inj Rehabil*. 2005, 11(2):34–49.

120. Israel JF, Campbell DD, Kahn JH, Hornby TG. Metabolic costs and muscle activity patterns during robotic- and therapist-assisted treadmill walking in individuals with incomplete spinal cord injury. *Phys Ther*. 2006, 86(11):1466–1478.

121. Cikajlo I, Matjacic Z, Bajd T. Development of a gait re-education system in incomplete spinal cord injury. *J Rehabil Med*. 2003, 35(5):213–216.

122. Field-Fote EC. Combined use of body weight support, functional electric stimulation, and treadmill training to improve walking ability in individuals with chronic incomplete spinal cord injury. *Arch Phys Med Rehabil*. 2001, 82(6):818–824.

123. Field-Fote EC, Tepavac D. Improved intralimb coordination in people with incomplete spinal cord injury following training with body weight support and electrical stimulation. *Phys Ther*. 2002, 82(7):707–715.

124. Bajd T, Andrews BJ, Kralj A, Katakis J. Restoration of walking in patients with incomplete spinal cord injuries by use of surface electrical stimulation—preliminary results. *Prosthet Orthot Int*. 1985, 9(2):109–111.

125. Bajd T, Stefancic M, Matjacic Z, et al. Improvement in step clearance via calf muscle stimulation. *Med Biol Eng Comput*. 1997, 35(2):113–116.

126. Ladouceur M, Pepin A, Norman KE, Barbeau H. Recovery of walking after spinal cord injury. *Adv Neurol*. 1997, 72:249–255.

127. Wieler M, Stein RB, Ladouceur M, et al. Multicenter evaluation of electrical stimulation systems for walking. *Arch Phys Med Rehabil*. 1999, 80(5):495–500.

128. Kim CM, Eng JJ, Whittaker MW. Effects of a simple functional electric system and/or a hinged ankle-foot orthosis on walking in persons with incomplete spinal cord injury. *Arch Phys Med Rehabil*. 2004, 85(10):1718–1723.

129. Bates A, Hanson N. *Aquatic Exercise Therapy*. Philadelphia: Saunders, 1996.

130. Haubert LL, Gutierrez DD, Newsam CJ, et al. A comparison of shoulder joint forces during ambulation with crutches versus a walker in persons with incomplete spinal cord injury. *Arch Phys Med Rehabil*. 2006, 87(1):63–70.

131. Melis EH, Torres-Moreno R, Barbeau H, Lemaire ED. Analysis of assisted-gait characteristics in persons with incomplete spinal cord injury. *Spinal Cord*. 1999, 37(6):430–439.

132. Delitto A, Snyder-Mackler L, Robinson A. Electrical stimulation of muscle: techniques and applications. In: Robinson J, Snyder-Mackler L, eds. *Clinical Electrophysiology: Electrotherapy and Electrophysiological Testing*. 2nd ed. Baltimore: Williams & Wilkins, 1995:121–153.

133. Hooker DN. Electrical stimulating currents. In: Prentice WE, ed. *Therapeutic Modalities for Physical Therapists*. 2nd ed. New York: McGraw-Hill, 2002:72–132.

134. Jacobs PL, Nash MS. Exercise recommendations for individuals with spinal cord injury. *Sports Med*. 2004, 34(11):727–751.

135. O'Sullivan SB. Strategies to improve motor function. In: O'Sullivan SB, Schmitz TJ, eds. *Physical Rehabilitation*. 5th ed. Philadelphia: F.A. Davis, 2007:471–522.

136. Wolfe G, Adams JM. Electromyography and electrical stimulation. In: Umphred DA, ed. *Neurological Rehabilitation*. 5th ed. St. Louis: Mosby Elsevier, 2007:1005–1035.

137. Prentice W. Proprioceptive neuromuscular facilitation techniques. In: Prentice W, ed. *Therapeutic Modalities for Allied Health Professionals*. New York: McGraw-Hill, 1998.

138. Schmitz TJ. Examination of the environment. In: O'Sullivan SB, Schmitz TJ, eds. *Physical Rehabilitation*. 5th ed. Philadelphia: F.A. Davis, 2007:401–467.

139. Adams J, Perry J. Gait analysis: clinical application. In: Rose J, Gamble J, eds. *Human Walking*. 2nd ed. Baltimore: Williams & Wikins, 1994:139–164.

140. Perry J. *Gait Analysis: Normal and Pathological Function*. Thorofare, NJ: Slack, 1992.

141. Perry J. Normal and pathological gait. In: Goldberg B, Hsu J, eds. *Atlas of Orthoses and Assistive Devices*. 3rd ed. St. Louis: Mosby, 1997:67–91.

142. Rancho Los Amigos Medical Center. *Observational Gait Analysis*. Downey, CA: Rancho Los Amigos Medical Center, 1996.

143. Edelstein JE. Orthotic options for standing and walking. *Top Spinal Cord Inj Rehabil*. 2000, 5(4):11–23.

144. Rasmussen AA, Smith KM, Damiano DL. Biomechanical evaluation of the combination of bilateral stance-control knee-ankle-foot orthoses and a reciprocating gait orthosis in an adult with spinal cord injury. *J Prosthet Orthot*. 2007, 19(2):42–47.

145. Barbeau H, Basso M, Behrman A, Harkema S. Treadmill training after spinal cord injury: good but not better. *Neurology*. 2006, 67(10):1900–1901, author reply 1901–1902.

146. Wernig A. Weight-supported treadmill vs over-ground training for walking after acute incomplete SCI. *Neurology*. 2006, 67(10):1900, author reply 1900.

147. Wernig A. Treadmill training after spinal cord injury: good but not better. *Neurology*. 2006, 67(10):1901, author reply 1901–1902.

148. Wolpaw JR. Treadmill training after spinal cord injury: good but not better. *Neurology*. 2006, 66(4):466–467.

149. Fisher B, Woll S. Considerations in the restoration of motor control. In: Montgomery J, ed. *Physical Therapy for Traumatic Brain Injury*. New York: Churchill Livingstone, 1995:55–78.

150. Umphred DA, Byl NN, Lazaro RT, Roller ML. Interventions for clients with movement limitations. In: Umphred DA, ed. *Neurological Rehabilitation*. 5th ed. St. Louis: Mosby Elsevier, 2007:187–281.

151. Carr J, Shepherd R. *Neurological Rehabilitation: Optimizing Motor Performance*. London: Butterworth-Heinemann Medical, 1998.

152. Davies P. *Steps to Follow: The Comprehensive Treatment of Patients with Hemiplegia*. 2nd ed. New York: Springer-Verlag, 2000.

CHAPTER 13

1. Boller F, Frank E. *Sexual Dysfunction in Neurological Disorders: Diagnosis, Management, and Rehabilitation*. New York: Raven Press, 1982.

2. Romano M. The physically handicapped. In: Gochros HL, Gochros JS, eds. *The Sexually Oppressed*. New York: Association Press, 1977:257–267.

3. Griffith ER. Sexual dysfunctions associated with physical disabilities. *Arch Phys Med Rehabil*. 1975, 56(1):8–13.

4. Kreuter M, Sullivan M, Siosteen A. Sexual adjustment and quality of relationships in spinal paraplegia: a controlled study. *Arch Phys Med Rehabil*. 1996, 77(6):541–548.

5. Richards E, Tepper M, Whipple B, Komisaruk B. Women with complete spinal cord injury: a phenomenological study of

sexuality and relationship experiences. *Sex Disabil.* 1997, 15(4): 271–283.

6. Bastanfar R, Crewe N. A qualitative study of the dating behaviors of men with spinal cord injury. *SCI Psychosoc Proc.* 2005, 18(2):76–82.

7. Foote J. Sex, sexuality, and fertility for women with spinal cord injury. *Top Spinal Cord Inj Rehabil.* 2003, 8(3):20–25.

8. Leibowitz R, Stanton A. Sexuality after spinal cord injury: a conceptual model based on women's narratives. *Rehabil Psychol.* 2007, 52(1):44–55.

9. Charlifue SW, Gerhart KA, Menter RR, et al. Sexual issues of women with spinal cord injuries. *Paraplegia.* 1992, 30(3):192–199.

10. Halstead L. Sexuality and disability. In: Krueger DW, ed. *Emotional Rehabilitation of Physical Trauma and Disability.* New York: Spectrum, 1984:232–252.

11. Harrison J, Glass CA, Owens RG, Soni BM. Factors associated with sexual functioning in women following spinal cord injury. *Paraplegia.* 1995, 33(12):687–692.

12. Siosteen A, Lundqvist C, Blomstrand C, et al. Sexual ability, activity, attitudes and satisfaction as part of adjustment in spinal cord-injured subjects. *Paraplegia.* 1990, 28(5):285–295.

13. Westgren N, Hultling C, Levi R, et al. Sexuality in women with traumatic spinal cord injury. *Acta Obstet Gynecol Scand.* 1997, 76(10):977–983.

14. White MJ, Rintala DH, Hart KA, et al. Sexual activities, concerns and interests of men with spinal cord injury. *Am J Phys Med Rehabil.* 1992, 71(4):225–231.

15. White MJ, Rintala DH, Hart KA, Fuhrer MJ. Sexual activities, concerns and interests of women with spinal cord injury living in the community. *Am J Phys Med Rehabil.* 1993, 72(6):372–378.

16. Levi R, Hultling C, Nash MS, Seiger A. The Stockholm spinal cord injury study: 1. Medical problems in a regional SCI population. *Paraplegia.* 1995, 33(6):308–315.

17. Fisher TL, Laud PW, Byfield MG, et al. Sexual health after spinal cord injury: a longitudinal study. *Arch Phys Med Rehabil.* 2002, 83(8):1043–1051.

18. Widerstrom-Noga EG, Felipe-Cuervo E, Broton JG, et al. Perceived difficulty in dealing with consequences of spinal cord injury. *Arch Phys Med Rehabil.* 1999, 80(5):580–586.

19. Sakellariou D. If not the disability, then what? Barriers to reclaiming sexuality following spinal cord injury. *Sex Disabil.* 2006, 24(2):101–111.

20. Althof SE, Levine SB. Clinical approach to the sexuality of patients with spinal cord injury. *Urol Clin North Am.* 1993, 20(3):527–534.

21. Cole T, Cole S. Sexual attitude reassessment programs for spinal cord injured adults, their partners and health care professionals. In: Sha'ked A, ed. *Human Sexuality and Rehabilitation Medicine.* Baltimore: Williams & Wilkins, 1981: 80–90.

22. Kirk S. Society and sexual deviance. In: Gochros HL, Gochros JS, eds. *The Sexually Oppressed.* New York: Associations Press, 1977:28–37.

23. Kreuter M, Sullivan M, Dahllof AG, Siosteen A. Partner relationships, functioning, mood and global quality of life in persons with spinal cord injury and traumatic brain injury. *Spinal Cord.* 1998, 36(4):252–261.

24. Tepper M. Sexuality and disability: the missing discourse on pleasure. *Sex Disabil.* 2000, 18(4):283–290.

25. Karp G, Klein SD, eds. *From There to Here.* Horsham, PA: No Limits Communications, 2004.

26. Griffith ER, Tomko MA, Timms RJ. Sexual function in spinal cord-injured patients: a review. *Arch Phys Med Rehabil.* 1973, 54(12):539–543.

27. Sipski M, Alexander C. Female sexuality after spinal cord injury: current knowledge and future directions. *Top Spinal Cord Inj Rehabil.* 1995, 1(2):1–10.

28. Cardenas D, Farrell-Roberts L, Sipski M, Rubner D. Management of gastrointestinal, genitourinary, and sexual function. In: Stover S, DeLisa J, Whiteneck G, eds. *Spinal Cord Injury: Clinical Outcomes from the Model Systems.* Gaithersburg, MD: Aspen, 1995:120–144.

29. Ferreiro-Velasco ME, Barca-Buyo A, de la Barrera SS, et al. Sexual issues in a sample of women with spinal cord injury. *Spinal Cord.* 2005, 43(1):51–55.

30. Bregman S, Hadley RG. Sexual adjustment and feminine attractiveness among spinal cord injured women. *Arch Phys Med Rehabil.* 1976, 57(9):448–450.

31. Cole T. Sexuality and the spinal cord injured. In: Green R, ed. *Human Sexuality: A Health Practitioner's Text.* Baltimore: Williams & Wilkins, 1979:243–263.

32. Ray C, West J. Social, sexual and personal implications of paraplegia. *Paraplegia.* 1984, 22(2):75–86.

33. Ekland M, Lawrie B. How a woman's sexual adjustment after sustaining a spinal cord injury impacts sexual health interventions. *SCI Nurs.* 2004, 21(1):14–19.

34. Corbet B. *Options: Spinal Cord Injury and the Future.* Denver: Hirschfeld, 1980.

35. Bonwich E. Sex role attitudes and role reorganization in spinal cord injured women. In: Deegan MJ, Brooks NA, eds. *Women and Disability: The Double Handicap.* New Brunswick, NJ: Transaction Books, 1985:56–67.

36. Miller S, Szasz G, Anderson L. Sexual health care clinician in an acute spinal cord injury unit. *Arch Phys Med Rehabil.* 1981, 62(7):315–320.

37. Cole T, Stevens M. Rehabilitation professionals and sexual counseling for spinal cord injured adults. *Arch Sex Behav.* 1975, 4(6):631–638.

38. Zupan M, Swanson T. *GIMP.* New York: Harper Entertainment, 2006.

39. Elliott S. Ejaculation and orgasm: sexuality in men with SCI. *Top Spinal Cord Inj Rehabil.* 2002, 8(1):1–15.

40. Langtry HD, Markham A. Sildenafil: a review of its use in erectile dysfunction. *Drugs.* 1999, 57(6):967–989.

41. Monga M, Bernie J, Rajasekaran M. Male infertility and erectile dysfunction in spinal cord injury: a review. *Arch Phys Med Rehabil.* 1999, 80(10):1331–1339.

42. Rampin O, Bernabe J, Giuliano F. Spinal control of penile erection. *World J Urol.* 1997, 15(1):2–13.

43. Smith EM, Bodner DR. Sexual dysfunction after spinal cord injury. *Urol Clin North Am.* 1993, 20(3):535–542.

44. Gott L. Anatomy and physiology of male sexual response and fertility as related to spinal cord injury. In: Sha'ked A, ed. *Human Sexuality and Rehabilitation Medicine.* Baltimore: Williams & Wilkins, 1981:67–73.

45. Weiss H. The physiology of human penile erection. In: Comfort A, ed. *Sexual Consequences of Disability.* Philadelphia: Stickley, 1978:11–24.

46. Rivas D, King S, Chancellor M. Male and female sexual dysfunction. *Top Spinal Cord Inj Rehabil.* 1996, 1(3):55–64.

47. McKenna KE. Neural circuitry involved in sexual function. *J Spinal Cord Med.* 2001, 24(3):148–154.

48. Courtois FJ, Macdougall JC, Sachs BD. Erectile mechanism in paraplegia. *Physiol Behav.* 1993, 53(4):721–726.

49. Crenshaw R, Martin D, Warner H, Crenshaw T. Organic impotence. In: Comfort A, ed. *Sexual Consequences of Disability.* Philadelphia: Stickley, 1978:25–35.

50. Geiger R. Neurophysiology of sexual response in spinal cord injury. *Sex Disabil.* 1979, 2(4):257–266.

51. Courtois FJ, Charvier KF, Leriche A, Raymond DP. Sexual function in spinal cord injury men. I. Assessing sexual capability. *Paraplegia.* 1993, 31(12):771–784.

52. Courtois FJ, Charvier KF, Leriche A, et al. Clinical approach to erectile dysfunction in spinal cord injured men. A review of clinical and experimental data. *Paraplegia.* 1995, 33(11):628–635.

53. Donovon W. Sexuality and sexual function. In: Bedbrook GM, ed. *Lifetime Care of the Paraplegic Patient*. New York: Churchill Livingstone, 1985:149–161.

54. Giuliano FA, Rampin O, Benoit G, Jardin A. Neural control of penile erection. *Urol Clin North Am*. 1995, 22(4):747–766.

55. Fitzpatrick WF. Sexual function in the paraplegic patient. *Arch Phys Med Rehabil*. 1974, 55(5):221–227.

56. Sonksen J, Chen D. Management of male infertility after spinal cord injury. *Top Spinal Cord Inj Rehabil*. 2002, 8(1):29–41.

57. Alexander MS, Bodner D, Brackett NL, et al. Development of international standards to document sexual and reproductive functions after spinal cord injury: preliminary report. *J Rehabil Res Dev*. 2007, 44(1):83–90.

58. Griffith ER, Trieschmann RB. Sexual functioning in women with spinal cord injury. *Arch Phys Med Rehabil*. 1975, 56(1):18–21.

59. Guyton A. *Human Physiology and Mechanisms of Disease*. 4th ed. Philadelphia: Saunders, 1987.

60. Vick R. *Contemporary Medical Physiology*. Reading, MA: Addison-Wesley, 1984.

61. Thews G, Vaupel P. *Autonomic Functions in Human Physiology*. New York: Springer-Verlag, 1985.

62. Sipski ML, Alexander CJ, Rosen R. Sexual arousal and orgasm in women: effects of spinal cord injury. *Ann Neurol*. 2001, 49(1):35–44.

63. Denys P, Mane M, Azouvi P, et al. Side effects of chronic intrathecal baclofen on erection and ejaculation in patients with spinal cord lesions. *Arch Phys Med Rehabil*. 1998, 79(5):494–496.

64. Tay HP, Juma S, Joseph AC. Psychogenic impotence in spinal cord injury patients. *Arch Phys Med Rehabil*. 1996, 77(4):391–393.

65. Benevento BT, Sipski ML. Neurogenic bladder, neurogenic bowel, and sexual dysfunction in people with spinal cord injury. *Phys Ther*. 2002, 82(6):601–612.

66. Courtois FJ, Gonnaud PM, Charvier KF, et al. Sympathetic skin responses and psychogenic erections in spinal cord injured men. *Spinal Cord*. 1998, 36(2):125–131.

67. Stein R. Sexual dysfunctions in the spinal cord injured. *Paraplegia*. 1992, 30(1):54–57.

68. Kuhr CS, Heiman J, Cardenas D, et al. Premature emission after spinal cord injury. *J Urol*. 1995, 153(2):429–431.

69. Sipski ML, Alexander CJ, Rosen RC. Physiological parameters associated with psychogenic sexual arousal in women with complete spinal cord injuries. *Arch Phys Med Rehabil*. 1995, 76(9):811–818.

70. Berard EJ. The sexuality of spinal cord injured women: physiology and pathophysiology. A review. *Paraplegia*. 1989, 27(2):99–112.

71. Sipski M, Alexander CJ, Gomez-Marin O. Effects of level and degree of spinal cord injury on male orgasm. *Spinal Cord*. 2006, 44(12):798–804.

72. Sipski ML, Alexander CJ, Rosen RC. Orgasm in women with spinal cord injuries: a laboratory-based assessment. *Arch Phys Med Rehabil*. 1995, 76(12):1097–1102.

73. Komisaruk BR, Gerdes CA, Whipple B. 'Complete' spinal cord injury does not block perceptual responses to genital self-stimulation in women. *Arch Neurol*. 1997, 54(12):1513–1520.

74. Jackson AB, Dijkers M, Devivo MJ, Poczatek RB. A demographic profile of new traumatic spinal cord injuries: change and stability over 30 years. *Arch Phys Med Rehabil*. 2004, 85(11):1740–1748.

75. National Spinal Cord Injury Statistical Center. Annual Report for the Model Spinal Cord Injury Care Systems. 2007, http://www.spinalcord.uab.edu. Accessed 12/15/08.

76. Brackett NL, Nash MS, Lynne CM. Male fertility following spinal cord injury: facts and fiction. *Phys Ther*. 1996, 76(11):1221–1231.

77. Ohl DA, Menge A, Sonksen J. Penile vibratory stimulation in spinal cord injured men: optimized vibration parameters and prognostic factors. *Arch Phys Med Rehabil*. 1996, 77(9):903–905.

78. Pryor JL, LeRoy SC, Nagel TC, Hensleigh HC. Vibratory stimulation for treatment of anejaculation in quadriplegic men. *Arch Phys Med Rehabil*. 1995, 76(1):59–64.

79. Seager SW, Halstead LS. Fertility options and success after spinal cord injury. *Urol Clin North Am*. 1993, 20(3):543–548.

80. Rutkowski SB, Geraghty TJ, Hagen DL, et al. A comprehensive approach to the management of male infertility following spinal cord injury. *Spinal Cord*. 1999, 37(7):508–514.

81. Sonksen J, Sommer P, Biering-Sorensen F, et al. Pregnancy after assisted ejaculation procedures in men with spinal cord injury. *Arch Phys Med Rehabil*. 1997, 78(10):1059–1061.

82. Denil J, Kuczyk MA, Schultheiss D, et al. Use of assisted reproductive techniques for treatment of ejaculatory disorders. *Andrologia*. 1996, 28(Suppl 1):43–51.

83. Nehra A, Werner MA, Bastuba M, et al. Vibratory stimulation and rectal probe electroejaculation as therapy for patients with spinal cord injury: semen parameters and pregnancy rates. *J Urol*. 1996, 155(2):554–559.

84. Yarkony G, Gittler M. Vibratory ejaculation for spinal-cord injured men. *Top Spinal Cord Inj Rehabil*. 1996, 1(3):82–87.

85. Matthews GJ, Gardner TA, Eid JF. In vitro fertilization improves pregnancy rates for sperm obtained by rectal probe ejaculation. *J Urol*. 1996, 155(6):1934–1937.

86. Lochner-Ernst D, Mandalka B, Kramer G, Stohrer M. Conservative and surgical semen retrieval in patients with spinal cord injury. *Spinal Cord*. 1997, 35(7):463–468.

87. Ohl DA, Sonksen J, Menge AC, et al. Electroejaculation versus vibratory stimulation in spinal cord injured men: sperm quality and patient preference. *J Urol*. 1997, 157(6):2147–2149.

88. Chen D, Hartwig DM, Rothe EJ. Comparsion of sperm quantity and quality in antegrade V retrograde ejaculates obtained by vibratory penile stimulation in males with spinal cord injury. *Am J Phys Med Rehabil*. 1999, 78(1):46–51.

89. Brindley G. Electroejaculation and the fertility of paraplegic men. *Sex Disabil*. 1980, 3(3):223–229.

90. Chung PH, Verkauf BS, Eichberg RD, et al. Electroejaculation and assisted reproductive techniques for anejaculatory infertility. *Obstet Gynecol*. 1996, 87(1):22–26.

91. Halstead LS, VerVoort S, Seager SW. Rectal probe electrostimulation in the treatment of anejaculatory spinal cord injured men. *Paraplegia*. 1987, 25(2):120–129.

92. Ohl DA, McCabe M, Sonksen J, et al. Management of infertility in spinal cord injury. *Top Spinal Cord Inj Rehabil*. 1996, 1(3):65–75.

93. Sedor JF, Hirsch IH. Evaluation of sperm morphology of electroejaculates of spinal cord-injured men by strict criteria. *Fertil Steril*. 1995, 63(5):1125–1127.

94. DeForge D, Blackmer J, Garritty C, et al. Fertility following spinal cord injury: a systematic review. *Spinal Cord*. 2005, 43(12):693–703.

95. Hamid R, Patki P, Bywater H, et al. Effects of repeated ejaculations on semen characteristics following spinal cord injury. *Spinal Cord*. 2006, 44(6):369–373.

96. Heruti RJ, Katz H, Menashe Y, et al. Treatment of male infertility due to spinal cord injury using rectal probe electroejaculation: the Israeli experience. *Spinal Cord*. 2001, 39(3):168–175.

97. Rutkowski SB, Middleton JW, Truman G, et al. The influence of bladder management on fertility in spinal cord injured males. *Paraplegia*. 1995, 33(5):263–266.

98. Siosteen A, Forssman L, Steen Y, et al. Quality of semen after repeated ejaculation treatment in spinal cord injury men. *Paraplegia*. 1990, 28(2):96–104.

99. Hirsch IH. Spermatogenesis following spinal cord injury. *Top Spinal Cord Inj Rehabil*. 1995, 1(2):27–43.

100. Taylor Z, Molloy D, Hill V, Harrison K. Contribution of the assisted reproductive technologies to fertility in males suffering spinal cord injury. *Aust N Z J Obstet Gynaecol*. 1999, 39(1):84–87.

101. Watkins W, Lim T, Bourne H, et al. Testicular aspiration of sperm for intracytoplasmic sperm injection: an alternative treatment to electro-emission: case report. *Spinal Cord.* 1996, 34(11):696–698.

102. Yamamoto M, Momose H, Yamada K. Fathering of a child with the assistance of electroejaculation in conjunction with intracytoplasmic sperm injection: case report. *Spinal Cord.* 1997, 35(3):179–180.

103. Chen SU, Shieh JY, Wang YH, et al. Pregnancy achieved by intracytoplasmic sperm injection using cryopreserved vasal-epididymal sperm from a man with spinal cord injury. *Arch Phys Med Rehabil.* 1998, 79(2):218–221.

104. Chung PH, Verkauf BS, Mola R, et al. Correlation between semen parameters of electroejaculates and achieving pregnancy by intrauterine insemination. *Fertil Steril.* 1997, 67(1):129–132.

105. Estores I, Sipski M. Women's issues after SCI. *Top Spinal Cord Inj Rehabil.* 2004, 10(2):107–125.

106. Baker ER, Cardenas DD. Pregnancy in spinal cord injured women. *Arch Phys Med Rehabil.* 1996, 77(5):501–507.

107. Craig DI. The adaptation to pregnancy of spinal cord injured women. *Rehabil Nurs.* 1990, 15(1):6–9.

108. Verduyn WH. Spinal cord injured women, pregnancy and delivery. *Paraplegia.* 1986, 24(4):231–240.

109. Wanner MB, Rageth CJ, Zach GA. Pregnancy and autonomic hyperreflexia in patients with spinal cord lesions. *Paraplegia.* 1987, 25(6):482–490.

110. Atterbury JL, Groome LJ. Pregnancy in women with spinal cord injuries. *Nurs Clin North Am.* 1998, 33(4):603–613.

111. Kobayashi A, Mizobe T, Tojo H, Hashimoto S. Autonomic hyperreflexia during labour. *Can J Anaesth.* 1995, 42(12):1134–1136.

112. Kaplan C. Special issues in contraception: caring for women with disabilities. *J Midwifery Womens Health.* 2006, 51(6):450–456.

113. Thornton CE. Sexuality counseling of women with spinal cord injuries. *Sex Disabil.* 1979, 2(4):267–277.

114. Leibowitz R. Sexual rehabilitation services after spinal cord injury: what do women want? *Sex Disabil.* 2005, 23(2):81–107.

115. Steger J, Brockway J. Sexual enhancement in spinal cord injured patients: behavioral group treatment. *Sex Disabil.* 1980, 3(2):84–96.

116. Eisenberg MG, Rustad LC. Sex education and counseling program on a spinal cord injury service. *Arch Phys Med Rehabil.* 1976, 57(3):135–140.

117. Romano MD, Lassiter RE. Sexual counseling with the spinal-cord injured. *Arch Phys Med Rehabil.* 1972, 53(12):568–572.

118. McAlonan S. Improving sexual rehabilitation services: the patient's perspective. *Am J Occup Ther.* 1996, 50(10):826–834.

119. Forsythe E, Horsewell JE. Sexual rehabilitation of women with a spinal cord injury. *Spinal Cord.* 2006, 44(4):234–241.

120. Kreuter M, Sullivan M, Siosteen A. Sexual adjustment after spinal cord injury (SCI) focusing on partner experiences. *Paraplegia.* 1994, 32(4):225–235.

121. Dunn M, Lloyd EE, Phelps GH. Sexual assertiveness in spinal cord injury. *Sex Disabil.* 1979, 2(4):293–300.

122. Corbet B, Dobbs J, Bonin B, eds. *Spinal Network: The Total Wheelchair Resource Book.* 3rd ed. Santa Monica, CA: Nine Lives Press, 2002.

123. Alexander MS, Alexander CJ. Recommendations for discussing sexuality after spinal cord injury/dysfunction in children, adolescents, and adults. *J Spinal Cord Med.* 2007, 30(Suppl 1):S65–S70.

124. Gatens C. Sexuality and disability. In: Woods NF, ed. *Human Sexuality in Health and Illness.* 3rd ed. St. Louis: Mosby, 1984:370–398.

125. Cole TM. Sexuality and physical disabilities. *Arch Sex Behav.* 1975, 4(4):389–403.

126. Szasz G. Sexual management. In: Ford J, Duckworth B, eds. *Physical Management for the Quadriplegic Patient.* 2nd ed. Philadelphia: F.A. Davis, 1987:377–396.

127. Taylor B, Davis S. Using the extended PLISSIT model to address sexual healthcare needs. *Nurs Stand.* 2006, 21(11):35–40.

128. Hale G, ed. *The Source Book for the Disabled: An Illustrated Guide to Easier More Independent Living for Physically Disabled People, Their Families and Friends.* New York: Paddington, 1979.

129. Denil J, Ohl DA, Smythe C. Vacuum erection device in spinal cord injured men: patient and partner satisfaction. *Arch Phys Med Rehabil.* 1996, 77(8):750–753.

130. Zasler ND, Katz PG. Synergist erection system in the management of impotence secondary to spinal cord injury. *Arch Phys Med Rehabil.* 1989, 70(9):712–716.

131. Deforge D, Blackmer J, Garritty C, et al. Male erectile dysfunction following spinal cord injury: a systematic review. *Spinal Cord.* 2006, 44(8):465–473.

132. Iwatsubo E, Tanaka M, Takahashi K, Akatsu T. Non-inflatable penile prosthesis for the management of urinary incontinence and sexual disability of patients with spinal cord injury. *Paraplegia.* 1986, 24(5):307–310.

133. Green B, Killorin W, Foote J, Sloan S. Complications of penile implants in spinal cord injured patients. *Top Spinal Cord Inj Rehabil.* 1995, 1(2):44–52.

134. Gianotten W, Bender J, Post M, Huing M. Training in sexology for medical and paramedical professionals: a model for the rehabilitation setting. *Sex Relat Ther.* 2006, 21(3):303–317.

135. Cole T, Cole S. The handicapped and sexual health. In: Comfort A, ed. *Sexual Consequences of Disability.* Philadelphia: Stickley, 1978:37–43.

136. Anderson C. Psychosocial and sexuality issues in pediatric spinal cord injury. *Top Spinal Cord Inj Rehabil.* 1997, 3(2):70–78.

137. Larsen E, Hejgaard N. Sexual dysfunction after spinal cord or cauda equina lesions. *Paraplegia.* 1984, 22(2):66–74.

138. Tepper M. Providing comprehensive sexual health care in spinal cord injury rehabilitation: implementation and evaluation of a new curriculum for health care professionals. *Sex Disabil.* 1997, 15(3):131–165.

139. Brashear D. Integrating human sexuality into rehabilitation practice. *Sex Disabil.* 1978, 1(3):190–199.

140. Higgins G. Sexuality and the spinal cord injured: treatment approaches. In: Krueger DW, ed. *Emotional Rehabilitation of Physical Trauma and Disability.* New York: Spectrum, 1984:253–265.

141. Kroll K, Klein E. *Enabling Romance: A Guide to Love, Sex and Relationships for the Disabled (And the People Who Care About Them).* Bethesda, MD: Woodbine House, 1992.

142. Pentland W, Walker J, Minnes P, et al. Women with spinal cord injury and the impact of aging. *Spinal Cord.* 2002, 40(8):374–387.

143. Neufeld JA, Klingbeil F, Bryen DN, et al. Adolescent sexuality and disability. *Phys Med Rehabil Clin N Am.* 2002, 13(4):857–873.

CHAPTER 14

1. Samson G, Cardenas DD. Neurogenic bladder in spinal cord injury. *Phys Med Rehabil Clin N Am.* 2007, 18(2):255–274, vi.

2. Suzuki T, Ushiyama T. Vesicoureteral reflux in the early stage of spinal cord injury: a retrospective study. *Spinal Cord.* 2001, 39(1):23–25.

3. Cardenas D, Farrell-Roberts L, Sipski M, Rubner D. Management of gastrointestinal, genitourinary, and sexual function. In: Stover S, DeLisa J, Whiteneck G, eds. *Spinal Cord Injury: Clinical Outcomes from the Model Systems.* Gaithersburg, MD: Aspen, 1995:120–144.

4. Ditunno JF Jr, Formal CS. Chronic spinal cord injury. *N Engl J Med.* 1994, 330(8):550–556.

5. Montgomerie JZ. Infections in patients with spinal cord injuries. *Clin Infect Dis.* 1997, 25(6):1285–1290.

6. Moy M, Amsters K. Urinary tract infection in clients with spinal cord injury who use intermittent clean self catheterisation. *Aust J Adv Nurs.* 2004, 21(4):35–40.

7. Chen Y, Roseman JM, DeVivo MJ, Funkhouser E. Does fluid amount and choice influence urinary stone formation in persons with spinal cord injury? *Arch Phys Med Rehabil*. 2002, 83(7):1002–1008.

8. Groah SL, Weitzenkamp DA, Lammertse DP, et al. Excess risk of bladder cancer in spinal cord injury: evidence for an association between indwelling catheter use and bladder cancer. *Arch Phys Med Rehabil*. 2002, 83(3):346–351.

9. Black K, DeSantis N. Medical complications common to spinal-cord injured and brain-injured patients. *Top Spinal Cord Inj Rehabil*. 1999, 5(2):47–75.

10. Consortium for Spinal Cord Medicine. *Neurogenic Bowel Management in Adults with Spinal Cord Injury*. Washington, DC: Paralyzed Veterans of America, 1998.

11. Chung EA, Emmanuel AV. Gastrointestinal symptoms related to autonomic dysfunction following spinal cord injury. *Prog Brain Res*. 2006, 152:317–333.

12. Harari D, Minaker KL. Megacolon in patients with chronic spinal cord injury. *Spinal Cord*. 2000, 38(6):331–339.

13. Anderson KD, Borisoff JF, Johnson RD, et al. The impact of spinal cord injury on sexual function: concerns of the general population. *Spinal Cord*. 2007, 45(5):328–337.

14. Bloemen-Vrencken JH, Post MW, Hendriks JM, et al. Health problems of persons with spinal cord injury living in the Netherlands. *Disabil Rehabil*. 2005, 27(22):1381–1389.

15. Levi R, Hultling C, Nash MS, Seiger A. The Stockholm spinal cord injury study: 1. Medical problems in a regional SCI population. *Paraplegia*. 1995, 33(6):308–315.

16. Pagliacci MC, Celani MG, Zampolini M, et al. An Italian survey of traumatic spinal cord injury. The Gruppo Italiano Studio Epidemiologico Mielolesioni study. *Arch Phys Med Rehabil*. 2003, 84(9):1266–1275.

17. Hicken BL, Putzke JD, Richards JS. Bladder management and quality of life after spinal cord injury. *Am J Phys Med Rehabil*. 2001, 80(12):916–922.

18. Oh SJ, Shin HI, Paik NJ, et al. Depressive symptoms of patients using clean intermittent catheterization for neurogenic bladder secondary to spinal cord injury. *Spinal Cord*. 2006, 44(12):757–762.

19. Consortium for Spinal Cord Medicine. *Bladder Management for Adults with Spinal Cord Injury: A Clinical Practice Guideline for Health-Care Providers*. Washington, DC: Paralyzed Veterans of America, 2006.

20. Yoshimura N, Chancellor MB. Neurophysiology of lower urinary tract function and dysfunction. *Rev Urol*. 2003, 5(Suppl 8): S3–S10.

21. Ugalde V, Litwiller S, Gater D. Bladder and bowel anatomy for the physiatrist. *Physical Medicine and Rehabilitation: State of the Art Reviews*. 1996, 10(3):547–568.

22. McGuire EJ, Morgan DM. Managing bladder disorders in patients with spinal cord injury. *Contemp Urol*. 2004, 16(2):12–26.

23. Chancellor MB, Rivas DA, Abdill CK, et al. Prospective comparison of external sphincter balloon dilatation and prosthesis placement with external sphincterotomy in spinal cord injured men. *Arch Phys Med Rehabil*. 1994, 75(3):297–305.

24. Chancellor M, Rivas D, Abdill C, et al. Management of sphincter dyssynergia using the sphincter stent prosthesis in chronically catheterized SCI men. *J Spinal Cord Med*. 1995, 18(2):88–94.

25. Rivas D, Abdill C, Chancellor M. Current management of detrusor sphincter dyssynergia. *Top Spinal Cord Inj Rehabil*. 1996, 1(3):1–17.

26. Dykstra DD. Botulinum toxin in the management of bowel and bladder function in spinal cord injury and other neurologic disorders. *Phys Med Rehabil Clin N Am*. 2003, 14(4):793–804, vi.

27. Royster R, Barboi C, Peruzzi W. Critical care in the acute cervical spinal cord injury. *Top Spinal Cord Inj Rehabil*. 2004, 9(3):11–32.

28. Young M, Bennett C, Razi S, Diaz F. Intermittent catheterization, indwelling catheters, reflex voiding: a review of outcomes and management options in spinal cord injury. *Top Spinal Cord Inj Rehabil*. 1996, 1(3):45–54.

29. McBride DQ, Rodts GE. Intensive care of patients with spinal trauma. *Neurosurg Clin N Am*. 1994, 5(4):755–766.

30. Wu Y, Chen D. Managing the neurogenic bladder in spinal cord injury. In: Yarkony G, ed. *Spinal Cord Injury: Medical Management and Rehabilitation*. Gaithersburg, MD: Aspen, 1994:41–57.

31. Benevento BT, Sipski ML. Neurogenic bladder, neurogenic bowel, and sexual dysfunction in people with spinal cord injury. *Phys Ther*. 2002, 82(6):601–612.

32. Francis K. Physiology and management of bladder and bowel continence following spinal cord injury. *Ostomy Wound Manage*. 2007, 53(12):18–27.

33. Gittler M. Acute rehabilitation in cervical spinal cord injury. *Top Spinal Cord Inj Rehabil*. 2004, 9(3):60–73.

34. Ku JH, Jung TY, Lee JK, et al. Influence of bladder management on epididymo-orchitis in patients with spinal cord injury: clean intermittent catheterization is a risk factor for epididymo-orchitis. *Spinal Cord*. 2006, 44(3):165–169.

35. Hansen RB, Biering-Sorensen F, Kristensen JK. Bladder emptying over a period of 10–45 years after a traumatic spinal cord injury. *Spinal Cord*. 2004, 42(11):631–637.

36. Hall MK, Hackler RH, Zampieri TA, Zampieri JB. Renal calculi in spinal cord-injured patient: association with reflux, bladder stones, and foley catheter drainage. *Urology*. 1989, 34(3): 126–128.

37. McGuire EJ, Savastano J. Comparative urological outcome in women with spinal cord injury. *J Urol*. 1986, 135(4):730–731.

38. Bycroft J, Hamid R, Shah PJ. Penile erosion in spinal cord injury—an important lesson. *Spinal Cord*. 2003, 41(11):643–644.

39. Trautner BW, Darouiche RO. Prevention of urinary tract infection in patients with spinal cord injury. *J Spinal Cord Med*. 2002, 25(4):277–283.

40. Matthews P. Elimination. In: Matthews PJ, Carlson CE, eds. *Spinal Cord Injury: A Guide to Rehabilitation Nursing*. Rockville, MD: Aspen, 1987:97–119.

41. Chang SM, Hou CL, Dong DQ, Zhang H. Urologic status of 74 spinal cord injury patients from the 1976 Tangshan earthquake, and managed for over 20 years using the Crede maneuver. *Spinal Cord*. 2000, 38(9):552–554.

42. Kraft C. *Bladder and Bowel Management*. Baltimore: Williams & Wilkins, 1987.

43. Rudy E. *Advanced Neurological and Neurosurgical Nursing*. St. Louis: Mosby, 1984.

44. Vaidyanathan S, Soni BM, Sett P, et al. Flawed trial of micturition in cervical spinal cord injury patients: guidelines for trial of voiding in men with tetraplegia. *Spinal Cord*. 2003, 41(12):667–672.

45. Chaviano A, Matkov T, Anderson C, et al. Mitrofanoff continent catheterizable stoma for pediatric patients with spinal cord injury. *Top Spinal Cord Inj Rehabil*. 2000, 6(Suppl):30–35.

46. Jamil F. Towards a catheter free status in neurogenic bladder dysfunction: a review of bladder management options in spinal cord injury (SCI). *Spinal Cord*. 2001, 39(7):355–361.

47. Chancellor M, Rivas D. Neuromodulation and neurostimulation in urology. *Top Spinal Cord Inj Rehabil*. 1996, 1(3):18–35.

48. Brindley GS, Polkey CE, Rushton DN, Cardozo L. Sacral anterior root stimulators for bladder control in paraplegia: the first 50 cases. *J Neurol Neurosurg Psychiatry*. 1986, 49(10):1104–1114.

49. Creasey G. Restoration of bladder, bowel, and sexual function. *Top Spinal Cord Inj Rehabil*. 1999, 5(1):21–32.

50. Yarkony GM, Roth EJ, Cybulski GR, Jaeger RJ. Neuromuscular stimulation in spinal cord injury. II: Prevention of secondary complications. *Arch Phys Med Rehabil*. 1992, 73(2):195–200.

51. Peckham P, Gorman P. Functional electrical stimulation in the 21st century. *Top Spinal Cord Inj Rehabil*. 2004, 10(2):126–150.

52. Creasey GH, Grill JH, Korsten M, et al. An implantable neuroprosthesis for restoring bladder and bowel control to patients with spinal cord injuries: a multicenter trial. *Arch Phys Med Rehabil*. 2001, 82(11):1512–1519.

53. Faghri P, Trumbower R. Clinical applications of electrical stimulation for individuals with spinal cord injury. *Clin Kinesiol*. 2005, 59(4):48–62.

54. Vastenholt JM, Snoek GJ, Buschman HP, et al. A 7-year follow-up of sacral anterior root stimulation for bladder control in patients with a spinal cord injury: quality of life and users' experiences. *Spinal Cord*. 2003, 41(7):397–402.

55. Kirshblum SC, Priebe MM, Ho CH, et al. Spinal cord injury medicine. 3. Rehabilitation phase after acute spinal cord injury. *Arch Phys Med Rehabil*. 2007, 88(3 Suppl 1):S62–S70.

56. Nomura S, Ishido T, Tanaka K, Komiya A. Augmentation ileocystoplasty in patients with neurogenic bladder due to spinal cord injury or spina bifida. *Spinal Cord*. 2002, 40(1):30–33.

57. Bennett J, Foote J, Green B, et al. Bladder augmentation: indications and long-term management. *Top Spinal Cord Inj Rehabil*. 1996, 1(3):36–44.

58. Scelza W, Shatzer M. Pharmacology of spinal cord injury: basic mechanism of action and side effects of commonly used drugs. *J Neurol Phys Ther*. 2003, 27(3):101–108.

59. Seoane-Rodriguez S, Sanchez R-Losada J, Montoto-Marques A, et al. Long-term follow-up study of intraurethral stents in spinal cord injured patients with detrusor-sphincter dyssynergia. *Spinal Cord*. 2007, 45(9):621–626.

60. Wheeler JS Jr, Walter JS, Chintam RS, Rao S. Botulinum toxin injections for voiding dysfunction following SCI. *J Spinal Cord Med*. 1998, 21(3):227–229.

61. Tabibian L, Ginsberg D. Transurethral collagen injection in neuropathic sphincter deficiency. *Top Spinal Cord Inj Rehabil*. 2003, 8(3):54–59.

62. Lynch AC, Antony A, Dobbs BR, Frizelle FA. Bowel dysfunction following spinal cord injury. *Spinal Cord*. 2001, 39(4):193–203.

63. Stiens SA, Bergman SB, Goetz LL. Neurogenic bowel dysfunction after spinal cord injury: clinical evaluation and rehabilitative management. *Arch Phys Med Rehabil*. 1997, 78(Suppl 3):S86–S102.

64. Van Wynsberghe D, Noback C, Carola R. *Human Anatomy and Physiology*. 3rd ed. New York: McGraw-Hill, 1995.

65. Guyton A. *Basic Neuroscience: Anatomy and Physiology*. Philadelphia: Saunders, 1987.

66. Ash D. Sustaining safe and acceptable bowel care in spinal cord injured patients. *Nurs Stand*. 2005, 20(8):55–64.

67. Frost F. Spinal cord injury: gastrointestinal implications and management. *Top Spinal Cord Inj Rehabil*. 1998, 4(2):56–80.

68. Kirshblum SC, Gulati M, O'Connor KC, Voorman SJ. Bowel care practices in chronic spinal cord injury patients. *Arch Phys Med Rehabil*. 1998, 79(1):20–23.

69. Cardenas DD, Farrell-Roberts L, Sipski ML, Rubner D. Management of gastrointestinal, genitourinary, and sexual function. In: Stover SL, DeLisa JA, Whiteneck GG, eds. *Spinal Cord Injury: Clinical Outcomes from the Model Systems*. Gaithersburg, MD: Aspen, 1995:120–144.

70. Slater W. Management of faecal incontinence of a patient with spinal cord injury. *Br J Nurs*. 2003, 12(12):727–734.

71. Garvin P. SCI neurogenic bowel care: nursing guidelines. *SCI Nurs*. 2005, 22(2):117–120.

72. Ayas S, Leblebici B, Sozay S, et al. The effect of abdominal massage on bowel function in patients with spinal cord injury. *Am J Phys Med Rehabil*. 2006, 85(12):951–955.

73. Haas U, Geng V, Evers GC, Knecht H. Bowel management in patients with spinal cord injury—a multicentre study of the German speaking society of paraplegia (DMGP). *Spinal Cord*. 2005, 43(12):724–730.

74. Branagan G, Tromans A, Finnis D. Effect of stoma formation on bowel care and quality of life in patients with spinal cord injury. *Spinal Cord*. 2003, 41(12):680–683.

75. Korsten MA, Fajardo NR, Rosman AS, et al. Difficulty with evacuation after spinal cord injury: colonic motility during sleep and effects of abdominal wall stimulation. *J Rehabil Res Dev*. 2004, 41(1):95–100.

76. King T, Green B. Neurogenic bladder in the patient with SCI: management challenges in the era of managed care. *Top Spinal Cord Inj Rehabil*. 2003, 8(3):60–74.

77. Hagglund KJ, Clark MJ, Schopp LH, et al. Consumer-assistant education to reduce the occurrence of urinary tract infections among persons with spinal cord injury. *Top Spinal Cord Inj Rehabil*. 2005, 10(3):53–62.

78. Vaidyanathan S, Soni B, Singh G, et al. Possible use of Bio-Derm external continence device in selected, adult, male spinal cord injury patients (letter). *Spinal Cord*. 2005, 43(4):260–261.

CHAPTER 15

1. *Uniform Federal Accessibility Standards*. Washington, DC: United States Access Board, 1984.

2. *Americans with Disabilities Act and Architectural Barriers Act Accessibility Guidelines*. Washington, DC: United States Access Board, 2004.

3. International Code Council. *American National Standard Accessible and Usable Buildings and Facilities* (ICC/ANSI A117.1-2003). Country Club Hills, IL: International Code Council, 2004.

4. Frechette L. *Accessible Housing*. New York: McGraw-Hill, 1996.

5. Architectural Barriers Act of 1968, 42 U.S.C. (As Amended through 1984). 1984:4151–4157.

6. *A Guide to Disability Rights Laws*. Washington, DC: United States Department of Justice, 2005.

7. Wylde M, Baron-Robbins A, Clark S. *Building for a Lifetime: The Design and Construction of Fully Accessible Homes*. Newton, CT: Taunton Press, 1994.

8. Mace R. *The Accessible Housing Design File*. New York: Van Nostrand Reinhold, 1991.

9. Kirchner C, Gerber E, Smith B. Designed to deter: community barriers to physical activity for people with visual or motor impairments. *Am J Prev Med*. 2008, 34(4):349–352.

10. Meyers AR, Anderson JJ, Miller DR, et al. Barriers, facilitators, and access for wheelchair users: substantive and methodologic lessons from a pilot study of environmental effects. *Soc Sci Med*. 2002, 55(8):1435–1446.

11. Rimmer JH, Riley B, Wang E, et al. Physical activity participation among persons with disabilities: barriers and facilitators. *Am J Prev Med*. 2004, 26(5):419–425.

12. Spivock M, Gauvin L, Brodeur JM. Neighborhood-level active living buoys for individuals with physical disabilities. *Am J Prev Med*. 2007, 32(3):224–230.

13. McClain L, Beringer D, Kuhnert H, et al. Restaurant wheelchair accessibility. *Am J Occup Ther*. 1993, 47(7):619–623.

14. McClain L, Todd C. Food store accessibility. *Am J Occup Ther*. 1990, 44(6):487–491.

15. Kroll T, Jones GC, Kehn M, Neri MT. Barriers and strategies affecting the utilisation of primary preventive services for people with physical disabilities: a qualitative inquiry. *Health Soc Care Comm*. 2006, 14(4):284–293.

16. Rimmer JH, Riley B, Wang E, Rauworth A. Accessibility of health clubs for people with mobility disabilities and visual impairments. *Am J Public Health*. 2005, 95(11):2022–2028.

17. Spivock M, Gauvin L, Riva M, Brodeur JM. Promoting active living among people with physical disabilities: evidence for neighborhood-level buoys. *Am J Prev Med*. 2008, 34(4): 291–298.

18. Borgenicht R, Hoffman M, Mustoe K, Vazquez A. *The ASSIST Guidebook to the Accessible Home: Practical Designs for Home Modifications and New Construction*. Salt Lake City, UT: ASSIST, 2005.

19. Davies T, Lopez C. *Accessible Home Design: Architectural Solutions for the Wheelchair User.* 2nd ed. Washington, DC: Paralyzed Veterans of America, 2006.

20. Hale G, ed. *The Source Book for the Disabled: An Illustrated Guide to Easier More Independent Living for Physically Disabled People, Their Families and Friends.* New York: Paddington, 1979.

21. Johnson PB. *Creation of the Barrier-free Interior.* Millville, NJ: A Positive Approach, 1988.

22. Steven Winter Associates. *Accessible Housing by Design: Universal Design Principles in Practice.* New York: McGraw-Hill, 1997.

23. Dobkin I, Peterson M. *Universal Interiors by Design: Gracious Spaces.* New York: McGraw-Hill, 1999.

24. Bostrom J, Mace R, Long M. *Adaptable Housing: A Technical Manual for Implementing Adaptable Dwelling Unit Specifications.* Washington, DC: Department of Housing and Urban Development, 1987.

25. Ford J, Duckworth B. *Physical Management for the Quadriplegic Patient.* 2nd ed. Philadelphia: F.A. Davis, 1987.

26. Bostrom J. Creating a workable kitchen. *Mainstream: Magazine of the Able-Disabled.* 1988, 12(7):25.

27. Center for Universal Design. *Fact Sheet 6: Definitions: Accessible, Adaptable, and Universal Design.* 2006, http://www.design.ncsu.edu/cud/pubs_p/docs/Fact%20Sheet%206.pdf. Accessed 08/13/08.

28. Jones M. *The Benefits of Universal Design in Housing to All Users.* Raleigh, NC: Center for Universal Design, North Carolina State University, 1995.

29. Consortium for Spinal Cord Medicine. *Preservation of Upper Limb Function Following Spinal Cord Injury: A Clinical Practice Guideline for Health-Care Professionals.* Washington, DC: Paralyzed Veterans of America, 2005.

Index